Periodontology
2nd edition

# Color Atlas of Dental Medicine

Editor: Klaus H. Rateitschak

Volume 1

# Periodontology

2nd revised and expanded edition

Klaus H. & Edith M. Rateitschak
Herbert F. Wolf
Thomas M. Hassell

Forewords by Roy C. Page and Hubert E. Schroeder
1382 Illustrations

Winner, Book Awards Competition
American Medical Writers Association
Physicians' Category, 1986 (1st edition)

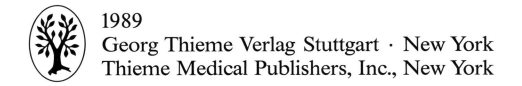

1989
Georg Thieme Verlag Stuttgart · New York
Thieme Medical Publishers, Inc., New York

## The authors:

Dr. Klaus H. Rateitschak
Professor and Chairman
Department of Cariology and Periodontology
and
Dr. Edith M. Rateitschak-Plüss
Senior Instructor
Department of Cariology and Periodontology
Dental Institute, University of Basle
Petersplatz 14, CH-4051 Basle
Switzerland

Dr. Herbert F. Wolf
Private Practitioner of Periodontics SGP
Instructor, Dental Institute, University of Basle
Löwenstraße 55, CH-8001 Zürich, Switzerland

Dr. Thomas M. Hassell
Professor and Chairman
Department of Periodontology, J-434
College of Dentistry, University of Florida
Gainesville, Florida USA 32610

**Library of Congress Cataloging in Publication Data**

**Periodontology. English**
Color Atlas of Dental Medicine / editor, Klaus H. Rateitschak ;
foreworks by Roy C. Page and Hubert E. Schroeder. – 2nd ed.
Adaption of: Parodontologie. 2nd. 1989.
Rev. ed. of: Color Atlas of Periodontology / Klaus H. Rateitschak
... [et al.] 1985.
Bibliography: p. Includes Index.
Contents: v. 1. Periodontology / Klaus H. Rateitschak ... [et al.]
1. Dentistry – Atlases. I. Rateitschak, Klaus H. II. Color Atlas
of Periodontology. III. Title.
[DNLM: 1. Periodontics – Atlases. WU 17 P257c]
RK287.P3713 1989
617.6'320754-dc20
DNLM/DLC
for Library of Congress

*Important Note:* Medicine is an ever-changing science. Research and clinical experience are continually broadening our knowledge, in particular our knowledge of proper treatment and drug therapy. Insofar as this book mentions any dosage or application, readers may rest assured that the authors, editors and publishers have made every effort to ensure that such references are strictly in accordance with the state of knowledge at the time of production of the book. Nevertheless, every user is requested to examine carefully the manufacturer's leaflets accompanying each drug in order to determine whether the dosage schedules recommended therein or the contraindications stated by the manufacturer differ from the statements made in the present book. Such examination is particularly important with drugs that are either rarely used or have been newly released on the market.

The 1st English edition of this book was published and copyrighted 1985 by Georg Thieme Verlag, Stuttgart, Germany.

Title of first English edition: Color Atlas of Periodontology
Title of the German editions: Parodontologie

| | |
|---|---|
| 1st German edition | 1984 |
| 1st English edition | 1985 |
| 1st French edition | 1986 |
| 1st Spanish edition | 1987 |
| 1st Japanese edition | 1987 |
| 1st Italian edition | 1988 |
| 2nd German edition | 1989 |
| 2nd English edition | 1989 |

© 1989 Georg Thieme Verlag, Rüdigerstraße 14,
D-7000 Stuttgart 30, Germany
Printed in Germany
Typesetting by G. Müller, Heilbronn
Reproductions by K. Porupsky, Stuttgart
Printed by K. Grammlich, Pliezhausen

Color Atlas of Dental Medicine

also available:

G. Graber
● Removable Partial Dentures

in preparation:

A. Geering, M. Kundert, C. Kelsey
● Complete Denture and Overdenture Prosthetics

Some of the product names, patents and registered designs referred to in this book are in fact registered trademarks or proprietary names even though specific reference to this fact is not always made in the text. Therefore, the appearance of a name without designation as proprietary is not to be construed as a representation by the publisher that it is in the public domain.

*Cover*
Computer-altered painting: Periodontal osseous destruction in right mandibular posterior segment. Probing the mesial bony pocket (CP 12 probe).

ISBN 3-13-675002-1 (GTV)
ISBN 0-86577-318-1 (TMP)      2 3 4 5 6

# Preface to the Second Edition

The first edition of this *Atlas* sold out shortly after its release. Numerous reprintings followed. The authors are now pleased to present this extensively revised and broadly expanded second edition.

Periodontology continues to grow in importance. While caries declines in the western world, this is not the case with the periodontal diseases. The treatment of gingivitis and periodontitis will therefore assume a more prominent role in the future.

A new edition of the *Atlas* was also necessary due to the rapid advances being made in periodontal research. These continuously provide new knowledge for the practitioner, who is confronted with decisions about when and to what degree periodontics should be integrated into the general practice of dentistry. In this regard, the *Atlas* plays the role of arbitrator between what is scientifically and theoretically possible and what is practical and realistic.

However, the incorporation of new knowledge into practice is only possible when older methods are discarded or when their significance is diminished. For example, the chapter on "Mucogingival Surgery" has been considerably shortened. Surgical treatment of recession was overdone for many years. On the other hand, many chapters were expanded and new ones were added, for example:

– New knowledge about etiology and pathogenesis of periodontitis
– New findings in epidemiology
– The Community Periodontal Index of Treatment Needs (CPITN)
– Expansion of the chapter "Types of Disease," with integration of new clinical cases, particularly in areas related to periodontology (oral pathology, systemic diseases, diabetes, Down Syndrome, AIDS etc.)

– More comprehensive presentation of *conservative therapy*, with emphasis on armamentarium and "step-by-step" procedure in actual clinical cases
– Systematization and comparison of standard periodontal surgical techniques, from the delicate ENAP (Excisional New Attachment Procedure) to the resective osseous surgery that is questioned today
– Expansion of interdisciplinary procedures (e. g., perio-endo, perio-prosthetics).

Finally, the future of our specialty is considered in a discussion of developing regenerative surgical techniques such as guided tissue regeneration.

In all, some 500 completely new and over 100 updated illustrations were integrated into this second edition. The complementary nature of text and figures, which was a hallmark of the first edition, has been enhanced here. We tried to increase the effectiveness of the *Atlas* by improving the visual appearance of the graphs, yet without neglecting the clarity of the text. The second edition contains a certain amount of repetition, some of which is intentional.

It is our hope that this second edition remains a *practical* periodontal atlas that reflects the current state of scientific knowledge.

This book is dedicated to our families, and to our friend, teacher and supporter, Dr. Hans R. Mühlemann, Professor emeritus.

Basle / Zurich / Gainesville, Summer 1989

Klaus H. & Edith M. Rateitschak
Herbert F. Wolf
Thomas M. Hassell

# Foreword to the First Edition

Roy C. Page, D. D. S., Ph. D.
Professor, Pathology & Periodontics
University of Washington, Seattle

Disease of the periodontium continues to be one of man's most widespread afflictions. These diseases are taking on an ever increasing importance in dentistry because of the decreasing prevalence of dental caries and the fact that they are prevalent in older people, a segment of our population that is rapidly increasing. Beginning with the early 1970s, there has been a virtual explosion in new basic information about all aspects of the periodontal diseases and this has led to major advances in our understanding. The rate of progress in acquiring new knowledge has greatly outstripped our capacity to integrate the new information into concepts about these diseases and into our methods of diagnosing and treating them. By and large, textbooks and monographs are out of date before they appear on the new book shelves, and all too frequently they fail to incorporate the new information or to apply it to clinical problems. This book is an exception.

The *Color Atlas of Periodontology* is different from existing textbooks and monographs in many ways. Indeed, it is not a textbook but it is far more than an atlas. It is a fresh approach in which the latest information has been integrated into already existing knowledge and presented in a highly effective, easy-to-understand manner using innovative diagrams, drawings, and clinical illustrations.

The publication has numerous strengths. A great deal of thought and planning appears to have been given to the selection of areas to be covered and to their sequencing. Coverage is extraordinarily complete, with sections on structural biology, pathogenesis, host response, epidemiology, diagnosis, therapy, adjunctive therapy, and maintenance. The book also includes sections on areas of dentistry related or allied to periodontics including endodontics, orthodontics, temporary stabilization, occlusal trauma and its management, medications frequently used in the course of periodontal therapy, and fixed and removable restorative treatment for periodontal patients.

The sections on structural biology, microbiology and host response are especially noteworthy because they are based on the most recent research findings and they are presented in a manner that even a beginning student can easily understand. An excellent selection of literature references has been provided. I also liked the section on diagnosis. All of the inflammatory diseases of the periodontium are included and documented using the latest terminology. This is accomplished without the inclusion of peripherally related oral lesions which would dilute and detract from the major diagnostic thrust.

The section on therapy constitutes about two-thirds of the book and is, without doubt, the most outstanding section. Coverage is unusually thorough. Every recognized method and procedure has been included beginning with oral hygiene, scaling, curettage and root planing, and extending through the entire range of resective and reconstructive procedures. For each procedure, the required instrumentation is illustrated, and an excellent clinical example has been chosen. Pretreatment clinical photographs and radiographs are provided along with a step-by-step illustration of the operative procedure and the postoperative results. Although there is a great deal of debate today concerning the relative merits of conservative versus the more extensive surgical methods of treatment, to their credit the authors of this *Atlas* have remained totally objective, showing no favoritism to one school of thought or another.

There has not previously been a comparable publication in the field of periodontology in the United States and there is unlikely to be another in the foreseeable future. The selection, organization, and sequencing of the information and the technical quality of this publication are unsurpassed. The book will be useful to undergraduate and graduate students, teachers, and practicing dentists and periodontists. It will in all likelihood become one of the most widely used and cited publications in our field.

# Foreword to the Second Edition

Hubert E. Schroeder, D.M.D., Dr. odont. h.c.
Professor and Chairman, Department of Oral Structural Biology
University of Zurich, Switzerland

The *Color Atlas of Periodontology,* first published 4 years ago, now reappears in an extensively revised and expanded second edition. Like its predecessor, but moreso, this is not a textbook in the usual sense of the term, nor is it merely a picture book of "case reports" and clinical situations. This book is a guide for practitioners of the periodontal healing arts, a detailed introduction to the rational practice of "causal therapy."

Although classical literature often provides a relatively clear view of the various diseases of the periodontium, only during the past 25 years has it become possible for periodontal scientists to re-evaluate this picture, and to describe and clarify the etiology and pathogenesis of these diseases. Today, the profession finds itself in the midst of an attempt to utilize the latest scientific discoveries for the improvement of its diagnostic and therapeutic skills. During a lifetime, the periodontium of a clinically healthy human usually undergoes various alterations that relate to physiological, functional, infectious or iatrogenic circumstances.

These alterations manifest themselves in atrophic tissue loss, in the cardinal symptoms of inflammation, in tissue destruction of varying severity and, ultimately, in tooth loss. The most common afflictions of the periodontal supporting structures are the various types of periodontitis, which are considered today as locally destructive, non-contagious infectious diseases. All types of periodontitis are caused primarily by anaerobic mixed infections, yet susceptibility to these bacterial infections may vary from individual to individual. The infecting bacteria take their origin as a supragingival plaque which extends apically onto the root surface, changing in composition subgingivally. The bacterial attack elicits inflammation, the development of periodontal pockets and abscess formation; the subsequent plethora of host defense mechanisms called into action eventually participates in destroying components of the tissues. Understanding of such host-pathogen relationships provides the framework for modern periodontal therapy which, so-based, can in many instances lead to clinically successful results.

This second edition of the *Atlas* by Edith and Klaus Rateitschak, Herbert Wolf and Thomas Hassell is one of the best, most comprehensive, most clinically relevant documentations on the subject of successful practical periodontics, which also illustrates the impact of related dental specialties – endodontics and prosthodontics, for example – upon the success of periodontal therapy. The strength of this book is to be found not only in the ideal integration of theoretical principles with practical considerations and the internal logic of the presentation, but also in the superb clinical photographs and schematic diagrams that weld this text into a coherent, systematic and thoroughly understandable entity. The fact that the authors provide both textual and illustrative emphasis on *prevention* underscores their basic intention, which is to advocate health maintenance. The more comprehensive presentation of the complex etiology, pathogenesis and the various types of periodontitis is welcome, as is the treatise on systemic disease such as AIDS, diabetes, trisomy etc. Every basic element of periodontal therapy is portrayed step-by-step by means of coordinated text and illustration; the crucially important elements of therapy are emphasized by repetition. Greatest emphasis is placed on conservative therapy, where intervention is kept to the minimum so as to preserve tissue wherever possible.

Each practitioner who peruses this book will come away with the current views of the pathogenesis of periodontal diseases and the essential elements of consequential periodontal therapy. Perhaps the periodontist, above all, will come to realize that for the modern practitioner the biomedical research laboratories in his profession are not merely ivory towers, not remote outposts from which an occasional crumb of a misleading message emanates. This volume is conclusive proof that many of the research findings from clinical as well as basic scientists have already had direct and immediate impact upon the practice of clinical periodontics today.

# Acknowledgements

The authors thank the following individuals who assisted in the preparation of this second edition:

Dr. Andreas Adler, Senior Instructor in the Department of Periodontology, Basle, for preparation of many of the intraoral photographs in this edition.

Dr. Arthur Hefti, Associate Professor of Periodontology, Gainesville, for contributions in the chapter "Etiology and Pathogenesis."

Dr. Roy C. Page, Professor of Periodontics and Pathology, Seattle, for his Foreword to the first edition.

Dr. Hubert E. Schroeder, Chairman of Oral Structural Biology, Zurich, for his contributions in the chapter "Structural Biology," and for his Foreword to the second edition.

We thank also these colleagues, who provided sage advice and practical suggestions:

Dr. Giorgio Cimasoni, Geneva; Dr. Erwin T. Egloff, New York; Dr. George Graber, Basle; Dr. Hans Graf, Berne; Dr. Markus Grassi, San Francisco / Berne; Dr. Bernhard Guggenheim, Zurich; Dr. Werner Iselin, Zurich; Dr. Alice Kallenberger, Basle; Dr. Niklaus P. Lang, Berne; Dr. Felix Lutz, Zurich; Dr. Benedict Maeglin, Basle; Dr. Michael Marxer, Lucerne; Dr. Jean-Marc Meyer, Geneva; Dr. Hans R. Mühlemann, Zurich; Dr. Paul W. Stöckli, Zurich.

Thanks also to the faculty and staff in the Department of Cariology and Periodontology, University of Basle Dental Institute; to the coworkers in the private practice of Dr. H. F. Wolf; and to the colleagues in the Department of Periodontology, University of Florida , who provided support, assistance and encouragement.

T. Hassell received support from USPHS grants DE-06671 and DE-07481 during preparation of this *Atlas*.

We would thank especially Ms. Censeri Abare (Gainesville) and Ms. Brigitte Kaiser (Basle) for preparation of the extensive manuscript, and Ms. Zita Baumann (Zurich) for her noteworthy organizational assistance.

Mr. Dieter Isch (Basle) is acknowledged for his work in preparing the black-and-white illustrations.

The concept for the first edition, by Mr. Bruno Kümin (Zurich), proved again in this second edition to be sound.

The new illustrations in this second edition were again prepared by Atelier Struchen and Partner (Zurich) from drafts created by H. F. Wolf.

The considerable production costs associated with preparation of the *Atlas* were defrayed in part by contributions from the following institutions, organizations and companies:

- Procter & Gamble Co., Cincinnati
- Elida Cosmetic Inc., Zurich
- Walter Fuchs Foundation, Basle
- Blend-A-Med-Research, Mainz
- Empress Publishers Inc., Bad Brückenau
- Colgate-Palmolive Inc., Zurich
- Gaba Inc., Therwil
- Trisa Toothbrush Co., Triengen

Not least of all we offer sincere thanks for the excellent cooperation we received from Thieme Publishers, especially Dr. D. Bremkamp, Mr. A. Menge and Mr. K.-H. Fleischmann during planning and execution of the work. Thanks also to Mr. W. Stahl (Reproanstalt Porupsky, Stuttgart) for his assistance with production. All of these gentlemen continually exhibited patience with and understanding for the authors' sometimes overzealous (not to say bizarre) ideas.

# Table of Contents

## Adjunctive Therapy

## Appendix

# Structural Biology

**1 Periodontium – Dictionary definition**

**periodontium** (per" e-o-don' she-um) [Lat. → *peri* around →, Gr. → *odous* tooth].

A *functional* system of different tissues, investing and supporting the teeth, including cementum, periodontal ligament, alveolar bone, and gingiva.

*Anatomically,* the term is restricted to the connective tissue interposed between the teeth and their bony sockets. Called also *Periosteum alveolare* [Lat.].

**periodontology** [Gr. → *logos*], the study of the periodontal diseases.

Knowledge of the normal morphology and structural biology of the periodontal tissues is a prerequisite for understanding pathology. Such knowledge also clarifies the goals of causal therapy: Elimination of pathogens, healing, and regeneration of structural and functional integrity.

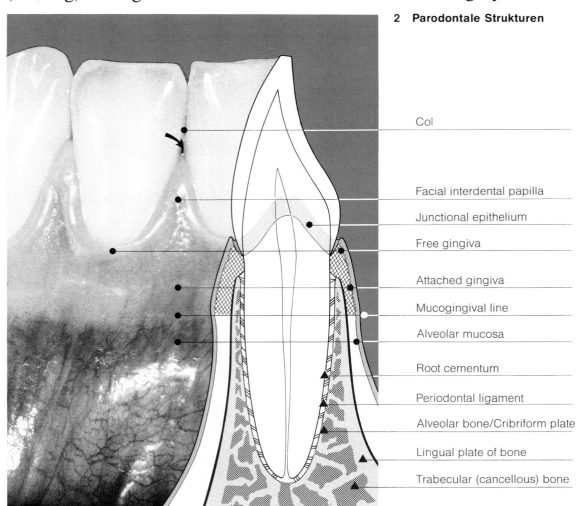

**2 Parodontale Strukturen**

Col

Facial interdental papilla

Junctional epithelium

Free gingiva

Attached gingiva

Mucogingival line

Alveolar mucosa

Root cementum

Periodontal ligament

Alveolar bone/Cribriform plate

Lingual plate of bone

Trabecular (cancellous) bone

# Gingiva

The gingiva is one portion of the oral mucosa. It is also the most peripheral component of the periodontium. Gingiva begins at the mucogingival line, and covers the coronal aspect of the alveolar process. On the palatal aspect the mucogingival line is absent; the gingiva here is a part of the keratinized, non-mobile palatal mucosa.

The gingiva ends at the cervix of each tooth, surrounds it and forms there the epithelial attachment by means of a ring of specialized epithelial tissue (junctional epithelium; compare p. 4). Thus the gingiva ensures continuity of the epithelial lining of the oral cavity.

The gingiva is demarcated clinically into the *free marginal* gingiva, ca. 1.5 mm wide; the *attached* gingiva, which may be of varying width; and the interdental gingiva, occupying the embrasures between adjacent teeth. Healthy gingiva is described as "salmon" or "coral" pink. Healthy gingiva is commonly pigmented in Blacks, and seldom also in Caucasians and Orientals.

Gingiva is firm in consistency and not mobile upon the underlying structures. The surface of gingiva is keratinized and may also exhibit an orange peel-like appearance called stippling (Schroeder 1987a).

### 3 Healthy gingiva in the person young
The free gingival margin courses parallel to the cementoenamel junction (CEJ). The gingival papillae fill the embrasures. A shallow linear depression, the gingival groove, can be observed in some areas, demarcating the free margin from the attached gingiva.

Courtesy F. Wolgensinger

*Right:* The radiograph depicts high interdental septa. The crest of alveolar bone is located ca. 1 mm apical to the CEJ.

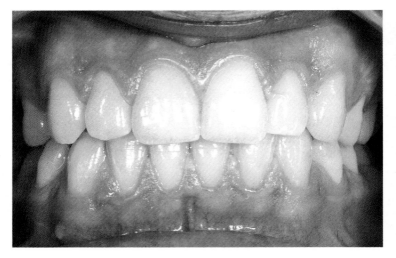
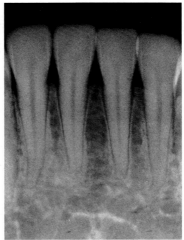

### 4 Healthy, lightly pigmented gingiva
The attached gingiva of this young Caucasian is deeply stippled and exhibits varying degrees of brownish pigmentation.

*Right:* This pigmentation results from the synthesis of melanin by melanocytes located in the basal layer of the epithelium. The melanocytes in this histologic section appear as brown spots.

Courtesy H. R. Mühlemann

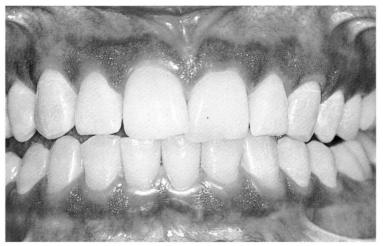
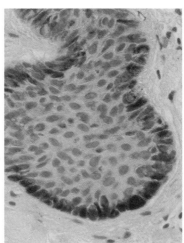

### 5 Healthy, deeply pigmented gingiva
Irregularly distributed, deep pigmentation in a 22-year-old Black without periodontal pockets. In the mandibular anterior area some of the papilla tips do exhibit mild recession.

*Right:* In the radiograph, the lamina dura is clearly visible. The alveolar crest is located ca. 2 mm apical to the cementoenamel junction and is somewhat more apical than in Figure 3.

Courtesy E. T. Egloff

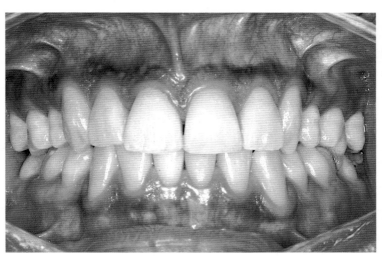
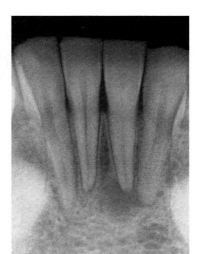

# Gingival Width

The attached gingiva becomes wider as a patient ages (Ainamo et al. 1981). It also varies considerably from tooth to tooth and among individuals. Although it was once believed that a minimum width of attached gingiva (ca. 2 mm) is necessary to maintain the health of the periodontium (Lang & Löe 1972), this view has been called into question in recent years (Wennström 1982, 1983, Dorfman et al. 1982, Wennström & Lindhe 1983 a, b).

# Col – Interpapillary Saddle

Apical to the contact area, the interdental gingiva assumes a concave form when viewed in labiolingual section (Fig. 8). The concavity, the "col," is thus located between the lingual and facial interdental papillae and is not visible clinically. Depending on the expanse of the contacting tooth surfaces, the col will be of varying depth and breadth. The epithelium covering the col consists of the marginal epithelia of the adjacent teeth (Cohen 1959, 1962; Schroeder 1986). In the absence of contact between adjacent teeth, the keratinized gingivae courses uninterrupted from the facial to the oral aspect.

| | | | | | | | | | | | | | | | | | |
|---|---|---|---|---|---|---|---|---|---|---|---|---|---|---|---|---|---|
| | | | | | | | | 6-6 | | | | | Max. facial | | | | |
| | | | | | | | | 4-4 | | | | | | | | | |
| | | | | | | | | 2-2 | | | | | | | | | |
| | | | | | | | | mm | | | | | Max. palatal | | | | |
| 8 | 7 | 6 | 5 | 4 | 3 | 2 | 1 | | 1 | 2 | 3 | 4 | 5 | 6 | 7 | 8 |
| 8 | 7 | 6 | 5 | 4 | 3 | 2 | 1 | | 1 | 2 | 3 | 4 | 5 | 6 | 7 | 8 |
| | | | | | | | | 2-2 | | | | | Mand. lingual | | | | |
| | | | | | | | | 4-4 | | | | | | | | | |
| | | | | | | | | 6-6 | | | | | | | | | |
| | | | | | | | | 2-2 | | | | | | | | | |
| | | | | ↑ | ↑ | | | 4-4 | | | ↑ | ↑ | Mand. facial | | | | |
| | | | | | | | | 6-6 | | | | | | | | | |

**6 Mean width of gingiva**
In the *maxilla* the *facial* gingiva in the area of the incisors is wide; it is narrow around the canines and premolars. On the *palatal* aspect the marginal gingiva blends without demarcation into the palatal mucosa.

In *the mandible* the *lingual* gingiva in the area of the incisors is narrow, but wide on the molars. On the *facial* the gingiva around the canines and the first premolars is narrow (arrow), but wide around the lateral incisors.

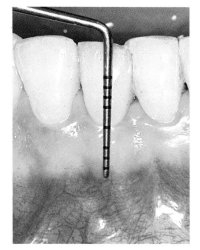 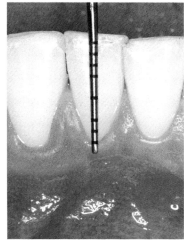

**7 Variability of gingival width**
The width of attached gingiva can vary dramatically. The three patients depicted here, all about the same age, exhibit gingival width varying from 1 to 10 mm in the mandibular anterior area.

*Right:* After staining the mucosa with iodine (Schiller or Lugol solution) the mucogingival line is easily visible because the non-keratinized alveolar mucosa is iodine-positive while the keratinized gingiva is not.

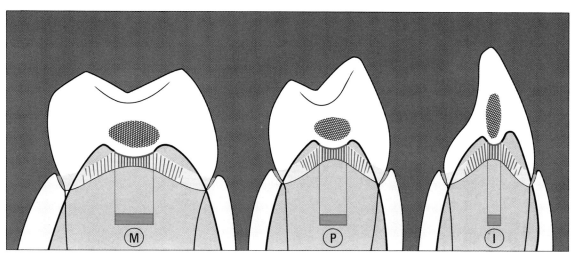

**8 Col – Interpapillary saddle**
The col consists essentially of a connection between the junctional epithelia (JE) of any two adjacent teeth. Tooth morphology, width of the tooth crowns and relative tooth position will determine the orofacial and the coronoapical extent of the contact surfaces (hatched) and therewith the breadth (2–7 mm, red bar), as well as the depth (0.1–2 mm) of the interpapillary saddle.

**I** = Incisor
**P** = Premolar
**M** = Molar

# Epithelial Attachment

### Junctional epithelium – Epithelial attachment – Gingival sulcus

The specialized junctional epithelium of the free marginal gingiva forms the epithelial attachment of gingiva to the tooth surface. This attachment is continuously being renewed throughout life (Schroeder & Listgarten 1977).

### Junctional epithelium

The junctional epithelium (JE) is approximately 2 mm in coronoapical dimension, and surrounds the neck of each tooth. At its apical extent it consists of only a few cell layers, more coronally it consists of some 15–30 cell layers. Subjacent to the sulcus bottom, the JE is about 0.15 mm wide.

The JE consists of two layers: basal, suprabasal. It remains undifferentiated and does not keratinize. The basal cells interface with the connective tissue via hemidesmosomes and the external basal lamina. Healthy JE has no rete ridges.

JE turnover rate is high (4–6 days) compared to oral epithelium (6–12 days; cf. Skougaard 1965, 1970).

**9   Marginal periodontium and gingiva in orofacial section**
The gingiva consists of three different tissues:

- Junctional epithelium
- Oral epithelium
- Lamina propria
  (connective tissue)

The *junctional epithelium* (JE) assumes a key role in maintenance of periodontal health: It creates the firm attachment of soft tissue to hard tissue; it is quite permeable, and thus serves as a pathway for diffusion of the metabolic products of plaque bacteria (toxins, chemotactic agents, antigens/mitogens etc.).

Even when the gingiva do not appear inflamed clinically, the JE is transmigrated by polymorphonuclear leukocytes (PMNs) moving toward the sulcus (see Etiology and Pathogenesis. p. 22).

The red arrows depict the migration of daughter cells of the basal layer toward the gingival sulcus.

The circled areas **A – B – C** are depicted in detail on page 5.

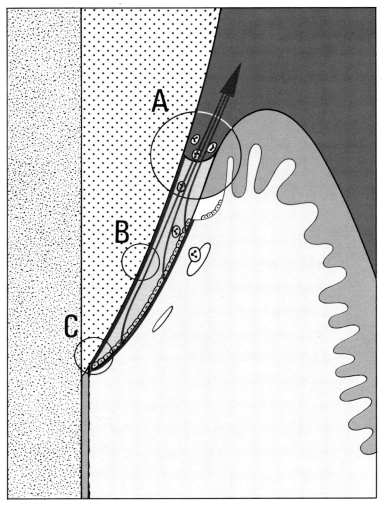

**Structure of the junctional epithelium (JE)**
   Height:           2 mm
   Coronal width:   0.15 mm

**A  Normal gingival sulcus (GS)**
   Histologic width: 0.15 mm
            Depth:   0–0.5 mm
   Clinical depth:   0.5–3 mm
            (dependent upon the penetration of the probe into the junctional epithelium; Fig. 292)

**B  Internal basal lamina (IBL)**
   "Epithelial attachment"
   Thickness: 350–1400 Å
   (1 Å = 0.0000001 mm)

**C  Apical extent of the junctional epithelium**

### Epithelial attachment

The epithelial attachment to the tooth provided by the JE consists of an internal basal lamina (IBL) and hemidesmosomes. The attachment of JE to hard tooth structure can occur on enamel, cementum or dentin in exactly the same manner. The basal lamina and hemidesmosomes of the epithelial attachment are structural analogs of their counterparts that comprise the junction between epithelium and subjacent connective tissue.

All cells of the JE are in continual coronal migration, even those cells in immediate contact with the tooth surface. Such cells must continually dissolve and re-establish their hemidesmosomal attachments. Between the basal lamina and the tooth surface, a 0.5–1 μm thick dental cuticle is frequently observed. This cuticle is probably a synthetic product of JE cells.

### Gingival sulcus

The sulcus is a narrow groove surrounding the tooth, about 0.5 mm deep. The bottom of the sulcus is made up of the most coronal cells of the junctional epithelium, which are constantly in the process of being sloughed. One lateral wall of the sulcus is made up of the tooth structure, the other wall is the non-keratinized oral sulcular epithelium (Lange & Schroeder 1971).

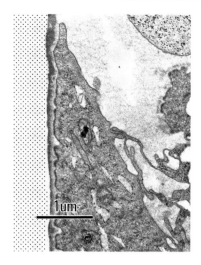

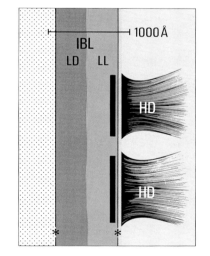

1 **Junctional epithelium**     **JE**

2 **Oral sulcular epithelium OSE**

3 **Connective tissue**        **CT**

4 **Gingival sulcus**          **GS**

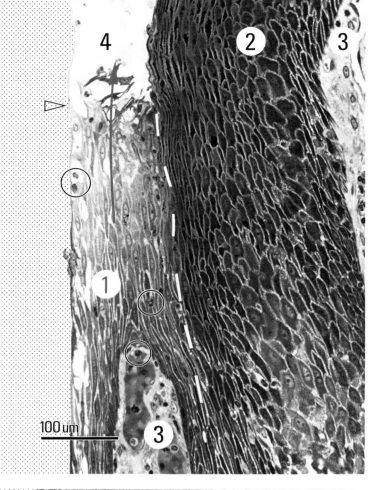

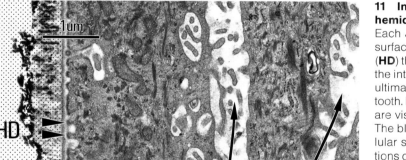

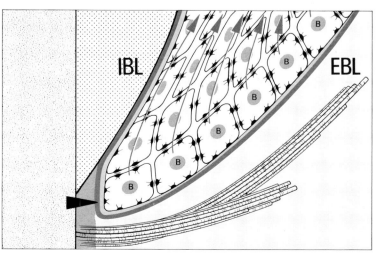

### 10 Gingival sulcus (GS) and junctional epithelium (JE)

In this histologic section, the spindle-shaped cells of the junctional epithelium (**1**) are oriented parallel to the tooth surface and are sharply demarcated (broken line) from the more deeply staining cells of the oral sulcular epithelium (**2**). All JE cells originate at the basal layer and migrate toward the sulcus bottom (**4**, red arrow) where they are sloughed into the sulcus. The basal layer can be 1.5–2 mm long, yet the sulcus bottom may be only 100–150 μm across, emphasizing the bottle-neck through which JE cells must pass.

Observe the polymorphonuclear leukocytes (circled), which emigrate from venule plexus in the subepithelial connective tissue (**3**) and transmigrate the JE.

*Left:* In the enlargement, a portion of the most coronal JE cell (cf. empty black arrow in lower power view) is shown still manifesting hemidesmosomes and an internal basal lamina attaching to the enamel surface.

TEMs courtesy *H. E. Schroeder*

### 11 Internal basal lamina and hemidesmosomes

Each JE cell adjacent to the tooth surface forms hemidesmosomes (**HD**) that enable the cell to attach to the internal basal lamina (**IBL**) and ultimately to the surface of the tooth. Remnants of enamel crystals are visible at the left (black spots). The black arrows indicate intercellular space between JE cells. Portions of three JE cells are observed (black dots).

*Left: The internal basal lamina* is comprised of two layers: the Lamina lucida (**LL**) and the Lamina densa (**LD**).

### 12 Most apical portion of the junctional epithelium

In a young, healthy patient the JE ends apically at the cementoenamel junction. Daughter cells of the cuboidal basal cells (**B**) migrate toward the sulcus (red arrows). If a JE cell comes into contact with the tooth surface, it establishes the attachment mechanism described above. The internal basal lamina (**IBL**) is continuous with the external basal lamina (**EBL**) around the apical extent of the JE (arrow).

Immediately below the JE, the first dentogingival collagen fiber bundles are seen.

# Connective Tissue Attachment

### Gingival and periodontal fiber groups – Root cementum

The connective tissue attachment structures provide the connection between teeth and their alveoli, between teeth and gingiva, as well as between each tooth and its neighbor. These structures include:

- Gingival fiber bundles
- Periodontal ligament fiber bundles
- Cementum
- Alveolar bone (see pp. 8 & 9)

### Gingival fiber bundles

In the supra-alveolar area, collagen fiber bundles course in various directions. These fibers give the gingiva its resiliency and resistance, and attach it onto the tooth surface subjacent to the epithelial attachment. The fibers also provide resistance to forces and stabilize the individual teeth into a closed segment (see also Fig. 14). The periostogingival fibers are also a component of the gingival fiber groups. These connect the attached gingiva to the alveolar process.

**13  Gingival and periodontal fiber bundles, cementum, alveolar bone**

The major portion of the connective tissue compartment of free marginal and attached gingiva is comprised of collagen fiber bundles (**A**). These splay from the cementum of the root surface into the gingiva. Other fiber bundles course more or less horizontally within the gingiva and between the teeth, forming a complex architecture (Figs. 14, 15). In addition to collagen fibers, one may also observe a small number of reticular (argyrophilic) fibers.

The periodontal ligament space (**B**) in adults is ca. 0.15–0.2 mm wide. About 60% of the space is occupied by collagen fiber bundles of ca. 4 μm thickness. The periodontal ligament fiber bundles traverse from cementum to the alveolar bone (**C**).

Approximately 28,000 fiber bundles may be detected in 1 mm² of cementum surface!

*Right:* Marginal gingiva. Fiber-rich connective tissue (**A**, blue), junctional epithelium and oral epithelium (red-brown).

Histology courtesy *N. P. Lang*

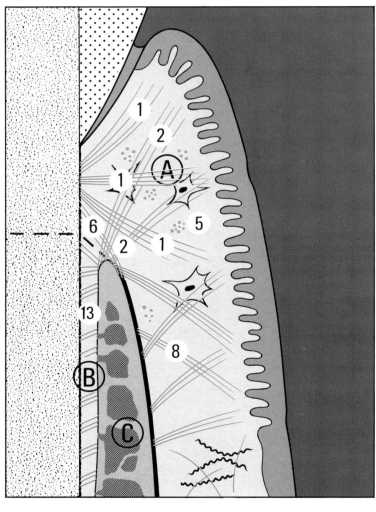

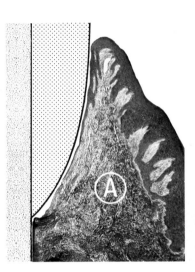

A  **Gingival fibers**

B  **Periodontal fibers**

C  **Alveolar bone**

### Periodontal ligament

The periodontal ligament (PDL) occupies the space between the root surface and the alveolar bone. The PDL consists of connective tissue fibers, cells, vasculature, nerves and ground substance.

The building block of a fiber bundle is the 40-70 nm thick collagen fibril. Many such fibrils in parallel arrangement make up a collagen fiber. Numerous fibers combine to form collagen fiber bundles. These collagen fiber bundles (Sharpey's fibers) insert into the alveolar bone on one end and into cementum at the other (Feneis 1952).

### Cementum

Various types of cementum cover the root (Schroeder 1986). Anatomically cementum represents a portion of the tooth; functionally however, it belongs to the tooth-supporting apparatus because the gingival and periodontal fiber bundles are anchored in it. Cementum becomes thicker from its coronal (50–150 μm) to its apical (200–600 μm) extent. In its apical third and sometimes in furcation areas, it contains viable cells. Lacunae up to 80 μm deep are often found in cementum (these may represent niches for bacteria and subsequent pocket formation (p. 135, Figs. 327 & 328).

Cementum is covered by a layer of "cementoid."

**Course of the gingival fiber bundles ...**
(see also Fig. 13 A)

1 Dentogingival
   – Coronal
   – Horizontal
   – Apical
2 Alveologingival
3 Interpapillary
4 Transgingival
5 Circular, Semicircular
6 Dentoperiosteal
7 Transseptal
8 Periostogingival
9 Intercircular
10 Intergingival

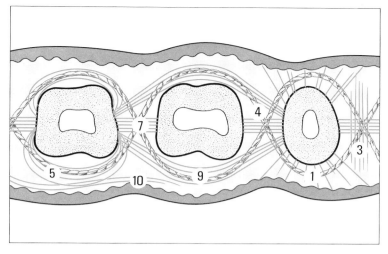

**Gingival fibers (A)**

**14  Fiber apparatus in horizontal section**
The course of the most important supracrestal (gingival) fiber bundles is depicted. The connections between teeth and gingiva as well as between individual teeth are clear. The numbers refer to the table (left) and also to Figure 13.

The course of *all* gingival fiber bundles is listed in the table (left).

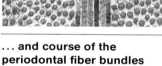

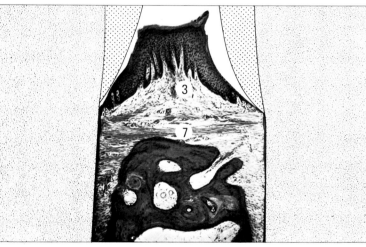

**15  Fiber bundles viewed in mesiodistal section**
In the interdental area the transseptal fiber bundles (**7**) serve to stabilize the arch in its mesiodistal dimension.

Histology courtesy *N. P. Lang*

*Left:* The basic element of fiber bundles is the *collagen fibril* (cut in cross- and longitudinal section). At the EM level collagen fibrils exhibit a regular 64 nm banding pattern (compare the wave length of blue light, 400 nm).

TEM courtesy *H. E. Schroeder*

**... and course of the periodontal fiber bundles**

11 Crestal
12 Horizontal
13 Oblique
14 Interradicular
15 Apical

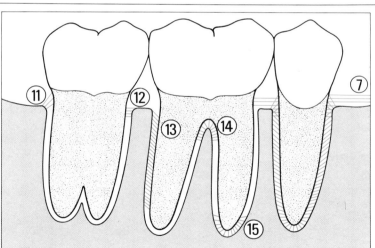

**Periodontal fibers (B)**

**16  Fiber apparatus in sagittal section**
The anchoring of a tooth in the alveolar bone is accomplished through the dentoalveolar fibers of the periodontal ligament.
   Occlusal forces are absorbed primarily by the oblique fibers, which course from bone to cementum (**13**). The remaining fiber bundles (**11, 12, 14, 15**) absorb and resolve forces that would tend to dislodge the tooth. All fibers resist forces of tipping and rotation.

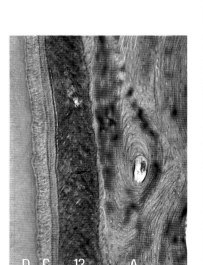

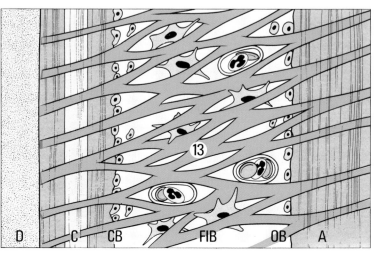

**17  Periodontal ligament (PDL) – Detail**
The collagen fiber bundles (**13**) are intertwined. Osteoblasts (**OB**) and cementoblasts (**CB**) occupy the surfaces of the adjacent tooth and bone, while numerous fibroblasts (**FIB**), vessels and nerve tissue are interspersed with the fiber bundles.

*Left:* The histologic section (Azan, x 50) depicts the fiber-rich periodontal ligament (**13**) and its relationship to dentin (**D**) / cementum (**C**) and the alveolar bone surface (**A**).

Histology courtesy *N. P. Lang*

# Osseous Support Apparatus

### Alveolar process – Alveolar bone

The *alveolar processes* of the maxilla and mandible are tooth-dependent structures. They develop with the formation of and during the eruption of the teeth and they atrophy for the most part after tooth loss.

Three structures of the alveolar process may be discriminated:

- Alveolar bone proper
- Trabecular bone
- Compact bone

Compact bone covers the alveolar process and it is thinner on its facial aspect. At the entrance to the alveoli it blends into the alveolar bone proper, which forms the alveolar wall and is approximately 0.1-0.4 mm thick. It is perforated with numerous small canals (Volkmann canals) through which blood and lymph vessels as well as nerves enter the periodontal space. Alveolar bone proper is seen as the lamina dura on x-rays.

Between the compact bone and the alveolar bone is the trabecular bone. Bone marrow spaces in the alveolar trabeculi contain mainly fatty marrow in adults.

**18   Bony support apparatus**
The tooth-supportive alveolar process consists of three different structures:

- **Alveolar bone (1)**
- **Trabecular bone (2)**
- **Compact bone (3)**

Alveolar bone and compact bone meet at the margin to form the alveolar crestal bone (arrow). In this region the alveolar process is often extremely thin, especially on the facial aspect, and unsupported by trabecular bone (cf. Fig. 23).

*Right:* Histologic section through the periodontium (H & E, x10).

On the right side of the picture the alveolar bone with its osteons and Haversian canal is visible. Bundle bone has been laid down adjacent to these structures on the periodontal aspect. The periodontal ligament contains cell-rich structures and a thin layer of cementoblasts (left).

Histology courtesy *H. E. Schroeder*

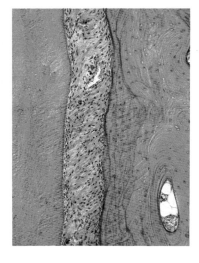

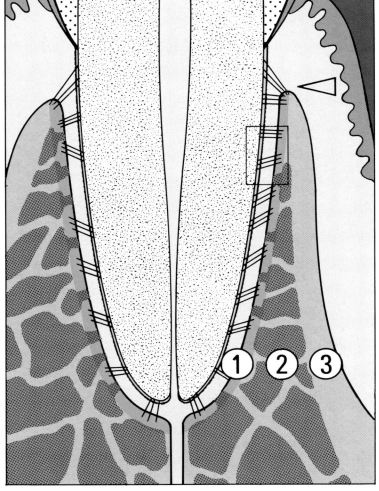

1  **Alveolar bone**
   – **Cribriform plate**
   – **Alveolar wall**
   – **Lamina dura** (radiograph)

2  **Trabecular bone**

3  **Compact bone**

**19 Mandibular alveolar process in sagittal section**
In this thin histologic section (H & E, x1) the elegant structure of the trabecular bone and the more or less large marrow spaces are visible. The alveolar bone proper is depicted as only a very thin, often partially broken line. The mandibular canal is visible at the lower left.

*Right:* In this transilluminated bone preparation it becomes clear that the alveolar bone is perforated by numerous small holes, as in a sieve (cribriform plate!).

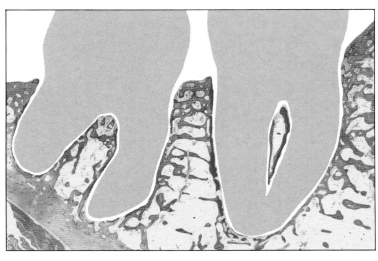

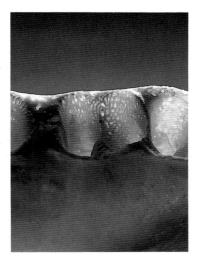

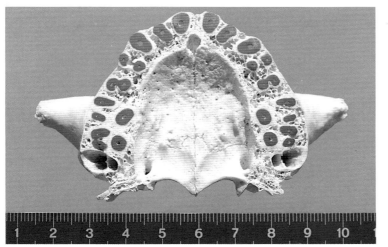

**Maxillary bone**

### 20 Maxillary alveolar process in horizontal section

The section is through the alveolar process and tooth roots at about the midpoint.

With the exception of the molar areas, the bone is thicker on the oral surface than on the facial. The trabecular bone is variably thick. Clearly visible is the varying mass of the bony interdental and inter-radicular septa, as well as the varying shapes of the root cross-sections.

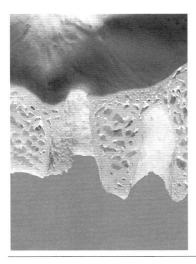
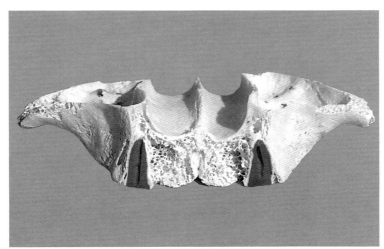

### 21 Maxilla – Frontal section

This section was cut through the plane of the canines, and it shows the relationship of the roots to the nasal sinuses. Clearly visible is the very thin bony layer on the facial surface of the roots (compare Fig. 20).

*Left:* The sagittal section shows how the root tips of premolars and molars sometimes extend into the maxillary sinuses. The alveolar bone may actually border directly on the sinus mucosa.

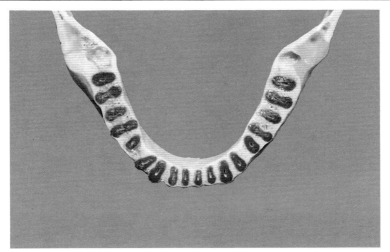

**Mandibular bone**

### 22 Mandibular alveolar process in horizontal section

The section represents a cut approximately halfway down the tooth roots. In contrast to the maxilla, the orofacial width of the mandibular alveolar process is considerably less. All roots exhibit an hourglass profile (proximal concavities).

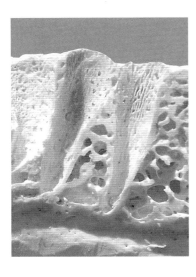
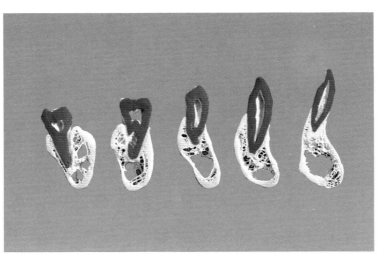

### 23 Orofacial section through the mandible

From right to left, an incisor, a canine, a premolar and two molars were sectioned. Impressive is the thin, tapered bony lamella on the facial aspect; it is impossible to distinguish between compact bone and alveolar bone proper.

*Left:* Sagittal section through the alveolar process and the alveoli. Especially in the molar area, the alveolar bone is traversed by numerous Volkmann canals.

# Blood Supply of the Periodontium

All periodontal tissues, but especially the periodontal ligament, have a copious blood supply even in the healthy state. This is due not only to the high metabolism of this cell- and fiber-rich tissue, but also to the peculiar mechanical/functional demands on the periodontium. Occlusal forces are resisted not only by the periodontal ligament and the alveolar process, but also by means of the tissue fluid and its transfer within the periodontal ligament space (hydraulic pressure distribution, dampening).

The most important afferent vessels for the alveolar process and the periodontium are:

– in the *maxilla,* the anterior and posterior alveolar arteries, the infraorbital artery and the palatine artery
– in the *mandible,* the sublingual artery, the mental artery, and the buccal and facial arteries.

Lymph vessels and nerves follow for the most part the blood vascular tree.

**24   Diagram of periodontal blood supply**
The periodontal ligament (**1**), the alveolar process (**2**) and the gingiva (**3**) are supplied by three vascular sources. These vessels exhibit frequent anastomoses. Within the periodontal ligament, the vascular network is especially dense, taking on the appearance and character of a thickly woven basket.

Adjacent to the junctional epithelium these vessels splay into a very dense *plexus* (**A**) with numerous venules. This may have some significance for immediate host defense against infection.

The oral epithelium contacts the subjacent connective tissue through a series of rete ridges. Each rete ridge of connective tissue contains *capillary loops* (**B**).

*Right* (**A**): In this tangential section of canine tissue, directly beneath the junctional epithelium, a dense *plexus of vessels* (**X**) is found even in health. Above the arrow one observes the most marginal vascular loops in the area of the adjacent oral sulcular epithelium. The vessels here are filled with a carbon-gelatin mixture (compare Figs. 98 & 101).

Courtesy *J. Egelberg*

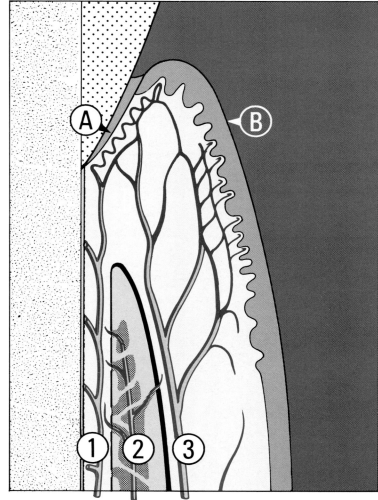
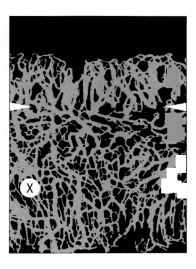

**Blood supply pathways**

**1 Periodontal**

**2 Alveolar**

**3 Supraperiosteal/ mucogingival**

**25   Fluorescence angiography – Vascular loops within the oral epithelium**
Following intravenous injection of 2 ml of sodium fluorescein solution (20%) the vessels (capillaries) subjacent to the oral epithelium can be rendered visible by UV-light. Some small vascular loops are visible in the connective tissue rete pegs (**B** in Fig. 24).

Courtesy *W. Mörmann*

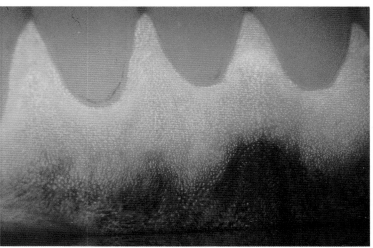

# Etiology and Pathogenesis

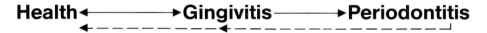

**Health** ←————→ **Gingivitis** ————→ **Periodontitis**

The most common diseases of the tooth supporting apparatus are plaque-induced, inflammatory alterations in the gingiva and the periodontium.

*Gingivitis* may persist for many years without progressing to periodontitis. With good oral hygiene and effective professional removal of plaque and calculus, gingivitis is completely reversible.

*Periodontitis* usually develops out of a more or less pronounced gingivitis. Periodontitis is only partially reversible (see Periodontal Healing, p. 136).

The reasons why gingivitis develops into periodontitis (or does *not*) are still incompletely understood. As with all opportunistic infections it appears that the proliferation of pathogenic microorganisms and their capacity to invade tissues, and above all the individual host response to such infections (resistance, immune status) are the determining factors (Listgarten 1986, 1987).

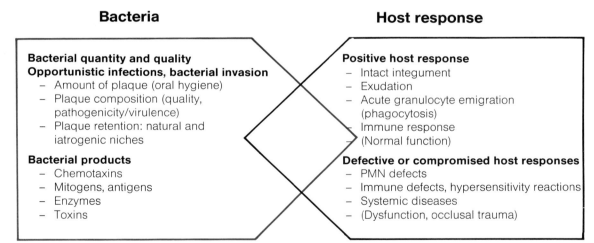

**Bacteria**

**Bacterial quantity and quality**
**Opportunistic infections, bacterial invasion**
- Amount of plaque (oral hygiene)
- Plaque composition (quality, pathogenicity/virulence)
- Plaque retention: natural and iatrogenic niches

**Bacterial products**
- Chemotaxins
- Mitogens, antigens
- Enzymes
- Toxins

**Host response**

**Positive host response**
- Intact integument
- Exudation
- Acute granulocyte emigration (phagocytosis)
- Immune response
- (Normal function)

**Defective or compromised host responses**
- PMN defects
- Immune defects, hypersensitivity reactions
- Systemic diseases
- (Dysfunction, occlusal trauma)

**26  Bacterial attack and host response**
The strength of bacterial attack depends on the virulence of the microorganisms, the amount and composition of plaque, ability of the organisms to invade tissues, and metabolic products.

The capacity of the host to respond to bacterial challenge (resistance, p. 25) will determine the severity of an ensuing gingivitis, the initiation of periodontitis, and the rapidity with which destruction of periodontal tissues proceeds.

An absolutely plaque-free condition in the oral cavity is unachievable, an illusion, and probably even unphysiologic. Nevertheless, gingival and periodontal health can be maintained if the accumulation of plaque is small and contains few virulent organisms (gram-positive, facultative anaerobes), and if an effective host response is mounted.

If the flora assumes a specific virulent (gram-negative) character inflammation and a pronounced immune response will be the result. A massive immune response represents not only defense mechanisms, but also destructive (cytotoxic) potential, especially in long-standing infection (pp. 25–30).

The products of bacteria that elicit inflammation are chemotaxins as well as mitogens, antigens and toxins.

If bacteria invade directly into tissue, it would be proper to speak of a true infection.

Bacterial enzymes and various toxins can probably cause tissue injury and destruction directly, without an immediate host response (inflammation). Bacterial products including hyaluronidase, chondroitin sulfatase, proteolytic enzymes as well as cytotoxins in the form of organic acids, ammonia, hydrogen sulfide and bacterial endotoxins (lipopolysaccharide, LPS) have been demonstrated in tissues.

## Accumulated Debris – Microbial Plaque

*Food debris* cling only lightly to the teeth and oral mucosa, and can be easily rinsed away with water.

*Food impaction* may occur in interdental spaces when fibrous foodstuffs become trapped, but can be removed mechanically (dental floss etc.).

*Microbial plaque* is a structured, resilient yellow-grayish substance that adheres tenaciously to teeth. It is composed of bacteria in a matrix of salivary glyco-proteins and extracellular polysaccharides including

glucans (e.g., dextrans, mutans) and fructans (e.g., levan). This matrix makes it impossible to rinse plaque away with water; it must be removed mechanically by means of hand instruments, the toothbrush or other oral hygiene aids. Supragingival plaque and subgingival plaque represent two distinct morphologic and micro-biologic entities.

One can distinguish between adherent and non-adherent subgingival plaque. The pathogenicity of bacterial strains within plaque varies considerably. Plaque adhering to the tooth surface can become calcified.

**27   Initial supragingival plaque colonization – Healthy appearing gingiva**
A disclosing agent reveals the initial, extremely thin layer of plaque.

The gingiva is still relatively free of inflammation as observed clinically. Gingival index (GI) and papilla bleeding index (PBI) scores are zero.

This initial accumulation of plaque is only a few cell layers thick and consists primarily of gram-positive cocci.

Gingival health can be maintained with this amount of plaque accumulation!

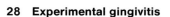

**28   Experimental gingivitis**
In 1965 Löe et al. published the classic experimental proof of the bacterial etiology of gingivitis. In plaque-free subjects with inflammation-free gingiva, plaque begins to accumulate if all oral hygiene is ceased. For the first few days this plaque is composed of *gram-positive* ⊕ cocci and rods, then later of filamentous organisms and finally of Spirochetes (*gram-negative* ⊖). Within a few days, a mild gingivitis ensues.

If the plaque is removed, the gingiva returns to a state of health.

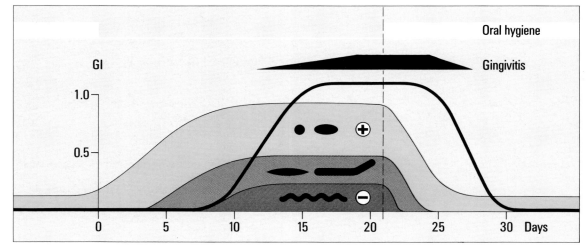

**29   Plaque accumulation – Gingivitis**
Whenever there is an accumulation of plaque, gingivitis will develop. As accumulation continues, the percentage composition of various organisms in plaque changes. Gram-negative anaerobes increase in frequency; these are more pathogenic than the earlier-appearing gram-positive cocci and rods. The gingiva reacts to both the quantitative and qualitative plaque changes with an inflammatory reaction (bleeding on probing) whose intensity may vary remarkably.

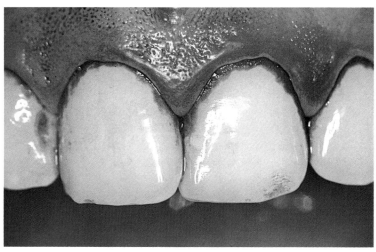

# Supragingival Plaque

### Accumulation – Alteration of composition

Within minutes to hours, a recently cleaned tooth is covered by a thin (0.1–0.8 μm) pellicle composed of salivary glycoproteins. Upon this pellicle, primarily colony-forming and gram-positive bacteria (*Streptococcus* and *Actinomyces* species) become established within 24 hours.

During the course of the next few days, the plaque increases in quantity as gram-negative cocci as well as gram-positive and gram-negative rods and filaments gain a foothold.

After three weeks, there is a significant increase in filamentous organisms, especially at the gingival margin (Listgarten et al. 1975; Listgarten 1976). The metabolic products of the plaque microorganisms provoke an elevated level of exudation and of PMN migration in the host tissues. This is the host's attempt to wall off invading bacteria. As gingivitis increases in severity, the junctional epithelium loses some of its resiliency, permitting the ingress of bacteria between the tooth and the epithelium. A gingival pocket develops.

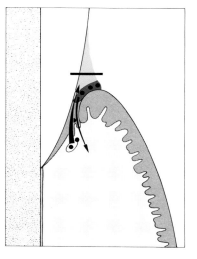

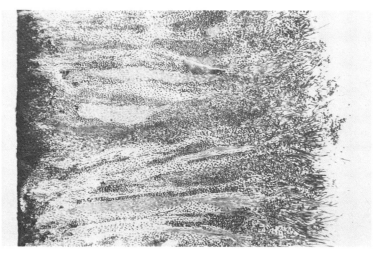

**30   One-week-old plaque – Metabolic interactions**
The newly formed plaque exhibits column-like structured colonies of coccoid organisms, with overlying rods and filaments.

*Left:* Interaction between host and plaque (blue, gram-positive; red, gram-negative). Increased migration of PMN's (thick arrow), with formation of a wall of leukocytes. Chemotactic substances from plaque (thin arrow).
The black horizontal line indicates the level from which the section of plaque was taken.

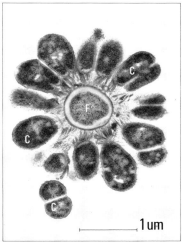

1 um

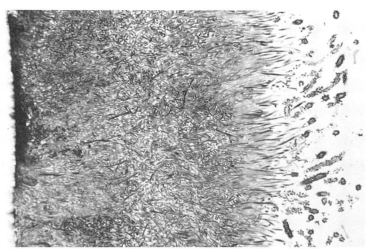

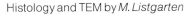

**31   Three-week-old plaque – "Corn cobs"**
The composition of the supragingival plaque has changed markedly. Filamentous organisms now predominate. Conspicuous forms resembling corn cobs are observed at the plaque surface.

*Left:* In this transmission electron photomicrograph, the structure of such a corn cob is revealed. At the center is a filamentous organism (**F**), surrounded by gram-positive cocci (**C**).

Histology and TEM by *M. Listgarten*

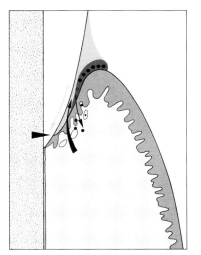

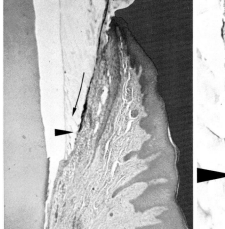

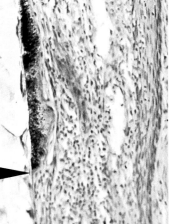

**32   Expansion of supragingival plaque – Gingival pocket**
Weakening of the attachment between tooth and JE allows initial apical migration of gram-positive plaque bacteria in a thin layer (compare black arrow). Gram-negative bacteria colonize subsequently, and a gingival pocket forms.

Histology courtesy *G. Cimasoni*

*Left:* Interaction between plaque and tissue. Gram-positive microorganisms are depicted as blue, with gram-negatives (red) adjacent to tissue.

## Natural Factors Favoring Plaque Retention

The most important naturally occurring plaque-retentive factors or "niches" include:

- Supra- and subgingival calculus
- Cementoenamel junction
- Tooth fissures and grooves
- Cervical and root caries
- Crowding of teeth in the arch
- Mouth breathing

*Calculus* represents a retentive site for vital, pathogenic bacteria because of its rough surface.

The *cementoenamel junction* also often exhibits retentive rough areas (including enamel "pearls" and projections).

*Carious lesions* may represent an enormous bacterial reservoir.

*Crowding of teeth* leads to increased accumulation of plaque because self-cleansing mechanisms are foiled and because oral hygiene is more difficult.

*Mouth breathing* leads to dehydration of the oral cavity, rendering the plaque tougher and stickier. The protective function of saliva is reduced.

**33  Supragingival calculus**
*Left:* Lingual surfaces of mandibular incisors and buccal surfaces of maxillary molars near the orifices of salivary glands often exhibit supragingival calculus.

*Right:* TEM of old supragingival calculus.
   Calcified plaque (**A**) close to the tooth surface (arrow). Calcification of plaque bacteria both *inter-* and *intracellularly*. Note cell-free accumulation of hexagonal *monocrystals* (**B**).

Courtesy *H. E. Schroeder*

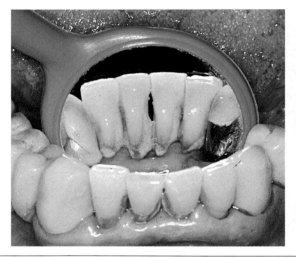
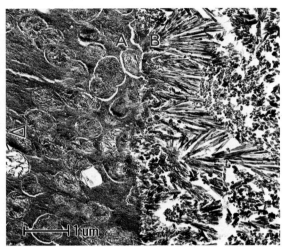

**34  Subgingival calculus**
*Left:* In this patient with long-standing periodontitis the gingiva has receded. Calculus that was formerly subgingival is now supragingival.

*Right:* Subgingival calculus is observed clinically after reflecting the gingival margin. Subgingival calculus is usually dark in color. It is also harder than the more loosely structured supragingival calculus. The cementoenamel junction is indicated by a dashed line.

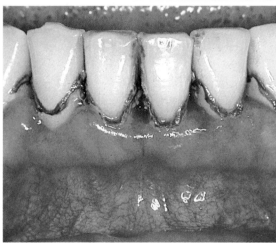
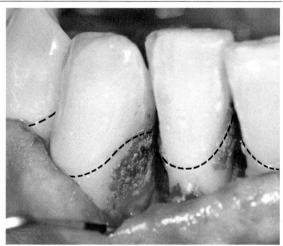

**35  Crowding**
*Left:* The lingually displaced mandibular incisors do not benefit from the natural self-cleansing action of the lower lip. Oral hygiene is also rendered more difficult.

**Enamel projection (+ pearl)**
*Right:* The furcation on this molar is filled by a projection of enamel that ends in a bulbous pearl. When a pocket forms in such an area, plaque control is particularly difficult.

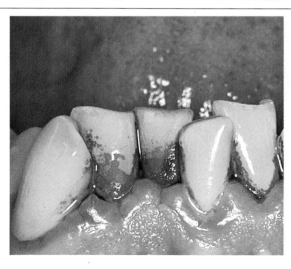
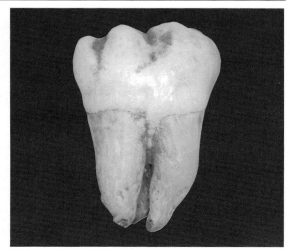

# Iatrogenic Factors Favoring Plaque Retention

Restorative dentistry – from a simple restoration to a full-mouth reconstruction – can do more harm than good to the patient's oral health if performed improperly. *Placing only optimum restorations is synonymous with preventive periodontics.*

*Fillings* that appear to be perfect clinically and macroscopically almost always exhibit deficiencies at the margins when viewed microscopically. Thus, when filling margins are located subgingivally they are always an irritation for the marginal periodontium (Renggli 1974, Hammer & Hotz 1979).

*Overhanging margins* of restorations and crowns accumulate additional plaque. Gingivitis ensues. The composition of the plaque changes. The number of gram-negative anaerobes (*Bacteriodes*), those mainly responsible for the initiation and progression of periodontitis, increases rapidly (Lang et al. 1983).

Gross iatrogenic irritants such as poorly designed *clasps* and *prosthesis saddles* may extert a direct traumatic influence on periodontal tissues.

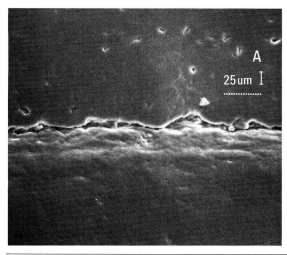

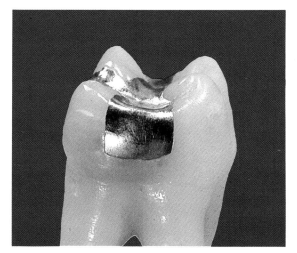

**36  Amalgam restoration**
A clinically acceptable proximal restoration.

*Left:* Viewed in the scanning electron microscope, a clearly visible margin defect is observed. Such a defect is a perfect niche for the accumulation of plaque.
**A** = Amalgam.
The white dots under the 25 μm legend are representative of the size of coccoid microorganisms (ca. 1 μm).

Courtesy *F. Lutz*

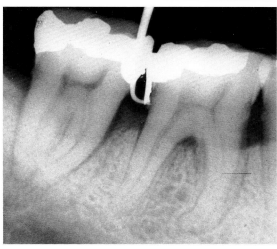

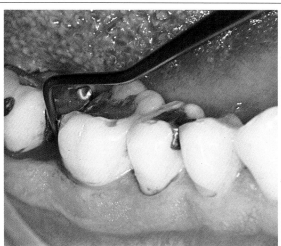

**37  Amalgam – Proximal overhang**
Gross overhangs such as this, located subgingivally, invariably lead to plaque accumulation and to gingivitis (note hemorrhage). The plaque accumulated beneath an overhang changes in its composition: Pathogenic gram-negative anaerobes (e. g., Bacterioides species) increase markedly in number.

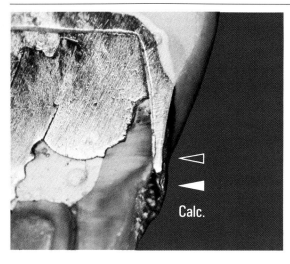

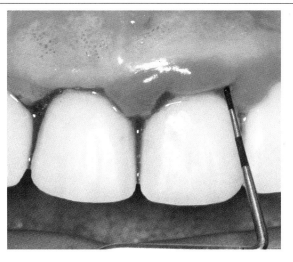

**38  Crown margin overhang and open margins**
*Right:* The cement that was used to cement this porcelain jacket crown has begun to extrude from the open margin. The massive retention of plaque between the crown and the prepared tooth leads to severe gingivitis with establishment of a pathogenic bacterial flora.

*Left:* Section through a porcelain-fused-to-gold crown with a margin that is both overhanging (arrows) and open. Darkly stained calculus (**Calc.**) is observed apical to the poor crown margin.

## Subgingival Plaque

### Adherent versus non-adherent flora

In the subgingival region it is possible to differentiate between *adherent* and *non-adherent* plaque. A dense plaque layer of varying thickness adheres to the tooth (root) surface. The composition of this adherent layer resembles the supragingival plaque associated with gingivitis: Some *gram-positive* cocci but primarily filaments and Actinomyces species. The adherent plaque can become mineralized to form subgingival calculus.

Near the soft tissue surface are observed freely moving, non-adherent bacterial accumulations comprised almost exclusively of gram-negative anaerobes: Motile and non-motile rods (Bacteroides species, especially *B. gingivalis*), Spirochetes and others. These non-adherent, partially motile, gram-negative, pathogenic anaerobes increase sharply in number in acute inflammatory lesions. They appear to play an important role in the progression of periodontitis (Listgarten 1976, Slots 1979, Page & Schroeder 1982, Lindhe 1983).

**39   Subgingival pocket flora**
On the tooth surface (left side of histologic section) is a thin layer of adherent, primarily gram-positive plaque bacteria (blue-violet).

Within the pocket exudate are observed larger loose accumulations of gram-negative anaerobic bacteria. Inset: Accumulations resembling test tube brushes also appear.

*Right:* Periodontal pocket. Adherent plaque shown as blue; non-adherent bacteria shown as red.

Histology courtesy *M. Listgarten*

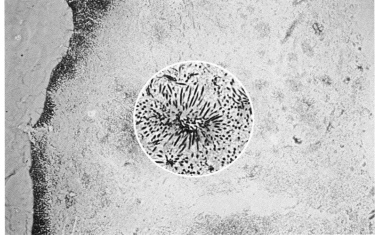
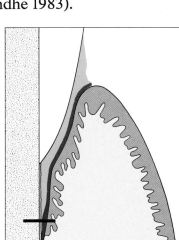

**40   Adherent plaque –
Root surface**
Within a pocket the root surface of a tooth manifesting periodontitis is covered with a densely intertwined bacterial colonization composed of many different bacterial forms (scanning electron photomicrograph).

Adherent plaque predominates, with an occasional motile organism from the non-adherent plaque.

The morphology of the bacteria permits neither a determination of the species nor any clues concerning pathogenicity.

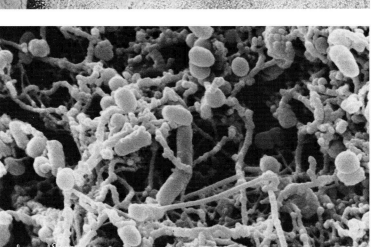

**41   Microorganisms of the non-adherent plaque**
In a streaked preparation (dark field) motile rods and Spirochetes predominate, while cocci and filaments are rare: Typical sign of an active pocket (exacerbation).

*Right:* Intact phagocytes (PMNs) in the pocket exudate do not lose their capacity for phagocytosis. Arrow depicts a Spirochete being engulfed.

Dark-field prints courtesy *B. Guggenheim*

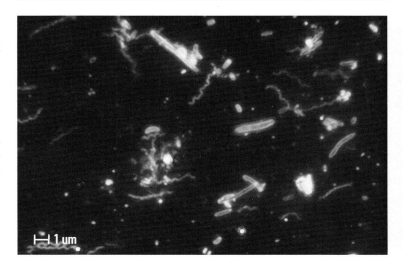
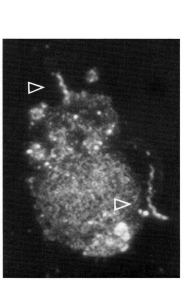

# Infection – Bacterial Invasion into Tissue?

In cases of periodontitis, especially the rapidly pro-gressive (RPP) and juvenile (LJP) forms, bacteria may traverse the pocket epithelium and invade the sub-epi-thelial connective tissue. This usually occurs only in the depth of a pocket where the organisms can avoid the massive inflammatory infiltrate that is located marginal-ly. It is probable that the invading bacteria secrete pro-tective leukotoxins that can momentarily either inhibit or neutralize the chemotactic substances guiding phago-cytic host defense cells (PMNs) to the area. Ultimately host defense cells *do* recognize and kill the bacteria.

If the number of invading organisms is small, necrotic areas will be left within the tissue; if the bacterial invasion is massive and acute, a purulent abscess with external drainage may be created (Frank 1980, Gillett & John-son 1982, Allenspach-Petrzilka & Guggenheim 1983, Genco & Slots 1984, Socransky et al. 1984, Nisengard & Bascones 1987, Saglie et al. 1988).

Whether the tissue damage is due primarily to direct toxicity of the bacteria or their products, or whether the destruction is caused by products of the host's own immune system, or both, remains unclear.

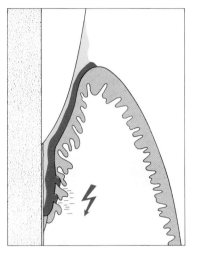

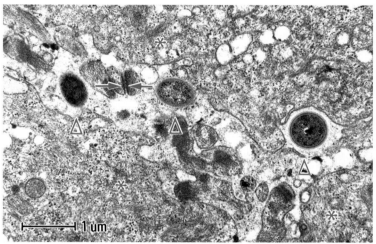

### 42 Bacteria in the pocket epithelium
During an exacerbation, bacteria (open triangles) traverse the wid-ened intercellular spaces of the pocket epithelium. Three epithelial cells (∗) and one desmosome (double arrow) are observed.

*Left:* Ulcerated epithelium is found in the depth of an active pocket. Bacteria are capable of penetrat-ing such epithelia to reach the connective tissue compartment. In this phase, components of the non-adherent subgingival plaque (red) assume prime importance.

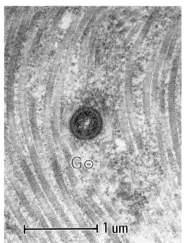

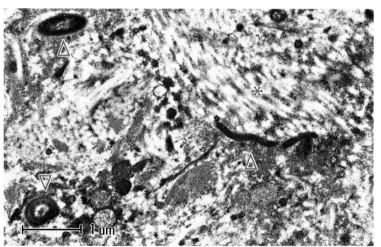

### 43 Bacterial invasion – Infection
In electron photomicrographs of *active* periodontal pockets, bacte-ria of various species are frequent-ly observed within the connective tissue (arrows). Tissue damage (∗ = degraded collagen) may result, or tissue may remain com-pletely healthy in appearance.

*Left:* A gram-negative bacterium (**G** ⊖) is observed in the midst of otherwise essentially intact colla-gen fibrils.

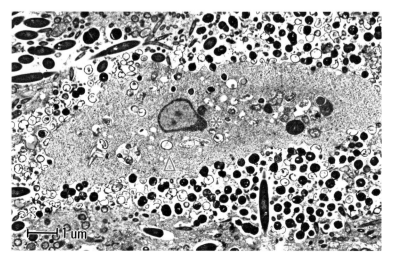

### 44 Necrosis – Suppuration
Almost the entire photomicrograph is filled by a dead phagocytic cell (∗). The cell contains phagosomes, some of which exhibit digested material (arrow).

The dead phagocyte is sur-rounded by dead bacteria and bacterial cell walls.

This pus must either be resorbed by the host tissue, or expelled.

TEMs courtesy *B. Guggenheim*

# Classical and Opportunistic Infection

## Classical infection

According to Koch's postulates, in a classical infection the defense capability of the host is overcome by a specific virulent strain of microorganism, which proliferates within the tissue and, as a result, provokes the host organism toward typical, reproducible symptoms of disease.

Examples of classic infectious diseases are diphtheria, tuberculosis and scarlet fever.

## Opportunistic infection

Opportunistic organisms are facultative pathogens. They are regularly found in the natural flora (e.g., in the oral cavity). They normally do not cause damage to the host. However, in certain situations (e.g., reduced resistance of the host) a selective proliferation of such facultative pathogens can occur. This situation is referred to as an infection with opportunistic organisms. Example: *Candida* infection in AIDS patients.

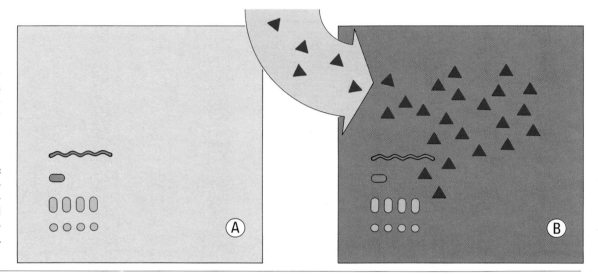

**45   Classical infection**

**A – Initial Situation**
Non-specific, "natural" colonization with gram-positive (blue) and a few gram-negative (red) microorganisms. The host is healthy (ecological balance).

**B – Infection**
An increased number of specific pathogenic microorganisms (violet triangles) penetrates the defense mechanism of the host and begin to proliferate. Tissue damage or disease is the consequence.

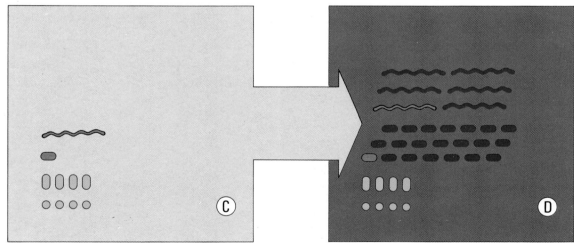

**46   Opportunistic infection**

**C – Initial Situation**
The same non-pathogenic flora is present, as in Figure 45 A.

**D – Infection/Shift**
Alterations in the micro-ecology and the general resistance of the host lead to a destabilization of the ecological balance. One or more species (Spirochetes, rods; red) react to this new situation with selective proliferation. In such increased numbers, these organisms can elicit tissue damage (disease).

## Specific plaque hypothesis

The *specific plaque hypothesis* states that specific virulent bacteria in plaque cause periodontitis (Slots 1986). These bacteria differ from other species on the basis of typical characteristics of pathogenicity and through their strongly increased presence in *acutely* diseased pockets. It is important to note that, according to the *specific plaque hypothesis*, these microorganisms constitute a minor component of "normal" (non-pathogenic) dental plaque in healthy subjects; only in *elevated numbers* do they become destructive.

## Non-specific plaque hypothesis

The *non-specific plaque hypothesis* relates periodontitis to a proliferating mixed infection that includes superinfection especially of the subgingival plaque. Host defense mechanisms do not mount an effective response (Theilade 1986). Specific bacterial *groups* (gram –) do play a role in disease activity.

Most recent research supports the non-specific plaque hypothesis as etiologic for adult periodontitis.

# Classified Microorganisms of the Plaque

About 300 species and sub-species of microorganisms can be isolated and characterized from plaque samples taken from the subgingival area (Moore et al. 1982 a, b; Slots & Genco 1984). Only very few of these are periodontal pathogens, and among these are the *black pigmented Bacteroides* (especially *B. gingivalis* and *B. intermedius*) and *Actinobacillus actinomycetemcomitans* (*Aa*). It is possible that several types of Treponema should also be listed under the rubric "periodontal pathogens."

Periodontopathic bacteria possess important biochemical characteristics that may account for their pathogenicity (Slots & Genco 1984). They are capable of colonizing root surfaces and pockets where they can maintain themselves within the microecology of the pocket flora. In addition to these properties, which are also shared by other bacteria, periodontal pathogens are also characterized by their ability to avoid the defense mechanisms of the host (leukotoxins) and to damage the periodontal tissues directly (endotoxins).

| Gram ⊕ positive | | Gram ⊖ negative | |
|---|---|---|---|
| Facultative anaerobes | Anaerobes | Facultative anaerobes | Anaerobes |
| **Streptococcus**<br>– S.mutans<br>– S.sanguis<br>– S.salivarius<br>– S.milleri<br>– S.mitis<br>**Micrococcus** | **Peptostreptococcus**<br>**Peptococcus**<br>**Streptococcus** | **Neisseria**<br>**Branhamella** | **Veillonella**<br>– V.alcalescens<br>– V.atypica<br>– V.parvula |
| **Actinomyces**<br>– A.naeslundii<br>– A.viscosus<br>**Bacterionema**<br>**Rothia**<br>**Nocardia**<br>**Lactobacillus**<br>– L.acidophilus<br>– L.casei<br>– L.fermentum | **Actinomyces**<br>– A.israelii<br>– A.odontolyticus<br>**Arachnia**<br>**Eubacterium**<br>**Propionibacterium**<br>**Bifidobacterium** | **Actinobacillus**<br>– A.actinomycetem-<br>comitans<br>**Capnocytophaga**<br>– C.gingivalis<br>– C.ochracea<br>– C.sputigena<br>**Eikenella**<br>– E.corrodens<br>**Haemophilus**<br>– H.segnis | **Bacteroides**<br>– B.gingivalis<br>– B.intermedius<br>– B.forsythus<br>– B.melaninogenicus<br>– B.loescheii<br>– B.denticola<br>– B.corporis<br>**Fusobacterium**<br>**Leptotrichia**<br>**Campylobacter**<br>**Selenomonas**<br>**Wolinella** |

| **Treponema**<br>– T. vincentii<br>– T. denticola<br>– T. socranskii | **Mycoplasma** | **Candida**<br>– C. albicans | **Entamoeba** | **Trichomonas** |
|---|---|---|---|---|

**47   Selection from the classified microorganisms**
Adapted from Slots 1976, 1979, 1986; Lindhe 1983.

●    **Cocci**

━    **Rods**

Light Blue: Gram +, aerobes
Dark Blue: Gram +, anaerobes

Light Red:  Gram –, aerobes
Dark Red:  Gram –, anaerobes

(The same color codes are used on pp. 20–21)

〰️ **Spirochetes and other microorganisms**

**Gram-positive bacterium**                   **Gram-negative bacterium**

Cytoplasmic membrane
Peptidoglycan

Periplasmatic space
(typical of gram-negatives)

Outer membrane
(proteins, lipids,
lipopolysaccharide LPS)

**48   Cell wall characteristics – Gram-positive bacteria (left)**
The peptidoglycan layer is much thicker than in the case of gram-negative microorganisms. Immunologically reactive teichoic acids are characteristic.

**Gram-negative bacteria (right)**
Over the cytoplasmic membrane and a periplasmatic space one observes a thin layer of peptidoglycan. A lipid bi-layer is linked with this layer, which contains lipopolysaccharide (**LPS**). LPS triggers the immune response and may damage tissue directly via endotoxin.

## Bacterial Flora and Types of Disease

All inflammatory periodontal diseases are caused by mixed infections (Theilade 1986). The qualitative composition of the microorganisms varies. Different plaque compositions are found between healthy and diseased periodontia, but also between any two patients with *identical* clinical periodontal conditions. Even in an individual periodontitis patient there will be various tooth surfaces and pockets with comparable attachment loss, which nevertheless reveal quite different bacterial populations (Theilade 1986). It is therefore incorrect to speak of any specific bacterial flora as the cause of gingivitis or periodontitis.

Exceptions to this general rule may be found in juvenile periodontitis and in ulcerative gingivitis. In the latter, treponemes (Spirochetes), *Fusobacterium, Bacteroides intermedius* and *Selemonas* are always found (Loesche et al. 1982, Falkler et al. 1987). In LJP the affected teeth (incisors and first permanent molars) are routinely colonized by *Actinobacillus actinomycetemcomitans* (Slots et al. 1980), but frequently also by Eikenella (Mandell 1984) and *Bacteroides gingivalis* (Tanner 1979).

### ● Healthy gingiva

A very thin, adherent layer of plaque that is often only a few cell layers thick can be associated with clinically healthy gingiva. It is even possible that these first gram-positive microorganisms occupy an "ecological niche" and therefore prevent proliferation and occupation by pathogenic organisms.

### ● Gingivitis
### ● Quiescent adult periodontitis (AP)

Considerably thicker supragingival plaque layers are observed in cases of gingivitis. Such *quantitative* accumulation of plaque plays an important role in the development of gingivitis. At the same time alterations in the *qualitative* composition of plaque flora become obvious. A gingivitis plaque is likely similar to that of a *quiescent,* slowly progressive adult periodontitis (AP).

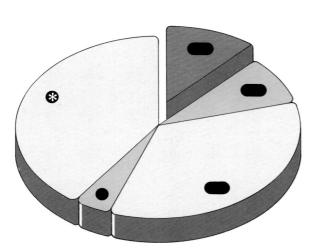

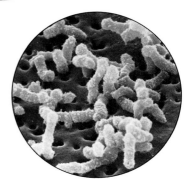

**49 Composition of plaque with healthy gingiva**
The size of the pie slices represents the percentage composition of classifiable cocci and rods. In the extremely thin plaque, gram-positive aerobic cocci and rods predominate (75%). These appear to be relatively non-pathogenic to the periodontal tissues.

Figure adapted from *Slots* 1979, *Lindhe* 1983

SEMs courtesy *B. Guggenheim*

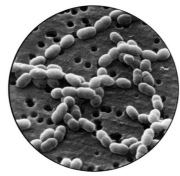

Streptococcus mutans (SEM)
*Streptococcus species*
*Actinomyces viscosus*
*Actinomyces naeslundii*
*Rothia dentocariosa*
*Bacteroides saccharolyticus*
*Capnocytophaga species*

**50 Composition of plaque in gingivitis and quiescent AP**
Especially in sites where plaque accumulates, gram-negative anaerobic organisms begin to predominate at the cost of gram-positive aerobic cocci and rods. In particular black pigmented types of *Bacteroides* and various forms of Spirochetes may become predominant.

Actinomyces viscosus (SEM)
*Actinomyces species*
*Streptococcus species*
*Bacteroides melaninogenicus*
*Capnocytophaga gingivalis*
*Eikenella corrodens*
(Spirochetes)

Although gingivitis and periodontitis are not specific infections, certain *groups of bacteria* are correlated with disease progression.

Healthy gingiva is usually associated with only a very thin, primarily gram-positive plaque. With increased plaque accumulation and an increase in gram-negative anaerobes, *gingivitis* must develop. If this persists for a certain time, the slowly progressive *adult periodontitis* (AP) can develop. In the case of *rapidly progressive* (RPP) and localized *juvenile periodontitis* (LJP),

particular gram-negative anaerobes appear to play an important role (Listgarten 1976; Van Palenstein-Helderman 1981; Lindhe 1983; Slots et al. 1986), in addition to the weakened host response.

The relationship between gram-positive and gram-negative microorganisms in the subgingival flora is different depending upon whether the disease is in an active phase or in quiescence. During an acute phase of AP, it is likely that the flora is indistinguishable from that of RPP in a young adult.

### ● Rapidly progressive periodontitis (RPP)
### ● Active adult periodontitis (AP)

In cases of RPP, and in the active phase of AP, the non-adherent subgingival plaque exhibits a markedly altered composition of the bacterial flora.

The supragingival plaque in RPP cases may be minimal, and is generally similar to the supragingival plaque found in the presence of healthy gingiva or gingivitis.

### ● Juvenile periodontitis (LJP)

In localized juvenile periodontitis (incisor-molar type) the subgingival, mobile, pathogenic plaque is similar in some aspects to that of the rapidly progressive form of the adult disease. Nevertheless, root surfaces rarely exhibit adherent microorganisms and calculus is therefore seldom observed.

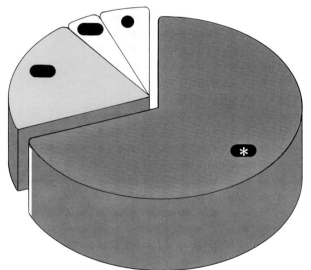

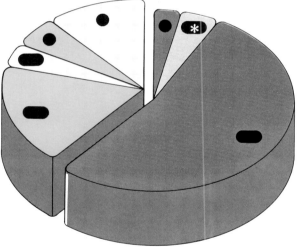

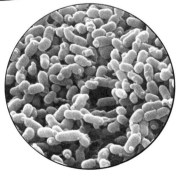

**51 Composition of plaque in RPP and active AP**
Almost three-quarters of the entire subgingival plaque consists of gram-negative anaerobic, partially motile rods and Spirochetes. Always found is *Bacteroides gingivalis,* which plays an etiologic role in the acute phases of RPP (and AP?).

**Bacteroides gingivalis (SEM)**
*Bacteroides intermedius*
*Actinobacillus actinomycetemcomitans*
*Fusobacterium nucleatum*
*Wolinella recta*
Spirochetes (*Treponema* species)

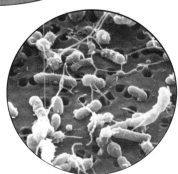

**52 Composition of plaque in LJP**
Considerably more than half of the microorganisms are gram-negative anaerobes.

Remarkable is the consistent presence of facultative anaerobic *Actinobacillus actinomycetemcomitans* (Aa), against which unusually high titers of circulating antibodies are found.

**Actinobacillus actinomycetemcomitans (SEM)**
*Capnocytophaga ochracea*
*Fusobacterium*
(Spirochetes)

# Histopathogenesis of Gingivitis and Periodontitis

The fine line demarcating healthy gingiva from gingivitis is difficult to discern. Even gingiva that appears quite healthy clinically will exhibit a few polymorphonuclear leukocytes within the junctional epithelium when viewed histologically. These PMNs have emigrated from the subepithelial vascular plexus and they end their journey by entering the gingival sulcus. Very small quantities of gingival sulcus fluid may therefore be considered physiologic (Cimasoni 1983).

Page and Schroeder (1976) described the temporal sequence of gingivitis and periodontitis development, based on their own research and a thorough literature review.

---

*Healthy gingiva* begins to exhibit the histologic features of the *"initial lesion,"* followed by an *"early lesion"* that persists for some time, and then an *"established lesion."* The clinically observable gingivitis in adults is always an established gingivitis, whose intensity, however, may vary considerably.

**Healthy gingiva**                    **Initial / Early gingivitis**

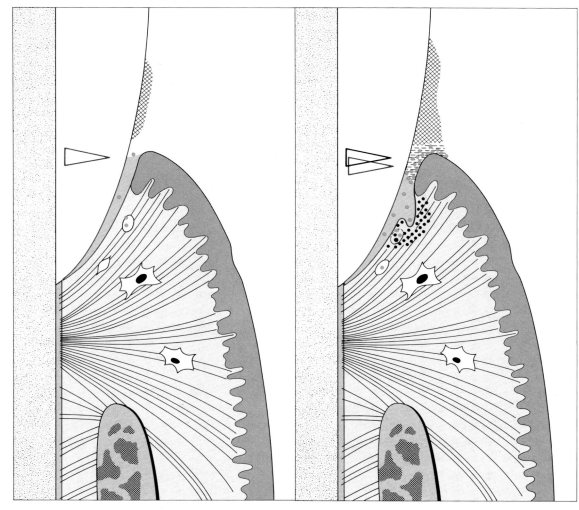

**53  Healthy gingiva**
Absence of plaque or very little accumulation (hatched area); normal junctional epithelium (pink); minimal sulcus depth (red arrow).

A few PMNs (blue dots) transmigrate the JE in the direction of the sulcus bottom. Dense collagenous fiber system; intact fibroblasts.

**54  Initial / Early gingivitis**
Early plaque accumulation. In the *initial* lesion, increased transmigration of PMNs (blue dots) within the JE.
   As the *early* lesion develops, the PMNs create a wall against the plaque bacteria within the slightly deepened sulcus (red arrow). A lymphocytic infiltrate (black dots) occurs in the subepithelial tissues.

| | | |
|---|---|---|
| **Plaque** | Little, primarily gram +, aerobic | Primarily gram +, aerobic |
| **Junctional epithelium/ Pocket epithelium** | Normal junctional epithelium without rete ridges | Initial alteration and lateral proliferation of the junctional epithelium in coronal region |
| **Vessels Inflammatory cells, infiltrate Exudate** | Few *PMNs* from subepithelial vasculature in junctional epithelium, very minimal exudate from the sulcus | Vasculitis, exudation of serum proteins, *PMN migration,* accumulation of *lymphoid cells,* very few plasma cells; appearance of immunoglobulins and complement |
| **Fibroblasts, connective tissue, collagen** | Normal | Cytopathic alterations of fibroblasts; collagen loss in infiltrated connective tissue areas |
| **Alveolar bone** | Normal | Normal |
| **Course of disease** | – | *Initial lesion* 2–4 days after plaque accumulation, *early lesion* 4–14 days |

The *initial* and *early lesions* are actually little more than histologic precursors for the established lesion in adults. In children, however, the "early lesion" can persist for extended periods of time.

The *established lesion* in adults can persist unchanged for years, perhaps even decades, without progressing to periodontitis. Adult gingivitis appears to be the result less of specific microorganisms than of plaque quantity and plaque products.

The progression of gingivitis into periodontitis (*pro-gressive lesion*), on the other hand, may well be due to some alteration of the pathogenic potential of the plaque (Van Palenstein-Helderman 1981, Figs. 26 & 43). Periodontitis may manifest clinically in various forms, which serve as the basis for their classification (cf. pp. 22–21, 86–97).

The histopathologic characteristics of the development of the gingivoperiodontal lesions are summarized in the table below.

**Established gingivitis**          **Periodontitis**

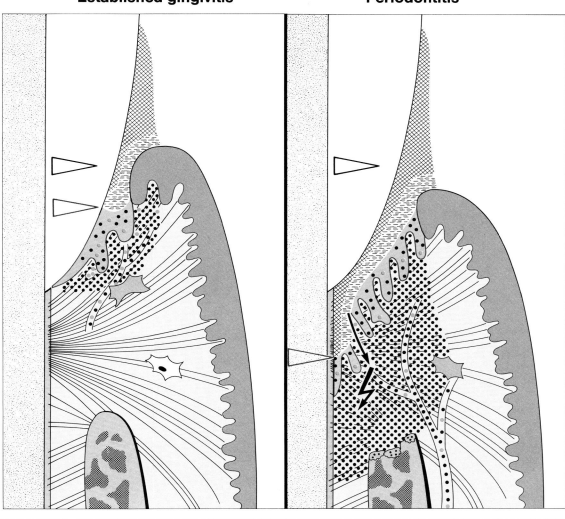

**55 Established lesion**
The gingiva responds to a massive accumulation of plaque. All of the characteristics of gingivitis are manifest but may be more or less pronounced both clinically and histologically. The gingival sulcus may actually be displaced somewhat apically (loss of *epithelial* attachment) as a consequence of the advancing front of accumulating plaque, resulting in the formation of a gingival pocket (distance between red and black arrows). There is *no* loss of connective tissue attachment. The differentiated inflammatory infiltrate protects the deeper structures.

**56 Periodontitis**
The most important histologic differences between gingivitis and periodontitis are bone resorption, apical proliferation and ulceration of the junctional (pocket) epithelium (red arrow indicates base of pocket), and progressive loss of connective tissue attachment (p. 24).

In acute (active) phases there may be bacterial invasion of the tissue, with resultant micro- or macro-abscess formation.

Adapted from *Page & Schroeder* 1982

| Gram + and gram – (in gingival pocket) | Adherent gram +, nonadherent gram – (in pocket) | **Plaque** |
|---|---|---|
| Lateral proliferation of JE, deepening of sulcus with formation of gingival pocket or pseudopocket | Apical proliferation of pocket epithelium, true pocket formation; ulceration of pocket epithelium | **Junctional epithelium/ Pocket epithelium** |
| Acute inflammatory alterations; *predominance of plasma cells; immunoglobulins in connective tissue, JE and gingival sulcus; increased sulcus exudate* | Acute inflammatory alterations as in gingivitis; *predominance of plasma cells;* copious exudate often suppurative; expansion of the inflammatory and immunopathologic reactions | **Vessels Inflammatory cells, infiltrate Exudate** |
| *Severe fibroblast injury, further loss of collagen, continued infiltration* | Further collagen loss in the infiltrated tissues, fibrosis in peripheral gingival regions | **Fibroblasts, connective tissue, collagen** |
| *Normal* | Loss of alveolar bone (attachment loss) | **Alveolar bone** |
| *Manifest 1–3 weeks after plaque accumulation; can persist for years without progressing* | Periods of quiescence and exacerbation. Progression: AP = slow; RPP & LJP = rapid | **Course of disease** |

# From Gingivitis to Periodontitis

### From reversible to irreversible

The progression of gingivitis into periodontitis is not completely understood. In terms of *pathomorphology*, the local interactions between attacker (microorganisms, bacterial products) and host defense (exudate, PMNs) are quite different in *gingivitis* and *periodontitis*.

In *gingivitis* the sulcus is normal or only slightly deepened, and the PMN-containing fluid flow through the junctional epithelium is parallel to the tooth surface, toward the sulcus. Junctional epithelial cells proliferate and move in the same direction. Thus, gingivitis can represent a stable situation. After removal of plaque, healing and tissue consolidation occur.

With *periodontitis,* bacteria reside on the root and in the pocket. Plaque and calculus form a barrier between tooth and adjacent soft tissues. The host defense reactions, which in principle are identical to those in gingivitis, now course perpendicularly toward the root surface. In the absence of therapy, spontaneous healing is no longer possible.

**57   Gingivitis with slightly deepened sulcus**
The products of the local (inflammatory) host defense course through the altered junctional epithelium toward the bottom of the gingival sulcus; these products are carried by the subepithelial infiltrate (light blue). The flow of exudate containing a large number of PMNs (blue, blue arrows) thus moves almost parallel to the tooth surface (red arrows = sloughing JE cells). The strength of the host response is sufficient to prevent microorganisms from migrating apically along the tooth surface: **Stable lesion.**

The position of the most coronal junctional epithelial cells attaching to the enamel remains constant (see marking, lateral empty arrow). If plaque is removed, gingivitis is reversible.

**Transition into ...**

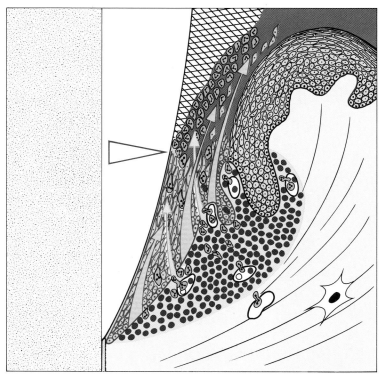
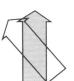

**58   ... Periodontitis**
Proliferation and apical expansion of bacterial plaque results in formation of a true periodontal pocket. Simultaneously a change in the direction of flow of the exudate occurs; it now flows from the infiltrate perpendicularly toward the plaque-covered tooth surface (blue arrows = exudate, PMNs; red arrows = sloughing JE cells). Spontaneous healing cannot occur. The epithelial attachment (empty arrow lower left) has been forced apically: **Progressive lesion.**

After root planing, tissue shrinkage and healing ("regeneration") occurs, but this phenomenon does *not* reconstitute original tissue architecture (Figs. 329–330; 948–949).

Adapted from *Schroeder & Attström* 1980, *Schroeder* 1983

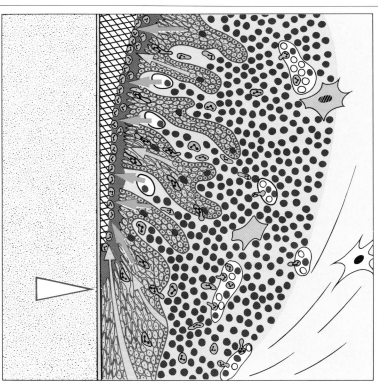

# Host Defense Possibilities

### Acute defense reactions

Foreign bodies such as bacteria, viruses or fungi which enter the organism encounter first a rapidly reacting, quite effective, but non-specific defense system. It can be recruited within a very few hours and consists primarily of cellular elements (granulocytes, PMN; macrophages, MΦ) as well as elements of the humoral complement system, activated via the alternate pathway.

### Adaptive defense reactions (immunity)

This second defense system is capable of recognizing foreign bodies specifically, differentiating them from host, and eliminating them. This remarkable ability of the immune system derives from the fact that information about any substance recognized as foreign antigen is stored in the lymphocytic, immunologic memory (T-cell memory), remains there, and can be called up as necessary.

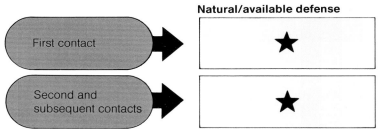 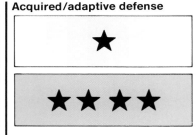

**59  Naturally occuring and acquired, adaptive defense**
*Natural* defense capability is non-specific and always available; it remains unaltered even in the face of repeated antigen contact.
  In contrast, *acquired immunity* is antigen-specific and reacts more strongly to continuing or repeated antigen contact.

Modified from *Roitt et al.* 1985

### Cells of the immune reaction

### Granulocytes – PMN

Each day an adult forms ca. $10^{11}$ (ca. 75 g) of neutrophilic granulocytes, which leave the ciculation after 10–20 hours and remain functional in tissue for an additional 1–2 days. The PMNs are the most important components of the acute defense against infection (phagocytosis, digestion). Enzymes from PMNs participate in foreign body defense by digesting phagocytozed particles; they can also damage host tissues. Phagocytosis, adsorption of opsonized, non-phagocytozable foreign bodies and bacterial toxins lead to exocytosis.

### Monocytes / Macrophages

The mononuclear phagocyte system consists of monocytes and tissue macrophages. Each day approximately $4 \times 10^8$ monocytes leave the circulation, differentiate into macrophages and, depending on location and function, remain active for up to 40 days. Macrophages can phagocytoze, but equally important is their secretion of various *enzymes* and monokines such as interleukin-1 or substances that influence osteoclast precursor cells.

Macrophages also function as regulators of the immune response (Figs. 60, 61).

### Lymphocytes: T-cells / B- and plasma cells

Lymphocytes are the key cells of the immune system. Approximately $2 \times 10^{12}$ of these cells exist in the host. In addition to host defense, these cells also provide immune surveillance and immune responses. There are two main classes:

1. *T-cells* perform numerous functions including:
– assistance in antibody production
– recognition and destruction of cells infected by virus
– activation of phagocytes, which then eliminate foreign bodies
– regulation of the extent and quality of the immune reaction.

The T-cell receptors serve for recognition of antigens. T-cells can become active in various functions after contact with antigen:

*T-helper cells* intensify not only the humoral B-cell response (antibody production), but also the T-cell mediated cellular reaction. Signal proteins such as Il-2 take part in these reactions.

*T-suppressor cells,* on the other hand, have inhibitory functions. A feedback mechanism is functional on T-helper cells.

*Cytotoxic T-cells* can damage foreign as well as host tissue.

2. *B-cells*. These carry antigen receptors in the form of immunoglobulins on their surfaces. Upon contact with antigen, they differentiate into antibody-producing plasma cells (Ebersole et al. 1987).

# Components of the Immune System

**60 Cellular and humoral elements in infiltrated pocket tissues**

| Cell type/Molecules | Characteristics | Function |
|---|---|---|
| **Polymorphonuclear granulocyte (PMN)**<br>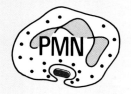 | – Differentiation, maturation and clonal expansion in bone marrow<br>– Lifespan: 2–3 days<br>– Ø 10–20 μm<br>– Fcγ-, C3-, C5-, CR-receptors<br>– Enzyme-containing granules<br>– Esterase-2 positive | – Diapedesis, chemokinesis<br>– Chemotaxis<br>– Adherence<br>– Phagolysosomes ⎫<br>– Degradation ⎭ **= phagocytosis**<br>– Microbicidal processes (= **cytotoxicity**)<br>– Release of microbicidal enzymes, neutral proteases, acid hydrolases etc.<br>– Release of arachidonic acid metabolites |
| **Complement system Cascade C1–C9** | – *Activation via classical pathway* (**CPW**) following aggregation of antibody with antigen (Ag/Ab complex)<br><br>– *Activation via alternate pathway* (**APW**) independent of antibody; microbial polysaccharides cleave C3 and lead to activation of C5 | – Immune adherence<br>– Increased capillary permeability<br>– Anaphylatoxin<br>– PMN chemotaxis<br>– Irreversible structural and functional membrane damage (= **cytotoxicity**)<br>– B-cell transformation |
| **Monocyte/Macrophage (MΦ)**<br>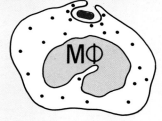 | – Differentiation, maturation and clonal expansion in bone marrow<br>– Lifespan: months<br>– Ø 12–25 μm<br>– Fcε-, Fcγ-, C3-receptors<br>– Esterase-1 positive | – **Phagocytosis, pinocytosis**<br>– Microbicidal processes (= **cytotoxicity**)<br>– Antigen processing and presentation<br>– Regulation of lymphocyte functions<br>– Production and release of biologically active substances: interferon, interleukin-1, prostaglandin, complement, lysosomal enzymes |
| **T-lymphocyte**<br>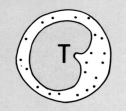 | – Stem cells from bone marrow, thymus-dependent maturation (**T**)<br>– Lifespan: months<br>– Ø 6–7 μm; activated 10 μm<br>– T-cell receptor<br>– Stimulation → lymphoblast<br>– T-surface antigens<br>– T4 on helper cells<br>– T8 on suppressor cells and cytotoxic cells | – **Cell-mediated immunity**<br>– T-helper cells: interaction with B-cells leads to antibody production<br>– T-suppressor cells: inhibit the B-cell response<br>– T-killer cells<br>– Lymphokines: lymphotoxins (= **cytotoxicity**) **IL** (Interleukin), **IFN** (Interferon), **MIF** (macrophage migration inhibition factor), **MAF** (macrophage activation factor = Interferon IFN) etc. |
| **B-lymphocyte/ Plasma cell**<br>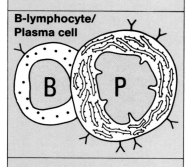 | – Stem cells from bone marrow (**B**), maturation in fetal liver, bone marrow, Peyer's patches<br>– Lifespan: months<br>– Ø 6–7 μm<br>– activated (plasma cell): Ø 10–15 μm<br>– Surface Ig as antigen receptor | – **Humoral immunity,** immunoglobulin synthesis<br>– B-lymphocyte: antigen-specific Ig of various classes<br>– Plasma cell: antigen- and class-specific Ig, monoclonal<br>– Mitogenic response, non-specific, polyclonal |
| **Antibody (AB) Immunoglobulin (Ig)**<br><br>Approx. mol. weight and %<br>**IgG** 150K 80%<br>**IgM** 900K 13%<br>**IgA** 300K 6%<br>**IgD** 185K 1%<br>**IgE** 280K 0.02% | – 5 classes: **IgA, IgD, IgE, IgG, IgM**<br>– Basic molecule: heavy and light polypeptide chains<br>– Fab-fragment with antigen binding regions<br>– Fc-fragment: complement activation, adherence to cell surface (opsonization) | – Antigen-antibody reaction: Ag/Ab complex<br>– Agglutination ⎫<br>– Precipitation ⎬ **= toxin neutralization**<br>– Opsonization ⎭<br>– **Cytotoxicity**<br>– Complement activation |

# Reciprocal Relationships Between Natural and Acquired Immunity

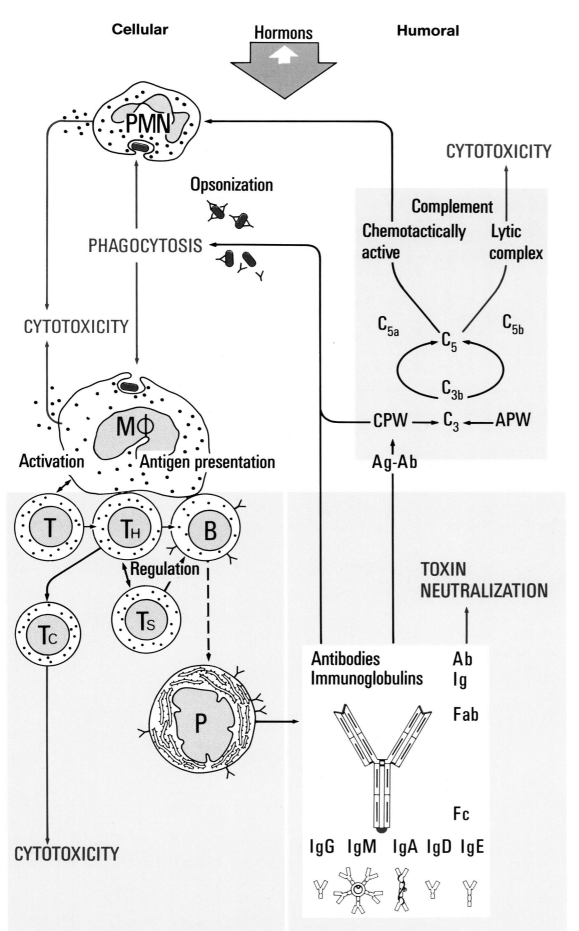

**Cellular**

**Hormons**

**Humoral**

PMN

Opsonization

PHAGOCYTOSIS

CYTOTOXICITY

CYTOTOXICITY

**Complement**

Chemotactically active

Lytic complex

$C_{5a}$  $C_5$  $C_{5b}$

$C_{3b}$

CPW → $C_3$ ← APW

Ag-Ab

M$\Phi$

Activation  Antigen presentation

T  $T_H$  B

Regulation

$T_C$  $T_S$

P

**TOXIN NEUTRALIZATION**

CYTOTOXICITY

Antibodies Immunoglobulins

Ab
Ig

Fab

Fc

IgG  IgM  IgA  IgD  IgE

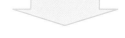

**61  Adaptive relationships**
Modified from *Roitt et al.* 1985

## Non-specific, natural immunity

**– PMN granulocytes**
Initial acute defense within the junctional epithelium and the sulcus (*phagocytosis*).
The PMN is short-lived. Upon death of the cell, lysosomal enzymes are released, which may damage host periodontal tissue (*cytotoxicity*).

**– Complement**
Earliest possible activation (antibody-independent) via the alternate pathway (**APW**). Subsequently dependent on antibodies, via the classical pathway (**CPW**). Products of this activation lead to cell lysis (membrane destruction: *cytotoxicity*).

**– Macrophages M$\Phi$:**
Phagocytosis. Secretion of enzymes and monokines. Macrophages regulate T- and B-cells (antigen presentation).

## Specific, adaptive / acquired immunity

**– T-Cells:** These are responsible for cell-mediated immunity. T-cells have activating (T-helper) and regulating (T-suppressor) functions and secrete various lymphokines.

**– B-lymphocytes/Plasma cells**
These are responsible for humoral immunity. Upon contact with antigen, B-lymphocytes differentiate into plasma cells that produce antibodies.

**– Immunoglobulins**
**IgG, IgM, IgA, IgD, IgE**

Immunoglobulins are seroproteins that specifically bind to those antigens by which they were activated.

# Acute Defense Mechanisms

### Normal function of polymorphonuclear leukocytes (PMNs)

Granulocytes in the circulating blood are attracted to a site of host defense via chemotactic mechanisms elicited by metabolic products of plaque microorganisms and by the invasion of these bacteria into tissue. PMNs initially adhere to the inner wall of the vessel ("pavementing"), then exit the vessel by migrating between endothelial cells into the tissue. The subsequent ameboid migration of PMNs is target oriented toward the particle to be phagocytozed. Recognition of the target is made easier when the foreign substances or bacteria are marked by opsonins. Examples of opsonins are the C3b fragment released upon complement activation and the Fc fragment of immunoglobulin G. When the receptor on the PMN comes into contact with the opsonized particle (adherence), the phagocytic process begins. Phagolysosomes begin to form within the PMN, and these fill with enzymes, which digest any phagocytozed microorganisms or other foreign substance.

**62 Polymorphonuclear granulocyte (PMN)**
This mature functional phagocytic cell has taken up several bacteria (arrows), which are killed in phagolysosomes. Portions of the PMN's segmented nucleus (**N**) are visible.

Upon the death of the short-lived PMN, the contents of its lysosomes are released and can inflict injury to host tissues.

TEM courtesy *H. E. Schroeder*

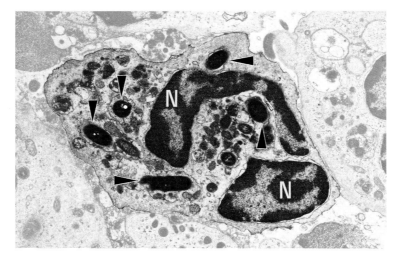

### Defects of polymorphonuclear granulocytes (PMN)

Defects of PMN function can significantly reduce host defense capabilities against infection. PMN functions that may be compromised include:

- Diapedesis
- Chemotaxis
- Adherence and phagocytosis
- Microbicidal activity

Systemic diseases characterized by *PMN defects* are well known (e.g., Lazy Leukocyte Syndrome, Chediak-Higashi Syndrome, Diabetes mellitus, chronic granulomatosis, Down Syndrome). These are usually accompanied by severe periodontal disease.

Granulocytes in most patients with prepubertal, juvenile (LJP) or rapidly progressive periodontitis (RPP) exhibit more or less severely compromised functions.

Host defense can be further compromised by the *"left shift"* of PMNs (young, immature cells), which is observed in all infections.

**63 Possible defects of polymorphonuclear granulocytes**
Defective phagocytes diminish acute defense capability. Normal PMN function may be blocked at various sites. Diapedesis may be impaired early on.

Chemotactic defects are most common, but inadequate adherence to bacteria, defective phagocytosis and impaired ability to digest engulfed substances may also occur.

Adapted from *Lindhe 1983*

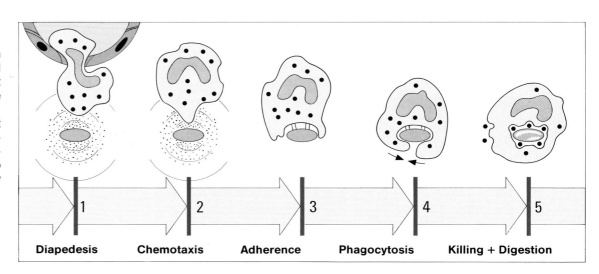

| 1 | 2 | 3 | 4 | 5 |
|---|---|---|---|---|
| **Diapedesis** | **Chemotaxis** | **Adherence** | **Phagocytosis** | **Killing + Digestion** |

## Acquired Immune Response

Upon first contact with an antigen (immunogen) certain defense cells are activated whose surface receptors (paratope) recognize the antigenic structures (epitope) most closely. Whether the result of this recognition is an *antibody response* (B-cells) or a *cell-mediated reaction* (T-cells) depends upon antigen presentation.

### Humoral immunity – B-cells

Remarkable differences can be observed between the primary and secondary antibody responses. Antibody synthesis following initial contact with an immunogen is delayed, mild and disappears quickly. The primary antibody response consists initially of antibodies of the IgM class, and this is followed by IgG antibodies with higher affinity for the immunogen.

The secondary response is characterized by earlier arrival and longer duration of antibody secretion (main-ly IgG). In addition much higher concentrations of antibody can be measured in circulation. Responsible for this typically enhanced and rapid immune response are the numerous memory cells.

### Cellular immunity – T-cells

Cell-mediated immunity describes an immune response that takes place for the most part without B-cell participation. In addition to the previously mentioned helper and suppressor cells, there exists an additional subgroup of T-cells, the cytotoxic lymphocytes. These possess immunologically specific receptors for epitopes of other cells and have the capability to destroy other cells. While antibodies can only neutralize *extracellular* organisms, the T-cells of the cell-mediated immune reaction are also effective against intracellular pathogens, especially viruses.

## Hypersensitivity Reactions

Immune responses that are excessive or that are not appropriate to the challenge are referred to as hypersensitivity reactions. These are cataloged into four main groups based on their pathogenesis; combined forms are very common. During hypersensitivity reactions, contact between the immune system and immunogens elicits a reaction which in some situations can lead immediately, or over time, to serious disease states and tissue damage. The reaction classes are depicted schematically in Figures 64–67. While types 1–3 are antibody-mediated, the delayed hypersensitivity reaction (type 4) is cell-mediated.

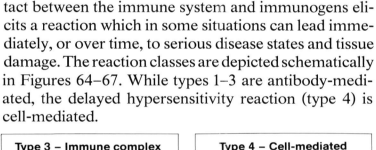

| Type 1 – Anaphylactic | Type 2 – Cytotoxic | Type 3 – Immune complex | Type 4 – Cell-mediated |

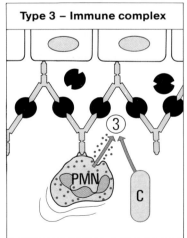
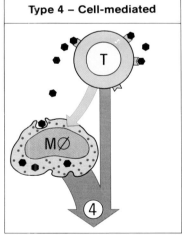

**64   Anaphylactic reaction**

Mast cells (**MA**) bind IgE (blue Y's) on Fc-receptors. Upon linking of IgE molecules by antigen (e. g., pollen) mast cell degranulation occurs with release of vasoactive amines (serotonin, histamine) and development of an inflammatory reaction (**1**).

*Examples:* Allergic asthma, hayfever, eczema.

**65   Antibody-mediated cytotoxic reaction**

This is elicited by antibodies that are targeted for cell surface antigens (host cells!).

The reaction (**2**) may lead either to antibody-dependent cell toxicity mediated by killer cells (**TK**), or by complement-mediated lysis (**C**, red).

*Examples:* Destruction of erythrocytes after transfusion; hemolytic diathesis of the newborn.

**66   Immune complex-mediated reaction**

If soluble antigen-antibody complexes form, platelet aggregation occurs and complement (**C**, red) is activated. Products of the complement cascade mobilize neutrophilic granulocytes (**PMN**), whose degranulation elicits tissue damage (**3**).

*Examples:* Serum sickness, Arthus reaction.

**67   Cell-mediated, delayed hypersensitivity**

This occurs more than 24 hr after antigen contact (e.g., viruses) and is mediated by T-cells (**T**) that had been previously sensitized to the antigen. Such T-cells release lymphokines (blue arrow), which recruit macrophages (**MΦ**) to the reaction site and activate them. These macrophages are responsible for the granulomatous reaction and for tissue destruction (**4**).

*Examples:* Contact sensitivity, tuberculin reaction.

Adapted from *Roitt* et al. 1985

# Attachment Loss

Attachment loss is the main symptom and the most significant event in the active phase of periodontitis. It includes the destruction of both supraalveolar and periodontal fiber apparatus as well as the adjacent portion of the alveolar bone (Schroeder 1983).

## Collagen fiber breakdown

Phagocytozing *neutrophilic granulocytes* constantly release granules that contain acid hydrolases (e. g., cathepsins) and neutral proteases such as elastase and collagenase. These degrade collagen as well as proteoglycans and fibrinogen.

Granulocytes are present in huge numbers during highly acute inflammation and in abscesses. When these cells burst within inflamed tissue, large quantities of the enzymes are released in a very short period of time.

*Mononuclear phagocytes* (macrophages) also participate in both acute and chronic inflammatory processes. Macrophage secretory products (e. g., acid hydrolases, lysozyme, neutral proteases) also influence the course of the inflammatory process.

## Destruction of bone

The details of the biologic mechanisms leading to localized destruction of alveolar bone remain poorly understood. Very few substances capable of mediating bone resorption have been demonstrated experimentally. Among these are the *prostaglandins,* especially PG-$E_2$, which are synthesized primarily by macrophages within inflamed tissues. A second group is the cytokines. These locally acting polypeptide hormones regulate the activities of various cells in the inflamed region. Known cytokines include the macrophage products interleukin-1 (Il-1) and tumor necrosis factor-$\alpha$ (TNF-$\alpha$), as well as $\gamma$-interferon (IFN) synthesized by lymphocytes. Bone resorption can also be initiated through the activation of the complement system.

Such mediators stimulate primarily the formation of new osteoclasts from precursor cells, or increase the resorptive capability of such cells. It is interesting that some mediators may also inhibit or otherwise modulate bone regeneration.

During acute phases direct stimulation of bone resorption is possible via bacterial lipoteichoic acids, peptidoglycans and lipopolysaccharide.

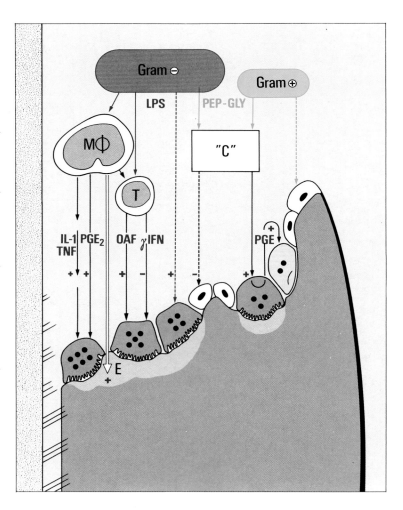

**68  Mechanisms of bone destruction**
Schematic representation of mechanisms active in local periodontal bone resorption.

The double arrow from the MΦ indicates enzymatic breakdown of *organic* bone matrix.

| | |
|---|---|
| **MΦ** | = Macrophage |
| **T** | = T-lymphocyte |
| **"C"** | = Activated complement system |
| **LPS** | = Lipopolysaccharide from gram-negative bacterial cell wall |
| PEP-GLY | = Peptidoglycan from bacterial cell wall |
| **Il-1** | = Interleukin-1 |
| **TNF** | = Tumor necrosis factor |
| **PG-E₂** | = Prostaglandin $E_2$ |
| **OAF** | = Osteoclast activating factor (cytokines, e.g., Il-1b) |
| **γ-IFN** | = γ-Interferon |

*Below:*
– Activated multinucleated osteoclast along a resorption site (acid resorption of the *mineral portion* of bone).
– Mononuclear osteoblast (inhibition of bone deposition).

# Cyclic Nature of Periodontitis

Throughout the history of the study of periodontal disease, periodontitis was always described as a more or less rapidly but *continuously* progressing chronic disease. This belief was based on the findings of epidemiologic studies, which had demonstrated increasing attachment loss with age (mean values per patient).

More recent investigations (Goodson et al. 1982, Socransky et al. 1984) have shown, however, that attachment loss seldom occurs evenly throughout the entire dentition and that it occurs *cyclically*. Loss of tooth supporting tissue actually occurs on individual teeth or even at individual sites of a tooth.

During acute, active destruction, gram-negative anaerobic bacteria come to predominate in the pocket. Direct microbial invasion into the tissues may occur. This leads to a massive host-defense reaction, with formation of micronecroses or purulent abscesses. The mechanisms of collagen destruction and bone resorption are activated (p. 30).

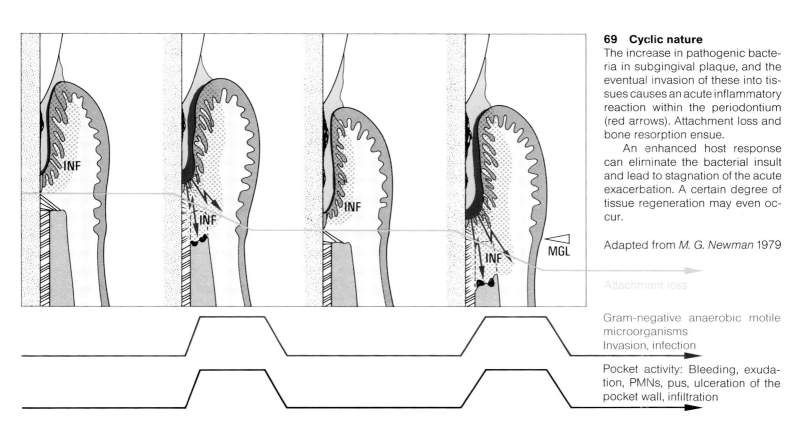

**69 Cyclic nature**
The increase in pathogenic bacteria in subgingival plaque, and the eventual invasion of these into tissues causes an acute inflammatory reaction within the periodontium (red arrows). Attachment loss and bone resorption ensue.

An enhanced host response can eliminate the bacterial insult and lead to stagnation of the acute exacerbation. A certain degree of tissue regeneration may even occur.

Adapted from *M. G. Newman* 1979

Attachment loss

Gram-negative anaerobic motile microorganisms
Invasion, infection

Pocket activity: Bleeding, exudation, PMNs, pus, ulceration of the pocket wall, infiltration

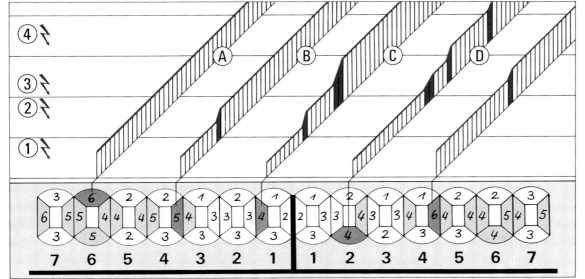

**70 Irregular, site specific attachment loss**
The periodontal pocket status (below) reveals moderate periodontitis with probing depths to 6 mm.

The majority of pockets can remain the same depth and inactive for years. However, at individual sites on some teeth, circumscribed symptoms of disease activity can occur (phases 1–4).

**A** Probing depth remains constant for years
**B** One acute phase, 1 mm loss
**C** Two acute phases,
1 mm + 2 mm loss
**D** Three acute phases, each with 1 mm loss

Adapted from *Socransky* et al. 1984

# Modifying Factors in Etiology and Pathogenesis

The bacterial insult and the host response to it may be modified by various cofactors that can determine the initiation and the clinical course of gingivitis and periodontitis.

| | |
|---|---|
| Local: | – Saliva quantity and composition |
| | – Mouth breathing |
| | – Mechanical, chemical, thermal, allergic and actinic irritation |
| | – Functional disturbances, occlusal trauma (clenching, bruxism), orofacial muscular parafunctions, parafunctions related to occupation |
| General: | – Severe systemic disease |
| | – Genetics, heredity |
| | – Endocrine disturbances |
| | – Medicaments |
| | – Nutrition |
| | – Age |

*Saliva* has a protective function. Salivary mucin (a glycoprotein) lines the oral mucosa as a protective film. Depending on flow rate and viscosity, saliva may exert a greater or lesser cleansing effect. The content of bicarbonate, phosphate, calcium and fluoride will determine salivary buffering capacity and its remineralizing potential. Secretory immunoglobulins (sIgA) as well as lysozyme, catalase, lactoperoxidase and additional enzymes help to determine the antimicrobial activity of saliva.

*Mouth breathing* leads to dehydration of the oral mucosa, cancelling the protective functions of saliva. Dryness allows plaque to cling even more tenaciously to the tooth surface.

*Exogenous irritants* of various types may be injurious to the oral mucosa, gingiva and periodontium:

*Mechanical* injuries resulting from eating or from improper use of the toothbrush or other oral health aids may elicit acute inflammatory reactions, which are usually of short duration. If periodontitis is already present, such irritation may elicit activity in a previously quiescent site.

*Chemical* irritations resulting from excessive concentration of locally applied medicaments or acids lead, like *thermal* effects, to damage to mucosa and gingiva, which is usually reversible. In more severe cases, necrosis may be the consequence.

*Allergic* reactions may exhibit a range of clinical manifestations from erythema to painful blistering.

These may be caused by topical medicaments, dentifrices, oral rinses, dental materials etc.

*Radiation burns* (actinic irritation) may occur subsequent to X-ray therapy for tumors in the head and neck area. Damaging consequences of such therapy are xerostomia and altered saliva composition that result from devastation of the salivary glands (Imfeld 1984). Only intensive radiation therapy will cause direct injury to mucosa or bone (hemorrhage, ulceration, osteoradionecrosis).

*Functional disturbances* (occlusal trauma) *cannot cause* either gingivitis or periodontitis. However, if an active periodontitis is already present, its progression may be accelerated by damaging and unphysiologic forces (see Function, p. 325).

Functional disturbances and orofacial muscle phenomenae *(oral parafunctions)* such as tongue thrusting, lip biting etc., as well as parafunctions related to one's occupation (e.g., playing a wind instrument, holding nails or pins in the teeth etc.), may lead to drifting of teeth, particularly in patients with periodontal disease.

*Severe systemic disease, genetic predisposition, disturbances in hormonal balance, as well as the side effects of drugs* that elicit or enhance gingivitis or periodontitis are dealt with in the chapter on Diseases of the Periodontium (p. 41).

*Nutrition* can influence the speed with which plaque accumulates and its composition. In extreme cases of nutritional deficiency the host response (immune status) against any marginal infection may be weakened. Of special importance in this regard are pronounced deficiencies of vitamins, minerals and trace elements, and particularly protein deficiency in poorly nourished individuals.

*Age* does not necessarily predispose one to periodontal diseases, although the histologically detectable biochemical alterations in connective tissue may be age related. It is worthy of note also that with increasing age the immune response is lessened. The host response to bacterial infection is reduced. Clinically, one may observe a certain involution of the healthy periodontium. This is, however, likely to be less an age-related phenomenon than the result of years of exposure to exogenous factors such as intensive oral hygiene, chronic inflammation, or iatrogenic irritants (Gorman 1967, Hansen 1973, Sauerwein 1983, Holm-Pedersen & Löe 1986).

# Epidemiology and Indices

*Descriptive* epidemiology deals with the occurrence, the severity and the distribution of diseases, as well as mortality in any selected population.

*Analytic* epidemiology seeks furthermore to discern the causes of a disease and to evaluate any public health consequences with regard to prevention and therapy (Frandsen 1984).

In periodontology, epidemiology is concerned with the prevalence of gingivitis and periodontitis as well as microbial plaque, which is the most important etiologic factor in this family of diseases. Today, not all of the results of classical epidemiologic studies performed over the last several decades are accepted entirely (p. 34). Such studies did not take into consideration the various forms of disease, symptoms of activity, and localization of the disease processes. These studies also failed to consider the treatment needs of the populations examined (Ainamo et al. 1982, Frandsen 1984, Listgarten 1988).

The distribution and severity of gingivitis and periodontitis, as well as plaque accumulation, are recorded in epidemiologic studies through the use of *indices*. Some of these indices are also useful for recording clinical findings in individual patients, and for diagnosis (plaque indices, bleeding indices), as well as for patient education and determination of treatment need (CPITN, Ainamo 1988, p. 35).

## Epidemiology of Gingivitis

Numerous epidemiologic studies have been performed, especially in children and adolescents. The reported morbidity figures range from very low to 100% (Page & Schroeder 1982, Stamm 1986). In addition, the severity of gingivitis varies greatly from study to study. Such differences result mainly from use of non-standard methods of investigation. Additional reasons for the large interinvestigation differences include the varying levels of oral hygiene (plaque control) within the populations examined, as well as geographic, social and ethnologic factors. The incidence and severity of gingivitis can vary within even a single population examined repeatedly at short intervals (Suomi et al. 1971, Page 1986). The

severity of gingivitis achieves its maximum in adolescents reaching puberty, then recedes somewhat, exhibiting a slight tendency to increase in adults as age increases (Stamm 1986).

The existence of gingivitis cannot be taken as evidence that periodontitis will eventually develop in an individual (Page & Schroeder 1982, Listgarten et al. 1985). The public health significance of gingivitis epidemiology may therefore be called into question.

In studies in which both gingivitis and plaque are considered, a clear relationship between oral hygiene and severity of gingivitis has emerged (Silness & Löe 1964, Koivuniemi et al. 1980, Hefti et al. 1981).

## Epidemiology of Periodontitis

From many nations of the world, numerous epidemiologic studies of periodontitis have been reported (Barmes 1984, Miller et al. 1987). The data from these studies – as in gingivitis – must be interpreted with caution since they present quite varying results. Particularly the figures concerning morbidity must be considered suspect. A figure of 100% incidence in a population can hardly be considered to be of public health significance if the attachment loss is minor and isolated to only a few interdental areas. Only data concerning the *severity* and the localization of the attachment loss will permit any meaningful statements (Miller et al. 1987).

Very few investigators have attempted to study the rapidity of attachment loss in a single population longitudinally over a course of years (Buckley & Crowley 1984) with simultaneous evaluation of the topography of attachment loss and its occurrence on individual teeth. In one large study, Löe and co-workers (1978) recorded the course of attachment loss over several years in one group of Norwegian students and academicians, and another group of laborers in a Sri Lankan tea plantation. The investigators then compared the findings from those two exceedingly different racial and socioeconomic groups. The results demonstrated that in the Norwegian group the "average" annual loss of attachment was 0.1 mm, while the Sri Lankan population exhibited 0.2–0.3 mm.

In general, epidemiologic studies seldom make any differentiation among:

1) Less frequently occurring forms of periodontal disease such as rapidly progressing periodontitis (RPP) of young adults and localized juvenile periodontitis (LJP)

2) The more widespread but slowly and intermittently progressive adult periodontitis (AP).

True forms of RPP are probably rare, representing only 2–5% of all cases. More exact data concerning LJP are available; in Europe about 0.1% of young persons are affected. Generally higher rates of morbidity have been reported from Asia and Africa (Saxén 1980, Saxby 1984, 1987, Kronauer et al. 1986).

Recently, following the recommendation of the WHO, epidemiologic studies of periodontitis evaluate more than just morbidity and severity of the disease. More often the treatment needs as well as the type of indicated therapy and the time required for it are also determined. For such investigations a new index was developed (Ainamo et al. 1982; p. 40): "Community Periodontal Index of Treatment Needs" (CPITN).

**71  Hamburg CPITN study – Treatment needs in 11,305 subjects (1987)**
**CPI Codes**

| **0** | Healthy | 3% |
| **1/2** | Bleeding/calculus | 37% |
| **3** | 3.5–5.5 mm pockets | 44% |
| **4** | 6+mm pockets | 16% |

**TN-Treatment Need**
About 84% of subjects could be treated by oral hygiene instruction (**TN I**) and scaling, (**TN II**), the remaining 16% required more involved therapy, including surgery (**TN III**).

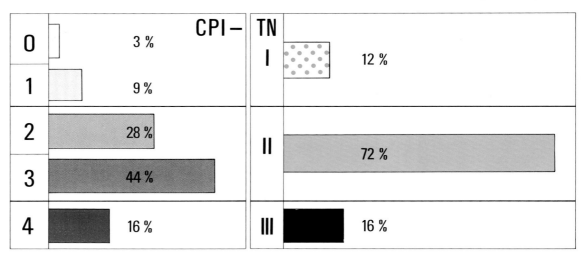

Initial field studies using the CPITN provided informative results (Ahrens & Bublitz 1987). In a large investigation of 11,305 subjects in Hamburg, only 2.8% were found to exhibit total periodontal health (code 0) and required no type of treatment. Nine percent exhibited bleeding on probing of the sulcus (code 1). In these patients only oral hygiene instruction was necessary. Calculus (code 2) was detected in 28% of the subjects and 44% had probing depths between 3.5 and 5.5 mm (code 3). These patients required supra- and subgingival scaling, which could be provided by auxiliary personnel such as the dental hygienist. Probing depths of 6 mm and deeper (code 4) were measured in only 16% of the subjects. These patients needed, in addition to scaling, more complex therapies such as root planing with anesthesia or surgical interventions. The latter could be undertaken only by a dentist or, in severe cases, by a periodontal specialist.

Other studies using the CPITN have provided similar results (Barmes & Leous 1986, Cutress 1986, Frentzen & Nolden 1987; Henne et al. 1988).

The CPITN is also useful in private practice for a cursory preliminary examination of a patient (Wolf 1987a).

# Indices

- **Plaque indices**
- **Gingival indices**
- **Periodontal indices**
- **Treatment needs indices**

## Value and possibilities for use

Alterations in the gingiva and the periodontium, as well as the main cause of these diseases (microbial plaque) may be assessed and quantitated through use of indices. These are useful primarily for epidemiologic studies, but may also comprise part of individual patient examinations.

Indices are numerical expressions of defined diagnostic criteria. Presence and / or severity of pathology are expressed by assessing a numerical value. In simplified indices, only the presence or absence of a symptom or an etiologic factor may be recorded as "yes" or "no." For example, after probing a gingival sulcus, a plus (+) signifies "bleeding," a minus (–) signifies "no bleeding."

A good index should be able to provide quantitative and qualitative expressions of the criteria under study. Furthermore, an index should be simple, objective, re-producible, quick and practical. It must exhibit validity, specificity, reproducibility and sensitivity. It should be easy enough for auxiliary personnel to use (e.g., dental assistant or hygienist) and should be amenable to statistical evaluation.

Although indices were developed *primarily for use in epidemiologic studies*, and continue to be used mainly for such studies, it has been difficult to achieve any degree of standardization among various international scientific groups. It is therefore often impossible to compare the results obtained in one epidemiologic study to those obtained in another investigation.

For the past several years, indices have come to be used *in the dental practice on individual patients*. The numerical quantitation of plaque and gingivitis can be performed particularly well. By recording indices throughout the course of a preventive program or a treatment regimen, it is possible to document success (or failure) objectively for both the practitioner and the patient. A change (e.g., improvement) in the index can also help to motivate a patient.

In the following pages, a few of the indices that are used internationally in epidemiologic studies are described briefly with emphasis on those that are well suited for use in the periodontal practice.

# Plaque Indices

A plaque index should provide a *quantitative* assessment. For *epidemiologic studies,* the relatively gross indices such as the plaque index (PI, Fig. 72; Silness & Löe 1964) are usually sufficient.

In private practice, on the other hand, the collection of a plaque or hygiene index is not intended to determine the average plaque accumulation, but to record the distribution of plaque in the oral cavity, i.e., to determine the *"plaque picture"* of an individual patient. Such a plaque index should also make it possible to record any improvements in cleaning efficacy during the course of therapy or during the recall interval. This is possible only through the use of an index that evaluates all tooth surfaces. Examples are the indices proposed by O'Leary (1972) and Lindhe (1983).

The following indices will be briefly presented:

- Plaque Index (PI, Silness & Löe 1964)
- Interdental Hygiene Index (HYG)
- Hygiene Index (HI: O'Leary et al. 1972, Lindhe 1983)

# Gingival Indices

Many indices have been developed for the evaluation and quantitation of gingivitis (Massler et al. 1950, Mühlemann & Mazor 1958, Löe & Silness 1963, Mühlemann & Son 1971, Carter & Barnes 1974, Saxer & Mühlemann 1975, Ainamo & Bay 1975, Lindhe 1983, Ciancio 1986).

For epidemiologic studies the relatively gross GI may be indicated.

For more individual studies, e.g., of smaller subject groups or in the dental practice, indices that utilize the symptoms of bleeding as the primary criterion are indicated.

Other indices that may serve the practitioner include the GI-S or the GBI, which record only bleeding on probing, without quantitating its intensity.

The following indices will be briefly presented:

- Gingival Index (GI, Löe & Silness 1963)
- Papilla Bleeding Index (PBI, Saxer & Mühlemann 1975)
- Gingival Index Simplified (GI-S, Lindhe 1983) which corresponds to the Gingiva Bleeding Index (GBI, Ainamo & Bay 1975)

## Plaque indices

### 72 Plaque Index (PI) of Silness and Löe

This index concerns *thickness* of plaque along the gingival margin; only this plaque plays any role in the etiology of gingivitis. To visualize plaque, teeth are dried with air. Plaque is not stained.

The PI is relatively time-consuming. It is indicated for *epidemiologic studies* in which the gingival index (GI) is recorded simultaneously. It is less useful for routine charting.

| Grade | | | Abbreviation | Grades/Codes |
|---|---|---|---|---|
| **0** | No plaque | | | |
| **1** | Thin film of plaque at the gingival margin, visible only when scraped with an explorer | | | |
| **2** | Moderate amount of plaque along the gingival margin; interdental space free of plaque; plaque visible with the naked eye | | | |
| **3** | Heavy plaque accumulation at the gingival margin; interdental space filled with plaque | | PI | 0–3 |

### 73 Interdental Hygiene Index (HYG)

This index records plaque-*free* surfaces as a percentage. It is thus similar to the Approximal Plaque Index (API) of *Lange* (1981), which records percent plaque accumulation.

After staining, a simple yes/no decision is made with regard to whether or not stained plaque is present (**+**) on the approximal surfaces or not (**–**).

The HYG is usually scored within a quadrant *from only one aspect,* i.e., from the facial or from the oral. This is also the case with the Papilla Bleeding Index (PBI, p. 37).

The HYG score is calculated as:

$$\textbf{HYG} = \frac{\text{number of plaque-free areas}}{\text{number of examined areas}} \times 100$$

The HYG is a sensitive index because small plaque quantity is also measured and because the index is scored in the interdental areas, which are in most cases not particularly well cleaned. The HYG is well suited for recording in *individual patients,* but less so for epidemiologic studies.

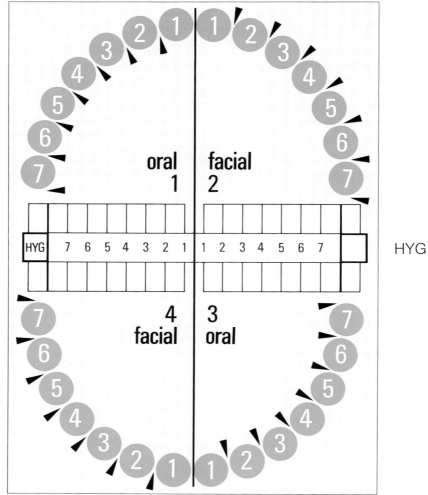

HYG      + or –

### 74 Hygiene Index (HI) – Recording plaque accumulation on all tooth surfaces

This most precise index involves measurement of plaque accumulation on *all four tooth surfaces* (facial, oral, mesial, distal).

With a simple yes/no decision the examiner can enter the presence (**+**) or absence of plaque into a simple chart and in doing so precisely ascertain the cleanliness of a dentition and express it as a percentage. For this index, plaque is stained with a disclosing agent. The HI was developed solely for use in *individual patients.*

HI      + or –

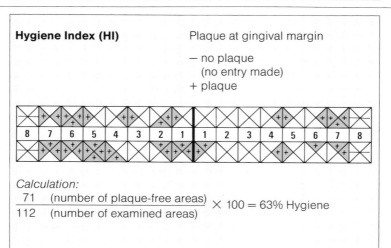

**Hygiene Index (HI)**     Plaque at gingival margin

— no plaque
  (no entry made)
+ plaque

*Calculation:*

$$\frac{71 \quad \text{(number of plaque-free areas)}}{112 \quad \text{(number of examined areas)}} \times 100 = 63\% \text{ Hygiene}$$

| Grades/Codes | Abbreviation | Grade | |
|---|---|---|---|
| | | **0** | Normal gingiva, no inflammation, no discoloration, no bleeding |
| | | **1** | Mild inflammation, slight color change, mild alteration of gingival surface, no bleeding |
| | | **2** | Moderate inflammation, erythema, swelling, bleeding on probing or when pressure applied |
| 0–3 | GI | **3** | Severe inflammation, severe erythema and swelling, tendency toward spontaneous hemorrhage, some ulceration |

## Gingival indices

### 75 Gingival Index (GI) of Löe and Silness

This index is used worldwide in epidemiologic studies and scientific investigations. The GI scores gingival inflammation from 0–3 on the facial, lingual and mesial surfaces of all teeth. The symptom of bleeding comprises a score of 2.

The GI is recommended for epidemiologic studies. It is less applicable for individual patients because the differences between the scoring levels are too gross.

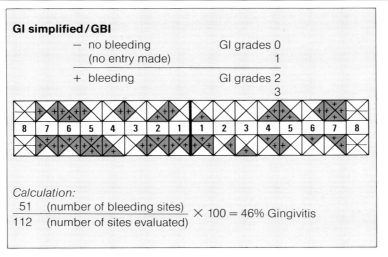

| | |
|---|---|
| 0–4 | PBI |

### 76 Papilla Bleeding Index (PBI)

The PBI discriminates four different degrees (intensities) of bleeding subsequent to careful probing of the gingival sulcus in the papillary region (interdental sampling, Figs. 78–81).

Probing is performed in all four quadrants. To simplify the recording of the PBI, quadrant 1 is probed only from the oral aspect, quadrant 2 from facial, 3 again from oral, and from the facial in quadrant 4 (see black arrows in diagram). Thus, the determinations are performed at the same sites where the interdental hygiene index (HYG, Fig. 73) is performed. Bleeding scores are entered into the chart (middle).

For use in the dental practice, several such forms may be arranged side by side. In this way findings recorded over a period of time can be conveniently compared. Any reduction in bleeding is an indication of a return to health of the gingiva. This will also be clear to the patient.

| | |
|---|---|
| + or − | GBI<br>GI-S |

**GI simplified / GBI**

| | | |
|---|---|---|
| − no bleeding<br>(no entry made) | GI grades | 0<br>1 |
| + bleeding | GI grades | 2<br>3 |

*Calculation:*

$$\frac{51 \;\; \text{(number of bleeding sites)}}{112 \;\; \text{(number of sites evaluated)}} \times 100 = 46\% \text{ Gingivitis}$$

### 77 Gingival Index Simplified (GI-S, Lindhe 1983) and Gingival Bleeding Index (GBI, Ainamo & Bay 1975)

Similar to the HI (Fig. 74) all four tooth surfaces are recorded as + or − for bleeding on probing.

Gingivitis incidence is calculated as a percentage of affected (bleeding) units.

Because over 100 individual sites must be evaluated in both the GI-S and the GBI, the indices are suited only for individual practice application on a routine basis, where they can be extremely beneficial (e.g., at recall appointments).

## Papilla Bleeding Index (PBI)

The PBI was developed for use in the private practice and not for epidemiologic studies. It is a *sensitive indicator* of the severity of gingival inflammation in individual patients. The PBI does not require a great amount of time, since only 28 measurement sites in the complete dentition are evaluated (Saxer & Mühlemann 1975).

The PBI has proven to be particularly useful for gauging success or failure during a course of periodontal therapy. While the patient watches in a mirror, the prac-

titioner can score the intensity of papillary inflammation. In this way, the PBI can also serve as an excellent method for motivating the patient toward good oral hygiene (Motivation, pp. 146–147). The patient can see when the gingival tissue bleeds, which helps him to realize where the diseased sites in his mouth are located.

Throughout therapy, repetitions of the PBI indicate to the patient any decrease in inflammation.

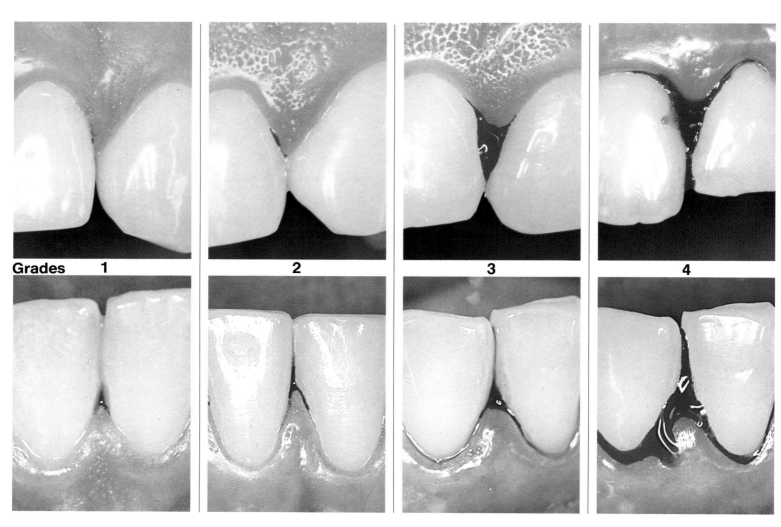

**Grades     1                    2                    3                    4**

**78   Grade 1 – Point**
20–30 seconds after probing the mesial and distal sulci with a periodontal probe, a single bleeding point is observed.

**79   Grade 2 – Line/Points**
A fine line of blood or several bleeding points become visible at the gingival margin.

**80   Grade 3 – Triangle**
The interdental triangle becomes more or less filled with blood.

**81   Grade 4 – Drops**
Profuse bleeding. Immediately after probing, blood flows into the interdental area to cover portions of the tooth or gingiva.

### Recording the PBI

Bleeding is provoked by sweeping the sulcus using a blunt periodontal probe under light finger pressure from the base of the papilla to its tip along the tooth's distal and mesial aspects.

*After 20–30 seconds,* when a quadrant has been com-

pletely probed, the intensity of bleeding is scored in four grades and recorded on the chart.

The sum of the recorded scores gives the *"bleeding number";* the PBI is calculated by dividing the bleeding number by the total number of papilla examined.

# Periodontal Indices

The determination of the severity of periodontitis through use of an index is really impossible. In contrast to a gingivitis index, which must only record the intensity of inflammation, any periodontitis index must, above all, measure the degree of loss of tooth-supporting tissues (attachment loss).

Periodontal indices find their most important use in epidemiologic studies. *In private practice,* a periodontal index *may* provide a quick overview of a patient's condition, but no index can ever replace a thorough individual examination (Gaberthüel 1987).

Many years ago numerous epidemiologic studies were performed using the *Periodontal Disease Index* (PDI) of Ramfjord (1959). More recently the CPITN is used in such studies. The CPITN is an index that combines measurement of the severity of disease as well as the necessity for treatment (Ainamo et al. 1982, Ahrens & Bublitz 1987).

## Periodontal Disease Index (PDI)

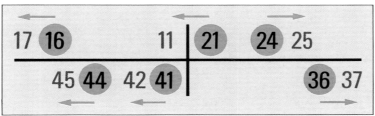

**82  Ramfjord teeth**
Ramfjord demonstrated that for epidemiologic purposes six teeth (red) could be taken as representative of the entire dentition. The substitutes for these six are shown on the chart in gray.

| Score | |
|---|---|
| **0** | No inflammation, no alterations in the gingiva |
| | **Gingiva** |
| **1** | Mild to moderate gingivitis at some locations on the gingival margin |
| **2** | Mild to moderate gingivitis of the entire gingival margin surrounding the tooth |
| **3** | Advanced gingivitis with severe erythema, hemorrhage, ulceration |
| | **Periodontium** |
| **4** | Up to 3 mm of attachment loss, measured from the cementoenamel junction |
| **5** | 3–6 mm of attachment loss |
| **6** | More than 6 mm of attachment loss |

**83  Periodontal Disease Index (PDI)**
The PDI contains a *gingivitis index* in scores 1, 2 and 3, and a measure of *attachment loss* independent of gingivitis, in scores 4, 5 and 6.
 The PDI is not indicated for private practice but for epidemiologic studies.

The *PDI* does not include examination of all 28 teeth (third molars are excluded in almost *all* indices), but rather a sample of six teeth that are representative of the entire dentition. These teeth were chosen so that each tooth type, both jaws and each quadrant are taken into account: teeth 16; 21, 24; 36; 41 and 44.

If one of these teeth is missing, its distal neighbor (17, 11; 25; 37; 42 or 45, respectively) may be substituted (Marthaler et al. 1971). The PDI evaluates these selected teeth for both gingivitis and attachment loss, with three gradations for each. For periodontitis grades 4, 5 and 6,

probing depth ("pocket depth") is not measured, rather the distance from the cementoenamel junction to the bottom of the pocket (attachment loss) is recorded.

An average PDI score (e.g., 2.8) *cannot* be taken to indicate that only gingivitis (to grade 3) is present, or whether attachment loss has already occurred on individual teeth. For example, mild gingivitis and slight attachment loss on individual teeth could lead to an average value below 3. Grades 1–3 and grades 4–6 should therefore be evaluated separately.

# Community Periodontal Index of Treatment Needs (CPITN)

The CPITN (p. 34) was developed in 1978 by the World Health Organization (WHO 1978, Ainamo et al. 1982) for epidemiologic studies. It is today the most often employed index. The major difference between the CPITN and other indices is that it determines not only the severity of gingivitis and periodontitis, but also provides data concerning the extent of therapy that is necessary. The examination is performed with a *special probe,* which serves more to determine what is normal (healthy) and what is abnormal (diseased) than to provide precise measurement of probing depths in millimeters. The CPITN is taken by *sextants.* A disadvantage of the CPITN is that attachment loss due to recession is not discerned.

In general only the highest score in any given sextant of teeth examined in adults is recorded. In the case of young patients (up to 19 years of age) and in epidemiologic studies the examination of one anterior tooth in the maxilla and the mandible, and the first permanent molars (or the second molars) is required (e. g., diagnosis of LJP!).

**84  CPI-codes and Treatment Needs (TN)**
**CPI:** The index scores (codes) describe the severity of disease, some aspects of the etiology (calculus), as well as symptoms such as bleeding upon probing. The absolute probing depth in mm is determined only secondarily; any gingival recession that might be present is not recorded at all.

**TN:** The index code prejudices the necessary treatment inasmuch as the absolute index score (4) does not correlate with the code from the "treatment package" (3). Codes 2 and 3 demand identical therapy!

| Code | | CPI – TN | | Treatment packages |
|---|---|---|---|---|
| **0** | Healthy | | | |
| **1** | Bleeding on probing | | **I** | Oral hygiene instruction (OHI) |
| **2** | Supra and/or subgingival calculus Iatrogenic marginal irritation | | **II** | I + calculus removal |
| **3** | Shallow pockets up to 5 mm | | | |
| **4** | Deeper pockets from 6 mm | | **III** | I + II + complex treatment |

**85  Index codes and special probe**
*Right:* The CPITN probe (Safident) has a small sphere on its end, 0.5 mm in diameter, and a black marking between 3.5 and 5.5 mm. Probes with markings at 8.5 and 11.5 mm are also available for use in practice.

*Left:* The CPI codes in schematic. The black marking is still partially visible during a probing at code 3, but disappears completely into the periodontal pocket at a code of 4.

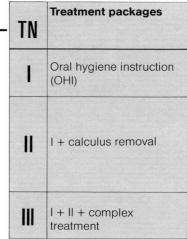

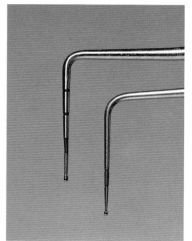

**86  CPITN in young adults to age 19 – Epidemiology**
Measurements are made around each of the six CPITN teeth, one in each sextant. The index codes are noted (teeth 17; 27; 37, and 47 are alternate teeth in case the first permanent molars are missing).

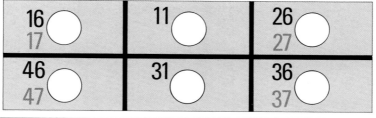

**CPITN**

**Epidemiology**

**Dental practice, to age 19**

**CPITN for adults**
All teeth are examined. Only the highest measured index code per sextant is recorded. The definition of the sextants is seen in the schematic.

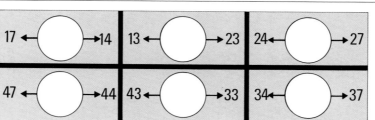

**Epidemiology**

**Dental practice, over age 19**

# Diseases of the Periodontium

The term "periodontal diseases" refers to inflammatory as well as recessive alterations of the gingiva and periodontium (Page & Schroeder 1982; AAP 1986 a, b; DGP 1987; Schroeder 1987 b).

*Gingivitis* and *periodontitis* are for the most part plaque-elicited diseases. In rare instances, systemic disorders may enhance these diseases or play a role in their etiologies.

## Gingivitis and Periodontitis

| Gingivitis |
|---|
| Periodontitis |
|   ● AP   Adult Periodontitis: Generalized but irregular, slowly progressing<br>  ● RPP  Rapidly Progressive Periodontitis: Generalized yet irregular,<br>          rapidly progressing<br>  ● LJP  Localized Juvenile Periodontitis: Localized to incisors and/or first<br>          permanent molars; rapidly progressive on these teeth<br>  ● PP   Pre-pubertal Periodontitis: Localized, generalized, rapidly progressing |
| ANUG/P  Acute Necrotizing Ulcerative Gingivitis/Periodontitis:<br>             Generally localized |

## Recession

This clinically inflammation-free, usually facially localized "retreat" of the alveolar bone and the gingiva, *termed recession,* is probably correlated with anatomy and morphology.

| Gingival recession<br>  ● localized<br>  ● generalized |
|---|

## Gingival and Periodontal Diseases, Local Etiology, without Participation of Systemic Factors

*Gingivitis* and *periodontitis* are elicited by micro-organisms via local opportunistic infections of the otherwise systemically healthy host. The rapidity of the attachment loss may be explained by the virulence of the microorganisms, their relative invasiveness and the toxicity of their metabolic by-products.

The remarkably variable individual defensive reaction of the host (immune status) to these infections plays a major role in determining the course of the disease. Defects of PMNs are known to occur ( cf. p. 42).

The causes of *recession* are not completely understood. The morphology of the facial alveolar bone, traumatic horizontal toothbrushing, and frenum pulls remain suspect.

# Gingival and Periodontal Diseases, Etiology Partially Local but with Systemic Involvement

Plaque-elicited gingival and periodontal diseases can be accentuated, enhanced or caused in part by hormonal disturbances, side effects of drugs, autoimmune diseases, anomalies of keratinization, dermatologic disorders, specific infections, injuries, allergies, poisons, metabolic disturbances, immune insufficiency (AIDS), inadequate nutrition, blood dyscrasias and severe genetically-determined general syndromes.

It is not possible to draw sharp demarcations between diseases of the gingiva and those of the mucosa (see also Lindhe 1983, Pindborg 1987).

---

● *The diseases listed below with a solid dot are represented in the clinical photographs that follow.*

## Primarily gingival changes

– *Hormonal complications:*
   ● Pregnancy gingivitis
   ○ "Pill" gingivitis
   ● Puberty gingivitis
   ○ Gingivitis menstrualis and intermenstrualis
   ○ Gingivitis climacterica

– *Side effects of drugs; gingival enlargement:*
   ● Phenytoin-induced gingival overgrowth
   ● Cyclosporine-A induced overgrowth
   ● Dihydropyridine-induced overgrowth
   ● Idiopathic fibrosis
   ● Epulis
   ● Neoplasm (tumors)

– *Autoimmune diseases, desquamative and bullous gingival alterations, keratinopathies, dermatologic diseases:*
   ● Pemphigoid (gingivosis)
   ● Pemphigus vulgaris
   ○ Epidermolysis bullosa
   ○ Erythema multiforme
   ● Lichen planus
   ● Parakeratotic lesions, pre-cancerous lesions
   ○ Dermatomyositis, scleroderma, psoriasis etc.

– *Specific infections:*
   ● Herpes
   ● Aphthae (?)
   ○ Toxoplasmosis
   ○ Actinomycosis
   ○ Candidiasis
   ○ Gonorrhea, syphilis etc.

– *Allergies:*
   ○ To medicines, metals, plastics etc.

– *Intoxications*

– *Injuries/burns:*
   ○ Mechanical, chemical, thermal, actinic

## Gingival *and* periodontal changes

– *Metabolic disturbances:*
   ● Insulin-dependent Juvenile Diabetes
   ○ Acatalasemia
   ○ Eosinophilic granuloma

– *Blood cell disorders:*
   ○ Preleukemic syndrome
   ● Panmyelopathy
   ● Leukemia
   ○ Cyclic neutropenia
   ○ Chronic neutropenia
   ○ Drug-induced agranulocytosis
   ○ Erythroblastic anemia

– *Immune deficiencies:*
   ● HIV-infections, AIDS

– *Inadequate nutrition:*
   ○ Pronounced ascorbic acid deficiency (scurvy)
   ○ Kwashiorkor (protein deficiency)

– *Genetically related general syndromes:*
   ● Down syndrome
   ● Papillon-Lefèvre syndrome
   ○ Chediak-Higashi syndrome
   ○ Hypophosphatasia (Rathbun syndrome)
   ○ Pelger-Huet nuclear anomaly

Genetically related general syndromes may lead to periodontitis in the *deciduous dentition* and in *prepubescent* children.

Defects of PMN granulocytes have been demonstrated in several of these syndromes. Disorders that weaken host defense mechanisms are likely the primary cause for the periodontitis that often accompanies systemic diseases.

# Gingivitis

**Plaque-induced gingivitis, chronic gingivitis**

Gingivitis is ubiquitous. It is a bacterially-elicited inflammation of the marginal gingiva (Löe et al. 1965). In the chapter "Etiology and Pathogenesis" (p. 11), the development and progression of gingivitis from *healthy* tissue to an *initial* lesion, then an *early* lesion and on to *established* gingivitis was described (pp. 22–23; Page & Schroeder 1976).

The only form of gingivitis observed clinically in *adults* is the established lesion, which can manifest varying degrees of severity. In *children,* however, the early lesion (gingivitis with predominance of T-cells) can persist for years.

Clinically and histopathologically it is possible to make a rather gross differentiation between mild, moderate and severe gingivitis. The amount of plaque accumulation, the types of microorganisms (virulence) and the reaction of the host (immune status) combine to determine the intensity of the inflammatory reaction.

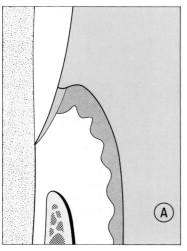 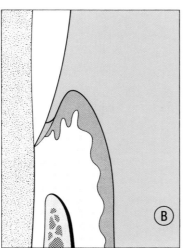 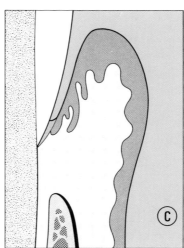

**87  Sulcus and gingival pockets**

**A Sulcus**
In healthy gingiva, a histologic sulcus of maximum 0.5 mm depth exists. During probing, the tip may penetrate the junctional epithelium up to 2 mm.

**B Gingival pocket**
Created when coronal junctional epithelium detaches from the tooth in gingivitis; no attachment loss.

**C Pseudopocket**
Created by gingival enlargement.

The fine line between healthy gingiva and gingivitis is difficult to discern. Even gingivae that appear healthy clinically will almost always exhibit a mild inflammatory infiltrate histologically. With increasing clinical and histologic inflammation, the basal cells of the coronal portion of the junctional epithelium proliferate laterally. The junctional epithelium becomes detached from the tooth, which permits apical movement of bacteria between the tooth and the epithelium, forming a *gingival pocket.*

If gingivitis is severe, edema of the tissues occurs and *pseudopockets* may develop.

Gingival pockets and pseudopockets are *not* true periodontal pockets by definition, because no apical proliferation of the junctional epithelium or loss of connective tissue attachment has occurred. Gingivitis may develop into periodontitis. Untreated, gingivitis can also persist over many years with variations in intensity (Listgarten et al. 1985). With treatment, gingivitis is completely reversible.

# Histopathology

The clinical and histopathologic pictures of established gingivitis are well correlated (Engelberger et al. 1983). The earliest mild infiltration of PMNs that occurs even in clinically healthy gingiva may be explained as a host response to the small amount of plaque that is present even in a clean dentition. Such plaque is composed of non-pathogenic or mildly pathogenic microorganisms, such as gram-positive cocci and rods.

As plaque accumulation increases, so does the severity of clinically detectable inflammation, as evidenced by the quantity of inflammatory infiltrate. It consists primarily of differentiated B-lymphocytes (plasma cells), with a smaller number of other types of leukocytes.

With increasing inflammation, more and more PMN granulocytes transmigrate the junctional epithelium. If the inflammatory process is not stopped, the junctional epithelium will take on the character of a pocket epithelium (p. 82; Müller-Glauser & Schroeder 1982).

**88  Healthy gingiva (left)**
Even in clinically healthy gingiva (GI = 0, PBI = 0), one can observe a very discrete sub-epithelial inflammatory infiltrate. Scattered PMNs transmigrate the junctional epithelium, which remains for the most part intact (H & E, x 10).

**89  Mild gingivitis (right)**
As clinical inflammation increases (GI = 1, PBI = 1), the amount of inflammatory infiltrate increases and collagen is lost in the area of infiltration (Masson stain, x 10).

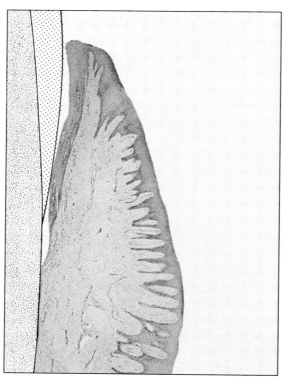
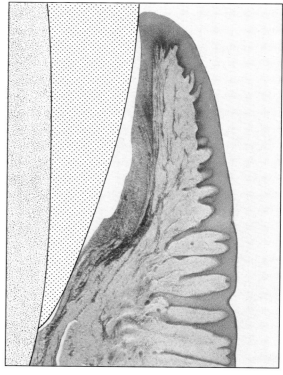

**90  Moderate gingivitis (left)**
When gingivitis is clinically apparent (GI = 2, PBI = 2), the infiltrate becomes heavier and more expansive. Collagen loss continues. The junctional epithelium proliferates laterally; a gingival pocket develops.

**P** = subgingival plaque
(Masson stain, x 10)

**91  Severe gingivitis (right)**
Pronounced edematous swelling (GI = 3, PBI = 3–4). The inflammatory infiltrate is expansive; collagen loss is pronounced. The junctional epithelium is transformed into a pocket epithelium (gingival pocket). Only in the apicalmost area are any remnants of intact junctional epithelium observed. Apical to the JE, the connective tissue attachment is intact (no loss of attachment; H & E, x 10).

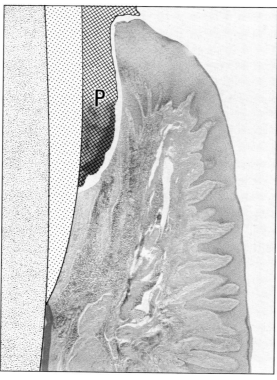
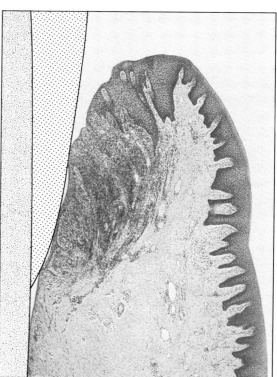

## Clinical Symptoms

- Bleeding
- Erythema (reddening)
- Edematous swelling
- Ulceration

The first clinical symptom of an established lesion is *bleeding* subsequent to careful probing. This hemorrhage is elicited by the penetration of a blunt probe through the disintegrating junctional epithelium and into the vascular sub-epithelial connective tissue. At this stage of the inflammatory process (PBI = 1), no gingival erythema may be visible clinically.

Symptoms of advanced gingivitis include profuse bleeding after sulcus probing, obvious *erythema* and simultaneous *edematous swelling*. In the most severe cases, spontaneous bleeding and eventually *ulceration* may occur.

Even severe gingivitis need not progress to periodontitis. With proper treatment, gingivitis is reversible; nevertheless, untreated gingivitis often evolves into a slowly progressing adult periodontitis (AP).

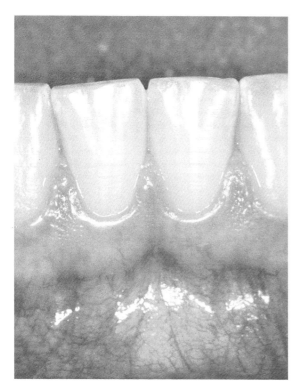

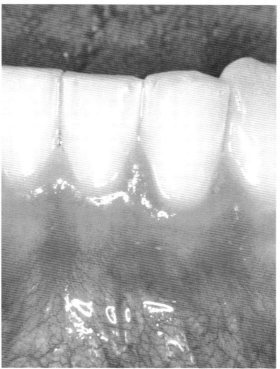

**92 Healthy gingiva (left)**
The gingiva is pale salmon pink in color and may be stippled. The narrow free gingival margin is distinguishable from the attached gingiva. After gentle probing with a blunt periodontal probe, no bleeding occurs.

**93 Mild gingivitis (right)**
Localized mild erythema and slight edema. Some of the former stippling is lost. Minimal bleeding after probing.

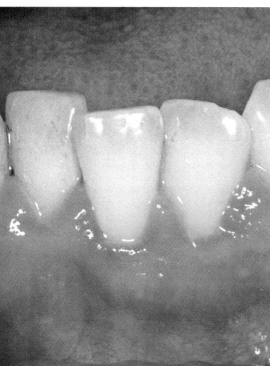

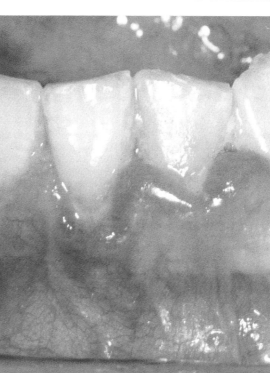

**94 Moderate gingivitis (left)**
Obvious erythema and edema. No stippling apparent; hemorrhage following probing of the sulcus.

**95 Severe gingivitis (right)**
Fiery redness, edematous and hyperplastic swelling; complete absence of any stippling; interdental ulceration, copious bleeding on probing, and spontaneous hemorrhage.

## Mild Gingivitis

A 23-year-old female came to the dentist for a routine check-up. She had no complaints and was not aware of any gingival problems, although in her medical history she indicated that her gingiva bled occasionally during toothbrushing. Her oral hygiene was relatively good. She had received toothbrushing instruction by a dentist once, but no subsequent instruction. The patient was not on any regular recall program. Calculus removal had been performed sporadically in the past during routine dental check-ups.

*Findings:*

| | |
|---|---|
| HYG, Hygiene Index: | 70% |
| PBI, Papilla Bleeding Index: | 1.5 |
| PD, Probing Depths: | ca. 1.5 mm maxilla |
| | ca. 3 mm mandible |
| TM, Tooth Mobility: | 0 |

*Diagnosis:* Gingivitis in initial stage
*Therapy:* Motivation, plaque and calculus removal
    *Recall:* Initially at 3 months, thereafter 6 months.
*Prognosis:* Very good.

**96 Mild gingivitis in anterior area**
In the maxilla, one observes no overt signs of gingivitis, except for a mild erythema.

In the mandible, especially in the papillary areas, slight edematous swelling and erythema can be detected (arrows).

*Right:* Radiographically there is no evidence of loss of supporting structure in the interdental bony septa. The maxillary incisors exhibit short roots.

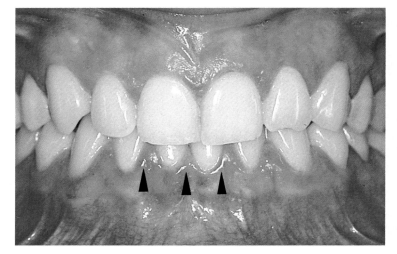 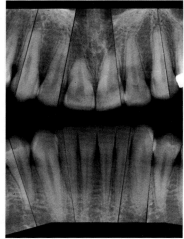

**97 Papilla Bleeding Index (PBI)**
After gentle probing of the papillary sulci with a blunt periodontal probe, hemorrhage of grades 1 and 2 occurs. This is a cardinal sign of gingivitis.

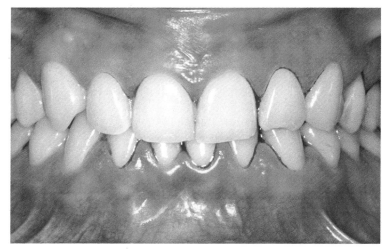

**98 Stained plaque**
Around the necks of the teeth and in interdental areas, small plaque accumulations are visible.

*Right:* Gingival vascular plexus (**X**) in the region of the junctional epithelium in mild gingivitis. Above the white arrows one observes the most marginal vascular loops in the area of the adjacent oral sulcular epithelium (**OSE**); compare Fig. 24 R).

Courtesy *J. Egelberg*

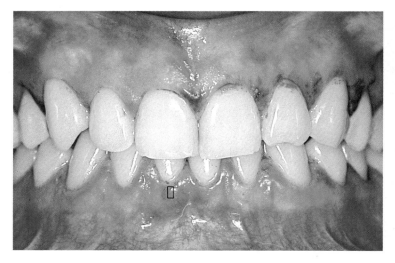 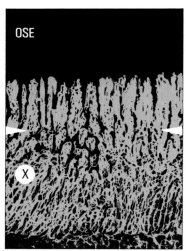

# Moderate Gingivitis

A 28-year-old female presented with a chief complaint of gingival bleeding. She "brushes her teeth," but has never received any oral hygiene instruction from a dentist or hygienist. Calculus had been removed only infrequently, and a professional debridement had never been systematically performed.

Generalized crowding of the teeth in both arches is evident, combined with an anterior open bite. These anomalies lessen any self-cleansing effects and make oral hygiene difficult. They may also increase the severity of gingivitis.

*Findings:*
HYG: 50%          PD: 3 mm in maxilla
PBI:  2.6 in maxilla          4 mm in mandible
      3.4 in mandible
TM:  0 in maxilla, 1 in mandible

*Diagnosis:* Maxilla, moderate gingivitis; mandibular anterior region, severe gingivitis with pseudopockets.

*Therapy:* Motivation, oral hygiene, plaque and calculus removal. After re-evaluation, possible gingivoplasty.

*Recall:* Every 6 months initially.

*Prognosis:* With patient cooperation, very good.

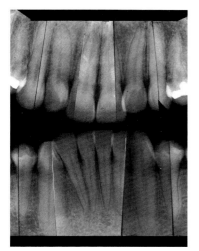
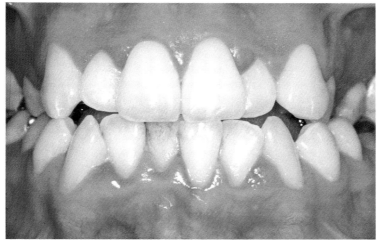

**99  Moderate gingivitis in anterior segments**
Erythema and enlargement of the gingiva. Symptoms are more pronounced in mandible than in maxilla.

*Left:* Radiographically there is no evidence of destruction of the interdental bony septa.

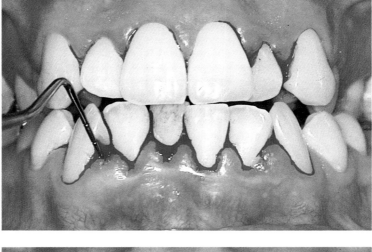

**100  Papilla Bleeding Index (PBI)**
The pronounced gingivitis that is particularly obvious in the mandibular anterior area is corroborated by the PBI. Bleeding scores of 3 and 4 are recorded after "sweeping" the sulcus with a periodontal probe in the papillary regions.

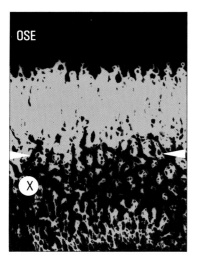
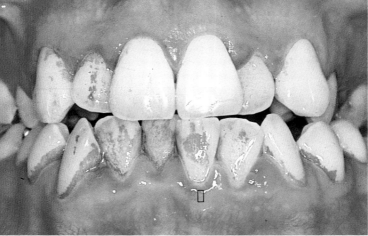

**101  Stained plaque**
Moderate plaque accumulation in the maxilla. In the mandible, heavier plaque, especially at the gingival margins.

*Left:* Vascular plexus of the gingiva (**X**) near the junctional epithelium with severe gingivitis (compare Fig. 24 R and 98 R).

Courtesy *J. Egelberg*

# Severe Gingivitis

A 15-year-old male was referred for evaluation and treatment of suspected juvenile periodontitis (LJP). The extremely pronounced gingivitis was, however, inconsistent with this diagnosis. Sulcus probing and radiographic examination revealed no attachment loss.

The patient practiced virtually no oral hygiene, stating that it was impossible to brush his teeth because his gingiva bleeds at the slighest touch. He had never received adequate motivation, nor any oral hygiene instruction, nor any treatment for his gingivitis.

*Findings:*
| | |
|---|---|
| HYG: 12% | PBI: 3.5 |
| PD:   Pseudopockets to 5 mm | TM: 0 |

*Diagnosis:* Severe gingivitis with edematous hyperplastic enlargement on the facial aspect of the anterior area; mouth breathing (?).

*Therapy:* Motivation, oral hygiene instruction, definitive debridement. Possible gingivoplasty.

*Recall:* Initially every 3 months.

*Prognosis:* With cooperation from the patient, good.

**102   Severe gingivitis**
The clinical symptoms of severe gingivitis such as erythema, edema and hyperplastic enlargement are observed. The anterior region is more severely affected (slight crowding, mouth breathing?).

Probing reveals no attachment loss. The base of the pseudopockets is not apical to the cementoenamel junction.

*Right:* Radiographically one observes no evidence of bone loss at the interdental septa, despite the severe inflammation.

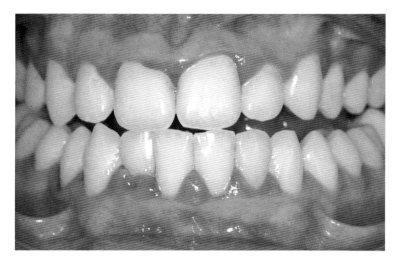
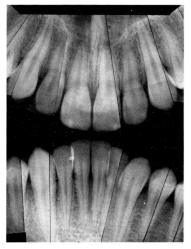

**103   Papilla Bleeding Index (PBI)**
Copious bleeding (PBI grade 4) occurs after sweeping the pseudopockets with a blunt periodontal probe.

The inflammation is somewhat milder in the premolar and molar regions.

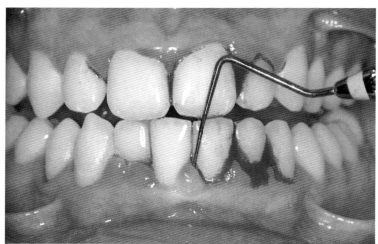

**104   Stained plaque**
Moderately heavy accumulation of supragingival plaque. Not visible is the expanse of the subgingival plaque in the pseudopockets.

The pronounced gingival inflammation, especially in the anterior region, anticipates significant plaque accumulation subgingivally. Subgingival plaque in pseudopockets, or a particularly pathogenic plaque could explain the clinical situation.

*Right:* The papilla between 21 and 22 is grossly enlarged, reddened and devoid of stippling.

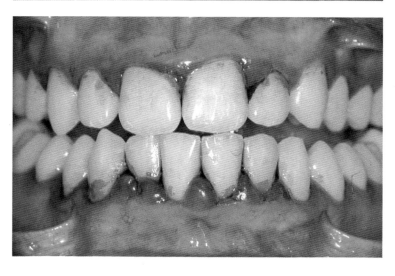
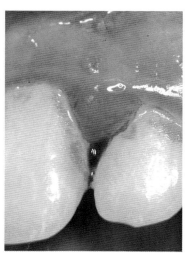

# Acute Necrotizing Ulcerative Gingivitis

**ANUG, Vincent's infection, trench mouth**

Acute necrotizing ulcerative gingivitis (ANUG) is a painful, rapidly progressive inflammation of the gingiva, which may enter a sub-acute or chronic stage. The disease seldom occurs as a generalized process nor is its severity always identical. It may be quite advanced in anterior teeth, while the premolars or molars are not affected at all or only mildly so. The reasons for this irregular appearance are unknown, but poor oral hygiene, locally predominating pathogenic bacteria and plaque-retentive areas likely are involved. Without treatment ANUG may progress to involve deeper periodontal tissues (p. 99).

Probing depths are usually shallow because gingiva propria is lost to necrosis as attachment loss proceeds. Secondary ulceration of other oral mucosal surfaces is rarely observed (Sabiston 1986, Claffey et al. 1986, Falkler et al. 1987).

*Caution:* Ulceration can represent an early oral symptom in HIV-positive patients and AIDS victims (cf. pp. 70–72; Greenspan et al. 1986, Robertson & Greenspan 1988)!

Next to simple gingivitis, ANUG is one of the most common diseases of the gingiva. Incidence figures ranging from 0.1–10% of the adolescent population have been reported.

The *etiology* of ANUG is not completely understood. In addition to plaque and a previously existing gingivitis, the following factors are suspected:

*Local Factors:*
- Poor oral hygiene
- Predominance of Spirochetes, *Bacteroides* and fusiform bacteria in the plaque
- Plaque-retentive areas (crowded teeth, overhanging restorations etc.)
- Smoking (local irritation from tar and other by-products of combustion)

*Systemic Factors:*
- Poor general health
- Fatigue or psychic stress
- Smoking (*nicotine* as a sympatheticomimetic and chemotaxin; Totti et al. 1984, Johnson & Engel 1986, Rivera-Hidalgo 1986)
- Age
- Season of the year (September/October & December/January; Škach et al. 1970)

The stereotypic ANUG patient is a young person who smokes heavily (tar and nicotine), exercises poor oral hygiene and is indifferent to his oral disease. He becomes interested in treatment only during painful exacerbations.

The *clinical course* is acute, with destruction of affected papillae within days. Even without treatment the acute phase may enter a remissive stage. Increased host resistance or self-treatment (e.g., rinsing with a disinfectant mouthwash) may be benefical in shortening the acute episode. Without professional treatment ANUG usually recurs, and may lead to periodontal involvement with attachment loss, especially in interdental areas (see pp. 99–100).

*Therapy* for initial cases should include debridement (ultrasonic), thorough cleansing with hydrogen peroxide, oral hygiene instruction and motivation. A recall appointment several days later is advisable for follow-up on the patient's home care.

For advanced or intractable cases, initial therapy can be supplemented with topical application of cortisone/antibiotic ointments. In severe cases with periodontal involvement, systemic penicillin, metronidazole (Flagyl) or ornidazole (Tiberal) may be used as adjunct therapy (Medicaments, p. 314).

## Histopathology

The clinical and histopathologic pictures in ANUG are correlated. The histopathology of ANUG is significantly different from of that of simple gingivitis.

As a consequence of the acute reaction, an enormous number of PMNs transmigrate the junctional epithelium in the direction of the sulcus and the col. In contrast to the situation in simple gingivitis, PMNs also migrate toward the oral epithelium and the tips of papillae, which undergo necrotic destruction. The ulcerated wound is covered by a clinically visible, whitish pseudo-membrane that consists of bacteria, dead leukocytes and epithelial cells, as well as fibrin. The tissue subjacent to the ulcerated areas is edematous, hyperemic and heavily infiltrated by PMNs. In long-standing disease, the deeper tissue regions will also contain lymphocytes and plasma cells. Within the infiltrated area, collagen destruction may proceed rapidly.

*Spirochetes and other bacteria often penetrate into the tissue* (Listgarten 1965, Listgarten & Lewis 1967).

**105   Papilla biopsy**
Affected papilla excised from a patient with mild ANUG resembling the clinical situation in Figure 107. The tip of the papilla and the tissue approaching the col have been destroyed by ulceration (**U**). The oral epithelium (**OE**, stained yellow) remains essentially intact. In the deeper layers of the biopsy one observes the red-stained intact collagen, while beneath the decimated papilla tip the collagen is largely obliterated (van Gieson, x 10).

The arrow indicates the section that is enlarged in Figure 106.

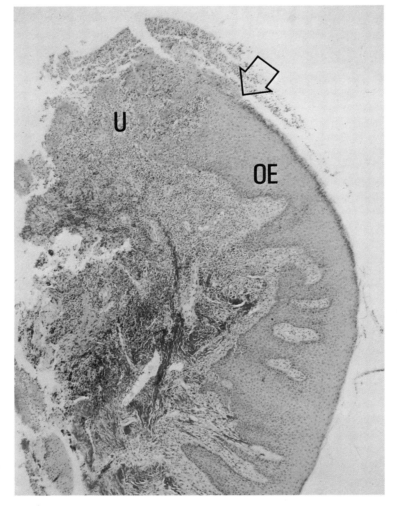

**106   Surface of the disintegrated tissue**
The upper portion of the figure exhibits thickly packed fusiform bacteria (**FUS**). Spirochetes present in the section are not visible with this staining technique, but the numerous **PMN**s are obvious. The brownish structures with weakly staining nuclei are dying epithelial cells (van Gieson, x 1000).

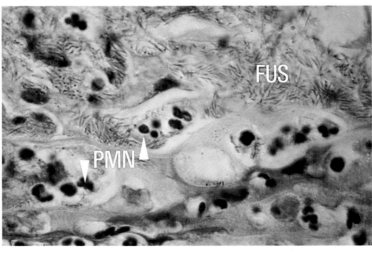

# Clinical Symptoms – Bacteriology

- Pain
- Necrotic destruction, ulceration
- Halitosis

The first clinical symptom of ANUG is *pain. Necrotic deterioration* of papilla tips begins in the col tissues in the interdental area, followed by destruction of the entire papilla and even portions of the marginal gingiva. It is not clear whether the gingival destruction is caused primarily by vascular infarction or by invasion (infiltration) of bacteria into the tissue. Without treatment, the osseous portion of the periodontal supporting apparatus can also become involved.

The patient with ANUG is characterized by a typical, insipid, sweetish *halitosis*. Generalized ANUG may be accompanied by fever and malaise; it can be differentiated from acute herpetic gingivostomatitis by the vesicular pattern (p. 69).

In only a few cases are depressed lesions on the cheeks, lips or tongue observed.

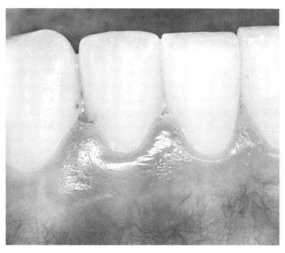

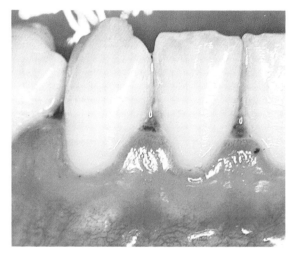

**107 Earliest symptom of ANUG (left)**
The most coronal portion of the papilla tip is destroyed by necrosis from the col outward. The defects are covered with a typical whitish pseudomembrane. The first pain may be experienced even *before* any ulcerations become visible clinically. ANUG should be diagnosed and treated in this early, reversible stage.

**108 Advanced stage of ulceration (right)**

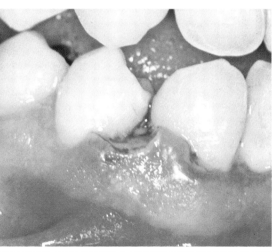

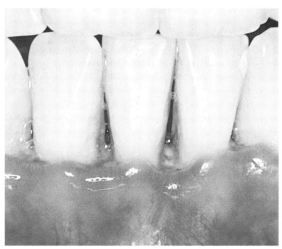

**109 Complete destruction of the papilla (left)**
Uneven involvement: Between the premolars there is no visible lesion, but areas of early necrosis can be seen on mesial and marginal aspects of the canine. Note the complete destruction of the papilla between canine and first premolar.

**110 Acute recurrence (right)**
The papillae are completely destroyed. The previous acute stage has led to reverse architecture of the gingival margin. Beginning osseous destruction: Periodontal involvement.

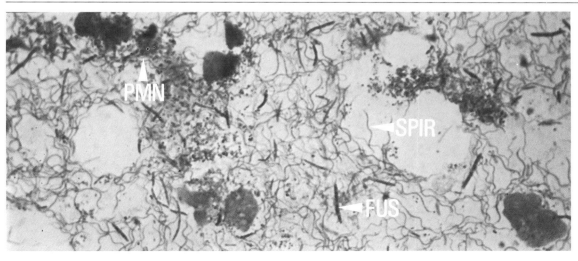

**111 Bacteriology – Smear of the pseudomembrane**
In addition to dead cells, granulocytes (**PMN**) and fusiform bacteria (**FUS**), enormous numbers of Spirochetes (**SPIR**) are visible (Giemsa, x 1000).

# Mild ANUG

A 19-year-old female experienced gingival pain and bleeding for three days.

*Findings:*
    HYG: 60%
    PBI:  3.2 in anterior segments
          2.6 in premolar and molar areas
    PD:   2–3 mm in interproximal areas
    TM:   0–1

*Diagnosis:* Acute necrotizing ulcerative gingivitis, localized, early stage.

*Therapy:* During the first appointment, careful debridement (ultrasonic), hydrogen peroxide rinses, oral hygiene instruction and motivation. The patient may be instructed to rinse at home with mild hydrogen peroxide solutions. At subsequent appointments, repeated motivation and home care instruction are provided, plaque and calculus are thoroughly removed by the dentist or hygienist. No systemic medications are indicated.

*Recall:* Short interval (information, OHI)!

*Prognosis:* With treatment and *patient cooperation,* good.

**112   Initial stage**
Initial acute ulcerative destruction of several papilla tips (arrows). Other papillae exhibit signs of mild inflammation, but no destruction.

*Right:* Radiographically one observes no evidence of resorption of interdental septal bone.

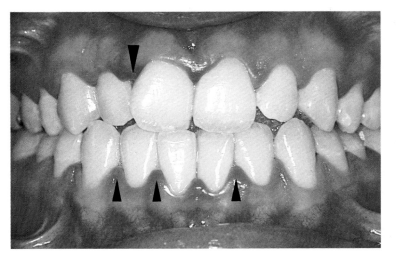
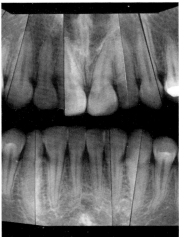

**113   Destruction of papilla tips in the maxilla**
Necrosis of the papilla between central and lateral incisors is apparent. Note simultaneous erythema and swelling, especially at the base of the papilla.
    Between the lateral incisor and the canine one observes the earliest signs of necrosis.
    Erythema of the papilla is noted between the two central incisors, but no clinically visible destruction. If the patient experiences pain when this area is probed gently, it is evidence that the necrotic process has already begun in the col area.

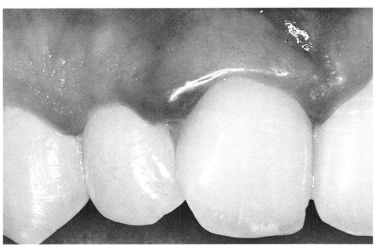

**114   Destruction of papilla tips in the mandible**
Each papilla exhibits signs of incipient ulceration, and each is already covered by a pseudomembrane consisting of fibrin, dead tissue cells, leukocytes and bacteria.

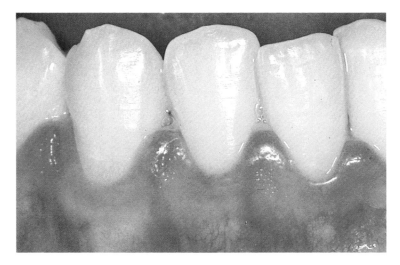

## Severe ANUG

A 16-year-old female presented with a chief complaint of severe pain, inflammation and bleeding of the gingiva. Identical symptoms had been experienced twice before at intervals of about three months. She treated the first acute episode herself with hydrogen peroxide rinses. She did not contact a dentist until this third incident.

*Findings:*

| | | |
|---|---|---|
| HYG: 10% | PBI: 3.8 | PD: Maximum 3 mm |
| TM: 1 | | interproximally |

*Diagnosis:* Severe generalized ANUG.

*Therapy:*

1. Careful debridement (ultrasonic), plaque and calculus removal, and topical application of antibiotic/cortisone ointment. Oral hygiene instruction and patient motivation. Re-evaluation; repeated oral hygiene instruction and patient motivation.
2. Gingivoplasty as appropriate.

*Recall:* At short intervals!

*Prognosis:* Good, but only with excellent patient cooperation. The chance of recurrence is high.

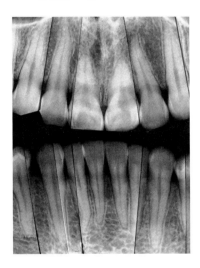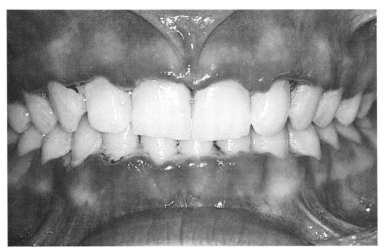

**115 Acute exacerbation of advanced, generalized ANUG**
Virtually all interdental papillae are destroyed to a greater or lesser degree. The ulceration has already spread to the facial marginal gingiva. The gingivae are fiery red and bleed spontaneously or at the slightest touch.

*Left:* The radiograph does not reveal any attack on the interdental bony septa.

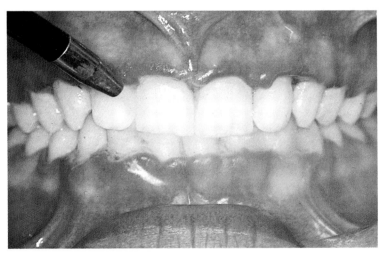

**116 Spraying away loose debris and the pseudomembrane**
Superficially located debris and the pseudomembrane can be easily removed from both teeth and gingiva by means of a water jet. Use of a spray for rinsing with a disinfectant will dramatically reduce the quantity of bacteria in the oral cavitiy.

The operator should wear eye protection when using a water spray for this purpose.

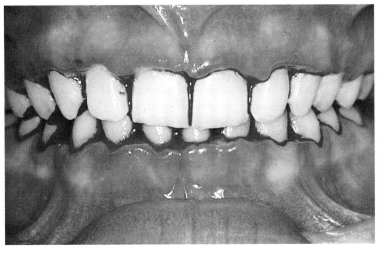

**117 Hemorrhage after spraying**
Heavy bleeding is provoked from the ulcerative gingiva by the water spray.

At this stage, the patient cannot be expected to perform efficient plaque control. Proper oral hygiene can be re-initiated only after successful treatment of the highly acute stage.

# Gingivitis Modulated by Hormones

Changes in the body's hormonal balance generally do not cause gingival inflammation, but can increase the severity of an already present gingivitis. For example, the insulin deficiency of Diabetes mellitus, as well as female sex hormones may often be associated with the progression of plaque-elicited gingivitis. One may distinguish:

- Puberty gingivitis
- Pregnancy gingivitis
- Gingivitis from the "Pill"
- Gingivitis menstrualis and intermenstrualis
- Gingivitis climacterica

### Puberty gingivitis

Epidemiologic studies have demonstrated that gingival inflammation during puberty is somewhat more pronounced when compared to the years preceding and succeeding puberty (Curilović et al. 1977, Koivuniemi et al. 1980, Stamm 1986).

If oral hygiene is poor and/or if the adolescent is a mouth breather, a typical gingival hyperplasia may ensue, especially in the maxillary anterior area (Figs. 102 & 729).

*Therapy:* Plaque and calculus removal, oral hygiene instruction and gingivectomy/gingivoplasty. Mouth breathing may require consultation with an appropriate medical specialist (ENT).

### Pregnancy gingivitis

This condition is *not* observed clinically in *every* pregnant woman! Even if oral hygiene is good, however, the gingivae will exhibit an elevated tendency to bleed (Silness & Löe 1964).

*Therapy:* Oral hygiene; recall every one to two months until breast feeding is discontinued.

### "Pill" gingivitis

A reaction of the gingivae to contraceptives generally occurs only after long-term, regular use (Lindhe & Björn 1967, Knight & Wade 1974, Pankhurst et al. 1981).

The symptoms include gingival hemorrhage, mild erythema and edema.

*Therapy:* Oral hygiene and possibly a switch to a different brand of oral contraceptive.

### Gingivitis menstrualis/intermenstrualis

This is exceedingly rare. Desquamation of gingival epithelium changes during the 28-day menstrual cycle, similar to vaginal epithelium. In exceptional cases the desquamation can be so pronounced that a diagnosis of "discrete" Gingivitis menstrualis or intermenstrualis may be made (Mühlemann 1952).

*Therapy:* Good oral hygiene to prevent secondary plaque-associated gingivitis.

### Gingivitis climacterica

This alteration of the mucosa is also rare. The pathologic alterations are observed less on the marginal gingiva than on attached gingiva and oral mucosa, which may appear dry and smooth, with salmon-pink spots. Stippling disappears and keratinization is lost. Patients complain of xerostomia and a burning sensation.

*Therapy:* Careful oral hygiene is necessary but may be painful. The patient should be instructed to use a soft-bristle toothbrush. Topical vitamin-A ointments or dentifrices, as well as locally applied anesthetics may be beneficial; in severe cases, systemic estrogen therapy.

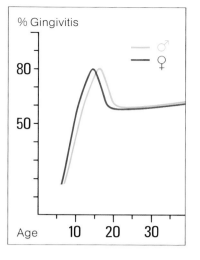

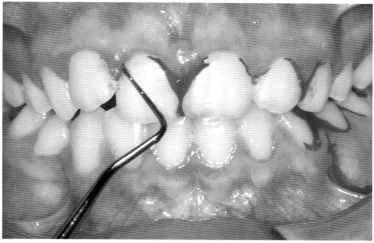

## Puberty

### 118   Puberty gingivitis
13-year-old female with severe hyperplastic gingivitis. Copious bleeding on probing. Plaque and mouth breathing were the main causes of the gingival inflammation. The pubertal hormonal surge may have been a cofactor.

*Left:* Morbidity of gingivitis in 10,000 persons. A peak is observed during puberty.

Adapted from *Massler* et al. 1950, *Stamm* 1986

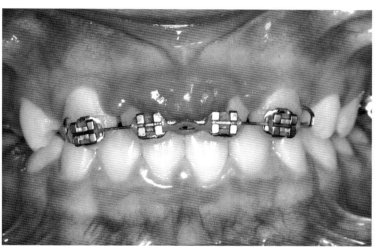

### 119   Puberty gingivitis, orthodontic treatment
A 13-year-old male patient lost his maxillary central incisors due to an accident. Gingivitis, possibly puberty-related, was present before the accident. Orthodontic means were used to move the lateral incisors mesially. This may have caused some extrusion of interdental tissue. In the absence of adequate plaque control, a severe inflammatory hyperplasia occurred between the lateral incisors.

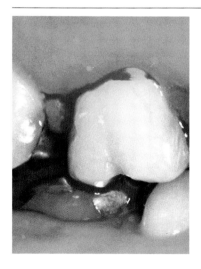

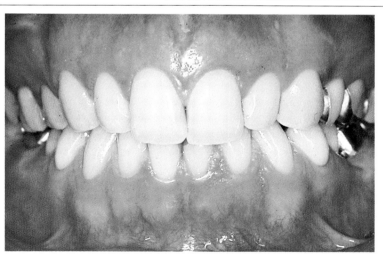

## Pregnancy

### 120   Mild pregnancy gingivitis
In this 28-year-old female, who is in her seventh month of pregnancy, a cursory inspection does not reveal symptoms of gingivitis in the anterior region. In the premolar and molar areas, however, a mild to moderate gingivitis is present.

*Left:* Copious hemorrhage occurs immediately after probing in the area of a defective restoration (plaque niche).

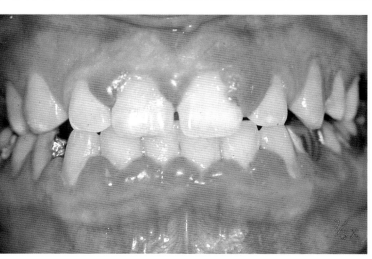

### 121   Severe pregnancy gingivitis
In this 30-year-old patient, moderate gingivitis was present even before her pregnancy.
     This photograph, taken during the eighth month, reveals severe inflammation and pronounced hyperplastic, epulis-like gingival alterations in the anterior segment.

## Severe Pregnancy Gingivitis, Gravid Epulis

This 24-year-old women was eight months pregnant. She presented complaining that she "bites the swollen gums" on the left side of her mouth. Clinical examination revealed a severe generalized gingivitis as well as the gravid epulis ("pregnancy tumor").

*Findings:*

HYG: 40%      PBI: 3.2      TM: 0–1

PD:   7 mm around teeth 34 and 35,
        otherwise generally 4 mm (pseudopackets)

*Diagnosis:* Severe generalized pregnancy gingivitis with large pyogenic granuloma near 34–35.

*Therapy:*

– *During the pregnancy:* Motivation, repeated oral hygiene instruction, plaque and calculus removal, gingivoplasty around 34 and 35 using electrosurgery.

– *After breast feeding is terminated:* Re-evaluation, further treatment planning.

*Recall:* Frequency depends on patient cooperation.

*Prognosis:* With treatment, good.

**122   Severe pregnancy gingivitis**
With poor oral hygiene, a pronounced gingivitis has developed during the last half of the pregnancy. A large epulis is observed buccally and lingually around the mandibular premolars.

*Right:* The histologic section (of gingiva, not the epulis; see black line) exhibits normal oral epithelium, a relatively mild inflammatory infiltrate and widely dilated vessels (H & E, x 40).

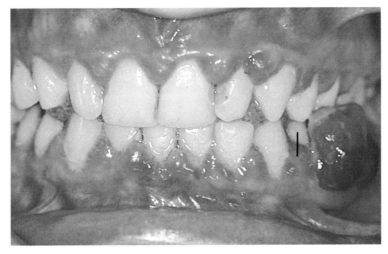 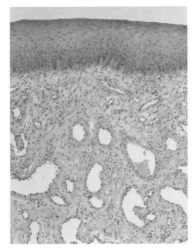

**123   Gravid epulis**
The surface of the epulis is ulcerated because the patient's maxillary teeth bite into the tissue during mastication. For this reason, the redundant tissue must be removed while the patient is still pregnant. Considerable hemorrhage may be expected during the surgery; therefore, electrosurgery is the treatment of choice.

*Right:* The radiograph depicts some horizontal loss of the crestal compact bone of the interdental septa.

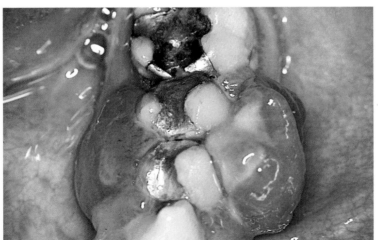 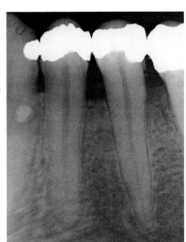

**124   Three months after gingivoplasty; two months post-partum**
Definitive periodontal therapy and treatment planning for restorative work that is sorely needed should begin at this time.

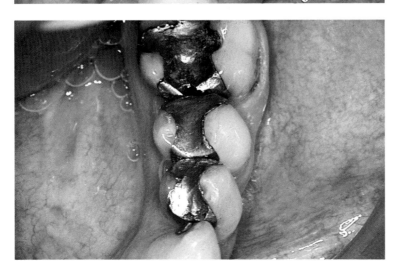

# Gingival Overgrowth
# Tumors
# Blood Dyscrasias

Swelling ("tumor") is one of the classical signs of inflammation in gingivitis and periodontitis. There are other types of gingival enlargement, however, whose etiologies are not linked directly or primarily with microbial plaque or hormonal imbalance.

Diseases of the hematopoietic system often are associated with severe gingival manifestations (Pindborg 1985, 1987). The following lesions and diseases will be briefly presented:

- Overgrowth elicited by drugs
- Benign tumors – Epulis, Fibrosis, Exostosis
- Malignant tumors
- Blood dyscrasias

### Overgrowth elicited by drugs

Some medications, whether applied locally or taken systemically, may elicit adverse side-effects in oral tissues. A classical example of this is the gingival enlargement and overgrowth caused by three classes of *systemic* medications:

- *Phenytoin* (hydantoin) has been used successfully since the late 1930s for treatment of seizure disorders (Merritt & Putnam 1938, 1939).

- *Dihydropyridines* (e.g., nifedipine) are used worldwide in the treatment of hypertension and post-myocardial syndrome.

- *Cyclosporine-A* is an immunosuppressive drug, first described by Borel et al. (1976). Cyclosporine has almost completely supplanted the classic immunosuppressive drug azathioprine and partially also cortisone, as drug of choice to prevent rejection of solid organ and bone marrow transplants.

- Several other systemic medications, albeit less frequently employed, may also elicit gingival overgrowth (e.g., the antiepileptic *sodium valproate* and the anticarcinogen *Bleomycin*).

### Benign tumors – Fibrosis, exostosis

Many different types of benign tumors may occur on hyperplasias of the gingiva, most commonly observed in the papillary area. It is possible to differentiate between granulomatous, giant cell, and fibrous epulis.

### Benign tumors – Fibrosis, exostosis

Many different types of benign tumors may occur on the gingiva, though these are not common. Such tumors should be distinguished from the swelling of simple gingivitis and the lesions of epulis, as well as from malignant tumors.

### Malignant tumors

Malignant tumors (e. g., carcinoma) occur relatively frequently in the oral cavity (p. 63), but rather more seldom directly on the gingiva or in the periodontium. Early recognition and diagnosis resides within the realm of responsibility of the dentist!

### Blood dyscrasias

Host response to challenge is significantly reduced during diseases of the hematopoietic system, particularly in leukemia. Severe manifestations of gingival and periodontal disorders often result.

# Phenytoin-Induced Gingival Overgrowth

Phenytoin prevents or reduces the severity of seizures associated with epilepsy (grand mal); it is ineffective in petit mal. Phenytoin is also often prescribed following neurosurgical operations or cranial trauma. The anticonvulsive effect is probably due to the inhibition of the spread of nerve potentials in the brain cortex.

*General* side effects of phenytoin are relatively minor. Some bone pathology may be observed after long-term therapy. The patient's mental capacity and reaction time may be negatively influenced.

The most important *oral* side effect is a pronounced, often secondarily inflamed *gingival overgrowth,* observed in about half of those treated, especially young patients (Hassell 1981). The overgrowth is caused by a subpopulation of gingival fibroblasts that produce excess connective tissue macromolecules.

*Therapy:* Motivation, repeated oral hygiene instruction, professional plaque and calculus removal. Once inflammation subsides, fibrous tissue can be excised. Lesions will recur if phenytoin ingestion is continued. Severity can be minimized by excellent oral hygiene.

**125   Mild phenytoin overgrowth**
Fibrous form of phenytoin overgrowth in a 19-year-old female patient with epilepsy, who had taken the medication for many years. She exhibited relatively good oral hygiene, which minimized secondary inflammation and thus kept gross enlargement and pseudopockets to a minimum.

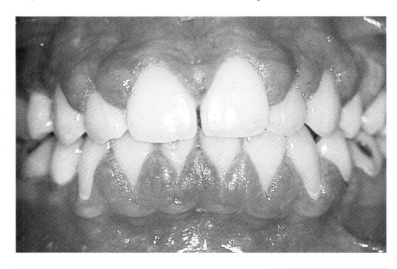

**126   Phenytoin –**
**Structure and chemical formula**
Phenytoin (diphenylhydantoin) is a 5,5-diphenyl-2,4-imidazolodinedione.

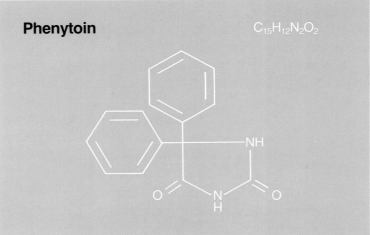

Phenytoin                    $C_{15}H_{12}N_2O_2$

**127   Severe phenytoin overgrowth, severe secondary inflammation**
This 44-year-old female patient had taken phenytoin on a chronic regimen for 6 years, since a neurosurgical procedure. She was mildly debilitated and therefore unable to perform adequate oral hygiene.

*Right:* There is radiographic evidence of bone resorption at the interdental septa.

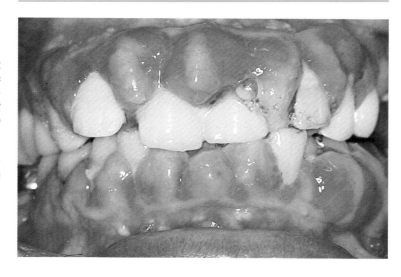

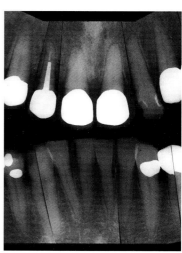

# Dihydropyridine-Induced Gingival Overgrowth

The substituted dihydropyridines (e.g., nifedipine, nitrendipine, felodipine) are calcium antagonists that reduce the influx of calcium ions into heart muscle and thereby reduce the strength of contraction as well as the vascular resistance. This reduces oxygen consumption by the heart while simultaneously increasing cardiac circulation. Thus, dihydropyridines possess both anti-anginal and anti-hypertensive effects. Some general side effects as well as interactions with other drugs are observed. In contrast to phenytoin, dihydropyridines are taken primarily by older patients (periodontitis?).

The most important *oral* side effect is an often pronounced, secondarily inflamed gingival overgrowth. The pathogenesis of the overgrowth is suspected to be similar to that observed in phenytoin-treated individuals (connective tissue accumulation), but an increase in acid mucopolysaccharides (ground substance) also appears to occur (Lucas et al. 1985, Barak et al. 1987).

*Therapy:* Following patient motivation, repeated oral hygiene instruction and initial therapy, severe lesions may be eliminated by gingivoplasty.

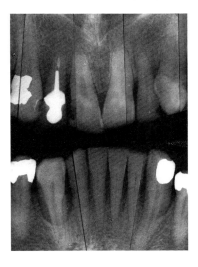
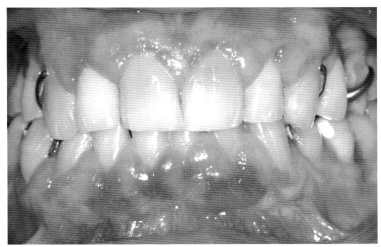

**128 Mild to moderate nifedipine overgrowth**
This 55-year-old male exhibits lesions of varying severity, with evidence of secondary inflammation. He had been taking "Adalat" (nifedipine) for two years because of his high blood pressure.

*Left:* The radiograph shows clearly that the gingival alterations are superimposed upon an existing periodontitis; the latter is *not* due to the drug.

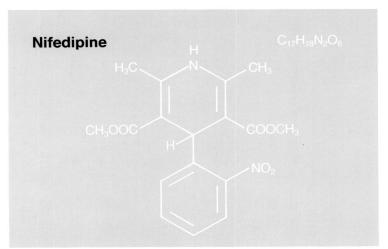

**129 Nifedipine – Structure and chemical formula**
This drug is a 1,4-dihydro-2,6-dimethyl-4-(2-nitrophenyl)-3,5-pyridine-dicarbonic acid dimethylester.

**Nifedipine** $C_{17}H_{18}N_2O_6$

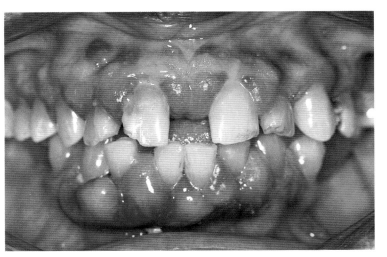

**130 Severe nifedipine overgrowth**
This 58-year-old female patient presented with severe, secondarily inflamed gingival overgrowth. The patient had taken "Procardia" (nifedipine) for four years.

# Cyclosporine-Induced Overgrowth

Cyclosporine-A is prescribed primarily following organ transplantation. The immune suppressive action of this drug ("Sandimmune") derives from the suppression of antibody production against *T-cell*-dependent antigens, the suppression of cell-mediated immunity, and interference with the production of lymphokines (IL-2, MIF etc.). There are numerous adverse side effects of cyclosporine; however, these are generally less severe than with the alternative immunosuppressive drugs. Side effects include lymphoma, hirsutism as well as *nephro-* and *hepatotoxicity.*

The *oral* side effect of cyclosporine is gingival overgrowth, which is often secondarily inflamed. The incidence and severity of the lesions are dose-dependent and correlated to blood levels of the drug.

*Therapy:* Oral hygiene and scaling will reduce inflammation and enlargement. Conservative therapy is effective when instituted before the cyclosporine regimen. In advanced cases, gingivoplasty may be indicated. *Organ transplant patients should receive comprehensive dental care beforehand* (Rateitschak-Plüss et al. 1983 a, b).

**131 Mild to moderate cyclosporine overgrowth**
This 45-year-old female began taking cyclosporine-A two years previously, following kidney transplantation. Gingival overgrowth is pronounced only in the mandible; secondary inflammation is in evidence.

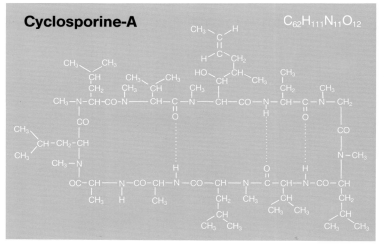

**132 Cyclosporine-A –
Structure and chemical formula**
The drug is a cyclic peptide (undecapeptide) consisting of 11 amino acids.

*Right: Tolypocladium inflatum* (formerly designated as *Trichoderma polysporum*) is the fungus from which cyclosporine was isolated during research on antibiotics.

SEM courtesy *R. Guggenheim*

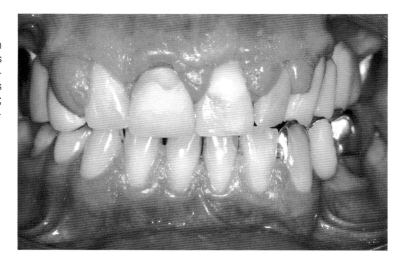

Cyclosporine-A

$C_{62}H_{111}N_{11}O_{12}$

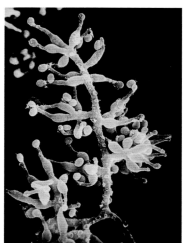

**133 Severe cyclosporine overgrowth – Overdosage**
Dramatic enlargements such as in this 51-year-old female are infrequently observed today. This patient had received approximately three times the dosage of cyclosporine that is common today. In addition, the patient exhibited poor oral hygiene.

*Right:* PMN granulocytes and plasma cells are observed histologically in the infiltrated subepithelial connective tissue (plaque-elicited, not pathognomonic for cyclosporine; H & E, x 400).

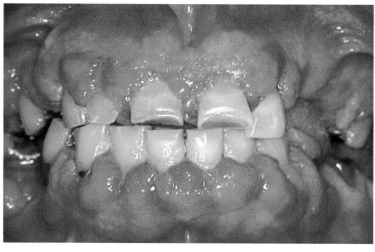

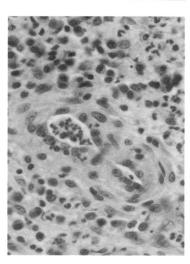

# Benign Tumors – Epulis

Gingival epulis represents a family of benign tumors, which can be differentiated from each other:

- Granulomatous epulis, pyogenic granuloma (includes gravid epulis; p. 56)

- Giant cell epulis

- Fibrous epulis

Giant cell epulis and granulomatous epulis may develop relatively quickly; fibrous epulis grows slowly. The etiology of such tumors is not completely understood, but marginal irritation is one likely cause. Some pathologists contend that giant cell epulis is the only *true* epulis. It is a fact that no histologic differences exist between fibrous epulis and fibromas in other areas of the oral cavity.

*Therapy:* Pyogenic granuloma and fibrous epulis can be removed by simple excision.

The giant cell epulis has a tendency to recur; following excision of such tumors, a gingival flap should be reflected, the tooth (and root) surfaces thoroughly cleaned and planed, and the bone filed.

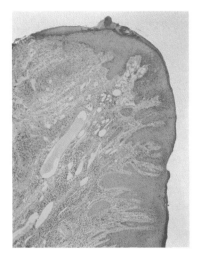
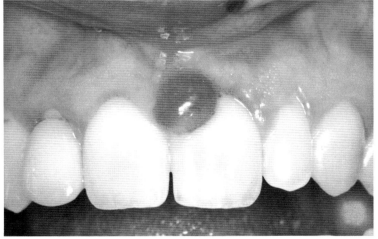

**134 Pyogenic granuloma, granulomatous epulis**
Localized, tumor-like, bright red, soft mass on the labial gingival margin in a 34-year-old female.

Epulis is usually seen in the papillary region, and less frequently, as in the present case, on the gingival margin. When probed or injured, the lesion exudes a copious mixture of blood and pus.

*Left:* The histologic view exhibits a loose granulation tissue filled with blood (H & E, x 40).

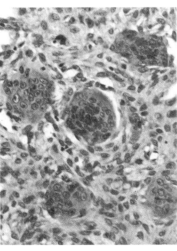
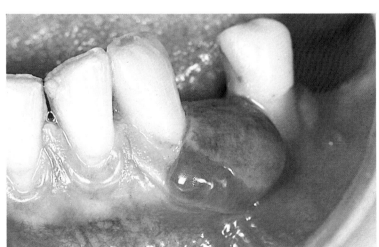

**135 Giant cell epulis – "True" Epulis**
Resembling clinically the granulomatous epulis, the giant cell epulis can only be diagnosed histologically. Such lesions can become very large and, as in this 50-year-old patient, can cause displacement of adjacent teeth.

*Left:* The histologic section reveals an inflammatory infiltrate including *multinucleated giant cells* in the subepithelial connective tissue (H & E, x 400).

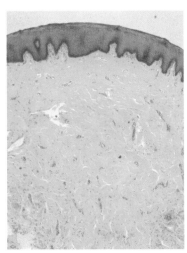
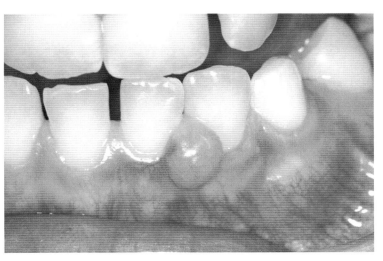

**136 Fibrous epulis**
This 45-year-old female exhibits a localized, fibrous, firm mass upon the gingiva between central and lateral incisors. The etiology of such lesions can seldom be ascertained.

*Left:* Histologically one observes an accumulation of fibrous connective tissue. If the mass becomes secondarily inflamed, a typical infiltrate can be expected.

Courtesy *B. Maeglin*

# Benign Tumors – Fibrosis, Exostosis

The list of benign tumors of the oral mucosa is long (Bhaskar 1986, Pindborg 1987). Mention will be made of only *gingival* tumors, as well as gingival and osseous lesions that must be distinguished from the plaque-elicited, inflammatory swellings (gingivitis) and epulis:

- Fibrosis
- Exostosis
- Verrucous hyperplasia, papilloma, hemangioma, gingival cysts, peripheral ameloblastoma, nevi

Fibrosis and exostosis may be localized or generalized on the gingiva. Their causes are for the most part unknown. Hassell and Jacoway (1981a, b) described a genetically determined (autosomal, dominant) form of gingival hyperplasia (Elephantiasis gingivae).

*Therapy:* True gingival hyperplasia (histologically determined) is treated by simple gingivoplasty. Osseous thickening can be reduced by osteoplasty following flap reflection. These procedures may also be combined (Fig. 138, right). Recurrence is, however, frequent.

**137    Hereditary gingival hyperplasia**

A 28-year-old man exhibited generalized gingival hyperplasia with regionally varying severity. His family history revealed that similar gingival alterations had been observed in his father (who today wears a complete denture). The hyperplasia occasioned pseudopockets, which act as niches for plaque accumulation and therefore can lead to secondary inflammation. Following surgical resection, such hyperplasia often recurs.

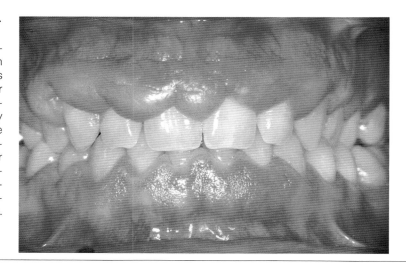

**138    Idiopathic gingival and bony thickening**

This 26-year-old female exhibited pronounced gingival *and* osseous thickening. The latter could be diagnosed by passing a sterile injection needle or probe through the hyperplastic soft tissue.

*Right:* The therapy consisted of a combined procedure including gingivoplasty and osteoplasty after flap reflection. Depicted is the suture closure of the flap, which was previously thinned by external gingivectomy.

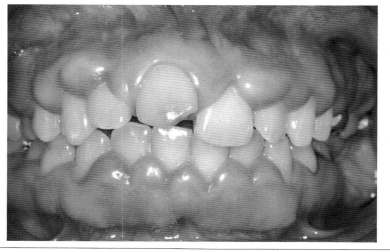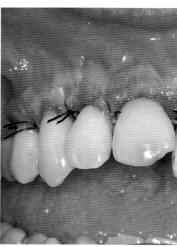

**139    Exostosis**

Exostosis is a harmless "idiopathic" thickening of bony tissue whose cause is unknown (bruxism?). Such bony lesions can be left untreated if they do not negatively influence function, well-being or periodontal health.

The maxillary right segment exhibits a particularly pronounced idiopathic osseous thickening, which could render oral hygiene more difficult.

Courtesy B. Maeglin

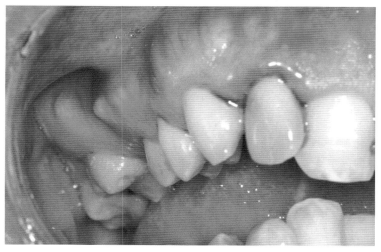

# Malignant Tumors

- Carcinoma

- Melanoma

- Sarcoma (chondrosarcoma, fibrosarcoma, rhabdomyosarcoma, lymphoma etc.)

Malignant epithelial and mesenchymal tumors are frequent in the oral cavity. In the Western world oral carcinoma accounts for 1–5% of all carcinoma. In Southeast Asia this figure may increase to 15–40% (Pindborg 1987). Malignant tumors are, however, seldom observed on the gingiva.

In addition to *primary tumors,* the gingiva may also be a recipient site for *metastases,* from the kidneys, lungs, prostate, breast or other organs.

*Therapy:* If there exists the slightest suspicion of malignancy, the patient should be referred immediately to the oral surgeon, who may elect to institute chemotherapy, radiotherapy or surgical excision. The dentist should avoid excessive manipulation of the mass, and must never attempt a biopsy!

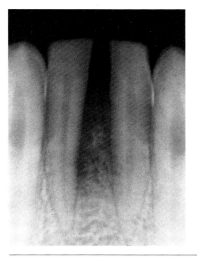
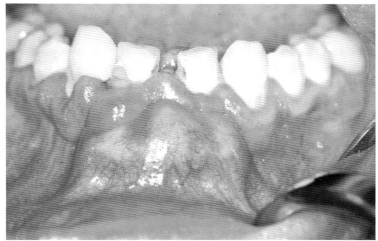

**140   Chondrosarcoma**
A 25-year-old female complained of a large swelling in the mandibular anterior area. The tumor extended from the gingiva into the oral mucosa and was ca. 2 cm wide. Histopathologic diagnosis: Highly differentiated chondrosarcoma.

The tumor was treated by radical surgery; metastases were not detected at the time of surgery.

*Left:* The radiograph reveals resorption of bone between the mandibular central incisors.

*Courtesy B. Maeglin*

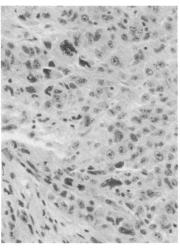
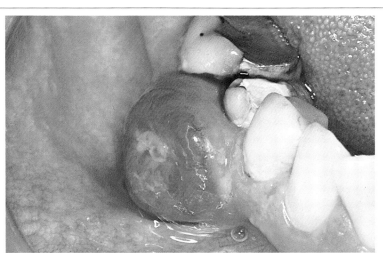

**141   Rhabdomyosarcoma**
A large, epulis-like swelling in a 38-year-old female was diagnosed by the pathologist as the rare malignant rhabdomyosarcoma. The tumor grows by invading the alveolar bone. Metastasis to other skeletal sites occurs rapidly.

*Left:* The histologic picture is one of growth of "strands" of the malignant tissue. Dramatic number of mitotic figures (H & E, x 400).

*Courtesy B. Maeglin*

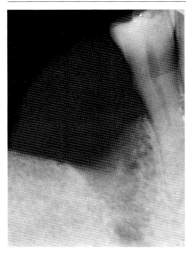
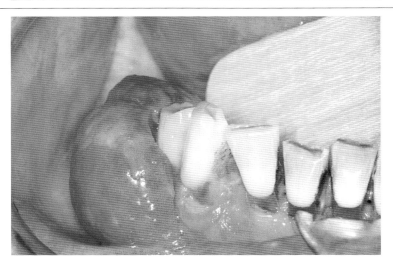

**142 Adenocarcinoma – Metastasis**
Poor wound healing occurred in a 63-year-old male after extraction of 45. A large swelling developed later in the right side of the mandible. Histopathologic diagnosis: Poorly differentiated adenocarcinoma. This was not a primary tumor, but a *metastasis* from the prostate.

*Right:* Poorly healing alveolus is visible in the radiograph. The soft tissue of the tumor is faintly visible.

*Courtesy B. Maeglin*

# Blood Dyscrasias

Malignant diseases of the hematopoetic system virtually always lead to a reduction in the efficacy of host defense. The balance between bacterial attack and immune response in the periodontal arena is likewise disturbed.

Those blood dyscrasias that may enhance gingivitis and periodontitis include:

- Acute and chronic myeloid leukemia
- Acute and chronic lymphatic leukemia
- Aplastic anemia

Leukemias are generalized, neoplastic overgrowths of the leukocytes and their precursor cells. Both qualitative as well as quantitative changes in the white cell picture occur. However, in sub- or aleukemically progressing leukemias (Schettler 1987) peripheral leukocyte counts may be normal or even reduced.

*Therapy:* The cure rate for leukemias, especially in younger patients, has increased dramatically in recent years due to chemotherapy and bone marrow transplantation. Depending on patient age and type of leukemia, over 50% of patients survive today.

**143   Acute lymphatic leukemia (ALL; AIDS patient)**
Rapidly progressing Burkitt-type leukemia (FAB classification L-3) in a 27-year-old *HIV-positive* female. Pallor of the attached gingiva, contour changes, heavy spontaneous hemorrhage.

It was not possible to determine absolutely whether the HIV infection already existed before the outbreak of the blood dyscrasia.

*Right:* Very severe lobulated hyperplasia in the maxillary right posterior region.

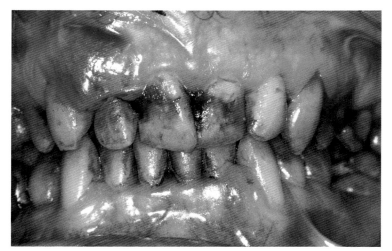 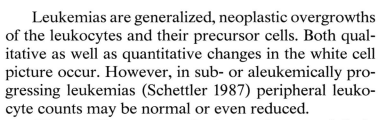

**144   Blood smear**
*Left:* Erythrocytes, lymphocyte, granulocyte.

*Right:* B-lymphocytes with empty vacuoles in the cytoplasm; crenated nuclei, with nucleoli; binucleated cells.
(May-Grünwald, x 1000)

◀ Healthy

Blood

ALL ▶

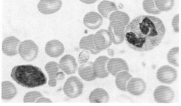 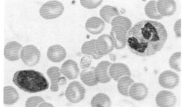 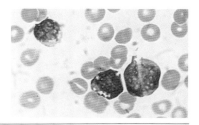

**145   Bone marrow**
*Left:* Various blood cell precursors; fatty marrow.

*Right:* "Empty bone marrow" with friable structure lacking precursor cells. Macrophages; increased fatty marrow.
(May-Grünwald, x 400)

◀ Healthy

Bone marrow

Aplastic anemia ▶

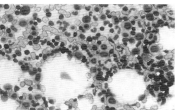 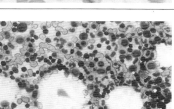 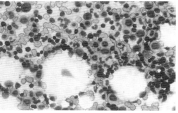 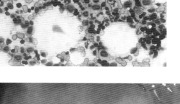 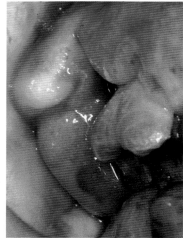 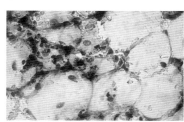

**146   Aplastic anemia**
This 17-year-old male suffered from severe aplastic anemia of unknown etiology; virtual complete lack of hematopoiesis. Severe hyperplastic gingival inflammation with spontaneous hemorrhage.

*Right:* In the area of teeth 12 and 13, vascular loops are evident throughout the thinned epithelium. Hemorrhage occurs at the slightest touch, or spontaneously.

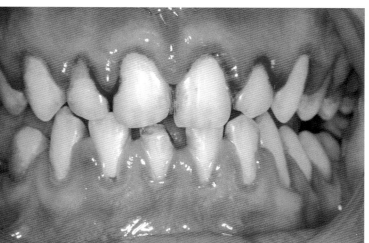 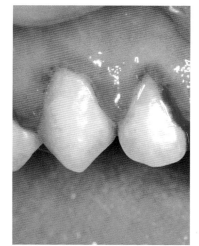

Courtesy B. Speck

# Autoimmune Diseases
# Anomalies of Keratinization
# Viral Infections
# HIV-Infection – AIDS

Autoimmune diseases are caused by an immune reaction to the body's own substances. Antibodies and/or sensitized lymphocytes that react with specific host antigens can be demonstrated. Among the oral manifestations of autoimmune disease are desquamative and bullous alterations of the gingiva and the oral mucosa.

Similarly, abnormalities of keratinization (Lichen planus, leukoplakia, precancerous lesions) and virus infections (Herpes) are often localized on gingiva and oral mucosa.

The AIDS virus does not directly elicit lesions in the oral cavity. However, because of the immune dysfunction, numerous opportunistic infections and neoplastic alterations may occur on the gingiva and oral mucosa of AIDS patients.

Several of the above mentioned types of lesions will be briefly described:

- Gingivosis, desquamative gingivitis/pemphigoid
- Pemphigus vulgaris
- Lichen planus
- Leukoplakia and precancerous lesions
- Herpetic gingivostomatitis
- HIV-Infection, AIDS

### Gingivosis, desquamative gingivitis

This is observed more often in women than in men. It can occur at any age, but is more common in middle-aged and elderly individuals.

### Pemphigoid

This lesion is most common in women beyond middle age. In addition to oral mucosa and gingiva, the conjunctiva and the pharynx are affected, less often also the skin.

### Pemphigus vulgaris

The lesions of Pemphigus vulgaris effect primarily elderly individuals, women more frequently than men. Skin and mucosa as well as gingiva and oral mucous membranes are affected.

### Lichen planus

This disease manifests in a large number of clinical pictures on skin and mucosa. It affects adults after age 30, men and women in equal number.

### Leukoplakia

Intraoral leukoplakia is quite common. In Sweden the morbidity was reported at 3.6% (Axéll 1976). Leukoplakia is more common in men than in women, and usually occurs in older individuals.

### Herpetic gingivostomatitis

This is a virus infection, which was previously described as a pediatric disease. Today it is acknowledged that young adults between 20–25 years may also be affected (Herrmann 1972).

### AIDS, acquired immune deficiency syndrome

AIDS is an infection caused by the *human immunodeficiency virus* (HIV; Gallo & Montagnier 1987, Koch 1987, Mann et al. 1988).

## Gingivosis/Pemphigoid

Mild forms of gingivosis (desquamative gingivitis) are characterized by slight gingival erythema. In more severe cases, epithelial desquamation occurs. If blister formation is also in evidence, the clinical descriptor is *pemphigoid.*

*Therapy:* True "causal" therapy is not possible. Therapy is therefore polypragmatic and symptomatic (pain medication and vitamin-A containing ointments). In severe cases (pemphigoid) topical (and systemic) corticosteroid preparations may be indicated.

## Pemphigus Vulgaris

Pemphigus vulgaris may effect the skin, as well as all mucosal surfaces and the gingiva.

With or without blister formation, the epithelial layer sloughs, leaving behind expansive and painful erosions. The histologic diagnosis may be substantiated by immunofluorescence serology and by identification of "Tzanck cells."

*Therapy:* Immunosuppressive drugs and systemic corticosteroids. The painful lesions can be treated topically and symptomatically with ointments containing cortisone and antibiotics.

**147   Gingivosis/desquamative gingivitis**
Severe erythema of the entire attached gingiva in this 62-year-old female. Epithelium can be easily separated from subepithelial tissues. Secondary gingivitis is elicited by plaque accumulation.

*Right:* Histology exhibits a thin oral epithelium devoid of rete ridges and not keratinized. The epithelium (**OE**) has separated from the underlying connective tissue (carbol fuchsin, x 100).

Courtesy H. R. Mühlemann

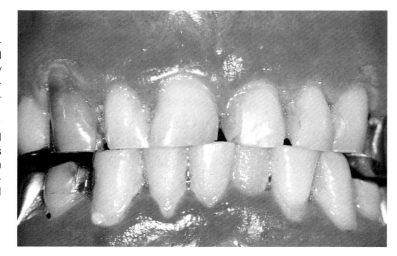 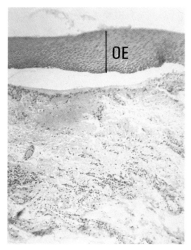

**148   Pemphigoid**
There are no strict criteria for clinical differentiation between gingivosis and pemphigoid. In this 54-year-old female, one observes a severe, marginally localized reddening of the gingiva. The patient reported recurring blister formation, especially on the lingual.

   The histologic picture is essentially identical to that of gingivosis (Fig. 147, right). The entire epithelium is dislodged from the underlying connective tissue (compare *intra*-epithelial dissolution in Pemphigus vulgaris).

Courtesy U. P. Saxer

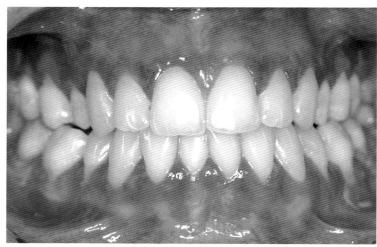

**149   Pemphigus vulgaris**
Fiery red gingiva with secondary effluorescences (burst vesicles). This 50-year-old female also manifested pronounced symptoms on her skin and on other areas of the oral mucosa.

*Right:* In the histologic section, it is clear that vesicle formation and sloughing of the superficial layer of gingiva occurs *intra*-epithelially. The basal cell layer remains attached to the connective tissue. **OE** = Oral epithelium (H & E, x 250).

Courtesy B. Maeglin

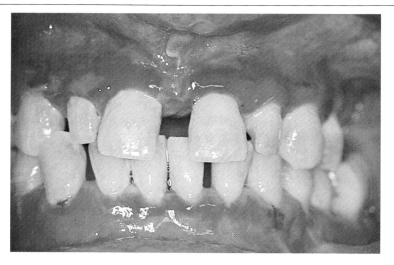 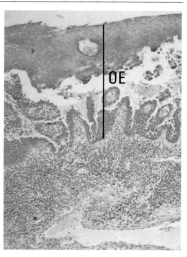

# Lichen Planus: Reticular and Erosive

Lichen (intertwined) is a general term for a family of similar-appearing yet differentiable skin and mucosal alterations (Lichen planus reticularis, erosivus, nitidus, pilaris, acutus, anularis, atrophicus, obtusus, pemphigoides, striatus, verrucosis etc.). Lichen occurs relatively frequently; morbidity figures of 0.2–1.9% of the adult population have been reported (Axéll 1976).

The symptoms of reticular lichen planus are milky-white, pebbly, hyperkeratotic effluorescences and/or net-like coatings, the so-called "Wickham's striae." The white lesions may also be expansive and resemble a leukoplakia. The affected mucosa may atrophy (atrophic form), and may subsequently erode (erosive lichen planus). In rare cases malignant transformation of erosive lichen planus has been described.

*Therapy:* There is no true causal therapy. The lesions should be monitored closely. Treatment for erosive forms includes systemic administration of corticosteroids, often combined with retinoids.

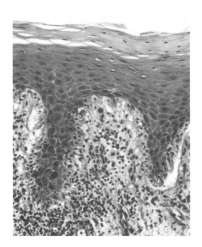
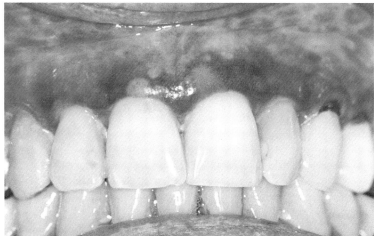
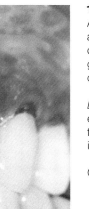

**150 Lichen planus**
A 42-year-old male presented with a whitish, hyperkeratotic, net-like coating (Wickham's striae) on the gingiva and oral mucosa, and secondary gingivitis.

*Left:* Histologically the epithelium exhibits rete ridges and hyperkeratosis. A subepithelial inflammatory infiltrate is visible (H & E, x 400).

Courtesy B. Maeglin

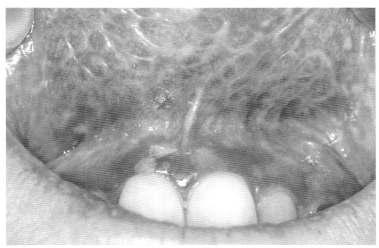

**151 Reticular lichen planus, "Wickham's striae"**
In addition to the red and whitish gingival lesions, the pronounced striae of this lesion are impressive, extending from the vestibular fold and covering the entire mucosa of the internal surface of the lip.

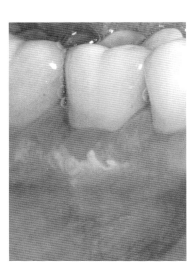
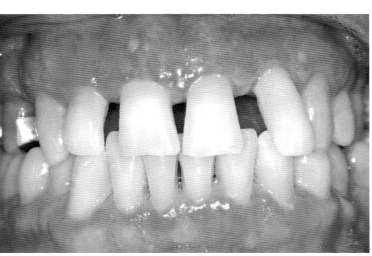

**152 Erosive lichen**
Red-whitish spots, some of which show initial erosions. Secondary plaque-induced gingivitis.

*Left:* The lesions extend over the entire gingiva to the molar area.

# Leukoplakia – Precancerous Lesions

Axéll et al. (1984) and Pindborg (1985) define leukoplakia as white spots "that cannot be classified as any other type of lesion, … except for the use of tobacco." The lesions are characterized histopathologically as hyperkeratotic epithelial thickening.

There are two distinguishable forms of leukoplakia: The more common *homogeneous* form and the *speckled* form (Bengel & Veltman 1986).

Leukoplakia may be localized to any area of the oral mucosa; gingival lesions are less common. The etiology is unknown, but a positive relationship exists between tobacco use and lesions on the floor of the mouth and palate. Smokers exhibit leukoplakia three times more frequently than non-smokers.

Secondary infections, e. g., Candida albicans, are common, as is transformation into precancerous lesions (10%).

*Therapy:* Biopsy for diagnosis, then vigilant observation. Mild cases may be treated with retinoids. Surgical intervention in pronounced cases where malignant transformation is suspected.

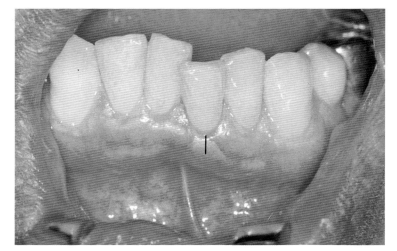 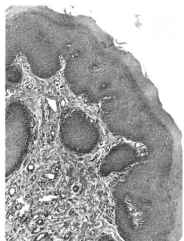

**153 Speckled leukoplakia**
In this 50-year-old female one observes very discrete, whitish lesions on the attached gingiva up to the free gingival margin. The etiology is unknown. The patient does not smoke.

*Right:* The histologic picture reveals slight thickening and hyperkeratosis of the gingiva (leukoplakia).

Courtesy *B. Maeglin*

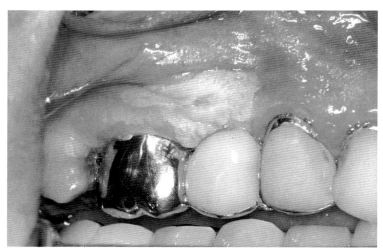

**154 Pronounced leukoplakia**
In this 65-year-old male cigarette smoker, expansive leukoplakia is observed on the attached gingiva near teeth 17, 16 and 15.

Courtesy *B. Maeglin*

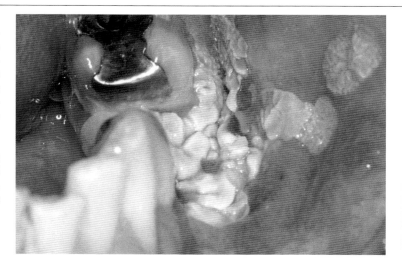 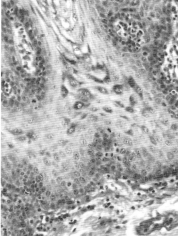

**155 Precancerous lesion**
The 40-year-old female had not noticed the leukoplakia. It transformed into a precancerous situation (verified histologically). The verrucous papillomatous lesions were localized to the gingiva in premolar and molar regions, the vestibulum and the cheek.

*Right:* The histologic section reveals epithelial acanthosis and keratinization of individual cells. At higher magnification numerous mitotic figures are observed.

Courtesy *B. Maeglin*

# Herpetic Gingivostomatitis

This viral infection is most commonly detected in children and in young adults between the ages of 20 and 25 (Herrmann 1972). Once primary infection has occurred, the patient experiences *fever* and painful swelling of the lymph nodes. Intraoral examination reveals an acute, painful gingivitis with blister-like aphthae, erosive lesions on the attached gingiva and not infrequently on the oral mucosa and lips as well. The differential diagnosis must include ANUG and common recurrent aphthous ulcer. The etiology is clear: Infection with *Herpes*

*simplex virus.* Predisposing factors include mechanical trauma, sun exposure, inadequate diet, hormonal disturbance and psychic trauma. The lesions generally disappear spontaneously within 1–2 weeks.

*Therapy: Topical* application of palliative ointments, and perhaps a plaque-inhibitory agent to prevent bacterial superinfection. Acyclovir preparations may be prescribed for topical and systemic use. In severe cases antibiotics may be used to combat any bacterial superinfection.

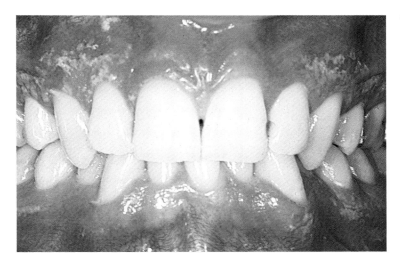

**156 Mild herpetic gingivostomatitis**
Whitish patches and erosive alterations, especially on the attached gingiva. This female patient exhibited good oral hygiene, very little plaque accumulation and hardly any signs of marginal inflammation. The possibility that the Herpes infection occurred secondary to a toothbrush injury cannot be ruled out.

Courtesy *N. P. Lang*

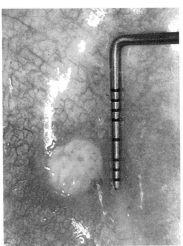
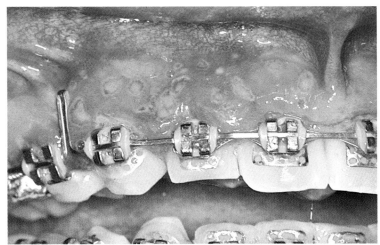

**157 Herpetic gingivostomatitis**
The patient's lack of oral hygiene coupled with the plaque retention fostered by orthodontic bands and wires led to gingivitis, which became superinfected with Herpes.

**158 Differential diagnosis: Solitary aphthous ulcer**
Whitish ulcer surrounded by fiery red mucosal tissue; often recurrent. Etiology is unknown. Solitary and multiple aphthae should not be confused with the effluorescences of Herpes!

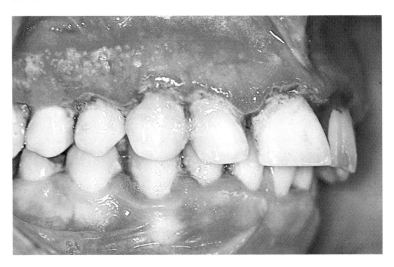

**159 Severe herpetic gingivostomatitis**
This 20-year-old male experienced fever and swollen cervical lymph nodes. A severe gingivitis was present even before the Herpes infection. This acute clinical picture is reminiscent of ulcerative gingivitis, which should be included in the differential diagnosis.

# HIV-Infection – AIDS

AIDS (Acquired Immune Deficiency Syndrome) is caused by the HIV 1 virus (*human immunodeficiency virus 1*). This immensely serious disease continues to spread worldwide, but precise data are lacking. According to calculations by Heyward and Curran (1988) 0.5–0.7% of the United States population (1–1.5 million persons) is already infected.

The *origin* of the disease is not completely clear. Retroviruses are well-known in the animal world. Approximately 70% of African green monkeys are infected with SIV (simian immunodeficiency virus), but without overt symptoms. Other monkey species (e.g., Macaques) do develop clinical Simian AIDS (SAIDS). Since the nucleotide sequence in SIV is 50% homologous with HIV 1, transfer of the retrovirus from animal to man cannot be excluded (Essex & Kanki 1988). It is at this time unknown, what percentage of HIV positive humans must be expected to actually reach stage 6 (WR classification, p. 71) and die of AIDS.

**160   Model of HIV**
The ca. 100 nm retrovirus consists of an external plasma membrane (phospholipids), from which "knobs" (glycoproteins) extend. The central ribonucleoprotein complex (RNP) contains the viral genome (RNA) and the reverse transcriptase.

*Right:*

**1 = RNA**
**2 = Reverse transcriptase**
**3 = Core (RNP) and "inner coat"**
**4 = External membrane with "knobs"**

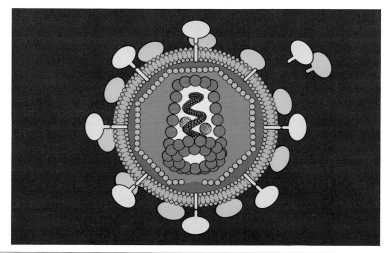 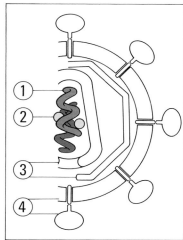

**WR stage 5**

**161   Gingivitis**
Atypical gingivitis in a young HIV-positive male (WR stage 5?). The free marginal gingiva exhibits extreme erythema. The attached gingiva shows spotty reddening, and even the mucosa appears abnormal, with above average erythema.

Courtesy J. R. Winkler

*Right:* ANUG-like gingivitis in a 22-year-old male (WR 5).

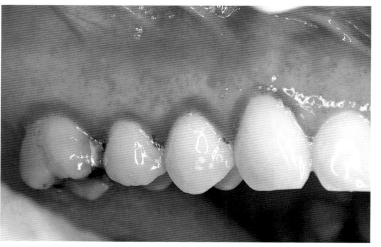 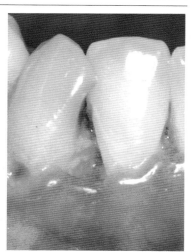

**162   Candidiasis**
The thrush infection on the palate of this 55-year-old female was the sole manifestation of her systemic AIDS infection. Candidiasis is the cardinal symptom for stage 5 in the WR classification.

This patient probably contracted the HIV infection after a blood transfusion.

Courtesy B. Maeglin

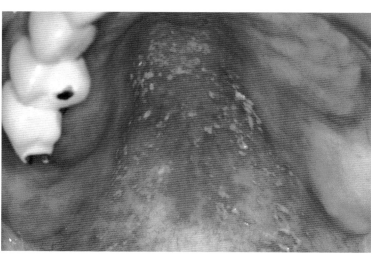

# HIV-Infection – Classification, Severity

Classification of the disease is made according to the "Walter Reed classification" (WR; Redfield et al. 1986, Redfield & Burke 1988). Six stages are distinguished (A–F):

A Detection of *HIV antibodies* or *HIV 1*. No symptoms, except transient episodes of fever.
B Chronic *lymphadenopathy* of months or even years duration.
C Subclinical immune system disturbances. Drop in T4 cells from normal 800 to $< 400/mm^3$ blood.

Duration of this stage: Ca. 18 months.
D Subclinical *immune defect*. Skin test for delayed hypersensitivity reveals partial (P) non-reaction. Duration: 2 years.
E *Candidiasis and other oral symptoms*. Skin test for delayed hypersensitivity completely (C) negative. Duration: 1–2 years.
F Severe systemic immune deficiency (AIDS), with opportunistic infections, tumor and severe periodontal disease (Figs. 166–167, p. 72). Most patients die within two years.

| Course of disease | | WR stage | (A) | (B) | **T4** | (D) | (E) | (F) |
|---|---|---|---|---|---|---|---|---|
| Exposure to HIV | ▶ | WR 0 | – | – | >400 | N | -- | – |
| Acute onset of infection | ▶ | WR 1 | + | – | >400 | N | – | – |
| Chronic lymphadenopathy | ▶ | WR 2 | + | + | >400 | N | – | – |
| T4 less than 400/mm³ Asymptomatic, subclinical immune defects | ▶ | WR 3 | + | ± | <400 | N | – | – |
| | ▶ | WR 4 | + | ± | <400 | P | – | – |
| Thrush, oral symptoms | ▶ | WR 5 | + | ± | <400 | C & + | | – |
| Opportunistic infections, AIDS | ▶ | WR 6 | + | ± | <400 | P/C | ± | + |

**163 "WR" – Walter Reed classification system* of progressive immune dysfunction**
WR is based on laboratory tests and clinical signs. Symptoms B – D/E must persist for at least 3 months.

Oral symptoms (WR 5) may appear only years after HIV infection or identification of the virus in blood, but this is still significantly earlier than full blown AIDS (WR 6).

*\* Walter Reed Army Institute of Research; Washington, D.C.*

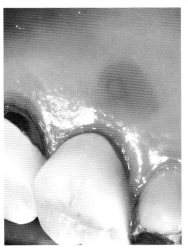
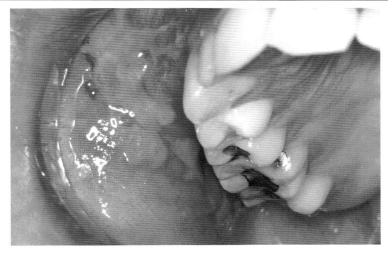

**WR stage 5**

**164 Herpes**
Severe herpetic lesion on the cheek in WR stage 5.

Courtesy *B. Maeglin*

*Left:* Localized, herpetic (aphtha-like) reddening on the palate in an HIV-positive female.

Courtesy *J. R. Winkler*

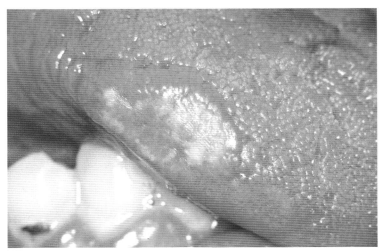

**165 Incipient "hairy leukoplakia"**
Lateral tongue border in an HIV-seropositive 43-year-old homosexual (WR stage 5). This rough leukoplakia of the tongue border is observed very frequently (15–20%) (*Greenspan et al.* 1986, *Reichart et al.* 1986). Severe forms are described as "hairy."

Courtesy *B. Maeglin*

# HIV-Infection – Oral Manifestations

Many symptoms of HIV infection appear in the oral cavity (Greenspan et al. 1986, Maeglin 1987, Grassi et al. 1987 a, Robertson & Greenspan 1988). According to the Walter Reed classification, such oral manifestations appear as pathognomonic only late, in stages 5 or 6.

The dentist may observe:
- Fungal infections
- Bacterial infections
- Viral infections
- Neoplasms
- Manifestations of unknown etiology

WR stage 5 may be characterized with Candidiasis and a peculiar form of gingivitis with atypical marginal erythema. Also frequently observed are Herpes infection, aphthous ulcer and hairy leukoplakia. Oral manifestations such as these must be diagnosed by the dentist at the earliest possible time.

In advanced WR stage 5, but especially in WR stage 6, the oral cavity often reveals opportunistic infections as well as sarcoma, carcinoma, oral manifestations of hematologic disorders, and extremely severe, ulcerative periodontitis.

## AIDS – WR stage 6

**166   ANUG-like periodontitis**
The patient with AIDS shows an ANUG-like severe, progressive periodontitis (*Winkler & Murray* 1987). The patient suffers severe pain ("deep" or osseous pain) and has a characteristic, unpleasant mouth odor.

Courtesy *J. R. Winkler*

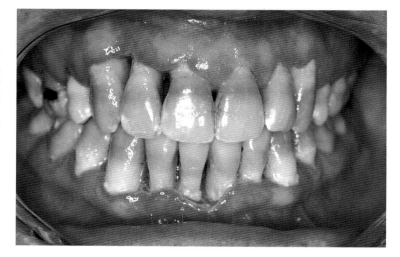

**167   Extreme ANUG-like periodontitis**
This man exhibited many systemic symptoms of severe, advanced AIDS; ANUG periodontitis was also diagnosed. The 26-year-old man complained of severe pain and spontaneous hemorrhage.

The patient died a few days after this photographic documentation.

Courtesy *T. Götsch*

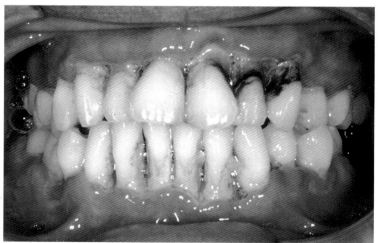

**168   Tumors associated with WR stages 5 and 6**

**Papilloma (left)**

**Kaposi sarcoma (middle)**

Courtesy *M. Grassi*

**Non-Hodgkin's lymphoma (right)**
This patient is *not* infected with HIV; however, identical lymphomas are frequently observed in AIDS patients.

Courtesy *B. Maeglin*

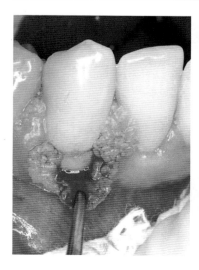
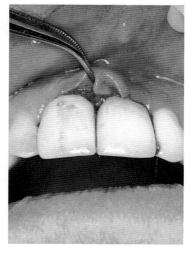
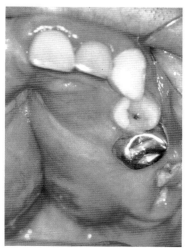

# Periodontitis

Periodontitis maintains its position as one of the widespread diseases of mankind. While caries morbidity, at least in the Northern hemisphere, is decreasing rapidly, the epidemiology of periodontitis exhibits only a slight tendency toward decreasing (Ahrens & Bublitz 1987, Miller et al. 1987, Lamezan & Rateitschak 1988).

Periodontitis is a disease of the tooth-supporting apparatus, caused by bacterial plaque accumulation. It usually develops from a pre-existing gingivitis; however, not *every* gingivitis develops into periodontitis. The quantity and virulence of microorganisms (pathogens) on the one hand, and host resistance factors (immune status) on the other hand are primary determinants for the activity and progression of periodontal destruction.

*Classification* of the various forms of periodontitis can be accomplished from two points of view: Etiology, microbiology = *dynamic pathobiology* (AAP 1986a, 1987a); clinical picture, course of disease = *pathomorphology.* In common international use today is the classification based on dynamic pathobiology (Page & Schroeder 1982, Schroeder 1987b). However, for practical clinical diagnosis, the degree of severity (pathomorphology) of each individual case must also be ascertained.

The current classification of periodontitis includes:

| | | |
|---|---|---|
| ● AP | Adult Periodontitis, slowly progressing periodontitis of adults | |
| ● RPP | Rapidly Progressive Periodontitis, periodontitis with a rapid clinical course in young adults | |
| ● LJP | Localized Juvenile Periodontitis, a rapidly progressive, localized periodontitis in young persons | |
| ● PP | Pre-pubertal Periodontitis, a very rapidly progressive periodontitis of the deciduous dentition | |

An additional form, *Refractory, rapidly progressive periodontitis,* also called "therapy-resistant periodontitis," has been described (AAP 1986a, b). It is not yet clear whether this form is a distinct disease entity or whether it is identical to RPP.

All of the above-noted forms of periodontitis exhibit pathologic changes in the periodontium *without* any accompanying systemic disease. Thus the "true" forms of periodontitis must be distinguished from the periodontal diseases that occur in conjunction with and resulting from systemic diseases (pp. 70–72, 102–108). Periodontitis as a symptom is usually the result of an immune deficiency resulting from the systemic disease; this may be related to non-specific host defense (PMN granulocytes) or to an adaptive specific immune reaction.

# Pathobiology – Forms of Periodontitis

With the exception of the exceedingly rare pre-pubertal periodontitis (PP), the various forms of periodontitis cannot always be distinguished from one another. For example, AP in elderly individuals with compromised immune capacity may suddenly take on the character of more aggressive forms of the disease. In such a case, AP may exhibit more frequent periods of disease activity and a pocket flora similar to RPP.

Such transitions may also exist between LJP and RPP. If, for example, localized osseous defects are diagnosed around the first permanent molars and/or anterior teeth soon after puberty, the diagnosis of LJP is clear. In the absence of treatment, as the patient ages other teeth are frequently also involved (Hormand & Frandsen 1979). In such cases LJP is very difficult to distinguish from RPP ("post-juvenile periodontitis").

*All* forms of periodontitis exhibit a clinical course with destructive (active) and quiescent periods. The factor(s) that trigger a transition from quiescence to active disease remain unknown.

## AP  Adult periodontitis / Slowly progressive periodontitis

This most common form of periodontitis begins between the ages of 30 and 40 years, with a gradual development, generally from a pre-existing gingivitis. The entire dentition may be equally affected. More often, however, the distribution of the disease is irregular, with more severe destruction primarily in molar areas but also in anterior segments. The gingivae exhibit varying degrees of inflammation, with "shrinkage" in some areas and fibrotic manifestations elsewhere. As was the case with incipient gingivitis, the plaque is composed primarily of gram-positive rods and cocci. This plaque provides the matrix for those organisms responsible for the progression of AP and also for subgingival calculus.

Exacerbations of AP occur at rather lengthy intervals. The disease leads to tooth loss only in much later years, or not at all.

*Therapy:* AP can be successfully treated by means of purely mechanical therapy, even if the patient's cooperation is *not* optimum.

## RPP  Rapidly progressive periodontitis of young adults

This relatively rare disease (Page et al. 1983 a) can begin immediately after puberty but is usually diagnosed initially between ages 20 and 30. Females are more frequently affected than males. In contrast to localized juvenile periodontitis (LJP), in RPP *all* teeth may be affected. Some authors have referred to RPP as *post-juvenile periodontitis*. Severity and distribution of attachment loss vary considerably. Acute exacerbations are followed by periods of relative quiescence. The etiology of the aggressive stages is to be found in the specific periodontopathogens (gram-negative anaerobes), which may actually invade the ulcerated pocket epithelium to some degree (infection).

*Therapy:* The majority of RPP cases can be successfully treated by means of mechanical therapy. Supportive chemotherapy (*metronidazole, orinidazole*) or antibiotic therapy (tetracycline) is recommended in this severe form of periodontitis.

| **169  Characteristics of AP – Periodontitis of adults** | | |
|---|---|---|
| **Clinical symptoms** | | |
| ● Morbidity | Ca. 70–80% of all adults (?) | |
| | Ca. 95% of all periodontal disease | |
| ● Initiation – Course | Ca. age 30 | |
| | Slow, "chronic" course | |
| ● Periodontal | – Involvement of all teeth, predisposition for localization at molars and anterior teeth | |
| | – Gingiva: Inflamed, fibrotic, with some shrinkage | |
| | – Alveolar bone: Irregular bone destruction around individual teeth | |
| ● Systemic disease | None | |
| **Blood cell defects** | *Neutrophilic granulocytes* | *Monocytes* |
| | – | – |
| **Bacterial infection** | Mixed infection. In *active* pockets frequently A. actinomycetemcomitans, B. gingivalis, B. intermedius, F. nucleatum | |
| **Inheritance** | Unknown (genetic predisposition?) | |

| **170  Characteristics of RPP – Rapidly progressive periodontitis** | | |
|---|---|---|
| **Clinical symptoms** | | |
| ● Morbidity | 2–5% of all periodontal disorders | |
| ● Initiation – Course | Between puberty and age 30, possibly preceded by LJP (post-juvenile periodontitis?) | |
| | Rapid cyclic course | |
| ● Periodontal | – Many or all teeth affected | |
| | – More or less pronounced gingival inflammation | |
| | – Horizontal and vertical bone loss | |
| | – Symptoms of pocket activity | |
| ● Systemic disease | None | |
| **Blood cell defects** | *Neutrophilic granulocytes* | *Monocytes* |
| Reduced chemotaxis | + + | + + |
| Elevated migration | + + | + + |
| **Bacterial infection** | Mixed infection | |
| | Specific preponderance of B. gingivalis, B. intermedius, A. actinomycetemcomitans (invasion), F. nucleatum, Spirochetes | |
| **Inheritance** | Sex-linked dominant (?) | |

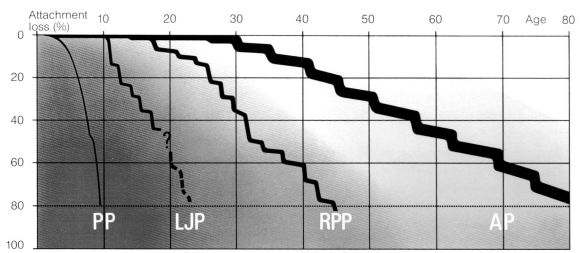

**171 Forms of periodontitis – Clinical course**

**AP** – Adult Periodontitis, slowly progressive periodontitis of adults

**RPP** – Rapidly Progressive Periodontitis, aggressive form of periodontitis seen in young adults

**LJP** – Localized Juvenile Periodontitis, a highly localized and rapidly progressing form of disease in young persons

**PP** – Pre-pubertal Periodontitis, rapidly progressing periodontitis in pre-pubertal individuals

## LJP  Localized juvenile periodontitis

This rare disorder occurs early and attacks the permanent dentition. LJP begins in puberty but is usually not diagnosed until several years later, often when lesions are discovered serendipitously on bite-wing radiographs. In the initial stages, incisors and/or first molars are affected in both maxilla and mandible. Later, other teeth may also be included in the disease process. Hereditary factors likely play a role. Girls are affected more frequently than boys. In its earliest stages, LJP seldom manifests as gingival inflammation. Patients exhibit normal appearing gingiva and very little supragingival plaque. The patient's serum contains high antibody titers to a bacterial leukotoxin that has the ability to injure PMNs.

*Therapy:* With prompt diagnosis and therapy consisting of vigorous mechanical debridement and systemic administration of *tetracycline,* the destructive process can be halted rather easily. Osseous defects may eventually regenerate.

## PP  Pre-pubertal rapidly progressing periodontitis

This exceedingly rare and rapidly progressive disease may be localized (usually to the deciduous molars) or generalized.

The *localized form* begins at ca. 4 years of age and is associated with only mild gingival inflammation in the presence of relatively little plaque.

The *generalized form* begins earlier, immediately after eruption of the deciduous teeth. It is associated with severe gingivitis; gingival recession is common. The attachment loss appears to be continuous rather than intermittent as with all other forms of periodontitis. Children with PP have frequent bouts of inner ear infection and infections of the respiratory tract (Page et al. 1983 a). Blood cell defects are commonly observed.

*Therapy:* The *localized* form can be halted through a combination of mechanical therapy and systemic antibiotics. The *generalized* form seems to be refractory to therapy.

---

**172  Characteristics of LJP – Localized juvenile periodontitis**

**Clinical symptoms**

| | | |
|---|---|---|
| ● Morbidity | 0.1% in young Caucasians 0.8% in young Blacks | |
| ● Initiation – Course | Ca. 13-year-olds, with onset of puberty rather rapid progression with active and quiescent periods | |
| ● Periodontal | – Only first molars and/or incisors affected – Gingiva often normal – Crater-like bone resorption | |
| ● Systemic disease | None | |

| **Blood cell defects** | *Neutrophilic granulocytes* | *Monocytes* |
|---|---|---|
| Reduced chemotaxis | + + | + + |
| Reduced phagocytosis | + | – |
| Defective receptors | + | – |

| **Bacterial infection** | Mixed infection Predominance of *A. actinomycetemcomitans* (Invasion!), Capnocytophaga species (?) |
|---|---|
| **Inheritance** | Autosomal recessive (Sex-linked dominant?) |

---

**173  Characteristics of PP – Pre-pubertal periodontitis**

**Clinical symptoms**

| | |
|---|---|
| ● Morbidity | Extremely rare (few documented cases) |
| ● Initiation – Course | Immediately after eruption of deciduous teeth |
| ● Periodontal Generalized type | – All teeth affected – Gingiva inflamed and hyperplastic |
| Localized type | – Very rare; individual teeth affected |
| ● Systemic disease | Susceptible to infections of the respiratory tract, otitis media, skin infections |

| **Blood cell defects** | *Neutrophilic granulocytes* | *Monocytes* |
|---|---|---|
| Adherence defect | + + | + |
| Chemotaxis defect | + + | + + |
| Receptor defect | + | + |

| **Bacterial infection** | Mixed infection Specific bacteria not demonstrated |
|---|---|
| **Inheritance** | Autosomal recessive |

Tables adapted from *Schroeder* 1987 b; *Page et al.* 1983 a/b, 1986

# Pathomorphology – Clinical Degree of Severity

Periodontitis is a general term. It includes various forms of inflammatory diseases, which differ in their dynamic pathobiology and to some degree also in their microbial etiology. The role played by host response also varies.

It may be trite, but it is necessary to state the fact that *all* forms of periodontitis *begin* at some point in time. They develop at various times during a patient's life, usually from a pre-existing plaque-elicited gingivitis. In the absence of treatment, the disease progresses, albeit at varying rates. It is therefore clear that during clinical data gathering, which leads to the diagnosis for an individual case, not only must the type of the disease be ascertained, it is also necessary to determine in what pathomorphologic stage the disease process currently exists or, in other words, how far attachment loss has progressed (AAP 1986a).

The practitioner therefore determines the prognosis and formulates a treatment plan on the basis of two diagnostic criteria: Type of disease and clinical degree of severity.

## Case diagnosis – Single tooth diagnosis

While it is usually possible to diagnose the type of periodontitis (AP, RPP, LJP, PP) for the entire dentition or for the individual patient, it is rather a more difficult matter to precisely define the clinical degree of severity. This situation results from the fact that periodontitis almost always progresses at different rates in different areas of the mouth, on different teeth, and even at different sites on individual teeth. Therefore any statement about "average" disease severity is usually meaningless.

The following pathomorphologic classification (degree of severity) cannot be understood as pertinent to the individual case (patient); it relates more to single tooth diagnosis as well as single tooth prognosis (pp. 128–129).

The reasons for the often quite irregular, localized destruction are not always clear (oral hygiene, localized specific bacteria, niches, function?).

In clinical practice we continue to use the terms mild, moderate and severe to describe the severity of periodontitis, although different authors, "schools," and periodontologic organizations use various synonyms for these different clinical manifestations of disease.

## Classification of clinical severity

- Mild (slight) periodontitis

- Moderate periodontitis

- Severe (advanced) periodontitis

## • Mild (slight) periodontitis

Initial attachment loss of one-quarter to one-third of the root length is observed radiographically. The bone loss picture is primarily horizontal because the bony septa in the coronal region are generally quite narrow, making pronounced vertical bone loss morphologically impossible (p. 77, Fig. 176). The (supra-alveolar) probing depths in the presence of normal gingival contour at about the level of the cementoenamel junction range from 4–5 mm (WHO: CPITN score <5.5 mm).

## • Moderate periodontitis

Attachment loss approaches the mid-point of the root. In addition to horizontal bone resorption, vertical defects are also in evidence (infrabony pockets). Probing depths (supra- or infrabony) of ca. 6–7 mm are observed. In slowly progressing periodontitis (AP), shrinkage (recession) of the gingiva may occur. This leads to shallower probing depths than the amount of attachment loss would anticipate.

Tooth mobility may be elevated. However, teeth with the above-described "moderate" attachment loss are often remarkably solid in their alveoli.

This mid-range degree of severity is not accepted in periodontal diagnosis by some authors.

## • Severe (advanced) periodontitis

Pronounced attachment loss occurs extending beyond the mid-point of the root, often in the form of vertical defects. Probing depths of 8 mm or more, usually infrabony, are the rule (WHO: CPITN score >5.5 mm). In slowly progressive advanced periodontal disease, more significant gingival shrinkage (recession) is usually in evidence (major differences between probing depths and attachment loss; pp. 88–89). Tooth mobility is elevated.

The *general* pathomorphologic classification of periodontitis described above attempts to provide a rough measure of the disease status through clinical examination. Such descriptions provide little information concerning the dynamics or the speed of progression of periodontitis.

For clinical use in determining prognosis and formulating the treatment plan, a thorough understanding of the dynamics of the course of disease is necessary, in addition to a good assessment of the disease severity around individual teeth. In severe cases, precise diagnosis and prognosis for strategically important abutment teeth is critical.

# Pockets and Loss of Attachment

Pocket formation *without* any loss of connective tissue attachment is seen in gingivitis in the form of the *gingival pocket* and the *pseudopocket* (p. 43).

A *true* pocket will exhibit attachment loss, apical migration of the junctional epithelium, and transformation of the junctional epithelium into a pocket epithelium (Müller-Glauser & Schroeder 1982). The *true* periodontal pocket may assume two forms:

– *Suprabony* pockets, resulting from horizontal loss of bone.

– *Infrabony* pockets, resulting from vertical, angular bone loss. In such cases the deepest portion of the pocket is located apical to the alveolar crest.

Whether pocket development is horizontal or vertical appears to be due to the thickness of the interdental septum or the facial and oral bony plates. True loss of attachment results from microbial plaque and the metabolic products of plaque microorganisms. The range and the effective radius of destruction is ca. 1.5–2.5 mm (Tal 1984; Fig. 176).

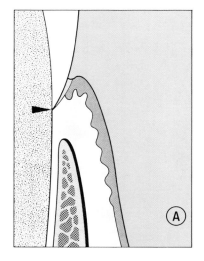
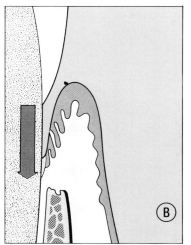
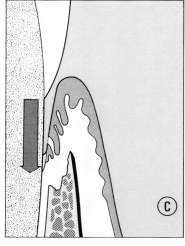

**174  Types of pockets**

**A  Normal sulcus**
Apical termination of the JE is at the cementoenamel junction (arrow; *no* pocket).

**B  Suprabony pocket**
Attachment loss; proliferating pocket epithelium. A remnant of junctional epithelium (pink) persists at the base of the pocket.

**C  Infrabony pocket**
Extends beyond the alveolar crest.

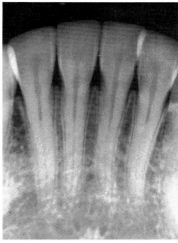
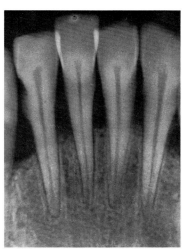
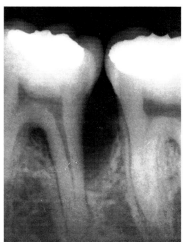

**175  No attachment loss, normal alveolar septa (left)**
Lamina dura remains intact.

**Horizontal bone loss (middle)**
Up to 50% loss of interdental septal bone.

**Vertical bone loss, furcation involvement (right)**
Severe bone loss distal to the first molar. The furcation of this tooth is also involved.

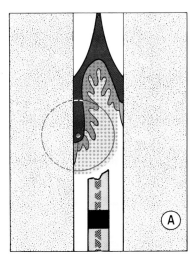
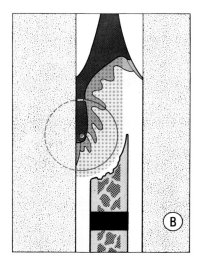
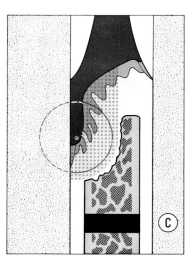

**176  "Range" of destruction = Contour of bone resorption**
The destructive process radiating from the plaque usually measures ca. 1.5–2.5 mm (red circles).
  The expanse (width) of the interdental septa therefore determines for the most part the type (morphology) of bone loss.

**A  Narrow** – Horizontal resorption

**B  Average** – Horizontal resorption, incipient vertical destruction

**C  Wide** – Vertical resorption, bony pocket

# Infrabony Pockets

The infrabony pocket (infra-alveolar vertical bone loss) may exhibit various forms in relation to the affected tooth (Goldman & Cohen 1980). Osseous defects are classified as follows:

– *Three-wall bony pockets* are bordered by one tooth surface and three osseous surfaces.
– *Two-wall bony pockets* (interdental craters) are bordered by two tooth surfaces and two osseous surfaces (one facial and one oral).

– *One-wall bony pockets* are bordered by two tooth surfaces, one osseous surface (facial or oral) and soft tissue.
– *Cup-shaped defects* represent a combined type of pocket, bordered by several surfaces of a tooth and several of bone. The defect surrounds the tooth.

The causes for this wide variation in pocket morphology and resorption of bone are myriad and cannot always be wholly elucidated in each individual case.

**177  Schematic representation of pocket morphology**

A **Three-wall** bony defect

B **Two-wall** bony defect

C **One-wall** bony defect

D **Combined** bony defect, crater-like resorption ("cup")

The walls of each pocket are shown in red.

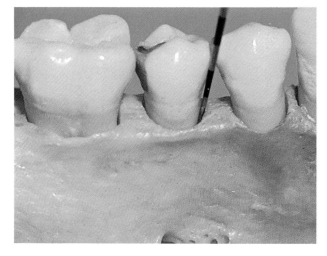

**178  Small 3-wall defect**
Early pocket formation on the mesial aspect of the second premolar. The color-coded probe (CP 12) measures a depth of ca. 3 mm. If gingiva were present, the total probing depth would be ca. 5 mm.

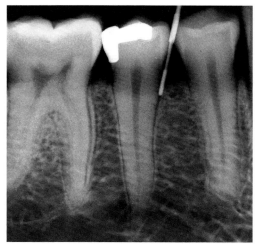

**179  Deep 3-wall bony pocket**
The periodontal probe descends almost 6 mm (measured from the alveolar crest) to the base of this 3-wall defect.

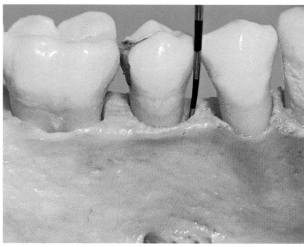

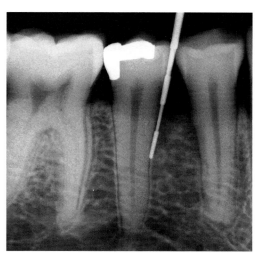

Mention was already made of the significance of bone thickness (p. 77). Since the bony septa between the roots become thinner coronally, the initial stage of periodontitis generally presents as horizontal resorption. The greater the distance between the roots of two teeth, the thicker will be the intervening septum, permitting the development of a vertical defect. In addition to such simple osseous morphology, other factors almost certainly play some role in the type of resorption:

- Local acute exacerbation elicited by specific bacteria in the pocket
- Local inadequate oral hygiene
- Crowding and tipping of teeth (plaque-retentive areas)
- Tooth morphology (root irregularities, furcations)
- Improper loading due to functional disturbances (?).

The morphology of the bony pocket is of importance in both prognosis and treatment planning. The amount of bone remaining will effect the chances of osseous regeneration after treatment.

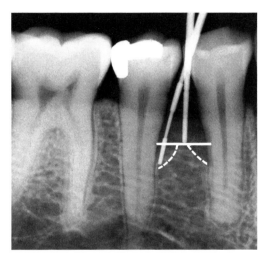
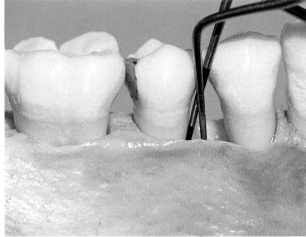

**180   2-wall bony pocket, interdental crater**
The coronal portion of this defect is bordered by only two bony walls (and two tooth surfaces). In the apical areas the 2-wall defect actually becomes *two* 3-wall defects (see probe tip left of interdental septum in radiograph, left).

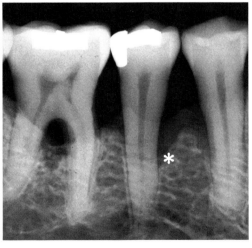
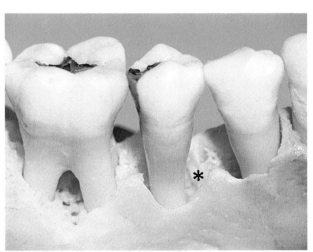

**181   One-wall bony pocket on the mesial of tooth 45**
Advanced bone loss in premolar/molar area. On tooth 45 the facial wall of bone is reduced almost to the level of the depth of the mesial pocket (∗). A portion of the lingual plate of bone (one wall) remains intact.
    The facial root surface and the interdental spaces could be covered with soft tissue to the cementoenamel junction, masking the defect clinically.

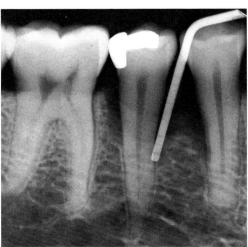
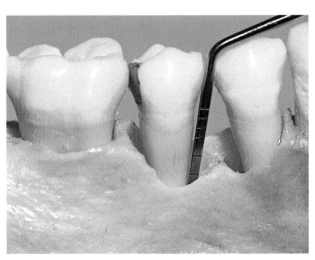

**182   Combined pocket, cup-shaped defect**
In the region of tooth 45, the apical portion of the osseous defect courses around the tooth, creating a "moat" or "cup" (Goldman probe *in situ*). The bony pocket is therefore bordered by several osseous and several tooth surface walls.

# Furcation Involvement

Periodontal bone loss in multirooted teeth presents a special problem when bi- or trifurcations are involved. Partially or completely open furcations tend to accumulate plaque (Schroeder & Scherle 1987). Exacerbations, abscesses, progressive loss of attachment and rapid deepening of periodontal pockets occur frequently, especially with through-and-through furcation involvement. In addition, open furcations are particularly susceptible to the development of dental caries.

Hamp et al. (1975) presented three degrees of furcation involvement, measuring horizontally.

In this *Atlas,* furcation involvement will be referred to according to *horizontal* measurements (cf. p. 118):

Class F 1: The furcation can be probed to a depth of 3 mm with the periodontal probe (F1).
Class F 2: The furcation can be probed to a depth of more than 3 mm, but is not through-and-through (F2).
Class F 3: The furcation is through-and-through and can be probed completely (F3).

**183 Classification of furcation involvement – Horizontal measurement**

**A F0:** Pocket at the mesial root, but without furcation involvement.
**B F1:** Furcation can be probed 3 mm in horizontal direction.
**C F2:** Furcation can be probed deeper than 3 mm.
**D F3:** Through-and-through furcation involvement.

Furcation involvement often occurs in conjunction with an infrabony defect.

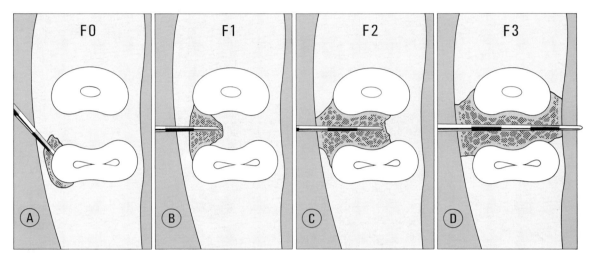

**184 No furcation involvement – Class F 0**
A ca. 5 mm deep suprabony pocket in the area of the buccal furcation.

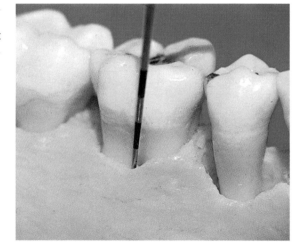
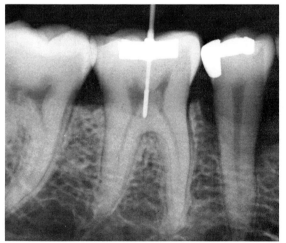

**185 Furcation involvement – Class F 1**
Using a curved, pointed explorer (CH 3) the buccal furcation can be probed to a depth of less than 3 mm. Probing is performed from both buccal and lingual aspects during clinical examination.

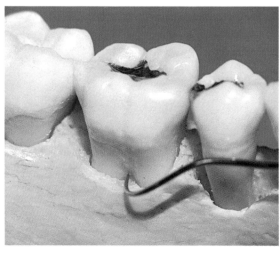
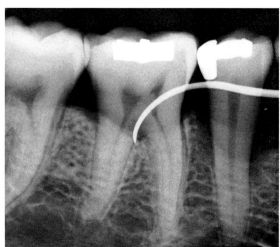

This classification of furcation involvement is applicable both in the mandible and in the maxilla, where it can rarely be diagnosed radiographically. In order to ascertain furcation involvement in the maxillary molars, probing must be performed from the buccal, distobuccal/palatal and mesiopalatal aspects.

*Vertical bone loss* in a furcation can also be classified (Subclasses A–C, Tarnow & Fletcher 1984); it is ascertained in mm from the roof of the furcation:

Subclass A: 1–3 mm
Subclass B: 4–6 mm
Subclass C: 7 + mm

*Therapy:* Class F1 and F2 furcation involvement may be successfully treated by root planing alone or by flap procedures (pp. 198–199).

Class F3 furcations are usually treated by means of hemisection or by resection of one root (pp. 265–272).

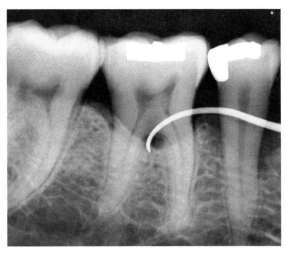
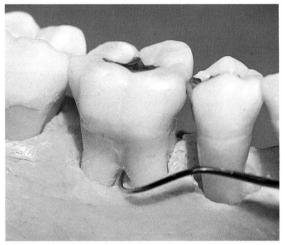

**186 Furcation involvement – Class F2**
The explorer can probe more than 3 mm into a furcation, which is not yet through-and-through.

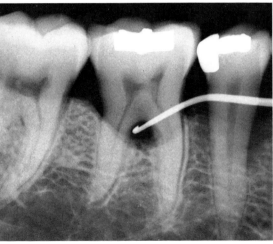
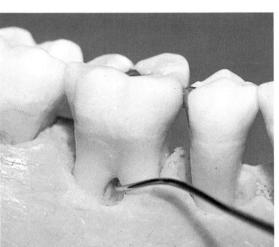

**187 Furcation involvement – Class F3, mild Subclass A**
Narrow, through-and-through bifurcation involvement in the face of relatively minor bone loss (blunt Nabers –2 explorer).

Less than 3 mm of bone loss in the vertical dimension; this corresponds to Subclass A.

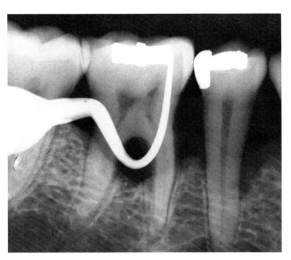
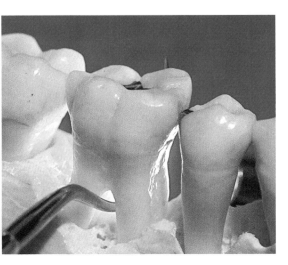

**188 Furcation involvement – Class F3, severe Subclass C**
Wide through-and-through bifurcation involvement in a case exhibiting severe horizontal and vertical bone loss (cowhorn explorer).

The vertical extent of the furcation exceeds 6 mm: Subclass C.

# Histopathology

The primary symptoms of periodontitis are attachment loss and pocket formation. *Pocket epithelium* has the following features (modified from Müller-Glauser & Schroeder 1982):

1. Irregular boundary with the subjacent connective tissue, exhibiting rete pegs; towards the periodontal pocket, epithelium is often very thin and partially ulcerated.
2. In the apicalmost region, the pocket epithelium becomes a very narrow junctional epithelium.
3. Transmigration of PMNs through the pocket epithelium.
4. Defective basal lamina complex on the connective tissue aspect.

Collagen is lost and inflammatory cells invade the subepithelial connective tissue compartment. In acute stages, pus formation and microabscesses occur. Bone is resorbed, and deeper osseous marrow is transformed into fibrous connective tissue.

**189 Suprabony pocket (left)**
Pocket epithelium with distinct rete ridges. In the apicalmost region (between the arrows) one observes intact junctional epithelium (exhibiting artifactual separation from tooth surface in this section). Subepithelial infiltrate extends into the area of the transseptal fibers (H & E, x 40).

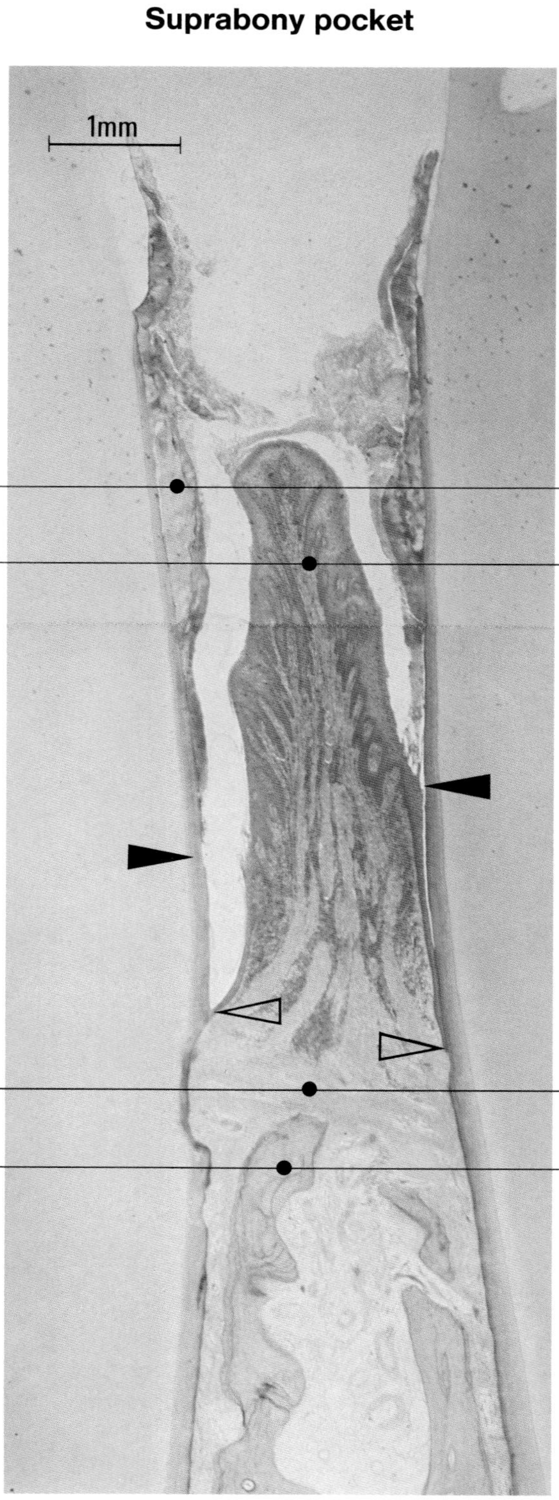

Plaque, calculus

Interdental papilla, col

Transseptal fibers

Alveolar bone

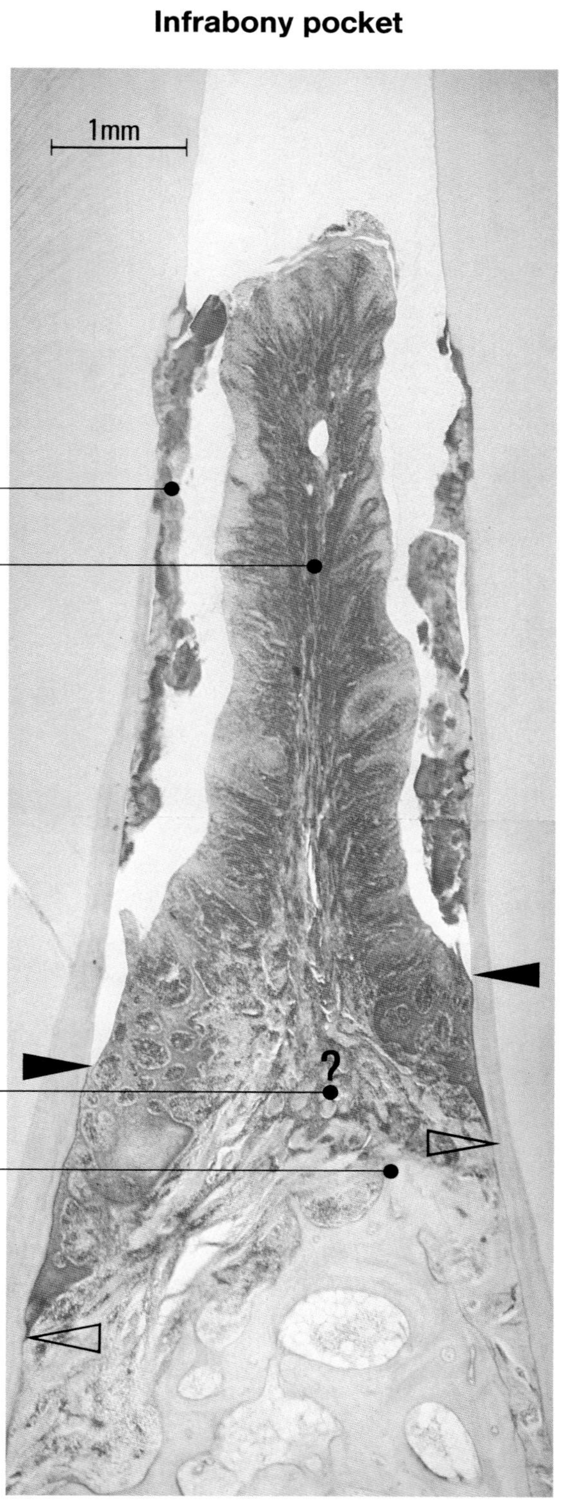

**190 Infrabony pocket (right)**
Intact junctional epithelium (open arrow) persists on the tooth (left), apical to the interdental bony septum. The pocket epithelium displays pronounced rete ridges and areas of ulceration. Inflammatory infiltrate extends into the periodontal ligament and marrow areas (H & E, x 40).

**Suprabony pocket**

**Infrabony pocket**

1mm

1mm

# Clinical and Radiographic Symptoms

The three *obligate symptoms* of periodontitis have been defined:

| | |
|---|---|
| 1 | **Inflammation (gingivitis)** |
| 2 | **True periodontal pockets** |
| 3 | **Bone resorption** |

(Attachment loss)

These primary symptoms can occur in varying degrees of severity and in different forms.

*Further symptoms,* listed below, can modifiy or complicate periodontal disease, but they may not be present in *every* case of periodontitis:

- Gingival swelling
- Pocket activity: bleeding, exudate, pus
- Pocket abscess, furcation abscess
- Fistula
- Gingival shrinkage (recession)
- Tooth migration, tipping, extrusion
- Tooth mobility
- Tooth loss

## Gingival swelling

Enlargement of the gingiva is a symptom of gingivitis that may remain if progression to periodontitis occurs.

If the gingiva is edematous or hyperplastically enlarged beyond the cementoenamel junction, attachment loss and pocket depth will be overestimated by the degree of swelling.

## Pocket activity

The *activity* of a pocket and the frequency of active episodes are of more importance than absolute pocket depth, especially with regard to treatment planning and prognosis. Bleeding on probing, presence of exudate, and suppuration after application of finger pressure are all signs that an active phase of periodontitis is in progress (Davenport et al. 1982). Such signs are especially frequent in cases of rapidly progressing periodontitis in young adults (RPP).

## Pocket and furcation abscesses

An additional symptom of active periodontitis is the pocket or furcation abscess. This develops during an acute exacerbation if necrotic tissue cannot be either resorbed or expelled ( for example, due to closure of the coronal gingiva above deep pockets, furcations and retentive areas). An abscess may also be the consequence of injury, for example biting upon hard, sharp foodstuffs, improper oral hygiene efforts (a broken toothpick), or iatrogenic trauma. In rare instances a periodontal abscess can develop into a submucosal abscess (parulis).

An abscess is one of the few manifestations of periodontitis that may elicit *pain.* If an abscess is expansive, extending to the apical region, the tooth may become sensitive to percussion. A painful abscess must be drained on an emergency basis, either by way of the pocket orifice itself or via incision through the lateral wall. An abscess may release spontaneously through a fistulous tract or at the gingival margin.

## Fistula

A *fistula* may be the result of spontaneous opening of an abscess if the gingival margin is sealed. If the underlying cause (active pocket) is not eliminated, the fistula may persist for an extended period of time without any pain. The orifice of a fistula is not always located directly above the acute process, and this can lead to improper diagnosis of the location of an abscess (probe the fistulous tract with a blunt probe!). Pulpal vitality of the tooth in question, and its neighbors, must also be checked, to ascertain possible endodontic complications.

## Gingival shrinkage (recession)

During the course of periodontal inflammation, especially the slowly progressive type (AP) gingival *shrinkage* may occur with time. Gingival shrinkage can also occur after spontaneous transition of an acute exacerbation into a chronic, quiescent stage, or following comprehensive periodontal therapy, or after drainage of abscesses. Whatever the cause, shrinkage leads to exposure of root surfaces. This type of gingival shrinkage should not be confused with true gingival *recession,* which can occur in the *absence* of clinical inflammation. True recession occurs without the formation of periodontal pockets and is most often observed on the facial aspect of roots. On the other hand, gingival shrinkage due to periodontitis may also be quite pronounced in the papillary regions.

If, as a result of shrinkage, the gingival margin is located apical to the cementoenamel junction, clinical probing of any pockets will underestimate the actual loss of attachment. True *attachment loss* must be measured from the cementoenamel junction to the base of the pocket.

## Tooth migration, tipping, extrusion

In advanced periodontitis additional clinical symptoms including migration and tipping of individual teeth or groups of teeth can occur. The result of such tooth movements is the creation of diastemata, which can be an esthetic problem, depending upon the expanse and location. There are many factors that could be responsible for tooth migration and it is not possible in every case to determine the specific cause. It is nevertheless clear that a compromised tooth-supporting apparatus is a prerequisite for tooth migration, tipping etc. Numerous other cofactors may also play a role: missing antago-

nists, functional occlusal disturbances, oral parafunctions (lip biting, tongue thrust etc.).

There has been speculation that a tooth exhibiting a deep pocket on one side and essentially intact periodontal fiber structure on the other side may migrate not so much as a result of pressure exerted by granulation tissue in the pocket, as by forces deriving from the still intact collagenous supracrestal fiber bundles in the healthy tissues. The fact that migrated teeth usually exhibit their unilateral pocket on the side opposite the direction of wandering would appear to support this hypothesis.

**191 Active pocket, suppuration (left)**
Pus exudes from a pocket on tooth 11 after finger pressure is applied.

**192 Pocket measurement: Probing depth = attachment loss (right)**
The measurement (8 mm) is made from the gingival margin, which in this case is still in its normal position at the cementoenamel junction (CEJ).

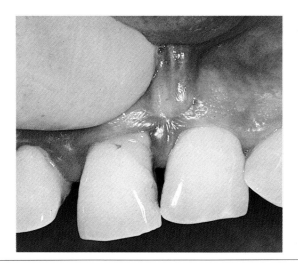
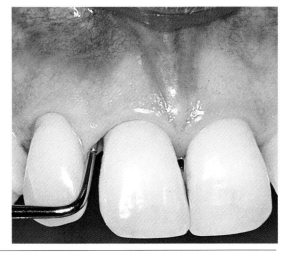

**193 Pocket measurement: Probing depth overestimates attachment loss (left)**
The measurement (7 mm) is made from the gingival margin, but the hyperplastic gingivae extend beyond the CEJ, creating a pseudopocket. The true attachment loss is 3 mm less than the probing depth.

**194 Pocket measurement: Probing depth underestimates attachment loss (right)**
The measurement (7 mm) is made from the gingival margin, but the true attachment loss is 10 mm.

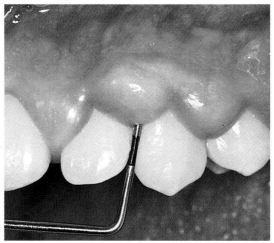
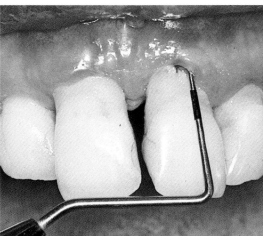

**195 Periodontal abscess**
Originating from a 12 mm pocket on the mesial aspect of the tipped, vital 47, an abscess has developed. The clinical view reveals an abscess just about to open spontaneously, directly through the attached gingiva; this is a somewhat atypical location for a fistula.

*Right:* The radiograph reveals a severe vertical bony defect on the mesial of 47.

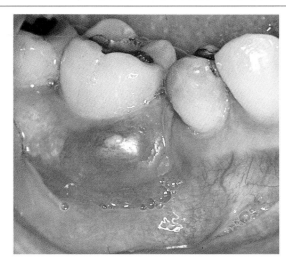
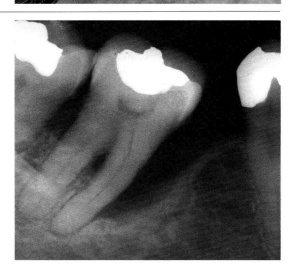

## Tooth mobility

Pathologically *increasing* tooth mobility is a symptom of severe, advanced periodontitis. This symptom must, however, be interpreted carefully because it can be influenced by numerous factors. Even in a healthy periodontium the teeth exhibit physiologic differences in mobility depending on number of roots, root morphology and root length (p. 326). Occlusal trauma can lead to increased tooth mobility even when the periodontal supporting structures are intact (pp. 330–331).

In cases of periodontitis, it is the quantitative loss of bone that is the primary determinant of tooth mobility, but superimposed occlusal trauma can increase tooth mobility still further. In such cases the combination of quantitative loss of tooth-supporting apparatus due to periodontitis, coupled with occlusal trauma, can lead to a continuously *increasing* (progressive) tooth mobility, which is very unfavorable in terms of single tooth prognosis.

## Tooth loss

The final "symptom" of periodontitis, the one which ultimately stops the disease process, is tooth loss. It seldom occurs spontaneously because extremely mobile teeth that are no longer functional are usually extracted prior to spontaneous exfoliation.

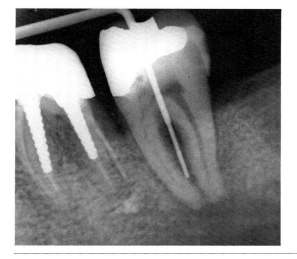

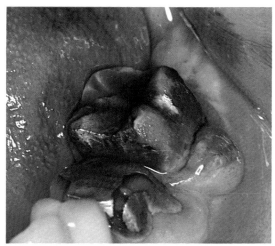

**196　Furcation abscess**
Originating from a deep (11 mm) pocket buccal to 37, an abscess has developed adjacent to the open furcation (Class F3).

*Left:* The radiograph depicts the probe (CP 12) in situ. The probe is inserted until intact bone is encountered; the inflamed soft tissue at the base of the pocket is easily traversed by the probe tip.

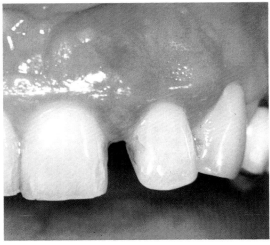

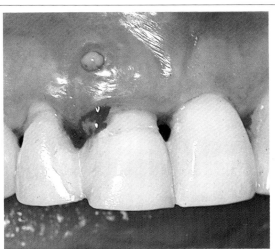

**197　Tooth migration (left)**
Creation of a diastema between teeth 21 and 22. The osseous septum between these teeth has been destroyed to the root apices. Granulation tissue, tension from intact periodontal fibers and oral parafunctions (e.g., tongue thrust) could have elicited the migration.

**198　Periodontal fistula (right)**
13 mm pocket on the distal of tooth 11, which is a candidate for extraction. After probing, pus escapes from both the fistulous tract and the gingival margin.

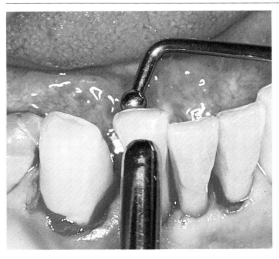

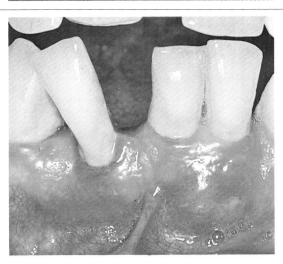

**199　Tooth mobility (left)**
Increased tooth mobility can be caused by functional disturbances and/or by periodontal attachment loss. Mobility is measured clinically by using two instruments or one instrument and the finger tip (p. 121).

**200　Tooth migration and tipping (right)**
Creation of a diastema by severe tipping of tooth 41 after loss of 42. Patient exhibits a heavy tongue thrust when swallowing.

## Adult Periodontitis (AP) – Mild to Moderate

This 51-year-old male had received restorative dental care at irregular intervals. The dentist had never performed any periodontal diagnostic procedures, nor any therapy. The patient himself complained of occasional gingival bleeding and calculus that disturbed him. He was unaware of any periodontal disease and felt he was completely functional in mastication.

*Findings:* See charting and radiographic survey (p. 87).
*Diagnosis:* Slowly progressing, mild to moderate adult periodontitis (AP).

*Therapy:* Motivation, oral hygiene instruction and follow-up initial therapy. After *re-evaluation,* modified Widman procedure at several sites. No systemic therapy. Possible bridges in mandibular posterior areas.
*Recall:* Every 4–6 months.
*Prognosis:* Even if the patient's cooperation is only average, the prognosis is good. In cases such as this, the dentist or periodontist is always "very successful."

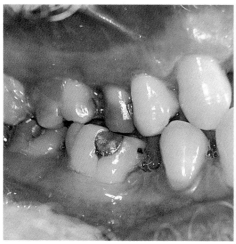 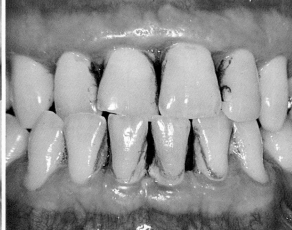 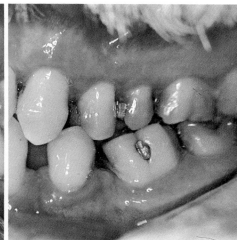

**201   Clinical picture (above)**
A cursory inspection reveals only mild gingivitis. The interdental papillae have shrunk. The mandibular first molars were extracted 30 years ago, with resultant slow tooth migration, tipping and the formation of diastemata. Recently the migration seems to have stabilized. Occlusion is far from ideal.

**202   Plaque disclosure, oral hygiene (right)**
The labial surfaces exhibit almost no plaque accumulation while the interproximal areas are filled with plaque and calculus.

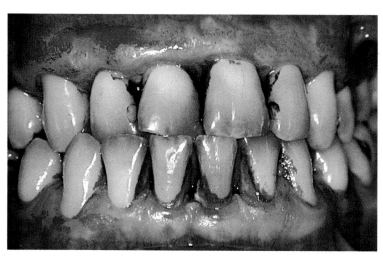

**203   Mandible during the flap procedure**
The facial crest of bone is somewhat bulbous but shows no signs of active destruction. Interdental 3 mm craters were detected. Treatment consisted solely of root planing, minor recontouring of the bulbous bony margin (osteoplasty) and repositioning of the flaps at the original location (no apical repositioning).

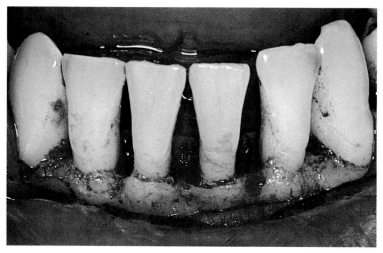

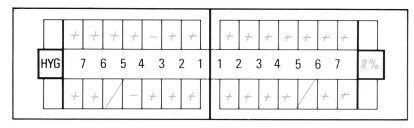

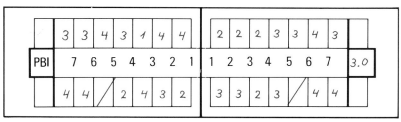

### 204 Hygiene Index (HYG) and Papilla Bleeding Index (PBI)

**HYG:** Oral hygiene is poor (8%). Almost all interdental spaces examined exhibit plaque.

**PBI:** All papillae bleed during performance of the PBI. The index is, indeed, very high (3.0).
These indices (HYG and PBI) were performed in the first and third quadrants only from the *oral* aspect, and in the second and forth quadrants from the *facial* (cf. pp. 36–37 and p. 126, Fig. 319).

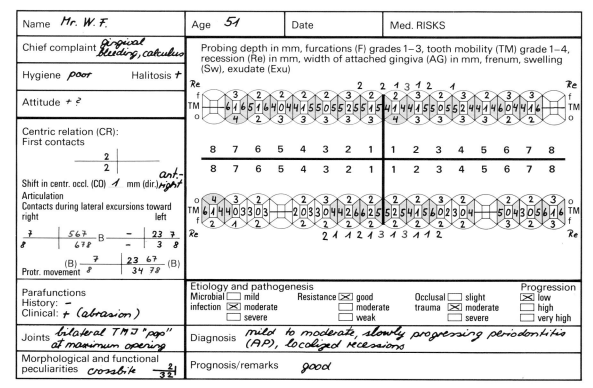

| Name Mr. W. F. | Age 51 | Date | Med. RISKS |
|---|---|---|---|

Chief complaint *gingival bleeding, calculus*

Hygiene *poor*    Halitosis +

Attitude + ?

Centric relation (CR):
First contacts
$\dfrac{2}{2}$

Shift in centr. occl. (CO) *1* mm (dir.) *ant.-right*

Articulation
Contacts during lateral excursions toward
right                                left

$\dfrac{7}{8}$ | $\dfrac{567}{678}$ B — $\dfrac{23\ 7}{3\ 8}$

(B) $\dfrac{7}{8}$ | $\dfrac{23\ 67}{34\ 78}$ (B)
Protr. movement

Parafunctions
History: –
Clinical: + (abrasion)

Joints *bilateral TMJ "pop" at maximum opening*

Morphological and functional peculiarities *crossbite* $\dfrac{2|}{3\,2|}$

Probing depth in mm, furcations (F) grades 1–3, tooth mobility (TM) grade 1–4, recession (Re) in mm, width of attached gingiva (AG) in mm, frenum, swelling (Sw), exudate (Exu)

Etiology and pathogenesis

| Microbial infection | ☐ mild ☒ moderate ☐ severe | Resistance ☒ good ☐ moderate ☐ weak | Occlusal trauma ☐ slight ☒ moderate ☐ severe | Progression ☒ low ☐ high ☐ very high |

Diagnosis *mild to moderate, slowly progressing periodontitis (AP), localized recessions*

Prognosis/remarks *good*

### 205 Periodontal charting – I

This periodontal chart (p. 126), which is used in many dental offices, has convenient places for recording probing depths, recession, furcation involvement and tooth mobility using numerical scores.

"Mr. W. F." exhibited uniform probing depths throughout, especially in the interdental areas. For an assessment of the true attachment loss, the mm measurements entered by "Re" (recession) must be considered; these indicate the amount of gingival shrinkage.

Tooth mobility (TM) is low (grade 0–2). Functional analysis reveals premature contact between the upper and lower right lateral incisors (crossbite, increased mobility). Disturbances in lateral excursion as well as in protrusion are also noted.

Complete information concerning the periodontal chart I and its use is presented on page 126 (Fig. 320).

### 206 Radiographic survey

The radiographs confirm the clinical observations: Localized, mild to moderate horizontal bone loss. Some of the restorative work is inadequate.

Most important is that the "strategically" important canines and molars will be easy to restore (no furcation involvement).

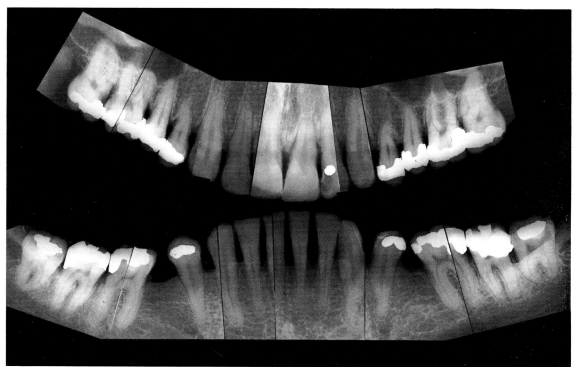

(*Note:* This is not a "panorama radiograph" in the usual sense of the term. Rather, this survey was prepared by cutting and fitting individual periapical radiographs into a unified whole. This practice provides a more detailed overview of each individual segment of the dentition than any available panoramic film.)

# Adult Periodontitis (AP) – Severe

This 61-year-old male patient "scrubbed" the maxillary anterior teeth using a horizontal motion. He had never received any oral hygiene instruction or demonstration; all other areas of the dentition were neglected. At his irregular visits to the dentist, only restorative procedures had been performed.

*Findings:* See chart and radiographic survey (p. 89).
*Diagnosis:* Moderate to severe adult periodontitis (AP). Gingival shrinkage in the maxillary anterior area.

*Therapy:*
1) *Immediate:* Extraction of 18, 17; 28; 46; root of 41 (the crown will be used as a temporary pontic by attaching it to adjacent teeth.
2) *Definitive:* Motivation, modification of oral hygiene technique, extraction of 26; 31. Definitive debridement and possible surgical procedures. Cast framework partial dentures.
*Recall:* Every 4–6 months.
*Prognosis:* For the teeth to be maintained and treated periodontally, the prognosis is good.

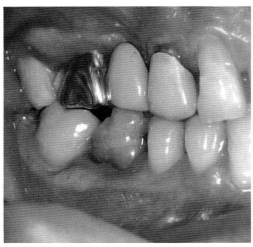 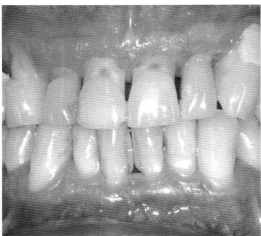 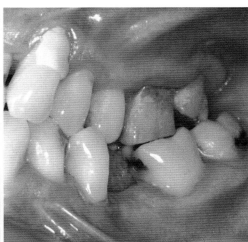

**207   Clinical picture (above)**
Noticeable in the maxillary anterior region are the severe gingival shrinkage and the wedge-shaped defects (hard-bristle toothbrush, abrasive dentifrice). Periodontal pockets in this region were "brushed away" by the patient!

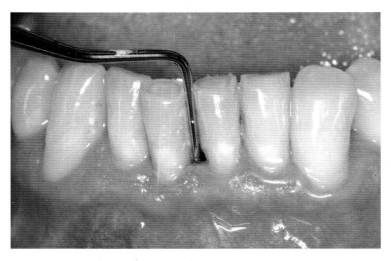

**208   Mandibular anterior probing depths (right)**
Probing of a 9 mm pocket on the mesial aspect of 41 provoked only slight bleeding. The cervical areas of the mandibular anterior teeth also exhibit massive abrasion due to improper toothbrushing.

**209   Retained root (41)**
Tooth 41 was no longer functional and had to be extracted. Its root, which had virtually no bony support remaining, was amputated and the natural crown was used as a temporary pontic by means of acid etched bonding to the adjacent teeth.

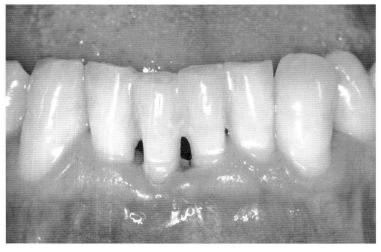

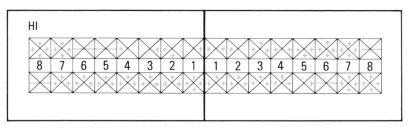

HI

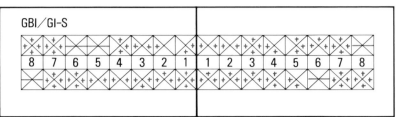

GBI/GI-S

**210  Hygiene Index (HI) and Gingival Bleeding Index (GBI)**

**HI:** Plaque is present on almost all tooth surfaces with the exception of the maxillary anterior and some facial surfaces in the mandibular anterior region (HI only 30.5%).

**GBI:** 74% of the pockets examined bled after gentle probing.

All teeth present were probed at all four surfaces (mesial, distal, facial, and oral; cf. pp. 36, 37 and p. 127, Fig. 321).

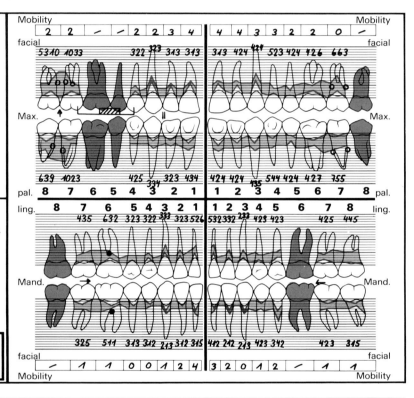

### Periodontal status

Name  Mr. M.D., age 61
Date

**Symbols for charting**
1. missing                         /
2. food impaction            ↑
3. open contact               ‖
4. mobility          0, 1, 2, 3, 4
5. bridge                        ▨
6. drifted/extrusion      D→I
7. beg. furcation exposure  ○
8. bifurcation exposed    ●
9. periapical area           ℺

### Etiology
non-specific bacterial infection

### Diagnosis
moderate to severe adult periodontitis (AP)

### Prognosis
fair to good on the teeth to be retained

**Systemic diseases?**
none

**211  Periodontal charting – II**
Using this modified "Michigan Chart" (p. 127), gingival contour, probing depths and attachment loss are represented visually.

Probing depths around each tooth are measured first from the facial aspect at mesial, mid-buccal and distal sites, then from the lingual aspect at three similar sites.

Because of the pronounced gingival shrinkage, the pockets in the anterior area are not very deep despite great attachment loss. All anterior teeth are highly mobile.

Complete information concerning the periodontal chart II and its use is presented on page 127 (Fig. 322).

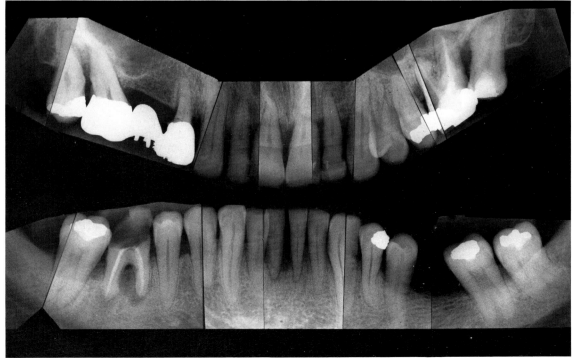

**212  Radiographic survey**
The radiographs reveal a very typical, irregular distribution of bone resorption; this is commonly observed in older patients with AP. While some teeth and/or some tooth surfaces have already lost all attachment, hardly any bone resorption is observed on the mandibular canines and the premolars. At tooth 46, the apical and periodontal lesions appear to communicate.

# Rapidly Progressive Periodontitis (RPP)

This 26-year-old female was referred from a general practitioner. Her chief complaint was mild pain and suppuration around teeth 35 and 36. From radiographs taken 3 and 6 years earlier the diagnosis of rapidly progressive periodontitis was readily made, and the severe migration of teeth 18 and 17 following extraction of 16 was obvious.

*Findings:* See charting and radiographs (p. 91).
*Diagnosis:* Rapidly progressive, moderate to severe periodontitis (RPP).

*Therapy:* Motivation and oral hygiene instruction. Initial therapy supported by systemic administration of metronidazole. Following *re-evaluation* additional therapy including flap surgery and extractions (retained third molars).
*Recall:* Absolutely every 2–4 months!
*Prognosis:* Questionable in the maxilla (RPP!); these teeth can only be maintained over the long term by frequent recall visits and excellent cooperation by the patient in home care. The prognosis in the mandible is somewhat better.

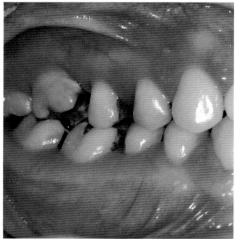 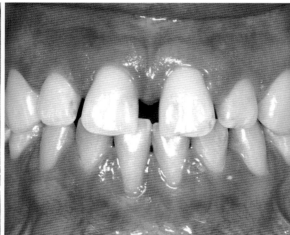 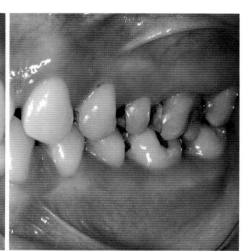

**213 Clinical picture (above)**
Erythematous gingiva with some edematous areas. These rather mild indications of inflammation belie the advanced stage of periodontitis: A typical RPP circumstance. Supragingival plaque accumulation on the facial surfaces appears slight.
The diastemata in the maxillary anterior region had become more pronounced in recent years.

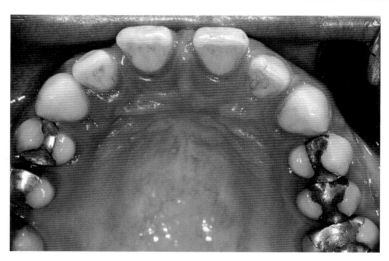

**214 Palatal view (right)**
Marginal inflammation; diastema formation anteriorly; defective amalgam restorations.

**215 Maxillary anterior probing depths**
An active pocket, 7–8 mm, is detected on the mesial aspect of tooth 11. A cursory inspection would likely not detect the extent of periodontal destruction.

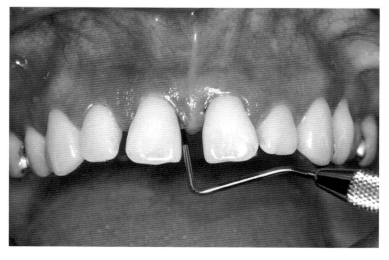

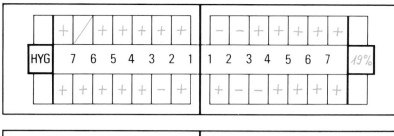

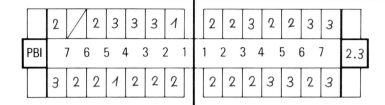

| HYG | 7 | 6 | 5 | 4 | 3 | 2 | 1 | 1 | 2 | 3 | 4 | 5 | 6 | 7 | |
|---|---|---|---|---|---|---|---|---|---|---|---|---|---|---|---|

*(HYG chart values: top row + / + + + + + / − − + + + + +; bottom row + + + + + − + / + − − + + + +)* 19%

| PBI | 7 | 6 | 5 | 4 | 3 | 2 | 1 | 1 | 2 | 3 | 4 | 5 | 6 | 7 | 2.3 |
|---|---|---|---|---|---|---|---|---|---|---|---|---|---|---|---|

*(PBI chart top row: 2 / 2 3 3 3 1 | 2 2 3 2 2 3 3; bottom row: 3 2 2 1 2 2 2 | 2 2 2 3 3 2 3)*

### 216 Hygiene Index (HYG) and Papilla Bleeding Index (PBI)

**HYG:** Although plaque accumulation appears minimal in the clinical picture (Fig. 213), after use of a disclosing agent, the HYG index reveals poor oral hygiene (19%).

**PBI:** More or less severe bleeding occurs at all papillary sites during recording of the PBI. The result is a high average bleeding value of 2.3.

---

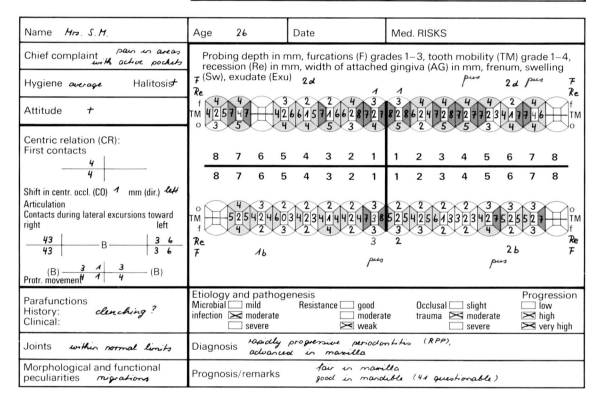

| Name | Mrs. S.M. | Age | 26 | Date | | Med. RISKS | |
|---|---|---|---|---|---|---|---|

**Chief complaint** pain in areas with active pockets

**Hygiene** average  **Halitosis** +

**Attitude** +

**Centric relation (CR):** First contacts  4 / 4

**Shift in centr. occl. (CO)** 1 mm (dir.) left

**Articulation**
Contacts during lateral excursions toward
right — B — left
43 / 43 | 3 6 / 3 6
(B) 3 1 / 3 (B)
Protr. movement 1 / 4

**Parafunctions** History: clenching? Clinical:

**Joints** within normal limits

**Morphological and functional peculiarities** migrations

Probing depth in mm, furcations (F) grades 1–3, tooth mobility (TM) grade 1–4, recession (Re) in mm, width of attached gingiva (AG) in mm, frenum, swelling (Sw), exudate (Exu)

**Etiology and pathogenesis**

| | | | | | Progression |
|---|---|---|---|---|---|
| Microbial infection | ☐ mild ☒ moderate ☐ severe | Resistance | ☐ good ☐ moderate ☒ weak | Occlusal trauma | ☐ slight ☒ moderate ☐ severe | ☐ low ☒ high ☒ very high |

**Diagnosis** rapidly progressive periodontitis (RPP), advanced in maxilla

**Prognosis/remarks** fair in maxilla, good in mandible (41 questionable)

### 217 Periodontal charting – I

Only one tooth (34) has a probing depth of less than 4 mm. Pockets between 4 and 8 mm are present on all other teeth. The attachment loss (AL) is especially advanced in the maxilla. Some of the deep pockets exhibit clear symptoms of activity.

Gingival recession is slight, except for tooth 41.

The degree of tooth mobility is consistent with the pattern of attachment loss. Except for a slight premature contact in centric relation, there exist no significant occlusal functional disturbances. To what extent the diastemata in the anterior area have been enhanced by clenching, possibly also by the tongue thrust habit cannot be determined with certainty.

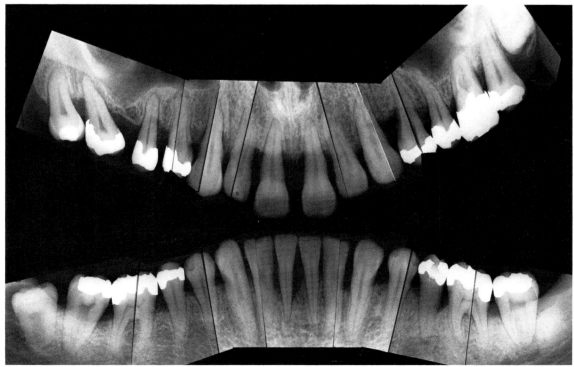

### 218 Radiographic survey

The pronounced bone loss is also evident in the radiographs, especially in the maxilla. Also obvious is the dramatic tipping of teeth 18 and 17 following extraction of the first permanent molar some six years previously.

# Rapidly Progressive Periodontitis (RPP) – Initial Findings ...

This female patient was only 22 years old. She complained of loosening of the maxillary central incisors and the space between teeth 11 and 12. She stated that gingival bleeding occurred from time to time during toothbrushing.

*Findings:*

HYG: 12%      PBI: 3.4

Probing depths, recession and tooth mobility, see Figure 220.

*Diagnosis:* Mild to moderate, localized severe, rapidly progressive periodontitis (RPP).

*Therapy:* Motivation and oral hygiene instruction. Definitive debridement. Following re-evaluation, periodontal surgery in all segments; modified Widman approach throughout, with full flap reflection in the maxillary anterior area. Extraction 38 and 48.

*Recall:* Never accomplished because patient moved.

*Prognosis:* With regular and short-interval professional *recall* and excellent patient cooperation in home care, the prognosis would have been good.

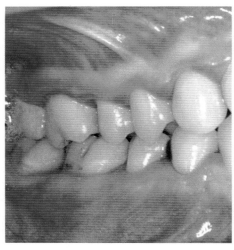 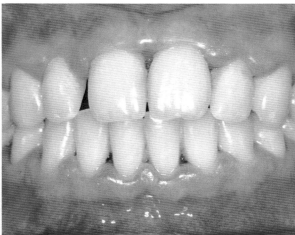 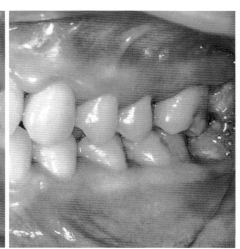

**219  Clinical picture (above)**
The gingivae exhibit shrinkage in the papillary regions, some hyperplastic areas and generalized inflammation.

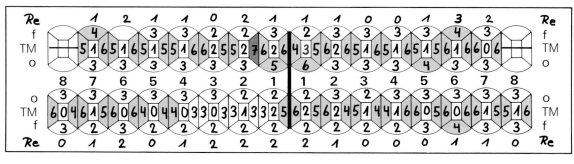

**220  Probing depths, gingival recession (Re) and tooth mobility (TM; right)**
Recession is minimal. Probing depths correspond well with attachment loss. Several teeth exhibit symptoms of pocket activity during probing.

**221  Radiographic survey**
Pronounced, irregular attachment loss is clearly visible in the maxilla, especially in the anterior segment.

In contrast, loss of tooth-supporting bone has been more regular in the mandible.

The relatively short roots on teeth 15 and 25 may be the result of previous orthodontic treatment.

Several carious lesions are evident.

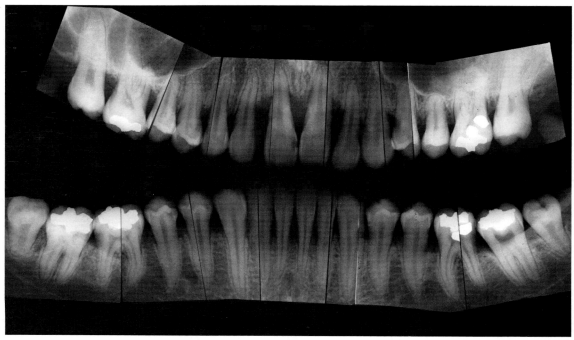

## ... and Findings 5½ Years Later

The indicated therapy (p. 92) led to an immediate improvement: Probing depths were reduced (shrinkage), pockets no longer exhibited symptoms of activity. The PBI was reduced to ca. 0.9, oral hygiene remained average (HYG: 60%). The diastema between teeth 11 and 12 began to close spontaneously.

After completion of the treatment, the patient left the country to spend time in an area with poor availability of dental care. She returned to our clinic only twice in the subsequent 5½-year period, during visits in her homeland. At both of these visits recurrence of periodontal pockets was evident; these were treated on an emergency basis by scaling and root planing, and on one occasion with systemic medication (metronidazole).

These attempts at treating the recurrence, in the face of virtual absence of maintenance therapy (recall) could *not* halt disease progression. The Hygiene Index (46%) and the PBI (2.1) had again fallen to unfavorable levels. The attachment loss continued on all teeth. A revised treatment plan including the unavoidable extractions and prosthetic therapy became necessary.

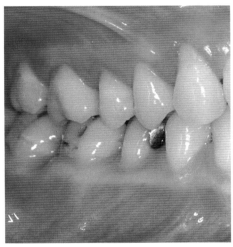
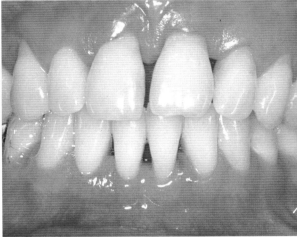
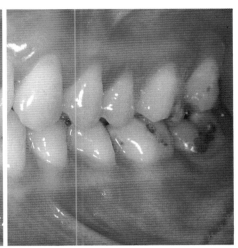

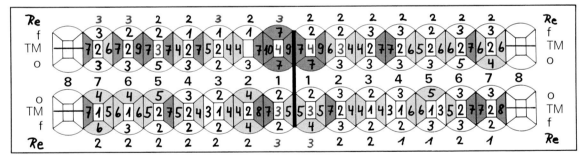

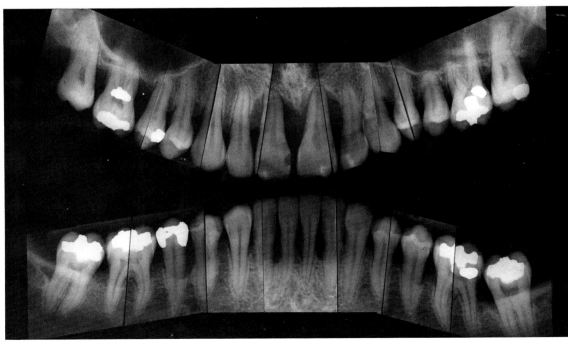

**222 Clinical picture after 5½ years (above)**
All teeth exhibit gingival shrinkage (previous periodontal treatment!). Recurrence of gingivitis and periodontitis with some active pockets.

**223 Probing depths, gingival recession (Re) and tooth mobility (TM; left)**
Despite the shrinkage of the gingival tissues, the pockets are considerably deeper than at the previous examination; the attachment loss is massive. Teeth 11 an 21 exhibit mobility of grade 4.

**224 Radiographic survey**
In comparison to the initial examination, the bone resorption is significantly more advanced in all segments of the dentition. Note especially the disease progression on teeth 15, 11; 21, 24, between 37 and 36, in the mandibular anterior segment and at tooth 45.

Teeth 11 and 21 exhibit virtually no bone support.

The comprehensive treatment plan must now include, in addition to repeated periodontitis therapy, extractions and prosthetic treatment (bridges or cast framework partial dentures).

# Juvenile Periodontitis (LJP) – Initial Stage

This 15-year-old female was referred from her private dentist because of "suddenly occurring" periodontal defects on all first permanent molars. Bitewing radiographs had been made periodically to check for dental caries, and gingival findings noted. Thus the localized osseous defects were not "accidental findings."

*Findings:* See charting and radiographs (p. 95).
*Diagnosis:* Incipient LJP. Typical involvement of first molars, with as yet no pocket formation around incisors.

*Therapy:* Improvement of interdental hygiene, especially in the molar areas. After initial therapy, modified Widman procedures with intensive root planing (direct vision!) on all involved molars. Possible filling of osseous defects with an implant material (?). Systemic medication with *tetracycline*.
*Recall:* Repeated professional tooth cleaning during the wound healing phase; subsequent 6-month recall.
*Prognosis:* Good.

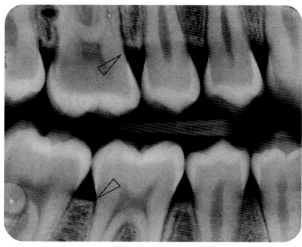

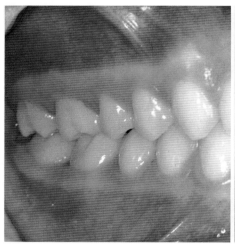

**225   Clinical picture – 15-year-old female (above)**
Caries-free dentition.
Upon cursory inspection the gingivae also appear healthy; however, numerous sites bleed after gentle probing.

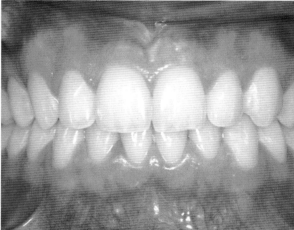

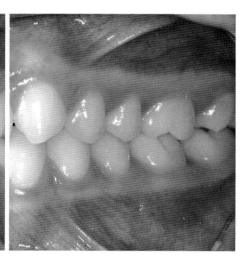

**226   Bitewing radiograph – Healthy 13-year-old (right)**
The radiograph reveals healthy interdental septa of compact bone around the first permanent molars (empty arrows).

**227   Bitewing radiograph – 15-year-old with LJP**
Two years later, obvious bony defects are visible mesial to 16 and distal of 46 (red arrows).
Virtually identical defects were also found on the contralateral side. *Early finding:* **LJP!**
The significance of regular clinical and radiographic screening in youngsters is clear.

*Right:* Osseous crater distolingual to tooth 46 during surgery.

Courtesy *U. Hersberger*

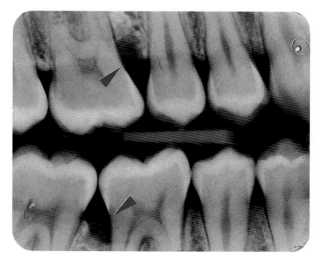

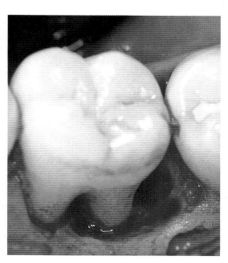

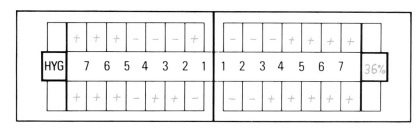

| | | | | | | | | | | | | | | | |
|---|---|---|---|---|---|---|---|---|---|---|---|---|---|---|---|
| | + | + | + | – | – | – | + | – | – | – | + | + | + | + |
| HYG | 7 | 6 | 5 | 4 | 3 | 2 | 1 | 1 | 2 | 3 | 4 | 5 | 6 | 7 | 36% |
| | + | + | + | – | + | + | – | – | – | + | + | + | + | + |

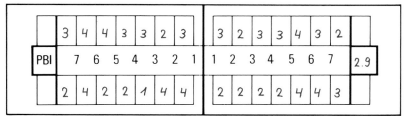

| | | | | | | | | | | | | | | | |
|---|---|---|---|---|---|---|---|---|---|---|---|---|---|---|---|
| | 3 | 4 | 4 | 3 | 3 | 2 | 3 | 3 | 2 | 3 | 3 | 4 | 3 | 2 |
| PBI | 7 | 6 | 5 | 4 | 3 | 2 | 1 | 1 | 2 | 3 | 4 | 5 | 6 | 7 | 2.9 |
| | 2 | 4 | 2 | 2 | 1 | 4 | 4 | 2 | 2 | 2 | 2 | 4 | 4 | 3 |

**228  Hygiene Index (HYG) and Papilla Bleeding Index (PBI)**

**HYG:** Only ten of the 28 interdental areas examined were free of plaque (–), despite the fact that the dentition appeared relatively clean upon cursory inspection (Fig. 225).

**PBI:** Even though the gingiva appeared healthy, the PBI (2.9) revealed a rather pronounced level of gingivitis.

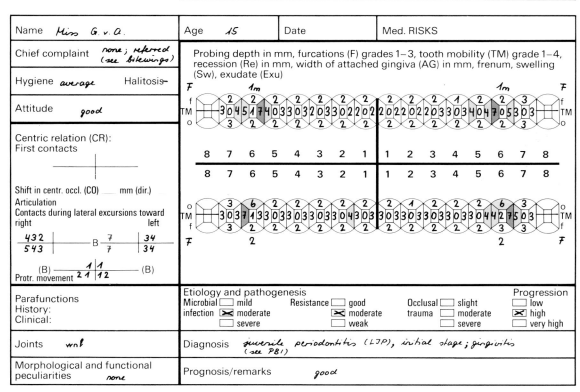

| Name  Miss G. v. a. | Age  15 | Date | Med. RISKS |
|---|---|---|---|
| Chief complaint  *none; referred (see bitewings)* | | | |

Probing depth in mm, furcations (F) grades 1–3, tooth mobility (TM) grade 1–4, recession (Re) in mm, width of attached gingiva (AG) in mm, frenum, swelling (Sw), exudate (Exu)

Hygiene *average*    Halitosis–

Attitude  *good*

Centric relation (CR): First contacts

Shift in centr. occl. (CO) ___ mm (dir.)
Articulation
Contacts during lateral excursions toward
right                                  left

432 / 543  —B— 7/7  34/34

(B) —— 1|1 —— (B)
Protr. movement  2 1 | 1 2

Parafunctions
History:
Clinical:

Joints  *wnl*

Morphological and functional peculiarities  *none*

**Etiology and pathogenesis**

| | | Progression |
|---|---|---|
| Microbial ☐ mild | Resistance ☐ good | Occlusal ☐ slight | ☐ low |
| infection ☒ moderate | ☒ moderate | trauma ☐ moderate | ☒ high |
| ☐ severe | ☐ weak | ☐ severe | ☐ very high |

Diagnosis  *juvenile periodontitis (LJP), initial stage; gingivitis (see PBI)*

Prognosis/remarks  *good*

**229  Periodontal charting – I**

All first permanent molars have probing depths up to 7 mm, which corresponds to about 5 mm of true attachment loss (see bitewing radiograph, Fig. 227).

The two maxillary first molars exhibit Class F1 furcation involvement from the mesiopalatal aspect.

There is no evidence at this time of pocket formation around the incisors, an area that is often affected in LJP patients.

The occlusion is normal, without parafunctions or occlusal trauma. Mobility of tooth 36 is slightly elevated.

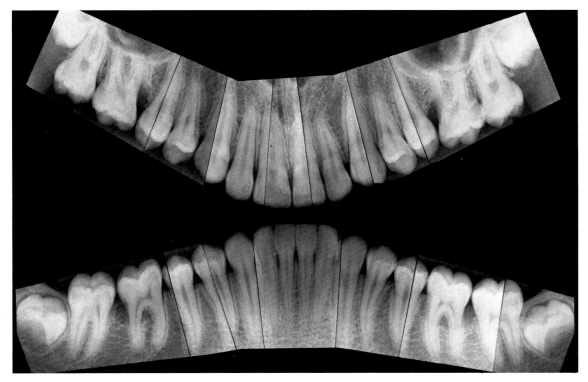

**230  Radiographic survey**

Routine periapical radiographs do not portray the osseous craters on the mandibular first molars as well as the bitewings (x-ray projection angle).

No bone loss is apparent on any teeth other than the first permanent molars.

# Juvenile Periodontitis (LJP) – Advanced Stage

A 21-year-old Black female student was referred to an oral surgeon for surgical extraction of an impacted third molar (38). The diagnosis of LJP was a serendipitous finding after radiographs were prepared. The patient had relatively good oral hygiene and little evidence of gingivitis.

*Findings:* See charting and radiographs (p. 97).
*Diagnosis:* Juvenile periodontitis with deep pockets on *typical* teeth (maxillary incisors and first molars).

*Therapy:* Oral hygiene instruction, modification of patient's technique; definitive debridement. Surgery (root planing with direct vision) and systemic tetracycline; extraction of 28 and 38.
*Recall:* Every three months.
*Prognosis:* Guarded on the seriously involved first permanent molars (furcation involvement). All remaining teeth are associated with a good prognosis.
This case has now been followed for *nine years*. The first permanent molars remain intact!

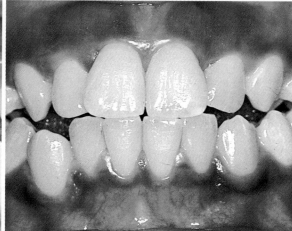

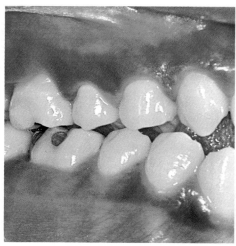

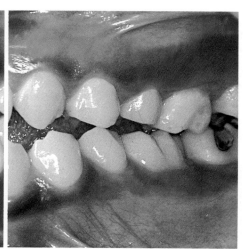

**231 Clinical picture (above)**
Pigmented gingiva. Very mild gingivitis in anterior area and posterior segments.
The type and severity of the disease process cannot be ascertained by a "quick look." An open bite is obvious in canine and premolar areas.

**232 Maxillary anterior area during flap procedure (right)**
9 mm of attachment loss can be seen in those areas typical for LJP: teeth 21 and 22.

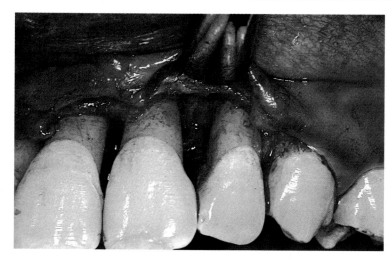

**233 Maxillary molars 26 and 27 during flap surgery**
The buccal roots of the first molar have practically no bone support. Note the crater defects and open trifurcation (Class F3).
Despite the serious periodontal involvement, the first permanent molars were retained. They have remained in function throughout the subsequent 9-year period.

*Right:* Initial radiographic view.

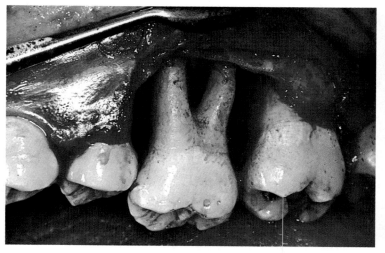

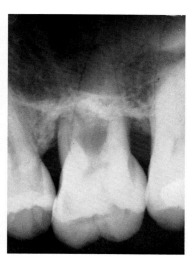

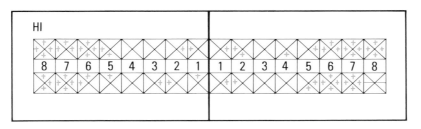

HI

| 8 | 7 | 6 | 5 | 4 | 3 | 2 | 1 | 1 | 2 | 3 | 4 | 5 | 6 | 7 | 8 |

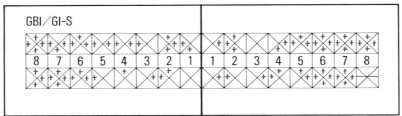

GBI/GI-S

| 8 | 7 | 6 | 5 | 4 | 3 | 2 | 1 | 1 | 2 | 3 | 4 | 5 | 6 | 7 | 8 |

### 234 Hygiene Index (HYG) and Gingival Bleeding Index (GBI)

**HYG:** The patient exhibits a hygiene index of 54.8% indicating that approximately one-half of all tooth surfaces are plaque-free. Plaque accumulation is observed mainly in the molar areas.

**GBI:** Gentle probing of the sulci/pockets resulted in bleeding at 58.2% of examined sites. The distribution of bleeding areas corresponded to the plaque accumulation.

## Periodontal status

Name *Miss M.D., age 21*
Date

**Symbols for charting**
1. missing    /
2. food impaction    ↑
3. open contact    ‖
4. mobility    **0, 1, 2, 3, 4**
5. bridge    ▨
6. drifted/extrusion    **D→I**
7. beg. furcation exposure    ○
8. bifurcation exposed    ●
9. periapical area    ⊛

## Etiology
*bacterial infection, particularly involving Actinobacillus actinomycetemcomitans (Aa); PMN defect?*

## Diagnosis
*localized juvenile periodontitis (LJP)*

## Prognosis
*good, except for 1st molars*

**Systemic diseases?**
*PMN defect?*

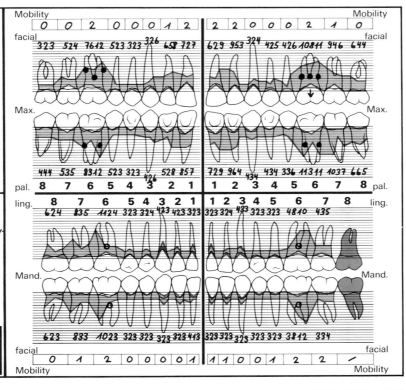

Mobility

| 0 | 0 | 2 | 0 | 0 | 0 | 1 | 2 | 2 | 2 | 0 | 0 | 0 | 2 | 1 | 0 |

facial

323 524 7612 523 323 326 652 727    629 953 324 425 426 10811 946 644

Max.

444 535 8312 523 323 528 857    729 964 434 434 336 11311 1037 665

pal.

| 8 | 7 | 6 | 5 | 4 | 3 | 2 | 1 | 1 | 2 | 3 | 4 | 5 | 6 | 7 | 8 | pal.

ling.

624 835 1124 323 324 423 423 323    323 324 423 323 323 4810 435

Mand.

623 833 1023 323 323 323 323 443    323 323 323 323 323 3812 334

facial

| 0 | 1 | 2 | 0 | 0 | 0 | 0 | 1 | 1 | 1 | 0 | 0 | 1 | 2 | 2 | ✓ |

Mobility

### 235 Periodontal charting – II

The gingival contour as shown on this modified "Michigan chart" reveals no gingival shrinkage or recession even on those teeth with severe involvement.

Probing depths up to 9 mm are present in the maxillary anterior region, and to 11 mm in maxillary molars, where furcation involvement is severe from all aspects (F3).

Bone resorption is less severe in the mandible. The anterior teeth reveal almost normal values. Only distal to the first permanent molar are 10–12 mm probings evident. Tooth 46 exhibited an F1 furcation involvement and tooth 36, F2.

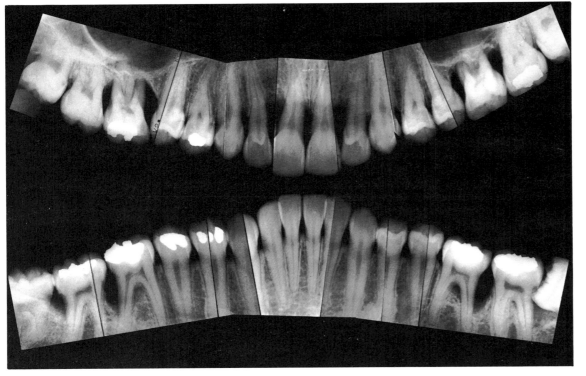

### 236 Radiographic survey

The radiographic picture of this advanced stage of disease reveals severe involvement of the maxillary anterior teeth and first permanent molars, which is typical for LJP. In this 21-year-old female, in whom LJP began during puberty, incipient osseous resorption has now also begun on other teeth:

| · 7 · 5 · · · · · | · · · · · 5 · 7 8 |
|---|---|
| 8 7 · · · · · · · | · · · · · · · · · |

Even in deep pockets there is no evidence of calculus accumulation. This is also typical of LJP.

# Pre-pubertal Periodontitis (PP)

This 2½-year-old boy was referred from his private dentist. The medical history, gathered from his parents (Japanese mother, Swiss father) revealed that the deciduous anterior teeth, with the exception of 61, had "fallen out" in the previous few months. The deciduous molars and canines in the maxilla were highly mobile, but there was no indication of resorption of their roots.

This case is difficult to classify in the absence of an identification of possible hematologic defects. Even though most of the teeth are affected, the relatively mild gingival inflammation and the absence of gingival hyperplasia speak against the generalized form (cf. p. 75). Laboratory studies should be performed to rule out hypophosphatasia (Rathbun).

---

*Findings:* See charting and radiographs.
*Diagnosis: Localized* pre-pubertal periodontitis (PP).
*Therapy:* Palliative or extraction (Page et al. 1983 b). Intensive periodontal preventive maintenance upon eruption of the permanent teeth.
*Prognosis:* Poor for the deciduous dentition, questionable for permanent teeth.

**237 Clinical picture – 2½-year-old child**
The maxillary anterior tooth 51 and all mandibular front teeth and the canines were lost spontaneously.

The gingivitis is unimpressive. Aphthous-like lesion in the lower left region.

*Right:* The radiograph clearly depicts the pronounced attachment loss on the anterior teeth, in the presence of complete roots. The pulp chambers appear to be above average in size.

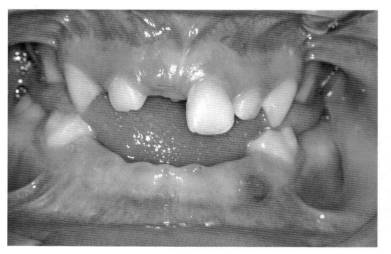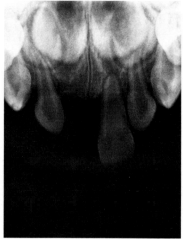

**238 Probing depths and tooth mobility**
Pocket probing was only possible on tooth 61, because the 2½-year-old boy was very sensitive and understandably impatient. All teeth exhibited elevated mobility. Teeth 54, 52; 61, 62, and 63 were highly mobile.

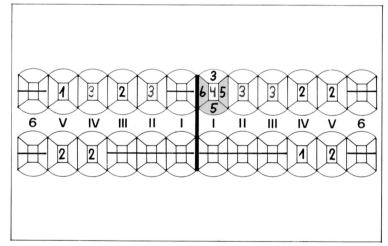

**239 Panoramic radiograph**
Irregular and in some areas extreme attachment loss is revealed on all maxillary deciduous teeth. The mandibular deciduous molars appear to be only slightly involved at this time.

Tooth 61, which was present in the clinical picture above (Fig. 237) was spontaneously exfoliated before the panoramic film was taken, some two weeks after the initial visit.

Courtesy *B. Widmer*

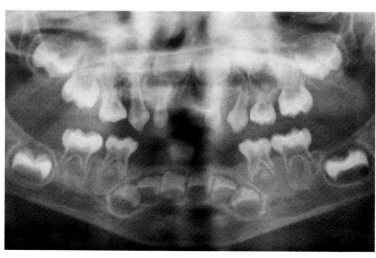

# ANUG / P (Ulcerative Periodontitis)

Acute necrotizing ulcerative gingivitis (ANUG) has already been described (p. 49). The local and systemic etiologic factors, as well as the histopathology of the gingival necrotizing form, are also applicable in *ulcerative periodontitis* (ANUG/P).

This bacterially elicited acute disease of the tooth-supporting structures (bone, periodontal ligament) always develops from a pre-existing ANUG. Its clinical course is one of periods of intensely active disease followed by quiescent periods of variable length.

ANUG/P has assumed greater importance in recent years because it is frequently observed as one of the oral symptoms of HIV-seropositive and AIDS patients (WR 5, 6; pp. 70–72).

*Therapy:* In the acute phase, careful plaque and calculus removal. Thereafter topical treatment with hydrogen peroxide rinses and application of antibiotic/corticosteroid ointments. After the pain has subsided, systematic mechanical initial periodontal therapy should be instituted (scaling and root planing).

In advanced cases surgery may be necessary as a final step to improve gingival contour.

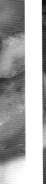
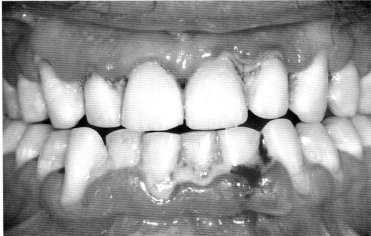

**Acute phase**

**240   ANUG/P (ulcerative periodontitis) – Second occurrence**
A 26-year-old male experienced an aggressive acute exacerbation for the second time. In addition to the pronounced gingivitis, attachment loss has occurred in the maxillary anterior and molar regions: *Acute ANUG/P.*

*Left:* Pronounced painful desquamative ulcer near tooth 18. The third molar was extracted after the acute exacerbation subsided.

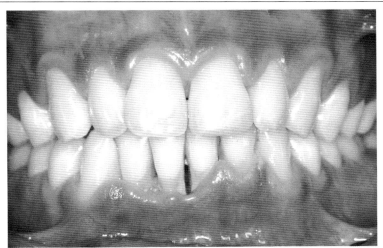

**Interval stages**

**241   Localized ulcerative periodontitis**
This 22-year-old male had experienced two acute exacerbations, neither of which were treated professionally. Presently the patient is free of symptoms: *Interval stage.*

*Left:* Advanced but discretely localized attachment loss in the mandibular anterior area. The interdental crater is a retention site for plaque and therefore represents an invitation to repeated exacerbation should any reduction in host resistance to infection occur.

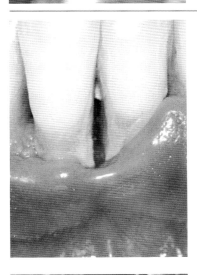
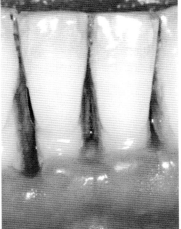
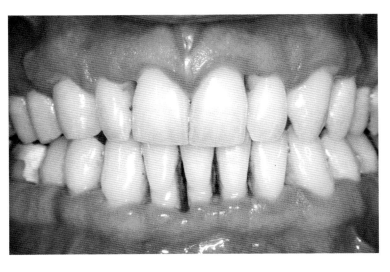

**242   Generalized ulcerative periodontitis**
This 30-year-old patient complained of "disappearing gingiva." He reported experiencing gingival pain many times during the past several years, but never sought professional care.

The now pain-free lesions vary extensively in degree of severity: *Interval stage.*

*Left:* In the mandibular anterior region, especially between teeth 41 and 42, attachment loss is advanced. Despite plaque and calculus accumulation, no symptoms of activity are evident.

# Ulcerative Periodontitis – Subacute Stage

A 28-year-old female complained of severe mobility of her mandibular anterior teeth. Off and on over a long number of years, she suffered from painful gingival inflammation, which had been treated only symptomatically. Periodontal debridement had never been performed. The patient is a heavy smoker.

*Findings:* See charting and radiographs (p. 101).
*Diagnosis:* Generalized, advanced ulcerative periodontitis with especially pronounced attachment loss in the mandibular anterior region.

*Therapy:* The treatment plan is very difficult to formulate at this point. Probably the lower anterior teeth must be extracted. The usual procedure is to wait until after initial therapy is complete before making the decision concerning which teeth to extract (molars?) and which to attempt to save by means of surgical intervention.
*Recall:* Every 3 months.
*Prognosis:* Average at best, and only then with excellent patient cooperation in home care.

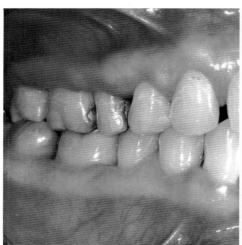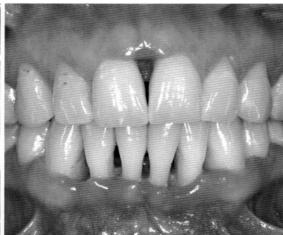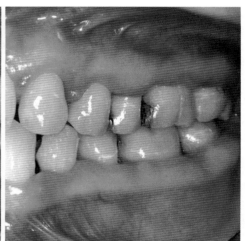

**243   Clinical picture (above)**
The ulcerous destruction of gingiva is painfully evident between teeth 11 and 21 as well as in the mandibular anterior area. The pronounced attachment loss in the molar segments would not be anticipated clinically (Figs. 247 & 248). Spontaneous hemorrhage and pain are minimal at this time: *Subacute stage.*

**244   Detail of maxilla – Papillary necrosis (right)**
The papilla between 11 and 21 was already destroyed during an acute episode. Currently an inactive crater about 5 mm deep exists.

**245   Detail of mandible – "Reverse gingival architecture"**
Intense reddening and formation of a pseudomembrane are indications that an acute phase is about to begin in the mandibular anterior segment. Pain occurs when the tissue is touched with a periodontal probe, and hemorrhage occurs after spraying.

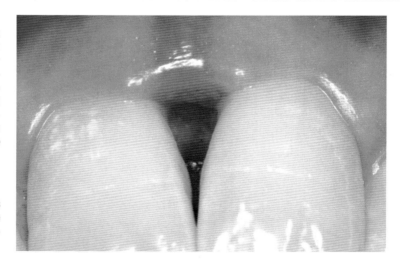

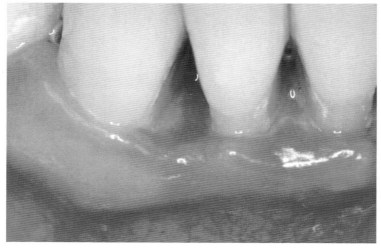

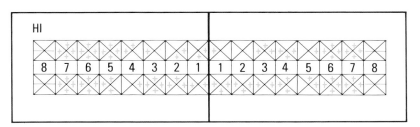

HI

| | | | | | | | | | | | | | | | |
|8|7|6|5|4|3|2|1|1|2|3|4|5|6|7|8|

### 246  Hygiene Index (HI) and Gingival Bleeding Index (GBI)

**HI:** Most tooth surfaces exhibit plaque after application of a disclosing solution; only 31% are plaque-free.

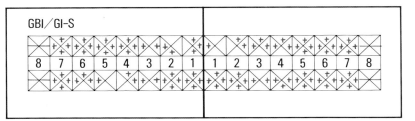

GBI / GI-S

| | | | | | | | | | | | | | | | |
|8|7|6|5|4|3|2|1|1|2|3|4|5|6|7|8|

**GBI:** Even though the *ulcerative* process in most areas of the dentition is in a clinically subacute stage, simple gingivitis is ubiquitous, as evidenced by bleeding after probing of sulci or pockets in 79% of sites examined.

## Periodontal status

Name  *Miss J. B., age 28*
Date

### Symbols for charting
1. missing                          /
2. food impaction              ↑
3. open contact                 ‖
4. mobility           **0, 1, 2, 3, 4**
5. bridge                            ▨
6. drifted/extrusion       **D→I**
7. beg. furcation exposure   ○
8. bifurcation exposed       ●
9. periapical area                Ⓠ

## Etiology
*"specific" bacterial infection*

## Diagnosis
*ANUG superimposed upon adult periodontitis*

## Prognosis
*relatively good on some individual teeth only*

**Systemic diseases?**
*none*

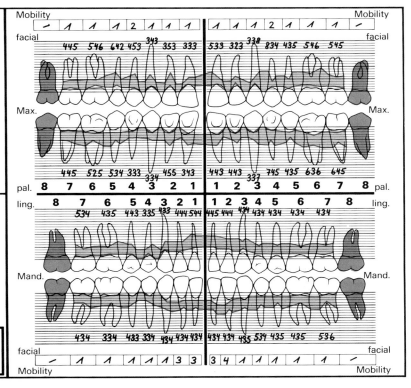

### 247  Periodontal charting – II
Especially in the mandibular anterior region, the charting reveals a picture that is typical for ANUG/P: As a consequence of necrotic destruction of the gingiva, the probing depths are considerably less than the actual attachment loss (pockets = red colored area between gingival margin and pocket bottom; cf. Radiographic survey, Fig. 248). This is especially true in the papillary regions where the necrotic process always begins and where the pathologic process is most aggressive throughout the course of the disease.

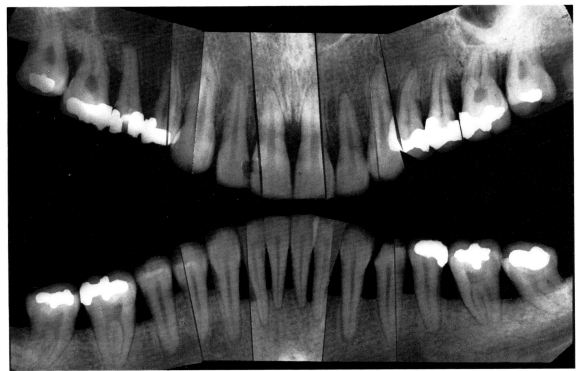

### 248  Radiographic survey
The severity and expanse of the severe periodontal destruction are depicted most dramatically in the radiographic survey. Teeth 31 and 41 exhibit virtually no remaining osseous support. On almost all other teeth, half to two-thirds of the tooth-supporting bone has been lost.

# Periodontitis Associated with Systemic Diseases
## Juvenile Diabetes

Many investigations of the relationship between diabetes and gingivitis/periodontitis have been published; however, the results of such studies have not led to consensus (see literature review in Gaberthüel and Curilović 1977, Saadoun 1980). Most authors found correlations between gingivitis/periodontitis and insulin-dependent juvenile diabetes (Belting et al. 1964, Schnetz & Franzen 1968, Cohen et al. 1970, Bernick et al. 1975, Ringelberg et al. 1977, Gislén et al. 1980, Cianciola et al. 1982, Wolf et al. 1987). One explanation for this could be the defects of polymorphonuclear granulocytes (PMNs) that are regularly observed in juvenile diabetes (Manouchehr-Pour et al. 1981a, b).

It is possible that the vascular pathology associated with diabetes (cf. retinoscopy, Fig. 253) may also play a role in terms of periodontal blood supply (Rylander et al. 1987), but this has yet to be proven.

*Case:* A 28-year-old male had developed severe, insulin-dependent juvenile diabetes at age 15. The associated periodontitis had never been treated.

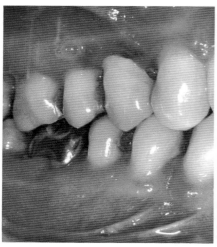 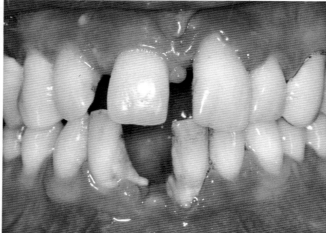 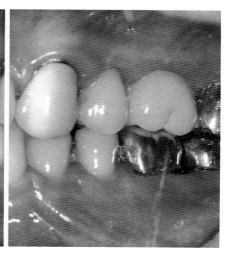

**249   Clinical picture (above)**
Localized acute inflammation of the gingivae, which exhibit some edematous swelling as well as areas of shrinkage. Plaque and calculus are abundant. Almost all of the deeper pockets exhibit signs of activity (pus).

**250   Probing depth, gingival recession (Re) and tooth mobility (TM, right)**
Immediately apparent is the extraordinarily irregular attachment loss. Probing depths in the interproximal areas range from 4 to 12 mm. Some teeth exhibit extreme mobility (cf. radiographic survey).

**251   Radiographic survey**
The radiographs confirm the clinical findings. Teeth 15, 14, 12; 21 and 32 must be extracted (see p. 103 for further treatment planning).

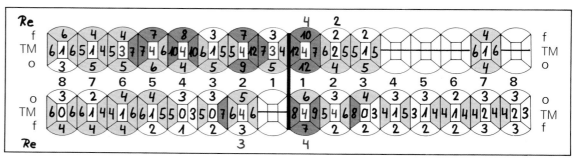

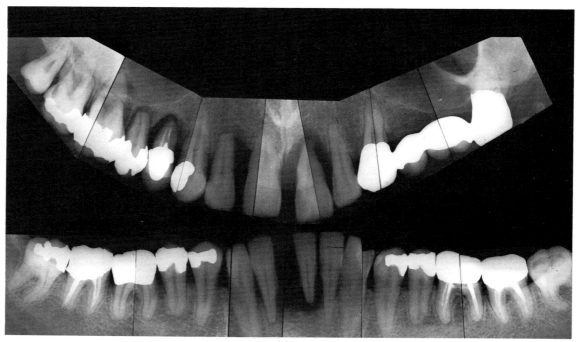

*Clinical findings:*
  HYG: 15%                PBI: 3.2
  Probing depths, gingival recession and tooth mobility are presented in Figure 250.
*Diagnosis:* Severe periodontitis that had progressed rapidly in a patient with juvenile diabetes.
*Therapy:* The treatment of periodontitis in patients with juvenile diabetes is more radical than in persons without systemic diseases.
  *Maxilla:* Extraction of all teeth with the exception of 13 and 23 (periodontal therapy); partial denture.

*Mandible:* Extraction of the remaining anterior teeth and the third molars.
Periodontal therapy on remaining teeth. Cast framework partial denture. Because of the poor prognosis and economic considerations, more involved reconstruction was not indicated.
*Recall:* Every 3 months.
*Prognosis of abutment teeth:* "Guarded" at best, in view of the proposed radical therapy.

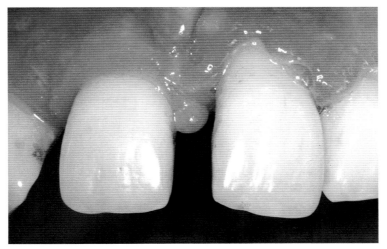

**252  Mandibular anterior area – Initial findings**
Diastemata had formed over the course of the previous years. Tooth 21 appears elongated, exhibits no bony support, is highly mobile and painful (radiographic survey, Fig. 251). It will be extracted along with the other teeth after a temporary removable partial denture is constructed.

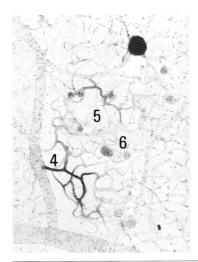
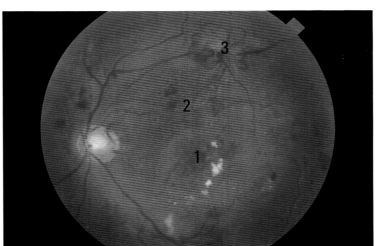

**253  Retinoscopy in diabetic retinopathy**
1 Yellow lipid bodies in the retina
2 Disseminated hemorrhage and microaneurysms
3 Neovascularization bundle due to ischemia

*Left:* Histologic view of diabetic retinal microangiopathy
4 Closure of a precapillary
5 Atrophic capillaries, cell-free zone
6 Microaneurysms

(Trypsin digestion,
Sudan III-hemalaun; x 25)

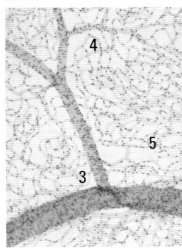
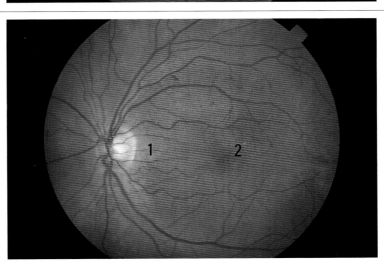

**254  Normal Retinoscopy, healthy eye**
1 Optic nerve papilla with exiting retinal vessels
2 Macula free of vasculature

*Left:* Normal histology of the retina
3 Retinal arterioles
4 Precapillaries
5 Capillaries

(Trypsin digestion, H & E; x 25)

Courtesy *B. Daicker*

# Periodontitis Associated with Systemic Diseases
## Down Syndrome, Trisomy 21, Mongolism

Trisomy 21 (Mongolism) carries the name of John Langdon *Down,* who first described the condition in detail in 1866 (Rett 1983, review by Reuland-Bosma & Van Dijk 1986, Rateitschak & Wolf 1987). The basis for the condition is a chromosomal aberration (Trisomy 21). This aneuploidy is the result of primary nondysjunction at meiosis, which is the cell division process for reproductive cells. Two homologues fail to dysjoin at the first meiotic division and two of the resulting gametes carry a double dose of the chromosome. Thus instead of a zygote containing one chromosome 21 from the male and one chromosome 21 from the female, the genotype of the zygote contains three chromosomes at position 21 (see karyotype, Fig. 258).

Mongolism occurs at a rate of one in about every 700 live births. It is likely, however, that the prevalence of mongolism will diminish significantly in the future as a result of increased use of ultrasound prenatal analysis and amniocentesis, as well as more liberal abortion laws (Schmid 1988).

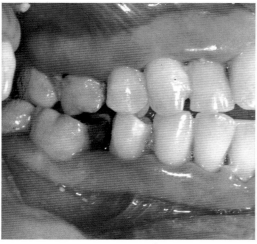
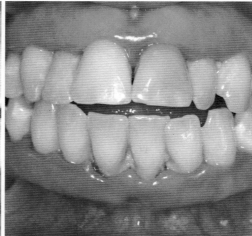
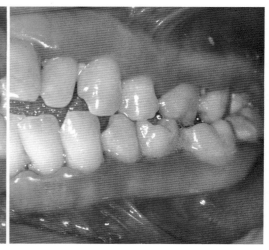

**255 Clinical picture (above)**
Poor plaque control, severe gingivitis, anterior open bite, cross-bite and end-to-end occlusion in molar regions.

**256 Probing depths and tooth mobility (TM, right)**
The deep pockets exhibit signs of activity. As a result of the massive attachment loss, all teeth exhibit varying degrees of mobility.

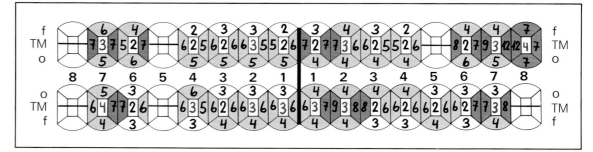

**257 Radiographic survey**
The radiographs corroborate the generalized profound attachment loss: Horizontal and in some areas vertical bone loss of 60–75%.

Widened periodontal ligament space anticipates the elevated tooth mobility.

Tooth 21 is non-vital and exhibits an apical radiolucency.

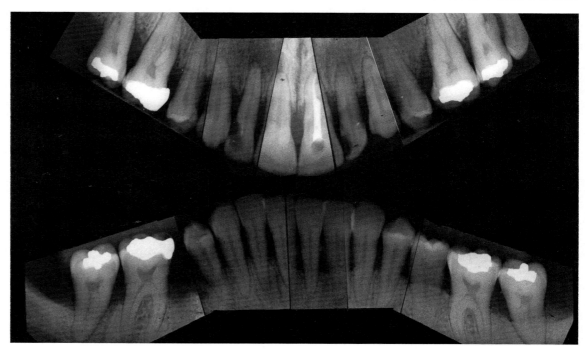

*Case:* This 27-year-old female has the mental development of a 6–7 year-old. She exhibited no cardiac defects. She grew up in her parent's home, is well cared for and can converse readily. For these reasons every attempt was made to maintain as many teeth as possible.

*Findings:*

   HYG: 0%           PBI: 3.8

   Probing depths and tooth mobility, see Figure 256.

*Diagnosis:* Severe periodontitis that has progressed rapidly in a patient with Down Syndrome.

*Therapy:* Professional debridement and oral hygiene instruction. (Trial: Toothbrushing by patient; interdental cleaning by mother).

Modified Widman procedures in all quadrants; extraction of teeth 17; 27, 28; 37 and 47.

*Recall:* Frequent, but brief appointments.

*Prognosis:* Patient cooperation will always be poor and plaque control will depend for the most part on her caretakers. The prognosis is therefore guarded.

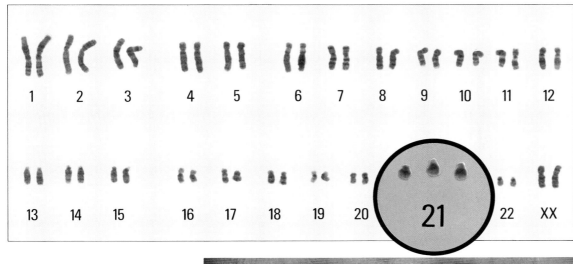

**258   Karyotype in Trisomy 21**
The abnormal chromosomal picture results from triplication of the small autosome 21. This "Trisomy 21" occurs in about 94% of all Mongoloid patients.

Courtesy *H. Müller*

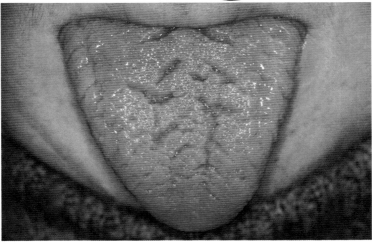

**259   Mongoloid symptoms – Scrotal tongue**
The deeply grooved tongue is one of the typical symptoms in Down Syndrome.

Mongoloid symptoms:

- **Scrotal tongue**
- **Ocular peculiarity**
- **Small head**
- **Stocky physique**
- **Short, soft hands**
- **Cardiac defects**
  One-third have a short life expectancy

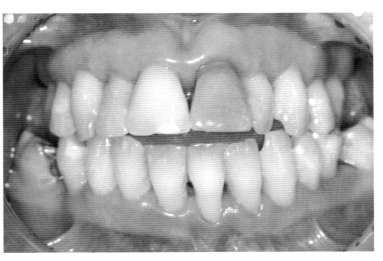

**260 Six months after treatment**
The entire dentition was treated by means of modified Widman procedures. The end result, six months after the final surgery, was an acceptable result in comparison to the initial situation.

A short-interval recall is recommended, and possibly also the use of a custom tray for daily application of gel (fluoride, chlorhexidine; cf. p. 284).

# Prepubertal Periodontitis Associated with Systemic Disease
## Papillon-Lefèvre Syndrome (PLS)

PLS is a rare, autosomal recessive genetic disease (Haneke 1979). Obligate symptoms include severe periodontitis and hyperkeratoses, usually localized to palms and soles of the feet, and other skin areas that commonly absorb minor trauma.

The deciduous teeth are lost prematurely in most cases. The permanent teeth are always periodontally involved. Immune defects, especially of PMNs, and an aggressive pocket flora (gram-negative anaerobes) are suspected etiologic factors, in addition to ectodermal and mesodermal defects.

Earlier therapeutic attempts were without success. However, more recently Preus and Gjermo (1987) reported that extraction of all primary teeth led to maintenance of the permanent teeth.

Tinanoff et al. (1986) extracted the already present permanent teeth in a 9-year-old PLS patient and were able to maintain the later erupting maxillary canines, premolars and third molars over the long term.

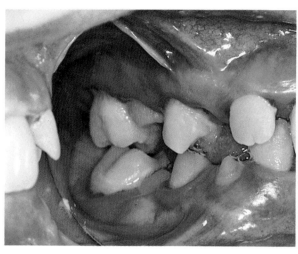 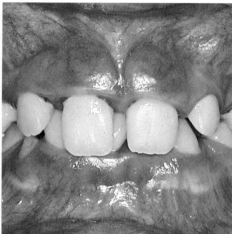 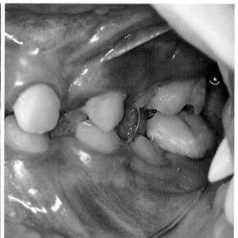

**261 Clinical picture (above)**
Severe gingivitis and periodontitis, plaque, spontaneous hemorrhage, exudate and suppuration. Abscess on the facial of 11 and 21. Poor occlusion, severe overbite. This young patient performed absolutely no oral hygiene, because he feared the spontaneous loss of his very loose teeth.

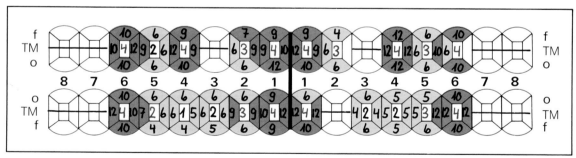

**262 Probing depths and tooth mobility (right)**
All of the deep pockets exhibit signs of advanced activity (pus).

**263 Radiographic survey**
The marked (∗) teeth are in the process of being exfoliated and will be extracted immediately.

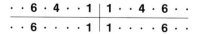
```
· · 6 · 4 · · 1 | 1 · · 4 · 6 · ·
· · 6 · · · · 1 | 1 · · · · 6 · ·
```

Periodontal destruction appears to begin immediately after eruption of the teeth, and subsequently progresses rapidly. Vertical defects (infrabony pockets) and Class F3 furcation involvement predominate.

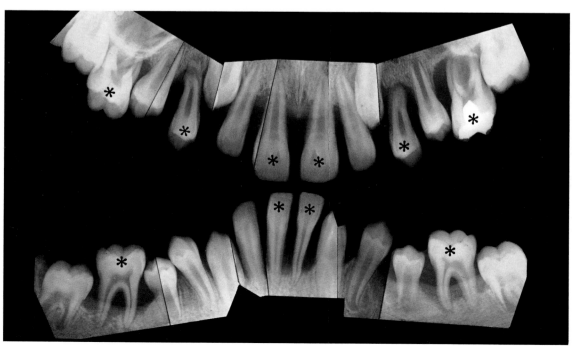

*Case:* A 9-year-old boy was referred from the pediatrician because of severe halitosis and extreme tooth mobility (Rateitschak-Plüss & Schroeder 1984).
*Findings:*

| HYG: 0% | PBI: 3.9 |
|---|---|

Probing depths, radiographic survey, tooth mobility and skin lesions: see Figures below.
*Special findings:* PMN defects, specific pocket flora (*Bacteroides* and Spirochetes).

*Diagnosis:* Acute, severe prepubertal periodontitis associated with PLS.
*Therapy:* Extraction of hopeless teeth (Fig. 263).
Periodontal therapy and simultaneous topical (chlorhexidine) and systemic (metronidazole/tetracycline) treatment; removable partial denture.
*Recall:* Very short check-up interval.
*Prognosis:* In this situation, virtually hopeless. Teeth that can be "saved" beyond puberty may be maintained over the long term (see next case, p. 108).

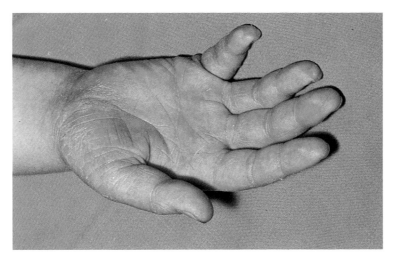

**Papillon-Lefèvre Syndrome (PLS) with palmar and plantar hyperkeratoses**

**264 Hyperkeratosis on palm of hand**
The hyperkeratotic area exhibits cracks and fissures, which are actually wounds that have occurred due to normal function. These heal poorly and slowly. The patient suffers from these palmar lesions mostly in winter.

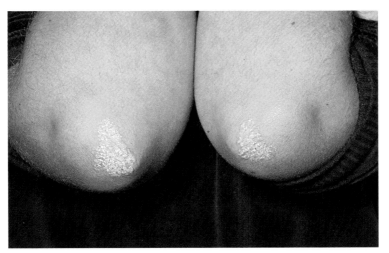

**265 Hyperkeratosis on elbows**

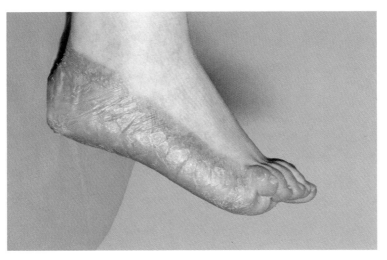

**266 Hyperkeratosis on sole and lateral border of foot**
The sharp line of demarcation between hyperkeratotic areas and normal-appearing skin corresponds to the outline of the shoe worn by this patient.
Minor trauma to the skin elicits this type of severe hyperkeratotic response. Dermatologists, too, can treat this disease only symptomatically.

# Papillon-Lefèvre Syndrome – "An Exception for Every Rule"

A 7-year-old girl was referred to the dental clinic because of severe mobility of her recently erupted permanent incisors and first molars. The patient remained under dental care for 24 years thereafter. As a teenager, the patient was reconciled to wearing cast framework partial dentures. At age eighteen, she underwent surgery to correct her mandibular prognathism (note osteosynthesis wires in radiograph, Fig. 269). At age 25 the remaining dentition was treated with splinted total reconstructions in mandible and maxilla, which were cemented temporarily.

*Diagnosis:* Acute, severe periodontitis in a case of Papillon-Lefèvre Syndrome (PLS).

*Course of the disease, and treatment:* In this exceptional case, it was possible to retain a large number of permanent teeth as a result of timely extractions, intensive periodontitis therapy, frequent recall and the excellent cooperation of the patient (Fig. 269).

It is worthy of note that the treatment rendered 24 years ago was purely mechanical and did not include the systemic tetracycline or metronidazole supportive therapy that would be common today.

**267    Radiographic and dental survey (7-year-old female)**
Erupted permanent teeth:

| | | | | | | | | | | | | |
|---|---|---|---|---|---|---|---|---|---|---|---|---|
| · · | 6 | · · · | 2 1 | 1 2 | · · · | 6 | · · |

··6···21 | 12···6··
··6···21 | 12···6··

The first permanent molars were exfoliated one year after eruption. The mandibular anterior teeth exhibit severe periodontitis.

The primary teeth were lost prematurely. All primordia teeth are present.

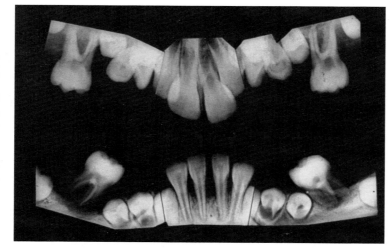

**268    Same patient age 31**
The patient smiles with her own teeth, which were deemed "hopeless" due to her Papillon-Lefèvre Syndrome when she was first examined 24 years previously. She displays advanced hyperkeratosis on both palms and painful cracks through the hyperkeratotic area on her heel.

The skin on the back of her hands is paper thin, hyperkeratotic, dry and visibly erythematous.

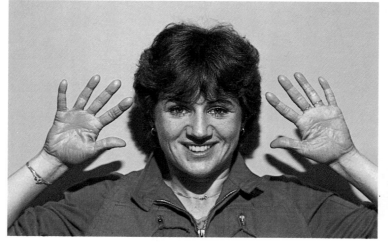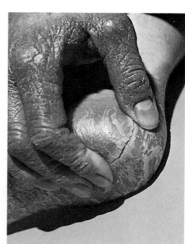

**269    Radiographic survey (31-year-old)**
Destructive periodontitis came to a halt after the patient traversed puberty. Total fixed reconstructions were seated upon abutments in both arches, where the 14 remaining teeth had been prepared:

87···3·|··3·5··8
87·54···|···45·78

This bridgework is seated only temporarily (Temp-Bond), and is periodically removed, cleaned and re-cemented.

Radiographs courtesy *U. P. Saxer*

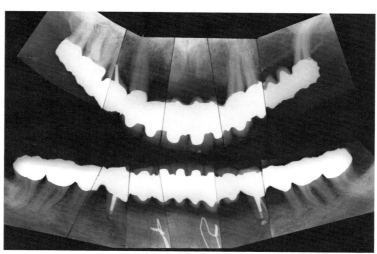

# Recession

**Attachment loss without infection (?)**

Gingival recession accounts for 5–10% of all attachment loss. Recession is defined as a seemingly inflammation-free clinical condition characterized by apical retreat of the facial and less often of the oral periodontium. Despite recession of the gingival margin, the interdental papillae usually fill the entire embrasure area in younger patients. Recession is usually localized to one or several teeth; generalized gingival recession is rare. Teeth exhibiting gingival recession are not mobile. The periodontal supporting structures are generally of excellent quality.

*Teeth are never lost due to gingival recession alone!*

If the patient's oral hygiene is inadequate, or if the recession reaches the movable oral mucosa, secondary inflammation may occur and eventually pocket formation (periodontitis) may ensue.

*Etiology:* The causes of recession have not been completely elucidated. It is probable, however, that a primary factor is purely the morphology and anatomy of the situation. The facial plate of bone overlying the root is usually very thin. Not infrequently the root surface is completely denuded of alveolar bone or exhibits *fenestrations* in the thin osseous lamella (Edel 1981, Löst 1984a). Complete absence of bone over the facial root surface is referred to as a *dehiscence*. This situation is most frequently observed on incisors, canines and premolars, and seldom on molar teeth (except the mesiobuccal root of maxillary first molars). Dehiscence is also frequently associated with tooth position anomalies such as buccoversion, supereruption etc. Despite the lack of a buccal plate of bone over the root, the gingival margin may maintain its normal position.

The recession is initiated as a consequence of the morphologic / anatomic situation and the following etiologic course:

– Improper, traumatic toothbrushing, e.g., horizontal scrubbing with excessive force (Smukler & Landsberg 1984; Mierau & Spinder 1984; Mierau & Fiebig 1986, 1987)
– Mild chronic inflammation that may be only slightly visible clinically (Wennström et al. 1987a)

– Frenum pulls, especially when fibers of the frenum attach near the gingival margin
– Orthodontic treatment (tooth movement labially; arch expansion; Foushee et al. 1985, Wennström et al. 1987a)
– Excessive periodontal scaling (care at recall!).

Bernimoulin and Curilović (1977) were unable to demonstrate that functional disturbances (bruxism) can elicit gingival recession. Controversy about the etiology of recession continues to cause heated discussion.

*Clinical picture:* In the following pages, recession is depicted schematically, on skull preparations and in clinical situations.

*Radiographically,* pure gingival recession localized to the facial surfaces of teeth *cannot be diagnosed.*

*Therapy:* With scrupulous and proper oral hygiene, recession can be brought to a halt without any further treatment. The vertical-rotatory brushing technique (modified Stillman, p.153) should be recommended.

Treatment for severe types of recession by means of mucogingival surgery is described in detail beginning on page 290. Such interventions are indicated if no attached gingiva is present or if proper oral hygiene cannot maintain an inflammation-free condition.

# Fenestration and Dehiscence of the Alveolar Bone

In a healthy periodontium the facial margin of the alveolar bone lies approximately 1–2 mm apical to the gingival margin, which courses near to the cemento-enamel junction. The facial aspect of the alveolar bone covering the root is usually very thin. As revealed by a flap operation or on a skull preparation, the coronal portion of the root often is not covered by bone (*dehiscence*) or there is *fenestration* of the facial bony plate. Towards the apex, the facial plate of bone becomes thicker and spongy bone fills the interval between facial and lingual cortical plates. In these thicker areas, recession generally stops spontaneously.

In *elderly* individuals, especially in those who have practiced intensive interdental hygiene for many years, recession of facial periodontal tissues may appear in combination with horizontal bone loss in the interdental area. In such cases, the interdental papillae usually also recede. Nevertheless, no *true* periodontal pockets are in evidence.

**270   Normal periodontium and various manifestations of recession as viewed in orofacial section**
The junctional epithelium is depicted in *pink* (no pockets); the mucogingival line is indicated (arrows).

**A**  Normal gingiva and bone
**B**  Parallel recession of bone *and* gingiva; *fenestration*
**C**  *Bony dehiscence* more pronounced than the gingival recession
**D**  Recession with formation of *McCall's festoons* (cf. Fig. 278)

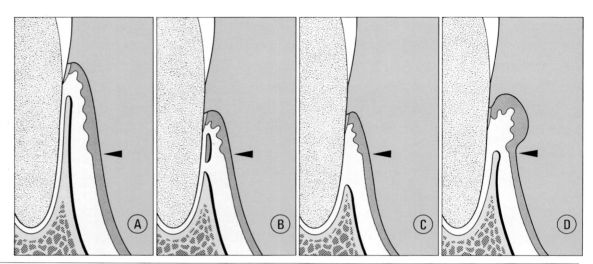

**Skull Observations**

**271   Fenestration (left)**
Adjacent to the fenestration on the facial aspect of tooth 13 (circled), dehiscences and primary horizontal bone loss in the interdental areas are visible.

**272   Dehiscence (right)**
A pronounced dehiscence that extends almost to the apex is observed on the facial of 13. The other teeth exhibit dehiscences of lesser severity. Generalized interdental bone loss is also in evidence.

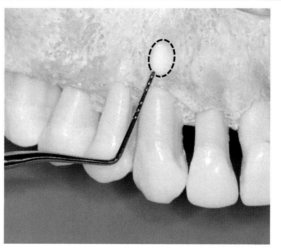
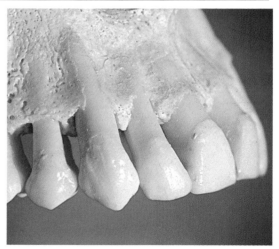

**Findings during surgery**

**273  Multiple fenestrations (left)**
In the course of an Edlan operation, large fenestrations became visible after reflection of the periosteum on teeth 16, 15, 13 and 12.

**274   Dehiscence on 13 (right)**
An unexpected osseous dehiscence was encountered during surgery. The dehiscence is more severe than the original gingival recession.

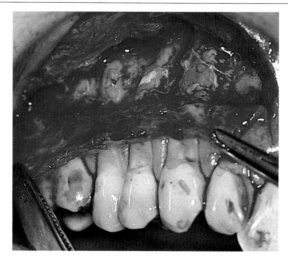
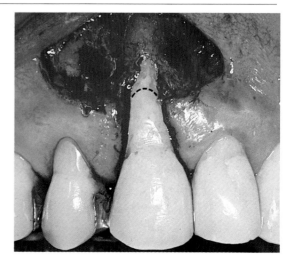

# Clinical Symptoms

- Gingival recession
- Stillman cleft
- McCall's festoon

The clinical manifestations of recession are numerous. Gingival recession usually begins with a gradual apical migration of the entire *facial aspect* of the gingiva, revealing the CEJ. Less frequently the first sign of recession is the relatively rapid formation of a small groove in the gingiva, a so-called *Stillman cleft*. This can expand into a pronounced recession. As a consequence of recession, the remaining attached gingiva may become somewhat thickened and rolled, a non-inflammatory fibrotic response known as *McCall's festoons*.

Esthetic considerations may prompt the patient to seek professional care if recession becomes pronounced in the maxillary anterior segment. As root surfaces are exposed, cervical sensitivity may also become a problem. Gingival recession is often observed on teeth that exhibit wedge-shaped defects near the gingival margin (Völk et al. 1987).

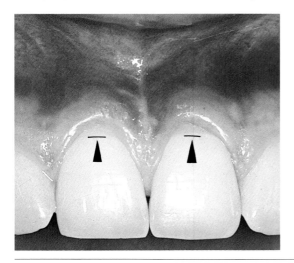

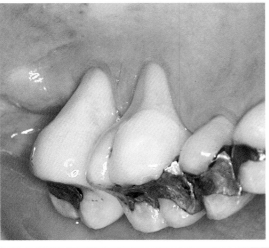

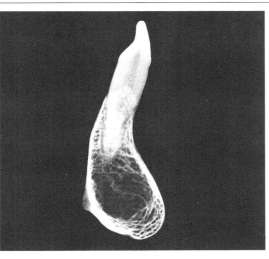

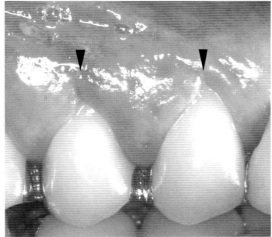

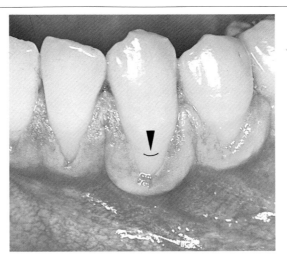

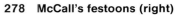

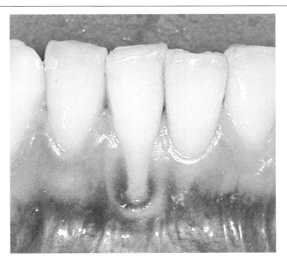

**275 Initial recession (left)**
The cementoenamel junction is marked in this view to demonstrate early gingival recession.

**276 Stillman cleft (right)**
Gingival cleft that is likely of traumatic origin. These may expand laterally and develop into gingival recession. The exposed root surface is often very sensitive, and is covered with plaque, which leads to secondary inflammation.

**277 Palatal recession (left)**
Due probably to tooth morphology and osseous anatomy, recession on the palatal or lingual surfaces is considerably less common than on facial surfaces.

**278 McCall's festoons (right)**
The attached gingiva in this case consists of nothing more than a collar-like, fibrous thickening. The arrow indicates the CEJ. This *may* be a tissue response to further recession beyond the mucogingival line. It is *not* an indication for mucogingival surgery!

Courtesy M. Ebneter

**279 Dehiscence of alveolar process (left)**
Orofacial section through an anterior tooth, as viewed in a radiograph. Remarkably little bone surrounds the tooth, facially and lingually.

**280 Severe localized recession (right)**
The root of this tooth has been denuded all the way down to the mucogingival line. The gingival margin is secondarily inflamed.

Following initial therapy, a mucogingival surgical intervention is indicated in this case (p. 307).

# Recession – Localized

A 26-year-old male presented to the clinic with a chief complaint of recession on his maxillary canines. His oral hygiene was impeccable; he claimed to brush his teeth four times a day. Neither a dentist nor a dental hygienist had ever observed his toothbrushing technique.

*Findings:*

HYG: 91%          PBI: 0.8

Figure 282 depicts probing depths, tooth mobility and areas of recession.

*Diagnosis:* Pronounced facial recession on canines. Initial generalized gingival recession.

*Therapy:* Instruction in the vertical-rotatory toothbrushing method (modified Stillman) using a soft toothbrush; repeated evaluation for gingival trauma.

Study models to document progression of gingival recession, should it continue. Mucogingival surgery should be considered only if the severity of the recession continues to increase.

*Recall intervall:* 6 months or longer.

*Prognosis:* good.

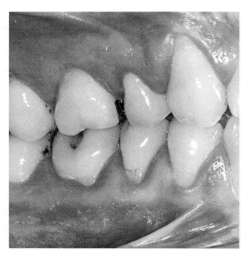
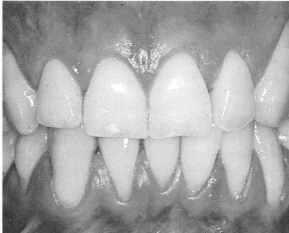
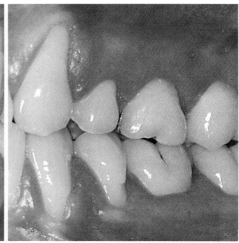

**281  Clinical picture (above)**
The recessions are of varying severity, with pronounced areas over the canines. The papillae still fill the interdental spaces. In the molar segments, mild marginal inflammation is noted. Tooth 35 exhibits a wedge-shaped defect.

**282  Probing depths, recession (Re), tooth mobility (TM; right)**

The classical recession is associated with neither pathologically deepened pockets nor elevated tooth mobility.

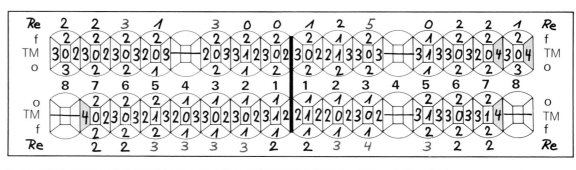

**283  Radiographic survey**
Facial osseous dehiscences are *not visible* on the radiograph. In young patients, no loss of interdental septal height is noted. Recession cannot be diagnosed using radiographs alone.

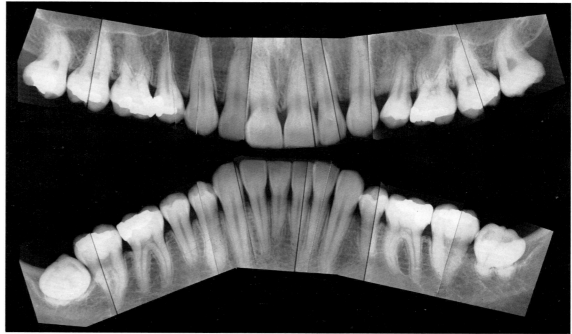

# Recession – Generalized

This 43-year-old female was worried that her teeth appeared to be getting longer. Wedge-shaped defects were in evidence on all canines and premolars; the patient experienced cervical sensitivity in these areas from time to time. She expressed the desire to have her "gum condition" treated if possible.

---

*Findings:*

HYG: 80%  PBI: 1.0
Probing depths, recession, TM: See Figure 285.
*Diagnosis:* Generalized, advanced facial recession. Mild

loss of periodontal supporting structure in interdental areas; shallow pocket formation but no hemorrhage.

*Therapy:* Change home care technique to vertical-rotatory brushing, modified Stillman; fabricate study models; monitoring at regular intervals of 3–6 months. If recession continues, mucogingival surgery with free gingival graft in mandible (p. 295).

*Recall:* 6 months or longer.

*Prognosis:* Good if secondary inflammation is avoided and proper oral hygiene is practiced.

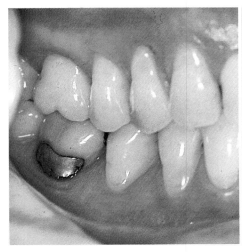
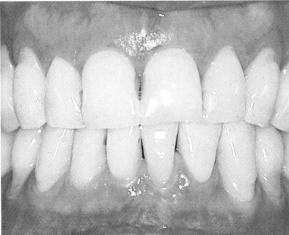
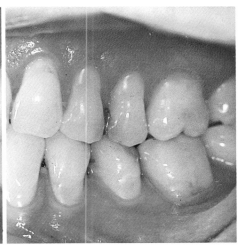

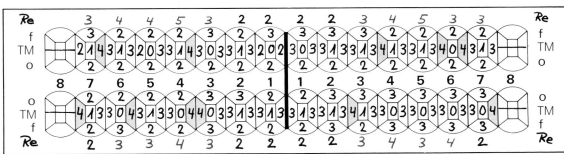

**284 Clinical picture (above)**
Generalized gingival recession is apparent in this middle-aged female. The interdental papillae have also receded slightly.

**285 Probing depths, facial recession (Re), tooth mobility (TM; left)**
In the mandibular premolar area, the facial attached gingiva is almost completely absent due to the gingival recession. In this area, attachment loss continued slowly despite changing the patient's brushing technique.

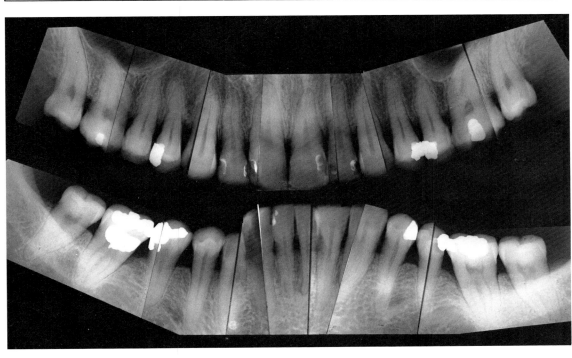

**286 Radiographic survey**
Mild generalized, horizontal reduction of interdental septal height is noted. The more advanced bone loss on the facial surfaces is not visible radiographically.

# "Destruction and Shrinkage" – Clinical Situations Resembling Recession

In addition to classic gingival recession, there are other forms of *clinically observable* attachment loss:
- *Recession of the entire periodontium in the elderly:* This condition is *not* the rule. It may be caused by mild chronic inflammation and shrinkage; it can be enhanced by improper (overzealous) toothbrushing technique or other iatrogenic irritation.
- *Recession with a superimposed secondary periodontitis:* This combination occurs seldom, because patients who practice proper oral hygiene usually exhibit neither plaque accumulation nor inflammation.
- *Destruction or shrinkage of the gingiva as a consequence of untreated periodontitis* (see also Symptoms of Periodontitis, pp. 84–85).
- *Condition following periodontal therapy:* "Long teeth," open interdental spaces and cervical sensitivity are often the uncomfortable consequences of treatment for advanced periodontal disease.

**287    Gingival shrinkage in an elderly man**
This 81-year-old man exhibited *no* periodontal pockets. The dentist had performed only restorative treatment.

The patient had taken care of the periodontal "treatment" by himself through vigorous brushing and a coarse diet (note wedge-shaped defects and abrasion).

Courtesy G. Cimasoni

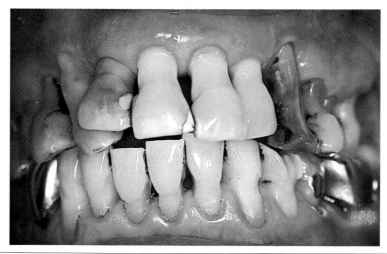

Similar clinical manifestations:
- at various ages
- with varying etiologies

81-year-old
---
Age

**288    "Recession" (shrinkage) in a case of untreated periodontitis**
This 32-year-old female with rapidly progressive periodontitis had 5–6 mm pockets in the interdental areas. In addition she exhibited 4–5 mm of gingival recession; thus, the true measure of *attachment loss* was 9–11 mm.

This uncommon degree of gingival recession appears to have been enhanced by improper toothbrushing technique (note wedge-shaped defects at cervical areas).

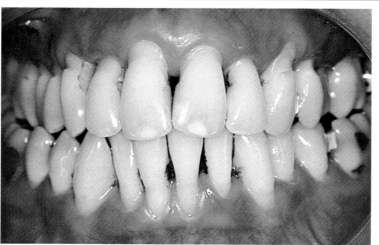

32-year-old
---
Periodontitis

**289    Clinical picture following periodontal therapy**
In this 36-year-old female with advanced, rapidly progressive periodontitis (9 mm pockets), the esthetic consequences of radical surgical intervention for treatment of the disease process are severe. The appearance is similar to advanced gingival recession.

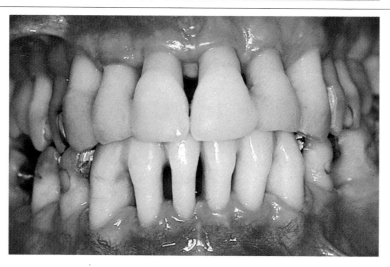

36-year-old
---
Therapy

# Charting – Diagnosis – Prognosis

## General Medical History

The examination of every patient must include a thorough medical history, which can be conveniently taken by means of a questionnaire. This is important for diagnosis of periodontal disease, for protection of the patient ("high risks," e.g., allergies, organ transplant, cardiac concern), and to prevent the spreading of dangerous infections (hepatitis, AIDS etc.).

## Specific History and Local Findings

Periodontal examination and data gathering provide information relative only to the clinical situation at the time of the examination. The course of the disease and its progression up to that time cannot be fully elucidated, nor can the future dynamics of the disease process be anticipated. For these reasons, the diagnosis and above all the prognosis must often be modified during therapy or at subsequent maintenance recall appointments (re-evaluation).

| Examination/Finding | Chart |
|---|---|
| **Compulsory examinations** | |
| Medical History ⟶ | Health questionnaire |
| Periodontal history ⟶ | Periodontal chart |
| Gingival inflammation (PBI, GBI/GI-S) ⟶ | Charts, rubber stamp |
| Plaque accumulation (HYG, HI) ⟶ | Charts, rubber stamp |
| Probing depths ⟶ | Periodontal chart |
| ⟶ Attachment loss ⟶ | Periodontal chart |
| Recession ⟶ | Periodontal chart |
| Furcation involvement ⟶ | Periodontal chart |
| Pocket activity (exudate, pus) ⟶ | Periodontal chart |
| Radiographic findings ⟶ | Radiographic status |
| Tooth mobility ⟶ | Periodontal chart |
| Minor functional analyses ⟶ | Periodontal chart |
| **Supplemental examinations** | |
| General medical examination ⟶ | Physician's report |
| Intraoral photography ⟶ | Photo status |
| Impressions for study models ⟶ | Study models, articulated if indicated |
| Sulcus fluid (SF) ⟶ | SF chart (measurements in 1/10 mm) |
| Microbial sampling from pocket ⟶ | Microscopic examinations (phase contrast) |
| PMN evaluation ⟶ | Laboratory report of PMN defect |
| Tissue biopsy ⟶ | Histologic evaluation & report |
| Major intraoral functional analyses (FA) ⟶ | FA chart |
| Major functional analyses including anatomically articulated casts ⟶ | Study models mounted in articulator, FA chart |

**290 Checklist of compulsory and supplemental exams**

### Compulsory

Periodontal charting cannot be performed properly using the dental charts commonly employed in general practice. A special periodontal charting page is required, often enhanced by additional charts for recording hygiene and gingival indices, functional analyses etc. Many such periodontal charting systems are commercially available. It is imperative that the *compulsory* examinations be systematically performed and recorded *for each tooth* in a logical and clearly arranged manner.

### Supplemental

In advanced cases, such as rapidly progressive or refractory periodontitis (RPP) and/or cases involving severe functional disturbances, it may also be necessary to record the optional findings as well (see chart, left). Which optional exam is to be performed will be determined by the individual situation.

# Probing Depth and Attachment Loss

The primary symptoms of periodontitis are loss of tooth-supporting tissues ("attachment loss") and formation of suprabony and infrabony pockets. Thus, the measurement of probing depths and loss of attachment is essential. The significance of these measurements is relative and not completely congruent with the anatomic-histologic relationships (Listgarten 1972, 1980, Armitage et al. 1977, Van der Velden & Vries 1980, Van der Velden 1986). The measurement of probing depths is nevertheless justified because "periodontal therapy" is often synonymous with "pocket therapy."

When a light force of 25 g is applied, the probe tip penetrates beyond the histologic bottom of the sulcus or pocket. In healthy gingiva, the histologic sulcus is about 0.5 mm deep, but the probe tip normally penetrates to a depth of 2.5 mm. If gingivitis or periodontitis are present, the tip of a periodontal probe may penetrate through the epithelium, through infiltrated and highly vascular connective tissue (with attendant hemorrhage) until resistance is met at the first intact collagen fibers that insert into cementum. Therefore, it is clear that the "probing depth" is also dependent upon the degree of health or

**291 Periodontal probes for measurement of probing depths**
The tip of the probe should be rounded and thin; the markings should be easy to read. Several examples of probe markings are:

1 **Michigan-O:** 3, 6, 8 mm
2 **CPITN:** 0.5, 3.5, 5.5
     (8.5, 11.5 mm)
3 **Williams:** 1, 2, 3, 5, 7, 8, 9, 10 mm
4 **CP 12:** 3, 6, 9, 12 mm
5 **GC-American:** 3, 6, 9, 12 mm

*Right:* Tips of the five periodontal probes listed above.

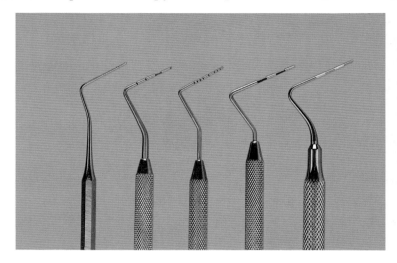
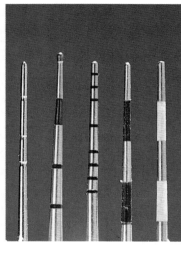

**292 Probing depth versus pocket depth**
This photomontage shows a periodontal probe (Michigan-O) in a shallow gingival pocket (cf. Figs. 294 & 294 L).

The pocket epithelium is perforated and the gingiva severely deflected. It is only the healthy collagenous fiber bundles and/or alveolar crest of bone that stop the probe tip from further penetration. The white arrow indicates the histologic bottom of the sulcus/pocket. The white open arrow represents the probing depth, determined in fact by the counterforce exerted by intact dentogingival fibers.

In diseased gingiva, the measurement error may be as much as 2 mm; in healthy tissues, less. This sort of error is not particularly important when performing the initial examination; however, for the "before and after" comparison, it may be of significance.

Courtesy *G. Armitage, N. P. Lang*

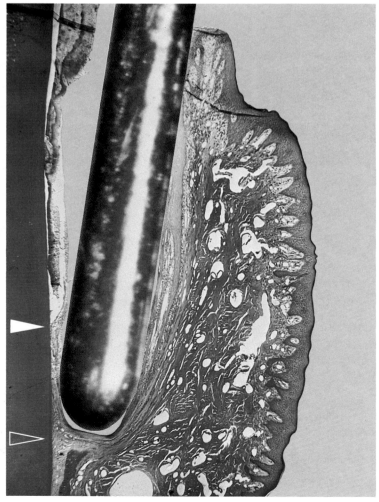

disease in the periodontal tissues. Probing depth will be 0.5–2.5 mm greater than the actual histologic pocket depth. For this reason it is more appropriate to speak of *probing depth* and not of *pocket depth*.

The measurement of probing depths provides information about attachment loss (AL; one may also speak of "attachment level") only when the gingival margin is at its normal location near the cementoenamel junction. Attachment loss will be underestimated if gingival recession has occurred, and overestimated if gingival enlarge-

ment is present. Clearly, true attachment loss must be measured from the CEJ and not from the gingival margin.

More important than the effective attachment loss is the expanse of the *remaining* attachment. This is directly dependent upon the length and thickness of the root, which determines the *area* available for insertion of collagen fibers, and can therefore only be appropriately estimated by combining clinical and radiographic observations.

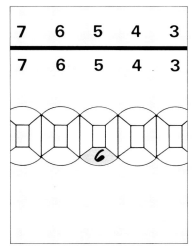

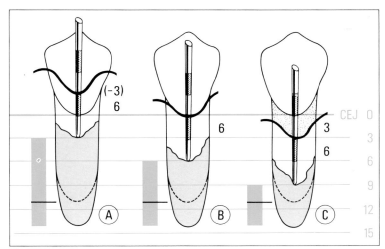

**293 "Probing depth 6 mm ..."**
This statement provides *no* information concerning attachment loss or how much attachment remains on a tooth (blue columns):

**A** 6 mm probing depth
 − 3 mm pseudopocket
 = 3 mm true attachment loss

**B** 6 mm probing depth
 = 6 mm true attachment loss

**C** 3 mm gingival recession
 + 6 mm probing depth
 = 9 mm true attachment loss

Root length may influence the clinical significance of AL.

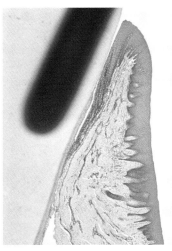

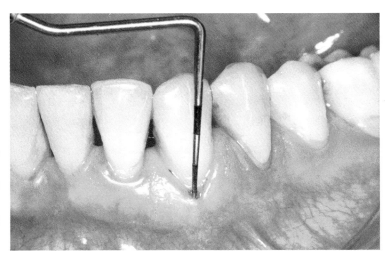

**294 "3 mm pocket"**
The probe tip extends beyond the sulcus bottom, penetrates the junctional epithelium and splits it. The internal basal lamina and several JE cell layers remain attached to the tooth. This splitting of the JE results in a reading of 3 mm for a "normal" sulcus depth.

The cellular turnover rate in the JE repairs such a split within 4–6 days by means of cell proliferation in the basal layer.
*Left:* The histologic picture with superimposed probe depicts the size relationships between junctional epithelium and periodontal probe.

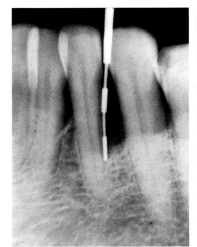

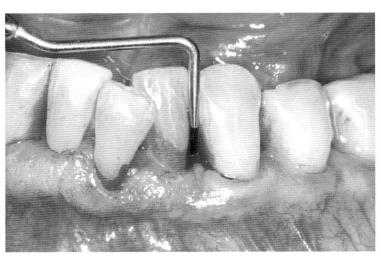

**295 "9 mm infrabony pocket"**
Even with light pressure (ca. 25 g) the probe penetrates beyond the bottom of the pocket and through the remaining junctional epithelium all the way to bone (advanced horizontal bone loss with incipient vertical defect formation).

*Left:* The probe tip has penetrated to the intact bone.

# Furcation Involvement – Root Irregularities

Treatment would be greatly facilitated if all tooth roots exhibited a round-oval profile! Very often, however, roots exhibit an hourglass shape. In the case of multirooted teeth, the practitioner must ascertain to what degree the furcation is involved by attachment loss. On the other hand one must also determine to what degree the individual roots are fused, a situation that often is accompanied by deep, narrow grooves along the root in the furcation area. Enamel projections and "pearls" in or near the furcation also deserve attention.

In addition, even the healthy root (*cementum*) surface is never smooth, rather it exhibits rough areas, and lacunae often occur in the apical region as well as in the furcations (Schroeder & Rateitschak-Plüss 1983, Schroeder 1986). In the presence of a periodontal pocket, root surface resorption may occur in the presence of granulation tissue.

The detection of such morphologic and pathologic peculiarities becomes more difficult as pocket depth increases and bone loss becomes more severe.

**296 Special probes for diagnosis of furcations and root irregularities**

- **CH 3:** Fine and pointed, paired left and right, curved. For surfaces and narrow grooves
- **Nabers 2:** Blunt, paired left and right, curved. For probing furcations
- **ZA 3:** Furcation probe. Similar to the Nabers 2, but with 3, 6 and 9 mm markings and color coding

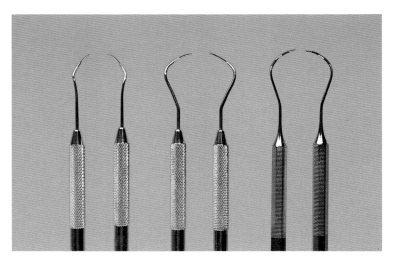

**Classification of furcation involvement: horizontal and vertical measurements (pp. 80–81)**

**Horizontal (Class F 1 – F 3)**

F 0 —
F 1 up to 3 mm
F 2 over 3 mm
F 3 through-and-through between two roots

**Vertical (Subclasses A–C)**

A up to 3 mm
B 4–6 mm
C 7 or more mm

**297 Section through maxilla**
This view, with the cut root surfaces colored red, clearly depicts the enormous variations in root morphology. The narrow furcations, root fusions and hourglass shapes of some roots can also be observed. The interdental and interradicular osseous septa are also of varying dimensions.

**298 Many forms of maxillary and mandibular molars (right)**
The roots were sectioned horizontally about 4 mm apical to the cementoenamel junction.

This view depicts clearly the variability of furcation areas as well as root fusions. It is easy to imagine the difficulties associated with root planing in such areas.

**299 Section through mandible**
Root morphology in the mandible is more uniform and less complicated than in the maxilla, but almost all of the roots exhibit some depressions labiolingually.

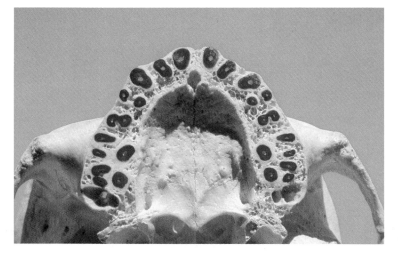

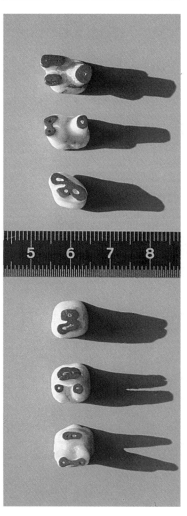

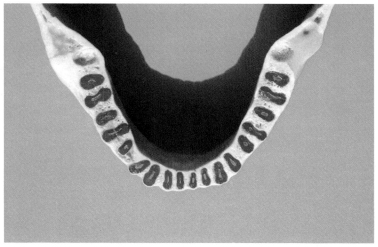

For diagnostic purposes, the blunt, straight periodontal probe alone is inadequate. Adjunct probes that are specially curved, blunt or pointed, are required.

It is important for the practitioner to ascertain the presence of root irregularities, because they represent potential plaque-retentive areas that must be dealt with during the course of periodontal therapy, for example during root planing. Furthermore when a flap procedure permits direct vision of the exposed root surfaces, the practitioner quickly realizes that Nature has even more morphologic fantasy than was perhaps apparent at the initial examination.

The radiograph can often provide additional evidence of root peculiarities, but cannot portray exactly the variations in root morphology that occur from tooth to tooth. The radiograph cannot replace a meticulous tactile examination of each root surface using a fine probe.

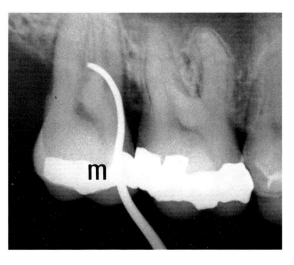
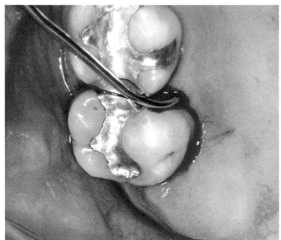

**Probing the trifurcation of tooth 17**

**300 "Mesial" furcation – m**
In the radiograph, no furcation involvement is visible. However, using a Nabers-2 probe it is possible to probe the interradicular area of tooth 17 via the mesial furcation.

The mesial furcation can only be probed with certainty from a mesiopalatal approach.

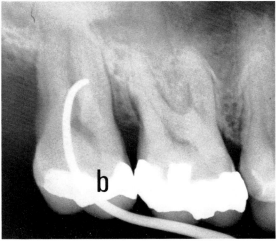
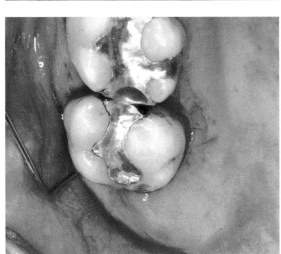

**301 "Buccal" furcation – b**
Through the narrow buccal furcation, between the mesiobuccal and distobuccal roots, the probe can also be guided into the interradicular area of the same tooth.

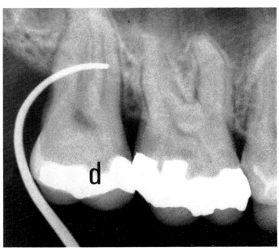
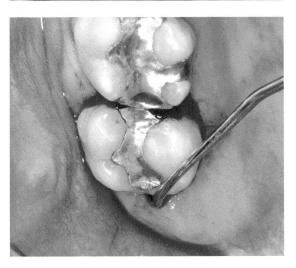

**302 "Distal" furcation – d**
When the second molar is the most posterior tooth in an arch, the distal furcation can be probed from either distobuccal or distopalatal approaches. As shown, the Nabers-2 probe achieves the interradicular area from the distal approach.

Thus, tooth 17 is shown to exhibit three different Class F3 furcation involvements: From the mesial, distal and buccal furca.

# Gingival Recession

Recession of the gingiva may be the primary reason a patient seeks dental care. Recession is easy to recognize during an examination of the oral cavity but a more objective assessment is required for recording recession in the patient's records. The extent of gingival recession is measured with the periodontal probe as the mm distance from the CEJ to the gingival margin. It also must be determined whether a normal sulcus or a pathologic pocket is present at the recession site. Pockets are rare in cases of pure gingival recession. The width of the remaining attached gingiva between the free gingival margin and the mucogingival line is of little consequence as long as no inflammation is present (Wennström 1982, 1987; Wennström & Lindhe 1983 a, b; Salkin et al. 1987).

However, a recession site where *no* attached gingiva remains is a significant observation, particularly when the mobile mucosa or frena extend directly to the gingival margin. The dentist also must clarify whether or not the recession is an esthetic problem for the patient.

**303 Attachment loss through recession – Toothbrush injury**
Recession on the facial surface of the canine is 5 mm (CEJ to gingival margin). The probe also extends 2 mm into the junctional epithelium. No attached gingiva remains in this area. Also absent is a McCall's festoon, which, if present, could be considered as a reparative attempt on the part of the host tissues.

*Right:* Bone loss on the facial surface cannot be diagnosed in a radiograph.

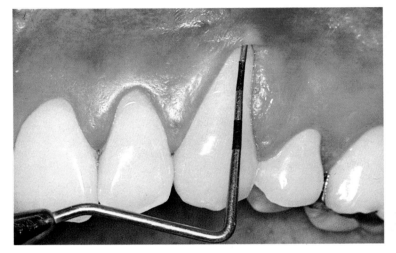 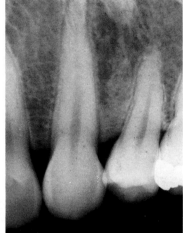

**304 Roll test**
Using a finger or a periodontal probe, the movable mucosa is pushed toward the recession site. This permits verification of presence or absence of attached gingiva, which will offer resistance. In this case, the mobile mucosa extends directly to the gingival margin.

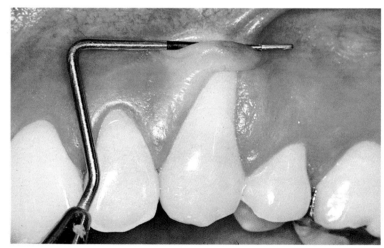

**305 Iodine test**
Gingiva and oral mucosa are painted with Schiller or Lugol solution (a solution of iodine and potassium iodide). The mucosa takes on a brown color because of its glycogen content, while the glycogen-free attached gingiva remains unstained. The iodine test depicted here reveals that *no* attached gingiva remains on the facial surface of tooth 23.

*Right:* Schiller's iodine solution.

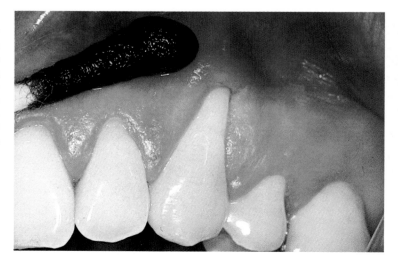 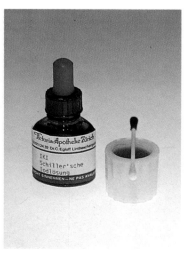

# Function – Tooth Mobility

A "mini" functional analysis can determine clinically the more important functional findings, such as premature contacts in retruded contact position, direction and extent of shifts during intercuspation, working side interferences, balancing side interferences, parafunctions (bruxism), TMJ changes, and habits such as lip biting, tongue thrust etc.

Parafunctions related to the patient's occupation should also be recorded, e. g., holding nails between the teeth, pencil biting, or playing a musical instrument.

The most important causes of elevated tooth mobility are *quantitative* loss of tooth-supporting structure due to periodontitis, and *qualitative* changes in the periodontal ligament due to occlusal trauma (Function, p. 325). It is important to differentiate between *increased tooth mobility* (stable increase; adaptation) and *progressively increasing tooth mobility* (unstable; pathologic). The degree of mobility should be entered in the periodontal chart (pp. 126–127).

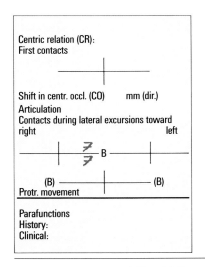

Centric relation (CR):
First contacts

Shift in centr. occl. (CO)        mm (dir.)
Articulation
Contacts during lateral excursions toward
right                                          left

(B) ——————————— (B)
Protr. movement

Parafunctions
History:
Clinical:

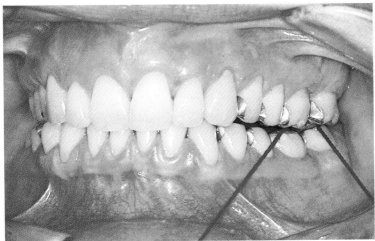

**306  Functional finding – Balancing contact**
During lateral excursion to the right, a heavy balancing side interference is noted between teeth 27 and 37; this is recorded in red on the chart (left). A thread will not pass between cusps on the balancing side during mandibular excursion.

*Left:* This finding is entered in section C of the periodontal chart (cf. Fig. 320). In periodontal patients the removal of such contacts is recommended (Function, p. 339).

## Severity of tooth mobility (TM)

**0 = Normal mobility**
   Physiologic mobility

**1 = Detectably increased mobility**

**2 = Visible mobility up to 0.5 mm**

**3 = Severe mobility up to 1 mm**

**4 = Extreme mobility**
   Vertical (axial) mobility, tooth no longer functional

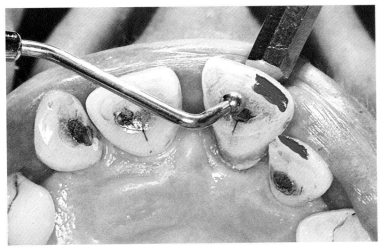

## Tooth mobility (TM)

**307  Tooth mobility test**
Increased tooth mobility is determined by applying a labiolingual force of approximately 500 g using two rigid instruments. As depicted here, the highly mobile tooth 21 can be displaced labially (note horizontal distance between the two red markings on teeth 21 and 22).

*Left:* Severity of tooth mobility is expressed using a scale of 0–4.

## Periotest – Degree of Attenuation (and tooth mobility?)

**– 8 through +9 = 0  physiologic mobility**

**10 through 19 = I  perceptible mobility**

**20 through 29 = II  visible mobility**

**30 through 50 = III  severe mobility**
   Tooth moves as a result of tongue or lip pressure

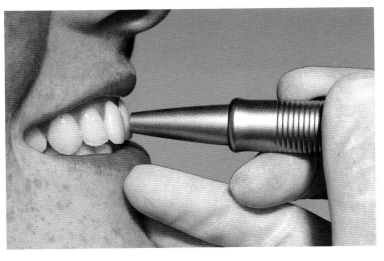

**308  Periotest**
In collaboration with the Siemens Company, *Schulte et al.* (1983, *Schulte* 1985) developed "Periotest," an instrument designed to measure the attenuation of implant abutments and natural teeth. Research is on-going to determine if this instrument may be used also to measure tooth mobility.

The tooth is percussed by a pestle 16 times (4 times per second). The degree of attenuation (scale range from – 8 through + 50) is recorded digitally and acoustically, then scaled into 4 degrees of tooth mobility (see table, left).

# Radiography

The clinical data described thus far *must* be supplemented by a radiographic examination. Comparative studies have shown that clinical measurement of probing depths and attachment loss does not always provide a complete and precise picture of the periodontal destruction. On the other hand, a diagnosis of periodontitis should never be made *solely* on the basis of radiographic findings. The two methods compliment each other (Schweizer & Rateitschak 1972).

## Extra- and intraoral radiographic techniques
*Screening – Panoramic radiography*

In recent years, great progress has been made in panoramic radiography. The slightly magnified film now provides a good overview of the dental structures, and often clarifies incidental observations (Fig. 310).
*Single Film Survey*

The panoramic film cannot yet completely replace the classical radiographic survey.

The parallel, right-angle technique using a long cone reveals the periodontal structures (Pasler 1985).

**Screening**

**309  Bitewing radiographs**
Depending upon the degree of caries activity bitewing radiographs are recommended every 1–2 years in children and adolescents. With the orthoradial technique used for bitewings, incipient proximal enamel lesions are detected earlier than with periapical radiographs.

When considering bitewing radiographs during periodontal diagnosis, the marginal bone should also be considered. Incipient juvenile periodontitis with typical bone loss in the region of the first permanent molars can be readily detected.

**Example:**

– **15-year-old:** Apparently healthy periodontium
– **20-year-old: LJP!**
  Osseous defect around the first permanent maxillary molar
– **25-year-old:** Progression of the untreated periodontitis, involvement of additional posterior segments: Post-juvenile periodontitis, transition to **RPP?**

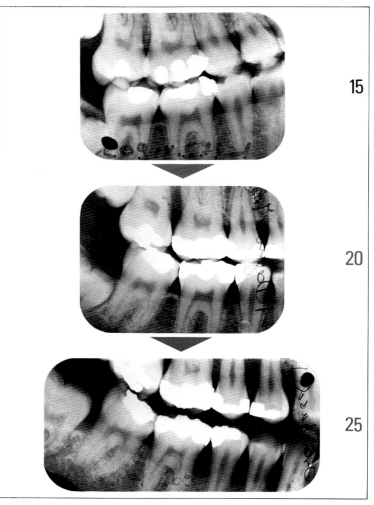

**310  Panoramic radiograph – Incidental finding**
Even though the diagnostic resolution of individual intraoral radiographs has not yet been achieved, the panoramic radiograph is of great value as a screening aid, especially in patients with a pronounced gag reflex. In terms of comprehensive dental care, any adjunct findings may be of significance in periodontology for diagnosis and treatment planning.

*Note:* Retained, severely impacted canine, large retention cyst (arrow).

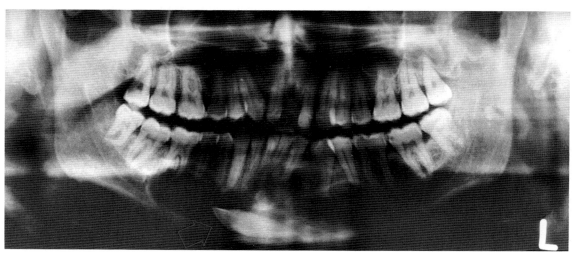

## Radiographic view of pathologic alterations and their causes

- *Distribution and localization of periodontal bone loss*
- Changes in the entire dentition
- On individual teeth (septa) and root surfaces
- *Type of bone loss*
- Resorption of alveolar margin
- Horizontal bone loss (with narrow septa)
- Vertical bone loss (with wide septa; p. 77)
- Vertical, cup-like bone loss

- *Extent of destruction*
- Distance from bone to the CEJ
- Furcation involvement
- Remaining attachment in relation to root length
- *Etiology of destruction*
- Supra- and subgingival calculus, iatrogenic irritants
- Tooth (root)-form and position (niches)

Radiographs depict destruction that has already occurred. Regular radiographic monitoring may clarify the dynamics of the course of disease.

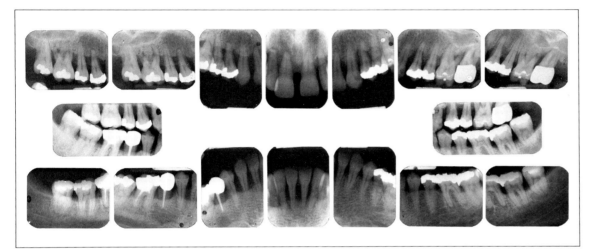

**Detailed radiographic findings**

**311 Radiographic survey for periodontal diagnosis**
At least 14 films are necessary for an unadulterated representation of all interdental and interradicular septa in a complete dentition.

This survey should be enhanced by two or four bitewing radiographs, especially in patients with restorations or crowns, in order to visualize iatrogenic factors most clearly.

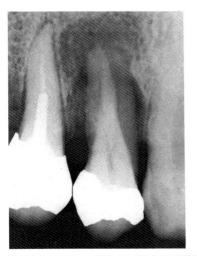
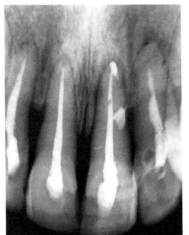
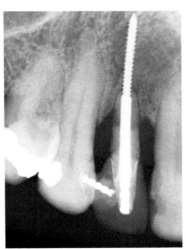

**312 Radiography – Special findings**
Endodontic problems are of special importance because, in combination with periodontal pathology, they can determine the fate of a tooth (cf. Endo-Perio, p. 311).

*Left:* Apical process, pocket abscess subsequent to pulpal necrosis.
*Center:* Periodontal bone loss extending on tooth 21 to near the region of a filled lateral pulpal canal.
*Right:* Transfixation screw (*Wirz* 1983) explains the low tooth mobility in the face of minimum osseous support.

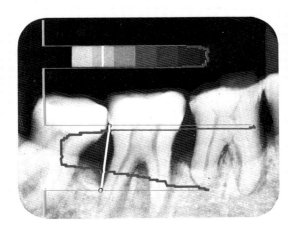

**313 The Future – Computer assisted radiographic evaluation**
Varying densities between two standardized films (e.g., findings before and after therapy) can be equalized by a computer, which will permit those sites with true differences to be discovered.

The film is scanned according to the gradation of gray. The measurement curve above shows the standardization using step-wise gradations (red portion above corresponds to the marked second field from the left). The measurements in a bony pocket are below.

# Photographic Survey and Study Models

Intraoral photography and study models are not obligatory for the examination of periodontitis patients. However, they may be useful for various reasons.

The *standardized photographic survey* (Bengel 1984, Wolf 1988) depicts the clinical picture visually in its natural colors and not merely in abstract numbers and indices as in the patient's chart. It can also be of use for the patient when changes occur during the course of therapy (reduction of inflammation, esthetics, tooth position, prosthetics, etc.; Freehe 1983). Intraoral photography also has forensic value.

*Study models* permit the measurement of the dental arch and the consideration of tooth form, tooth position and occlusion. Comparison of models over longer periods of time can demonstrate progressive tooth migration and recession; however, true functional analysis for prosthodontic treatment planning with individual maxillary and mandibular models simply placed one upon the other is not possible. These types of analyses and planning can only be accomplished following registration of interarch relationships on the patient and transfer of the relationships to an articulator.

**314 Photographic survey – Standardized**
The minimum survey (upper row of pictures) consists of three pictures: right side (**1**), anterior (**2**) and left side (**3**) with the mouth closed.

A survey including six pictures is more informative, and includes occlusal views of the maxilla (**4**) and the mandible (**6**) as well as an anterior view with the mouth open (**5**).

*Right:* Logos for the six standard photographs (*Wolf* 1988).

**Magnification:**
**2/3 x:** Photos 1, 2, 3 and 5
**1/2 x:** Mirror photos 4 and 6.

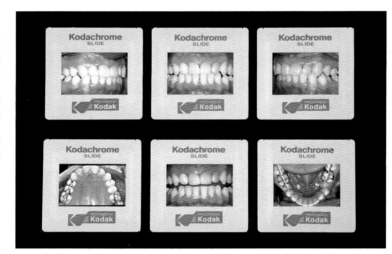
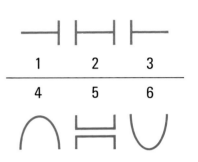

**315 Photographs ...**
Intraoral photography permits recording above all the color, form and structure of the facial gingival and the teeth. Tooth shape (mass) can be evaluated only on some teeth because of the perspective.

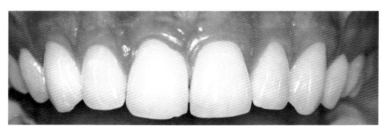

**... Versus study models**
In contrast to photography, the study model can be examined from all aspects (facial, oral, occlusal) in proper perspective. However, texture and color (e.g., inflammatory changes) cannot be evaluated.

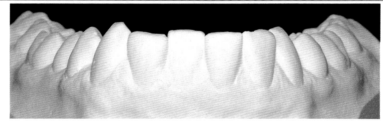

**316 Study models**
Study models are generally fabricated using dental stone and an alginate impression in a universal tray. Models permit the consideration of the course of the marginal gingiva as well as the shape and position of the teeth.

Since functional disturbances (occlusion, articulation) are of secondary importance in terms of the etiology of inflammatory periodontal diseases, stone models are usually not necessary for diagnosis in uncomplicated cases.

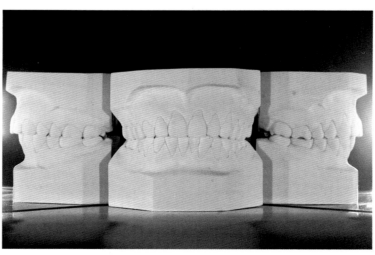

## Microbial Pocket Diagnosis – Dark-Field Microscopy

Based upon new scientific evidence, it was recommended several years ago that in addition to clinical and radiographic examinations for periodontitis (static summation of previous disease activity) the composition of the actual subgingival flora be ascertained during data gathering (Keyes 1978 a, b; Socransky 1977; Newman & Socransky 1977; Slots 1977; Listgarten & Helldén 1978; Evian 1982; Singletary et al. 1982; MacPhee & Muir 1986). This type of examination can be performed following removal of plaque specimens from the pocket directly in the dark-field or phase-contrast microscope.

Direct observation in the microscope is relatively simple and can be easily performed in the dental operatory. The method permits differentiation of subgingival microorganisms according to morphologic criteria and their mobility. Thus, in terms of diagnosis, conclusions about their pathogenic potential are possible to some degree.

The transfer of the microscopic picture of many motile bacteria onto a TV monitor in the operatory may have a significant *motivation effect* for the patient in addition to its value in diagnosis (Fig. 348).

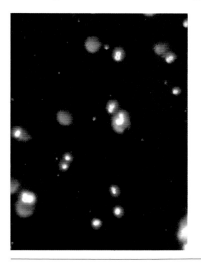 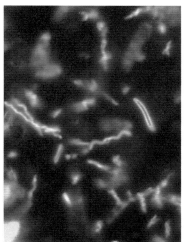 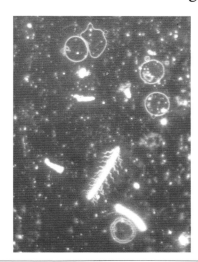

**317 Smears of bacteria viewed in dark-field of varying stages of pocket activity**

*Left:* **"Inactive pocket" – Cocci**
In addition to the non-classifiable particles, cocci dominate in an overall small number of bacteria.

*Center:* **"Active pocket" – Mobile rods and spirochetes**
These microorganisms and the higher density of bacteria characterize the "active" phase.

*Right:* **"Special Findings"**
In addition to cocci and rods, a "Centipeda periodontii" is visible.

## Bacterial Cultures – DNA Tests

The preparation of cultures makes possible the isolation and identification of specific cultivable bacterial species from subgingival plaque. This is in contrast to dark-field microscopy, wherein only the differentiation of morphotypes is possible. Using these methods (Slots 1975) and the immunologic and genetic engineering techniques that have increased the sensitivity of the methods, selective substrates have been used to identify and demonstrate the more interesting bacterial strains such as *Actinobacillus actinomycetemcomitans (Aa)* as well as Bacteroides species *(B. gingivalis, B. intermedius)*,

*Capnocytophaga, Eikenella corrodens,* and *Fusobacterium.*

The problem of how to successfully sample anaerobes clinically has never been solved satisfactorily; however, the problem can be avoided using modern methods which require *no* living bacteria but only their genetic material (DNA). Combined recombination tests for *Aa* and *Bacteroides* ($DMD_X$-test) are already commercially available (Hammond 1983, Dzink et al. 1985, Slots et al. 1986). The usefulness of these methods for the practitioner is doubtful however in light of the questionable nature of the "specific plaque hypothesis."

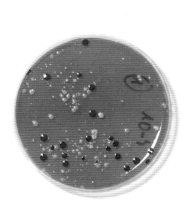 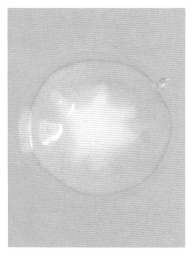 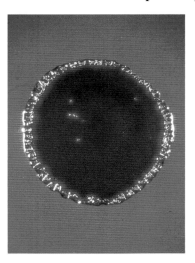

**318 Anaerobic bacterial culture on a blood-agar plate**
*Left:* Various bacterial colonies on a blood agar plate incubated under anaerobic conditions for 10 days. In addition to the black-pigmented *Bacteroides* colonies, many other bacterial colonies are visible.

*Center:* **Actinobacillus actinomycetemcomitans**
This colony exhibits the typical star-structured center.

*Right:* **Bacteroides colony**

# Diagnostic Charting – Chart Series I ...

Observations made during examination of the periodontium must be recorded in writing, schematically, radiographically and sometimes photographically or through use of study models. Such records are critical for treatment planning and for establishing a prognosis.

Diagnostic charting is also necessary for patient information and for the re-evaluation of a case following initial therapy, as well as for final evaluation and later comparisons.

Charts vary from school to school and even from practice to practice; in some countries, insurance com-

panies require the use of certain types of charts. Although it doesn't matter which particular chart the practitioner elects to employ, we present several possibilities for the recording of clinical observations:

I: Easy-to-use charts with numerical entries for:
– Interdental hygiene (HYG)
– Papilla bleeding index (PBI)
– A periodontal chart for the more important periodontal findings

**319   Charts for HYG and PBI – Measurement techniques**

**HYG:** Plaque in proximal areas is scored from the oral aspect in quadrants 1 & 3, from facial in 2 & 4.

*Right:* Plaque present (**+**)

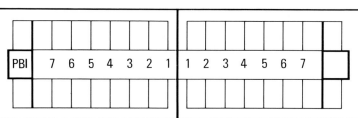

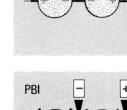

**PBI:** Observation of bleeding (inflammation) in the papillary region is made on the same measurement sites (cf. p. 37).

*Right:* The bleeding intensity is recorded in four degrees of severity (cf. p. 38).

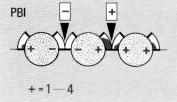

+ = 1 – 4

**320   Periodontal chart – I**
Universally applicable chart (Basle School, modified by Gressly; cf. pp. 87, 91, 95).

**A   Medical history**

**B   Periodontal findings**
Probing measurements in millimeters. Colors used in this *Atlas:*

   **0–3** mm = no color
   **4–6** mm = light red
   **7 +** mm = dark red
   **TM** = tooth mobility

Note spaces for recording recession (**Re**), furcation involvement (**F**), gingival width (**AG**) etc.
The actual attachment loss (**AL**) can be *calculated* from the probing depths and recession measurements.

**C   Functional findings**

**D   Etiology, diagnosis and prognosis**

**Measuring probing depth**
The bottom of the pocket is "sounded" continuously with the periodontal probe. The greatest values detected "mesially – facially – distally – orally" are recorded in the chart (4 values).

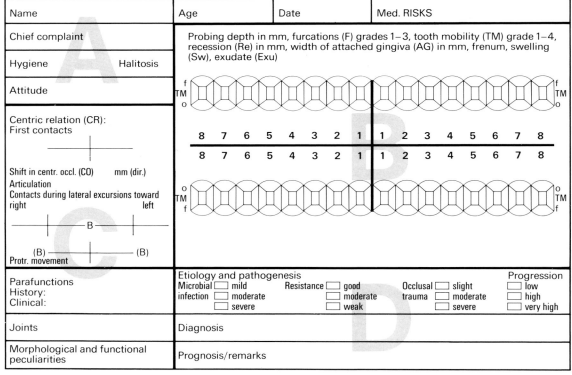

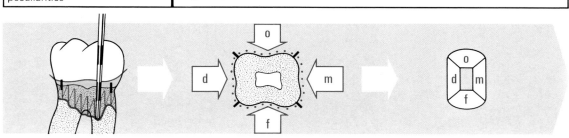

# ... and Chart Series II

II: This more comprehensive chart depicts:
- Plaque accumulation (Hygiene Index, HI)
- Observation of bleeding upon probing (Gingival Bleeding Index, GBI, as well as Gingival Index Simplified, GI–S
- A periodontal chart in which important findings can be recorded by sketching.

The gingival contour and the probing depths measured from the gingival margin are drawn in. This graphic representation of the clinical situation aids in visualization of the pathomorphologic situation.

## Diagnosis

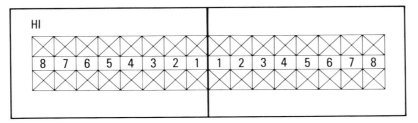

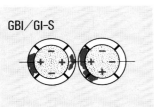

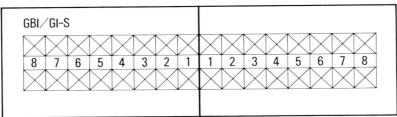

**321  Charts for HI and GBI/GI-S – Measurement**

**HI:** Presence or absence (yes/no decision) of plaque on all four tooth surfaces.
*Left:* Plaque along the gingival margin, independent of its expanse (**+**).

**GBI/GI-S:** The sulcus is probed completely around the tooth. If bleeding occurs within 30 seconds, the measurement is scored as positive.
*Left:* The four measurement sites per tooth in the chart. Bleeding (**+**) scored independent of intensity.

---

### Periodontal status

Name
Date

**Symbols for charting**
1. missing     /
2. food impaction    ↑
3. open contact    ‖
4. mobility    **0, 1, 2, 3, 4**
5. bridge
6. drifted/extrusion    **D→I**
7. beg. furcation exposure   ○
8. bifurcation exposed   ●
9. periapical area   ⊗

### Etiology

### Diagnosis

### Prognosis

**Systemic diseases?**

**322  Periodontal chart – II**
(e.g., University of Michigan, modified; cf. pp. 89, 97, 101)

**A  Legend** (symbols) for filling out the chart

**B  Periodontal findings**
Course of the gingival margin and probing depths are entered precisely in millimeters. This provides an excellent *picture* of the pattern of attachment loss.

**C  Etiology, diagnosis, prognosis**
The most important etiologic factors are recorded and a summary diagnosis is made. Statements concerning the prognosis are always subject to change.
Any systemic diseases that may be of consequence for the pathogenesis (host response) or for the therapeutic procedures are noted.

**Measuring probing depth**
The depth of the pocket is sounded continuously with the probe. The greatest values of the measurements of facial (mesiofacial – facial – distofacial) and oral (mesio-oral – oral – disto-oral) are noted (6 values are entered).

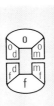

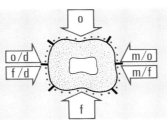

## Diagnosis

The recording of the general medical history, the special (local) dental history and all individual findings on the teeth and periodontium leads to the *diagnosis*. A differentiation should be made between the *overall periodontal diagnosis* (type and course of disease) and the periodontal single-tooth diagnosis (localized attachment loss, activity/inactivity).

Consideration of the clinical findings and the diagnosis then leads to a *prognosis,* which can be only temporary at this early stage. As with diagnosis, the prognosis is established for the entire case as well as for individual teeth (e.g., abutment teeth).

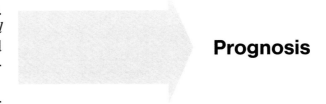

**Prognosis**

### General periodontal diagnosis

The general diagnosis is made for the entire patient:

- *Gingivitis*
  acute, chronic; hyperplastic; hormonal or complicated by medications; as a secondary manifestation of or caused by systemic disease
- *Periodontitis* (type, dependent upon age):
- – AP, RPP, LJP, PP
- – as a manifestation of systemic disease etc.
- *Recession*

The *general periodontal diagnosis* represents only the disease type present in the *patient*. However, it is rarely observed that gingivitis or periodontitis or even recession is generalized or equally severe throughout the dentition. Much more often one observes, for example, severe pathologic alterations on individual teeth, while others are only mildly involved, and others exhibit no pathology whatever.

**323   Chart for "single-tooth diagnosis"**

In addition to the periodontal diagnosis for the entire dentition (type of pathology and "average" diagnosis), each tooth should be considered individually. The recording of single-tooth diagnosis in a chart depicts visually the distribution of involvement and provides guidelines for the therapeutic emphasis.

– **Gingivitis**
– **Periodontitis, mild**
– **Periodontitis, severe**
– **Furcation involvement**

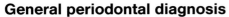

| | 8 | 7 | 6 | 5 | 4 | 3 | 2 | 1 | 1 | 2 | 3 | 4 | 5 | 6 | 7 | 8 |
|---|---|---|---|---|---|---|---|---|---|---|---|---|---|---|---|---|
| Gingivitis | | | | | | | | | | | | | | | | |
| Periodontitis, mild | | | | | | | | | | | | | | | | |
| Periodontitis, severe | | | | | | | | | | | | | | | | |
| Furcation involv., F1–3 | | | | | | | | | | | | | | | | |
| **Diagnosis for individual teeth** | 8 7 6 5 4 3 2 1 | | | | | | | | 1 2 3 4 5 6 7 8 | | | | | | | |
| | 8 7 6 5 4 3 2 1 | | | | | | | | 1 2 3 4 5 6 7 8 | | | | | | | |
| Gingivitis | | | | | | | | | | | | | | | | |
| Periodontitis, mild | | | | | | | | | | | | | | | | |
| Periodontitis, severe | | | | | | | | | | | | | | | | |
| Furcation involv., F1–3 | | | | | | | | | | | | | | | | |

### Periodontal "single-tooth diagnosis"

Every periodontal survey as well as the charts for plaque accumulation and inflammation (bleeding, pp. 126–127) include single-tooth findings in addition to an overview of the entire case; for example, probing depths around each tooth on 4–6 sites are measured and noted, or even drawn in schematically. Thus on the classical periodontal survey charts of a patient, each tooth individually may be considered and its individual diagnosis expressed in words.

Lindhe (1983) proposed the use of a special chart in which each tooth has to be considered individually in terms of the pathology surrounding it, for example various intensities of gingivitis and/or periodontitis.

Table 323 presents, similarly, relevant or determinant criteria for single-tooth diagnosis of importance for therapy.

# Prognosis

Determining the prognosis for a new periodontitis patient is difficult, and depends on a myriad of factors. A *provisional prognosis*, made after the initial examination and diagnosis, frequently must be modified during the course of treatment. Modifying factors would include degree of patient cooperation and dexterity, and the reaction of the host to treatment in terms of wound healing and capacity for regeneration. These factors are difficult to assess at the outset of treatment.

Generally speaking, slowly progressing adult periodontitis (AP) carries a good prognosis, while the less common rapidly progressive periodontitis of young adults (RPP) has a less favorable prognosis.

The case prognosis is based on consideration of the *prognosis for each individual tooth (maintainable, doubtful, hopeless)*.

## General prognostic factors
## Local prognostic factors

Of considerable value during formulation of a prognosis is a systematic approach and consideration of both *general* and *local* factors that impact positively or negatively on the case.

### General prognostic factors
- Systemic health, host resistance, immune status
- Heredity
- Etiology and type of periodontitis
- Age in relation to attachment loss
- Regularity of periodontal recall
- Patient's desires, demands, and ability to be motivated (don't overtreat!)

### Local prognostic factors
- Amount and bacterial composition (virulence) of plaque
- Speed of plaque formation, independent of quality and intensity of oral hygiene
- Depth and localization of pockets
- Furcation involvement (degree of severity)
- Activity of pockets
- Expanse of attachment loss
- Remaining attachment (root length)
- Type of bone loss: horizontal or vertical
- Tooth and root morphology, tooth position anomalies (plaque-retentive areas)
- Tooth mobility in relation of amount of bone loss
- Tooth mobility in relation to occlusal trauma

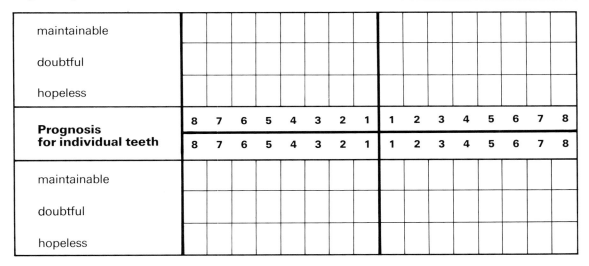

| | | 8 | 7 | 6 | 5 | 4 | 3 | 2 | 1 | 1 | 2 | 3 | 4 | 5 | 6 | 7 | 8 |
|---|---|---|---|---|---|---|---|---|---|---|---|---|---|---|---|---|---|
| maintainable | | | | | | | | | | | | | | | | | |
| doubtful | | | | | | | | | | | | | | | | | |
| hopeless | | | | | | | | | | | | | | | | | |
| **Prognosis for individual teeth** | | 8 | 7 | 6 | 5 | 4 | 3 | 2 | 1 | 1 | 2 | 3 | 4 | 5 | 6 | 7 | 8 |
| maintainable | | | | | | | | | | | | | | | | | |
| doubtful | | | | | | | | | | | | | | | | | |
| hopeless | | | | | | | | | | | | | | | | | |

**324   Chart for "single-tooth prognosis"**
A prognosis must be established for each individual tooth:

- **maintainable**
- **questionable**
- **hopeless**

It is worthy of consideration that an apparently hopeless tooth that is still in function and painless need not *a priori* be sentenced to extraction.

The single-tooth prognosis should be re-evaluated and revised following initial therapy.

## Periodontal "single-tooth prognosis"

The diagnosis of a case and the compilation of various single-tooth prognoses (strategically important abutment teeth) lead to a total case prognosis and will determine whether the comprehensive therapy will be *radical* or *conservative*, or perhaps only *palliative*.

If the prognosis is poor, especially in cases of rapidly progressive, advanced, active disease in a patient who cannot be motivated adequately, the practitioner must consider whether performing periodontal therapy is rational at all. In some cases it may be *better to perform extractions and treat the case prosthetically.*

# Prevention

## Maintenance of Health – Prevention of Disease ...

... are the noblest goals of modern medicine! For the patient, prevention is more comfortable, simpler to perform and, last but not least, less costly than treatment. The cost "explosion" in all disciplines of diagnostic and therapeutic medicine is enormous. It is scarcely possible to finance such costs regardless of whether socialized medicine or private insurance or direct payment by patients is invoked. Such ethical, social and scientific facts demand that we move toward prevention.

## General Medical and Oral Prevention

Prevention should benefit every socioeconomic segment of society and every age group. Children and young persons in particular should be exposed to preventive measures. At the same time, they must be educated as to the importance of their own responsibility in personal health care. Over the long term, it is really the patient's own desires and persistence that must keep his preventive orientation and behavior alive. This can only be expected if his doctor (dentist), medical auxiliaries, clinic personnel, public institutions etc. continually make known the possibilities and the enormous importance of prevention and thereby motivate the patient toward maintenance of health. Only through a coordinated massive effort can preventive goals be achieved. In general medicine there are many examples of pathogenic influences that are known to the layman. Preventive behavior is encouraged worldwide: Don't smoke, drink less alcohol, watch your diet, exercise more. However, too many people seldom go beyond making good resolutions.

In a similar manner, *oral* preventive measures including proper nutrition and good oral hygiene are acknowledged as important, but are also too often not carried out persistently over the long term. In addition, the life expectancy continues to increase; elderly individuals appear to be more difficult to motivate and they tend, generally, to lose some abilities in thinking and memory as well as manual dexterity (p. 362).

Successful oral prevention demands the recognition and elimination of all irritants that could damage the oral structures. Simultaneously, all possible attempts should be made to elevate the level of host resistance to the pathogenic agents or situations. The great successes in caries prevention may be traced to some degree to such elevation of host resistance, through fluorides. In addition one must consider the reduction of sugar composition, and plaque control by means of effective oral hygiene procedures.

## Prevention of Periodontitis

In recent years it has been demonstrated in well documented studies that prevention of periodontitis can be successful if performed consistently and appropriately (Axelsson & Lindhe 1977, 1981 a, b; Axelsson 1982). However, since it is as yet impossible to effect any elevation in host resistance (e. g., an influence on the immune response against marginal infection), such successes can only be achieved through local, mechanical measures. Prevention of gingivitis and periodontitis is similar to caries prevention in terms of patient motivation as well as recognition and removal of plaque by means of effective oral hygiene procedures performed at least once daily. The goals of plaque control are prevention of gingival margin infection, prevention of gingivitis and prevention of the initiation of periodontitis. The immediate future does not hold a "chemical toothbrush;" chemoprevention for long-term use remains an utopic goal. While effective plaque-inhibiting rinsing solutions are known (e. g., chlorhexidine), all are associated with side effects that prohibit regular long-term use.

In addition to oral hygiene by the patient, professional tooth cleaning (pp. 161–178) must be performed at regular intervals depending upon the susceptibility (resistance) and the hygiene status (plaque and calculus formation) of the patient. Prevention of periodontitis is and remains primarily in the realm of *individual* prevention.

From a somewhat broader perspective, prevention of periodontal disease encompasses several additional measures that are also targeted toward elimination of plaque, but indirectly. Included under this heading are elimination of natural plaque-retentive areas (crowding, etc.) and above all the elimination of iatrogenic irritants. An overhanging restoration or a poorly adapted crown margin make oral hygiene in the interdental area impossible. Dental floss is ineffective in such cases; it tears and becomes lodged in the defective restoration. The possibility for satisfactory hygiene in an individual patient must be created by the dentist and his auxiliary personnel. Efficient oral hygiene leading to freedom from plaque will only be possible if crown and restoration margins are supragingival, free of overhang and free of defects. The junction between filling material and tooth substance must be smooth.

The dentist's efforts in prevention of periodontal disease must, however, go beyond the correction of restorative inadequacies that represent plaque-retentive areas. The dentist must fabricate and insert only restorations and reconstructions that enhance prevention, wherever possible with supragingival margins. Perfect operative and prosthodontic dentistry is an important component of preventive periodontics.

An additional component of periodontal prevention is maintenance of the successes achieved by periodontal therapy. Proper maintenance prevents re-infection. If total freedom from plaque is an utopian goal, reality lies in defining for each patient an individual optimum level of hygiene (Hygiene Index) that can be maintained over the years. This will be dependent upon the patient's degree of motivation and above all the recall frequency. Many investigators have demonstrated that the gingival and periodontal condition does not deteriorate if the recall interval, which is established for each individual patient, is adhered to rigorously (Ramfjord et al. 1975, 1982; Rosling et al. 1976 a; Axelsson & Lindhe 1981 a, b; Axelsson 1982).

The prevention of dental pathology cannot be taken lightly. It requires time – considerable time – both from the patient *and* from the therapist. This investment of time is usually under-estimated; such underestimation can lead to a less than effective and consistent pursuit.

Effective preventive measures for gingivitis and periodontitis are identical to the "Initial Therapy" regimen described in detail on pages 145–178.

# Therapy of Periodontal Diseases

## Gingivitis and Periodontitis ...

... are elicited by plaque microorganisms. The intensity of the inflammation and the speed of periodontal destruction are determined on the one hand by the types of microorganisms and their interactions, and on the other hand by the immunologic response of the host to the opportunistic mixed infections (pp. 11–32).

The defense mechanisms of the host have as yet proved impossible to influence either in a preventive sense or therapeutically. Nevertheless, many investigators continue to state that the immune response of a host could be enhanced by medicines, nutrition, life styles etc.; in terms of periodontal pathology, however, such hypotheses have not yet been verified.

The maintenance of periodontal health and the therapy of gingivitis and periodontitis are to date therefore only possible through the reduction or *elimination of the causative microorganisms* from the tooth and root surfaces.

## Periodontitis: Goals and Concepts of Therapy

Clinical treatment of periodontitis patients has undergone certain changes over the years and decades as a result of the ever-increasing understanding of its etiology and pathogenesis. Early on, the primary treatment modality was surgical elimination of pockets (symptomatic treatment). Today "causal" therapy is targeted toward the elimination of supragingival plaque and subgingival microflora, toward the reduction of inflammation and the healing of defects.

*Theoretically,* this goal could be achieved through two basically different concepts:

---

**Medicinal therapy**

---

**Mechanical/instrumental/local therapy**

---

At first glance, *medicinal therapy* would appear to be a logical procedure, as with other bacterially elicited diseases.

In fact, disinfectants, e.g., chlorhexidine, are already in routine use *topically* as rinsing solutions.

In terms of *systemic treatment,* antibiotics (tetracycline) and other chemotherapeutic agents (metronidazole, ornidozle) could be prescribed. Because of their side effects and/or the possibility of resistant strains, sensitization etc., such medicaments should only be used for short time periods and only under well delineated indications. In some specific cases, they may serve as an adjunct to local treatment (pp. 314–318).

*Mechanical/instrumental therapy* remains today in the foreground. It can be categorized in two different concepts:

---

**"Closed" therapy – Scaling**

---

**"Open" therapy – Surgery plus scaling**

---

*Closed treatment* consists of debriding the tooth and root surfaces of plaque and calculus as well as root planing *without* reflecting a soft tissue flap. Thus, this form of therapy is rendered *without direct vision,* using only the sense of touch.

*Open therapy* is performed subsequent to the reflection of a gingival flap, *with direct vision*. The shape of the flap and its reflection is generally nothing more than a means to an end, and not actual therapy.

Open and closed treatment can be combined with each other or performed one after the other depending upon the severity of disease or the accessibility of the root surfaces. However, the one hundred percent elimination of all microorganisms is not guaranteed with *certainty* with any modality of therapy (Löst 1986, Rateitschak 1986, Vouros et al. 1986).

The course of periodontitis therapy therefore includes the following sequence of events:

1 **Initial therapy**
   **(hygiene phase, causal therapy)**
2 **Surgical therapy (corrective phase)**
3 **Maintenance therapy (maintenance phase)**

The goal of the sequence of therapeutic measures is a "clean tooth," a clean, biocompatible root surface.

## Therapeutic Success

The term "success" (or "failure") subsequent to treatment for periodontitis can be interpreted in many ways. A "healing success scale" ranging from wishful thinking to achievable treatment results would include:

**\*\*\*\* Complete regeneration**

**\*\*\* Healing of the pockets**

**\*\* Cessation of attachment loss**

**\* Elimination of inflammation**

**\*\*\*\*** *Complete restoration/regeneration of all lost tissues ("four-star healing"):*
This type of regeneration is only achieved following successful treatment of gingivitis (without attachment loss). The treatment of periodontitis generally does *not* lead to total regeneration of all diseased tissues.

**\*\*\*** *Pocket elimination via healing/repair:*
In the marginal soft tissues this results in formation of a long junctional epithelium and approximation of connective tissue to the root surface. In the apical regions, regeneration of bone, cementum and periodontal ligament ("true new attachment," partial "reattachment," pp. 136–137) occurs, along with shrinkage of the marginal tissues.

This "three-star healing" subsequent to periodontitis therapy should be regarded today as successful therapy and a desirable result.

**\*\*** *Cessation of attachment loss at its current position:*
This amounts to a stoppage of the progression of attachment loss in areas where pockets were in evidence, possibly by means of a long junctional epithelium. Inactive, shallow marginal pockets could remain. Tissue shrinkage does occur. In the case of very advanced periodontitis the therapist must often be satisfied with this type of "two-star healing." In such cases, at regular recall appointments the practitioner should check for symptoms of renewed pocket activity especially in residual pockets (reinfection), which would demand additional therapy.

**\*** *Elimination of the inflammatory processes (bleeding):*
This involves a reduction of the severity of inflammation and a certain degree of tissue shrinkage, without any periodontal tissue regeneration. Relatively deep, but inactive, residual pockets remain.

A "one-star healing" may nevertheless be viewed as a partial success. Such "success" descends into failure, however, if the pocket is re-colonized and reinfected with resultant renewed inflammation.

In addition to these primary goals of therapy, periodontal treatment also strives to achieve:

- improvement of gingival (and also osseous) contour, which simplifies plaque control
- creation of optimal functional occlusal relationships
- stabilization of mobile teeth (function).

## Recession ...

... has many causes. These are generally not characterized as pathology. If recession progresses continuously toward the mucogingival border, the consequences may be serious (pp. 109–113).

If a minimal width of attached gingiva remains, a simple adjustment in the patient's oral hygiene may stop the progress of recession (Mierau & Fiebig 1987; Wennström & Lindhe 1983 a, b).

In very advanced cases, in the absence of attached gingiva and with simultaneous marginal inflammation, mucogingival surgical procedures are routinely effective (p. 289).

# Therapy – Problems

The principle of periodontitis therapy is simple: Thorough cleaning of tooth and root surfaces. However, in practice it is associated with many problems:

- the irregular contour of the *pocket*
- the *micromorphology* of the roots and furcations, especially cellular cementum, cementicles, lacunae and resorptions (Schroeder & Scherle 1987)
- the *macromorphology* of the root with narrow furcations, root fusions, ridges, grooves etc.

Rarely is the depth of a periodontal pocket identical at all sites around the tooth. Usually some areas of the tooth are more involved than others.

The natural root surface is rough, especially in areas with cellular cementum and in furcations. It often exhibits cementicles and enamel pearls, and even in health some lacunae are observed (Schroeder & Rateitschak-Plüss 1983, Schroeder 1986, Holton et al. 1986). Cleaning of such plaque-retentive areas by means of root planing is difficult and time-consuming.

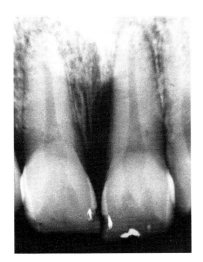

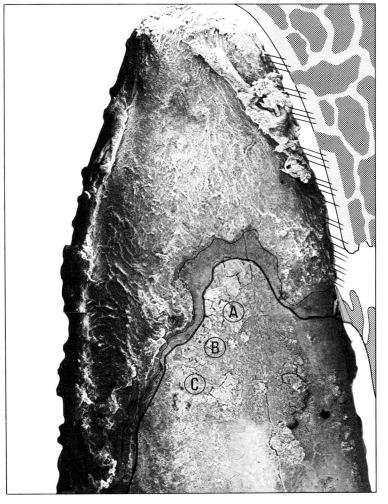

**325  Mesial view of the pocket contour in an actual case**
The left central incisor has a very deep pocket on its mesial aspect, while only minimum attachment loss is evident on the distal aspect (cf. radiograph, left).

The junctional epithelium that persists at the base of the pocket is marked in red. Its course is irregular and at one location is even "undercut" in the apical region. Toward the palatal aspect (left in scanning electron photomicrograph) periodontal structures can still be observed. In the center of the picture, the wall of the pocket represented by the bacteria-coated root surface is visible.

The difficulty for mechanical therapy becomes clear: On the one hand the bottom of the pocket must be achieved, and on the other hand any remaining soft tissue attachment must not be destroyed.

At the sites marked **A, B** and **C** the structures depicted below were observed.

*Left:* Radiograph. Tooth 21 was extracted. Its mesial root surface is depicted in this SEM photo (center).

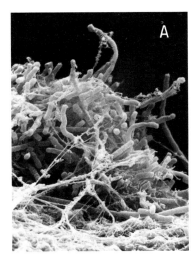
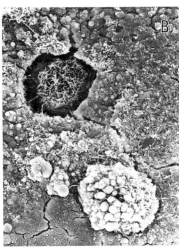
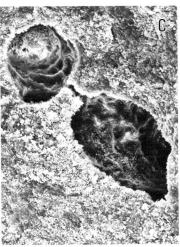

**Root surface in area of the pocket**

**326  Adherent plaque (A)**
Upon the root surface, which represents one wall of the pocket, a thick layer of adherent plaque is found.

**327  Lacuna filled with bacteria (B)**
This indentation (upper left) probably existed before the disease process reached this site.

**328  Empty lacuna on the root surface (C)**

SEMs courtesy *H. E. Schroeder*

# Periodontal Healing
# Reattachment – New Attachment

In recent years, the dental profession has moved away from the more radical treatment modalities (surgical pocket elimination) in cases of periodontitis. The primary goals of therapy today are elimination of the etiology by scaling and root planing, and enhancement of healing in diseased tissues. Numerous research studies performed during the last several years have provided answers to questions concerning whether or to what extent healing is possible in the form of reattachment or regeneration (cf. Schroeder 1983, Polson 1986, Karring 1988). Healing may be classified as:

1 Epithelial reattachment

2 Epithelial regeneration (new attachment)

3 Connective tissue reattachment

4 Connective tissue regeneration (new attachment)

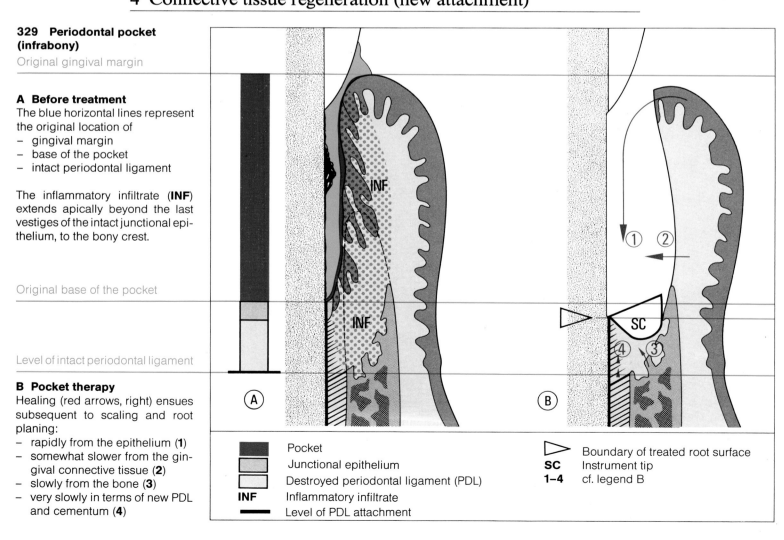

**329 Periodontal pocket (infrabony)**

Original gingival margin

**A Before treatment**
The blue horizontal lines represent the original location of
– gingival margin
– base of the pocket
– intact periodontal ligament

The inflammatory infiltrate (**INF**) extends apically beyond the last vestiges of the intact junctional epithelium, to the bony crest.

Original base of the pocket

Level of intact periodontal ligament

**B Pocket therapy**
Healing (red arrows, right) ensues subsequent to scaling and root planing:
– rapidly from the epithelium (**1**)
– somewhat slower from the gingival connective tissue (**2**)
– slowly from the bone (**3**)
– very slowly in terms of new PDL and cementum (**4**)

Pocket
Junctional epithelium
Destroyed periodontal ligament (PDL)
**INF** Inflammatory infiltrate
Level of PDL attachment

▷ Boundary of treated root surface
**SC** Instrument tip
**1–4** cf. legend B

## Epithelium

1. *Reattachment of epithelium (diseased or healthy) does not occur;* any healing or repair results from activity in the basal cell layer.

2. *Epithelial regeneration* ("new attachment," de novo formation) usually occurs after all types of successful periodontal treatment. Epithelial daughter cells resulting from mitotic activity quickly cover the connective tissue wound surface and develop into a new "long" junctional epithelium with a basal lamina and hemidesmosomes along the root surface (Listgarten 1976). The new epithelium generally covers the entire length of the treated pocket; this may explain why some investigators have observed new epithelial tissue *apical* to new bone that has formed (Caton & Nyman 1980; Stahl et al. 1982, 1983; Magnusson et al. 1983).

## Connective tissue

3. *Connective tissue reattachment* may be expected only in the most apical regions (infiltrated but *not infected*) subjacent to the junctional epithelium, where no mechanical treatment (root planing) has been performed. It is in these areas that remnants of periodontal ligament fibers and intact root cementum remain (see 3 in Figs. C and D, below; Listgarten & Rosenberg 1979; Nyman et al. 1982 a, b; Isidor et al. 1985).

4. *Connective tissue regeneration* (new attachment): Formation of new cementum with insertion of newly generated connective tissue fiber bundles may be expected after traditional therapy only in the deepest areas of the pocket, if at all (see 3 B in Fig. D).

Connective tissue accumulating postsurgically parallel to the root surface but not inserting into new cementum probably derives from gingival fibroblasts and not from periodontal ligament cells (see 3 A in Fig. D, below; Caton et al. 1980).

Whether or not conditioning the root surface (acid-etch, fibronectin etc.) or covering of the root with barriers (Millipore filters etc.) can enhance true connective tissue attachment during healing remains under study (Ririe et al. 1980, Cole et al. 1981, Polson & Proye 1983, Stahl et al. 1983, Badersten 1984, Bogle et al. 1985, Gottlow et al. 1986).

## Alveolar bone

New bone formation, whether detected radiographically or through a re-entry procedure, is not evidence of true periodontal regeneration with newly formed PDL and cementum (Listgarten 1980). This would have to be demonstrated histologically.

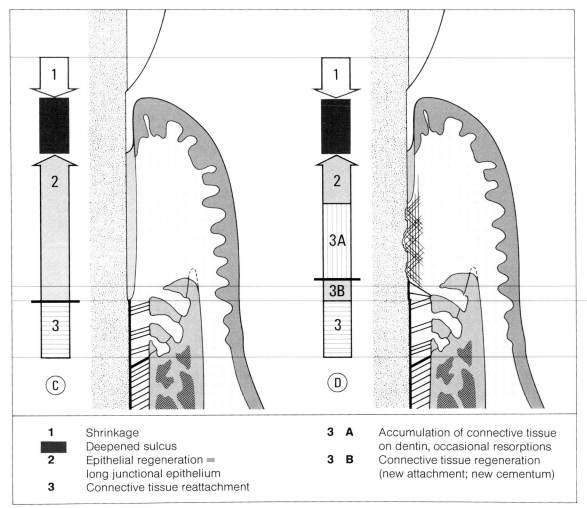

**330  Types of healing**
Healing can occur by generation of a new junctional epithelium (**2**), by connective tissue accumulation (**3 A**), connective tissue regeneration (*new attachment,* **3 B**), or connective tissue *reattachment* (**3**).

**C  Long junctional epithelium**
During the healing process the tissues shrink (**1**), cells of the oral epithelium grow out, contact the tooth surface and develop into a new junctional epithelium (**2**). This new JE continues apically until the first connective tissue fibers embedded in cementum are encountered (**3**).

Boundary of treated root surface

**D  Connective tissue accumulation, periodontal regeneration**
In coronal areas, healing occurs as described under C. Apical to the new junctional epithelium (**2**), collagen fibers approximate the root surface. Resorption of hard tissues is possible (**3 A**).

Formation of new cementum with inserting fibers (**3 B**) occurs seldom in the apical area.

In the most apical region of the treated area, reattachment of residual fibers may occur (**3**).

| | | | |
|---|---|---|---|
| **1** | Shrinkage | | |
| ■ | Deepened sulcus | **3 A** | Accumulation of connective tissue on dentin, occasional resorptions |
| **2** | Epithelial regeneration = long junctional epithelium | **3 B** | Connective tissue regeneration (new attachment; new cementum) |
| **3** | Connective tissue reattachment | | |

# Treatment Planning – Sequence of Treatment

Following any necessary emergency procedures, a thorough clinical examination and determination of prognosis, a case presentation is made. The patient is informed about the diagnosis, severity of disease, the necessity for treatment and the phases of treatment. During the case presentation the dentist should begin to gather the subjective signs indicating the patient's desire to cooperate.

The approximate time course for the proposed therapy and the expected costs are also discussed.

The *treatment plan* depends upon the following factors:

– medical history, clinical findings and diagnosis
– the patient's own wishes (don't overtreat!)
– the patient's interest level and degree of cooperation
– case prognosis
– financial wherewithal of the patient if there is no insurance or other third party coverage.

**331  Basic treatment plan**
Almost all periodontal therapy, regardless of the disease type, follows a similar general course.

**1. Initial therapy**
Creation of hygienic relationships in the oral cavity through the combined efforts of the dentist, the dental auxiliaries and the patient.

Subgingival scaling can then be performed. Fuctional disturbances are eliminated. The patient's cooperation is definitively ascertained.

After *re-evaluation,* one or the other of the following ensue ...

**2. Surgical intervention**
Correction of morphologic problems that persist after initial therapy, and treatment of the root surface with direct vision.

**3. Maintenance phase (recall)**
The recall interval is determined for the most part by the patient's level of cooperation and motivation, by the success of the active therapy, and by the type and degree of severity of the original periodontal disease process.

**A.** *Negative findings at re-evaluation*
If the patient's level of home care is insufficient or if the initial therapy did not achieve the expected goals, initial therapy may be repeated.

**B.** *Positive findings at re-evaluation*
If initial therapy alone has led to control of the periodontitis and if no morphologic problems are evident, the patient moves directly into the recall phase.

**C.** *Recurrent periodontitis*
If signs of active periodontitis are detected during a recall appointment, the patient's oral hygiene is monitored and the dentist may elect to re-institute initial therapy.

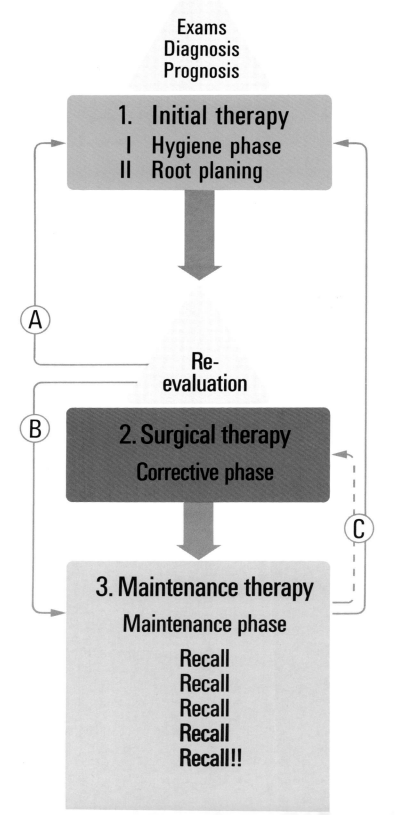

Exams
Diagnosis
Prognosis

**1.  Initial therapy**
**I  Hygiene phase**
**II  Root planing**

Ⓐ

Re-
evaluation

Ⓑ

**2. Surgical therapy**
**Corrective phase**

Ⓒ

**3. Maintenance therapy**
**Maintenance phase**
**Recall**
**Recall**
**Recall**
**Recall**
**Recall!!**

**Checklist of periodontal therapy**

– history and clinical examination
– diagnosis
– emergency treatment
– case presentation
– information and motivation
– provisional prognosis
– temporary treatment plan

**Initial therapy I – Hygiene**
– oral hygiene instruction
– supragingival debridement
– elimination of iatrogenic irritants
– elimination of plaque-retentive areas

**Initial therapy II – Root planing**
– subgingival scaling and root planing (+/– curettage)
– functional therapy I

– temporary restorations
– endodontic therapy
– orthodontic therapy
– temporary splinting

**Re-evaluation**
– definitive prognosis
– definitive treatment plan

**Surgical therapy – Corrective phase**
– ENAP – Open curettage
– modified Widman flap
– fully reflected flaps
– combined operations
– special surgical procedures
– gingivectomy/gingivoplasty
– mucogingival surgery
– postoperative care

– functional therapy II
– temporary restorations
– definitive restorations

**Maintenance therapy – Recall**
– check for pocket activity
– re-motivation, re-instruction
– plaque and calculus removal

– treatment of recurrent disease

# Schematic Plan for Therapy of Periodontal Diseases of Varying Severity

The five diagrams below demonstrate how the length, intensity and frequency of treatment can vary dramatically, depending on the type of disease being treated. In every case, initial therapy consisting of local debridement, oral hygiene instruction (OHI) and motivation is performed, while surgical intervention is reserved for only more advanced cases of periodontitis.

Systemic medication is employed as an adjunct to local therapy only in resistant and rapidly progressive disease (RPP), as well as in juvenile periodontitis (LJP).

**Symbols for planning and treatment**

△ Comprehensive data gathering and re-evaluation

△ Regular check-ups

| Appointments for initial therapy

| Appointments for surgery

| Postoperative care

R 1 First recall
Maintenance therapy

⬤ Systemic chemotherapy (as adjunct)

CHX Topical chemotherapy (Chlorhexidine)

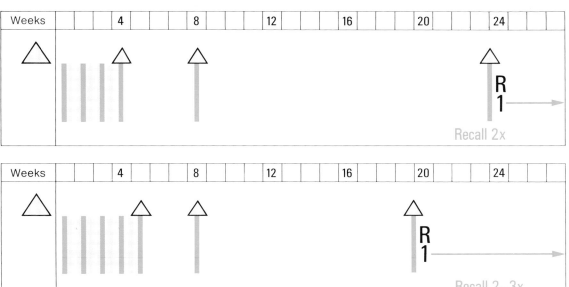

**332 Time frame for therapy (five examples)**

**1 Gingivitis**
Successful therapy for gingivitis usually requires only a few appointments for motivation, OHI and debridement. At the first recall shortly after treatment, the definitive recall interval is determined.

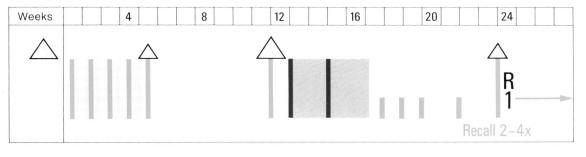

**2 Mild, slowly progressive periodontitis**
Periodontal disease in its initial stage does not require substantially more comprehensive treatment than does simple gingivitis. Debridement and root planing can be accomplished as therapy for the initial attachment loss. Recall 2–3 times per year.

**3 Moderate, slowly progressing periodontitis**
Following initial therapy, two procedures in specific arch segments are planned in this case. Immediately thereafter postoperative care in the form of repeated cleaning is provided. First recall at 2–3 months postoperatively, then a regular recall interval of 2–4 times per year.

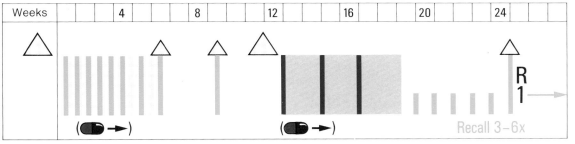

**4 Severe, rapidly progressive periodontitis**
Initial therapy can require 8–10 appointments. Subsequently three surgical sessions with appropriate follow-up are planned. Both phases are supported by systemic administration of antibiotics. The recall interval is very short, e.g., every 3 months.

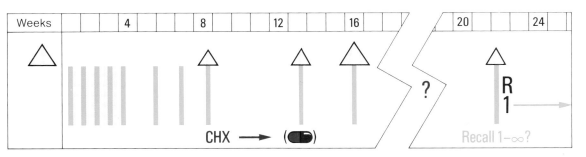

**5 Most severe, "hopeless" periodontitis**
Poor patient cooperation will hamper success. When the chances of success appear dim after initial therapy has already begun, treatment may have to be abandoned. Treatment in such cases simply involves frequent recall and palliative therapy.

# Individual Planning

In the preceding pages the basic treatment planning and the course of therapy for patients with gingivitis and/or periodontitis were presented. In contrast to other disciplines in dentistry (e.g., prosthodontics), the course of therapy in periodontology is, in principle, always the same:

---

### 1  Initial therapy
Hygiene, scaling, root planing

---

### 2  Corrective phase
Periodontal surgery, orthodontics, prosthetics

---

### 3  Maintenance phase
Recall, treatment of recurrent disease

---

These phases of treatment, however, may be weighted quite differently in individual patients. Also, in addition to the periodontal planning and treatment, all of the other necessary dental treatments must be simultaneously planned, and it must be determined whether they will be performed before, during or after periodontal therapy ("comprehensive dentistry," cf. Lang 1988).

## Treatment *before* systematic periodontal therapy

The medical history will reveal any contraindications to dental treatment. Any necessary medical treatment must be instituted prior to periodontal therapy.

Immediately thereafter, all dental emergencies should be dealt with. Abscesses must be drained, hopeless teeth must be extracted and, if necessary, temporary prostheses must be fabricated (esthetics, function).

Prior to actual periodontal therapy, any necessary endodontics is performed, especially in cases of acute apical involvement or questionable multirooted teeth. It must be determined whether any teeth must be extracted for non-periodontal reasons, e.g., periapical lesions.

Carious lesions must be filled *temporarily* in every case (e.g., glass ionomer cement). When it becomes clear that a carious tooth is maintainable from the periodontal standpoint, operative treatment can be carried out definitively.

Teeth that are severely elongated or tipped or have migrated or that create functional disturbances or esthetic problems should be dealt with by morphologic odontotomy. Oral mucosal abnormalities must be diagnosed and treated before periodontal therapy.

**333  Quadrants – Sextants**
Mechanical / instrumental periodontal therapy is usually planned for *quadrants* (**1–4**) or *sextants* (**S1–S6**) for either the right or left side of the dentition.

In very severe cases only two or three teeth may be treated at a single appointment; on the other hand in mild or moderate cases, two quadrants or up to three sextants may be treated during one appointment. Whenever possible, the patient should be left, after surgery, with one non-treated side (chewing function).

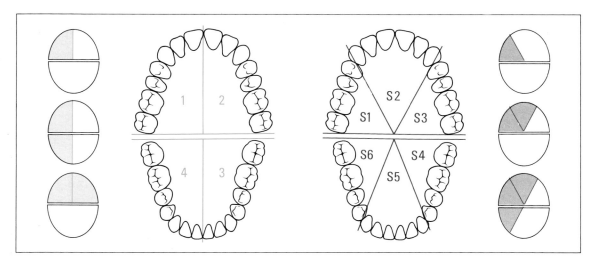

## Treatment *during* periodontal therapy

Generally speaking, during the course of systematic periodontal therapy, no other (e.g., reconstructive) treatments are performed. However, during a waiting period, e.g., between conclusion of initial therapy and re-evaluation, definitive operative treatment on certain teeth may be performed.

## Treatment *following* periodontal therapy

Definitive removable or fixed prosthetic reconstructions should be undertaken only *after* periodontal therapy. In every case, a waiting period (consolidation) of several months should occur between termination of periodontal therapy and initiation of definitive reconstructive dentistry.

## Detailed planning of the periodontal therapy

The actual periodontal therapy must be planned in detail for each individual patient. Depending upon the severity of the case, the age of the patient and his physical and psychological constitution (and the wishes of the patient), periodontal therapy is carried out in smaller or larger steps. Subsequent to gross debridement, patient motivation and oral hygiene instruction, subgingival scaling and root planing are performed. Necessary surgery is accomplished by *sextant* or *quadrant*.

# Emergency Treatment

Many periodontitis patients are not aware of their disease. Only when an acute exacerbation occurs do they seek out a dentist. Periodontal emergencies should be handled immediately after the medical history is taken (anticoagulants? focal infection? allergies?).

A succinct clinical and radiographic examination must also be performed for such emergency patients, most of whom present with pain. The consequences of more radical or conservative treatment should be discussed briefly with the patient.

Examples of periodontal emergency situations and treatment include:

| |
|---|
| Topical medicinal and mechanical therapy (ANUG/P) |
| Treatment of acute, suppurating pockets |
| Opening periodontal abscesses |
| Immediate extraction of hopelessly mobile teeth that cannot be maintained |
| Treatment of accidental periodontal trauma |

Periodontitis with superimposed acute *necrotizing ulcerative gingivitis* (ANUG/P) is painful and progresses very rapidly. Treatment is often instituted on an emergency basis. Careful instrumentation and application of topical agents generally bring relief within a few hours and a reduction of the acute situation. *Caution:* Ulceration may be a symptom of HIV-seropositivity (WR stages 5 & 6).

*Active suppurating pockets* generally are not painful if drainage is established at the gingival margin (exception: abscess). Such pockets represent an exacerbating inflammatory disease process, which leads to rapid attachment loss. They must be treated immediately with application of rinsing solutions; mechanical cleansing must eventually also be instituted.

*Periodontal abscesses* are usually very painful. They must be drained immediately. This can usually be accomplished via probing from the gingival margin.

In the case of molars with deep pockets or furcation involvement an abscess that penetrates the bone may develop subperiosteally. These cannot always be reached via the gingival margin, and must be drained by means of an incision.

*Immediate extractions:* Acute pain is not an indication for immediate extraction. Extractions should be reserved for teeth that cannot be maintained or are highly mobile or which cause the patient undue discomfort. In the case of anterior teeth, for esthetic reasons, extractions should be avoided when possible, or an immediate temporary should be prepared.

*Acute, endodontic/periodontal processes* have a more favorable prognosis if the primary problem is of endodontic origin. The root canal should be treated first, subsequently the pocket (pp. 311–313).

*Accidental periodontal trauma* usually requires immediate splinting, subsequent to any necessary reimplantation or repositioning of the tooth. If a traumatized tooth already exhibits periodontal destruction, its maintainability should be carefully evaluated.

**334 Emergency situation: Acute necrotizing ulcerative gingivitis (ANUG)**
The severe pain in the acute stage permits only a very careful peripheral attempt at cleansing.

Following gentle debridement with 3% hydrogen peroxide, a combined cortisone/antibiotic ointment may be applied with cotton pellets or a blunt cannula.

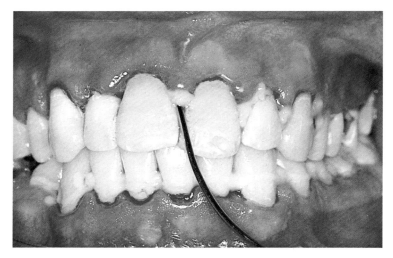

**335 After emergency treatment – Subacute stage**
Several days after gentle topical application of medicaments and emergency debridement the signs of active ANUG have subsided.

Treatment by means of systematic subgingival scaling can now proceed. A gingivoplasty may be indicated subsequently.

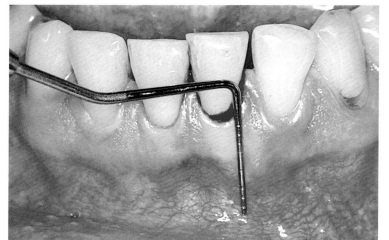

**336 Emergency situation: Localized acute pocket**
Tooth 31 is vital and should be maintained despite the 10 mm pocket. Very little pus has formed; drainage via the gingival margin appears possible. The tooth is slightly percussion sensitive. Prior to systematic mechanical treatment the tooth is treated on an emergency basis with topical application of a medicament.

*Right:* The radiograph reveals that about one-fourth of the root is still anchored in alveolar bone.

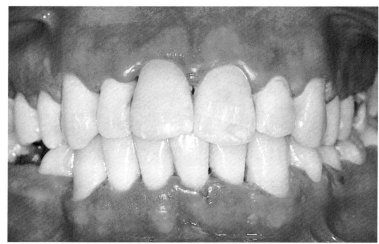

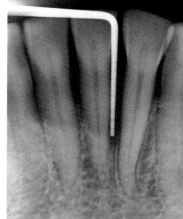

**337 Emergency treatment using local medicament, and follow-up**
As an emergency measure the pocket was first rinsed thoroughly with chlorhexidine and then filled with achromycin ointment (3%). Once the acute symptoms subside, a thorough root planing can be performed.

*Right:* Eight weeks after emergency therapy, the gingiva has shrunk somewhat. Probing depth is now only ca. 3 mm.

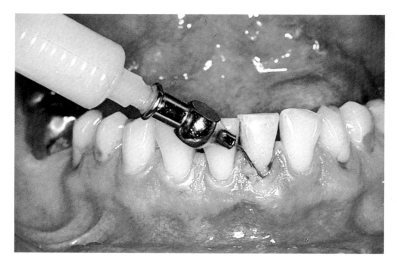

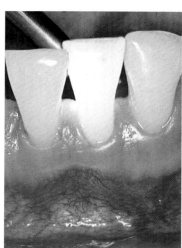

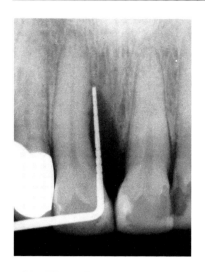
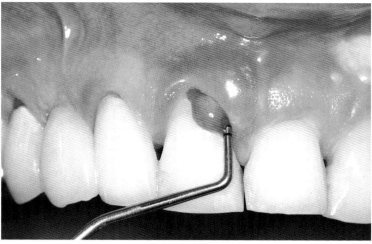

### 338 Emergency situation: Pocket abscess – Drainage from pocket
Originating from a deep pocket mesial to tooth 11, a periodontal abscess has formed. Copious pus exudes when the pocket is probed.

*Left:* The radiograph depicts the periodontal probe inserted to the bottom of the osseous defect.

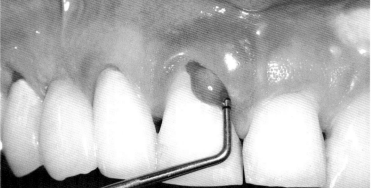

### 339 Emergency treatment using topical medicament
The abscess has opened via the gingival margin. The pocket is first thoroughly rinsed (0.9% NaCl, CHX etc.), then filled with an antibiotic-containing ointment.

Once the acute symptoms have subsided definitive therapy including closed or open root planing can be undertaken.

*Left:* Radiograph 6 months after definitive therapy: New bone formation is apparent.

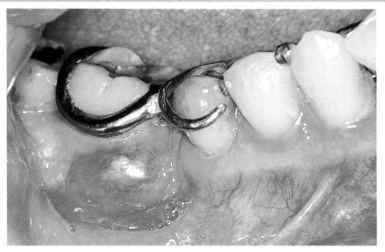

### 340 Emergency situation: Pocket abscess – Buccal drainage
Originating from the deep infrabony pocket mesial to the tipped tooth 47, an abscess has developed. The buccal gingiva is distended as the abscess is about to penetrate the mucosa.

Tooth 47 is an abutment for a removable partial denture that is ill-fitting.

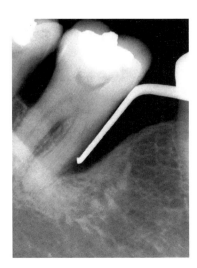
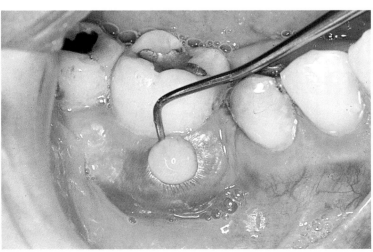

### 341 Abscess – Drainage
As soon as the mucosa was touched gently with a probe, the abscess opened immediately and pus exuded.

*Left:* In the radiograph one observes the deep mesial periodontal pocket with a hoe scaler in situ. Since the furcation appears not to be involved it is possible to consider maintaining this tooth, which is an abutment for a removal partial denture.

**342 Emergency situation in posterior segment:
Hopeless molar (37)**
Pus exudes spontaneously from the deep distal pocket and the buccal furcation around tooth 37. The tooth is vital, highly mobile and painful to the slightest touch.

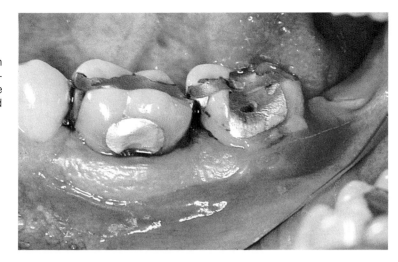

**343 Radiograph of 37 before extraction**
The periodontal probe can be inserted almost to the root apex in the deep facial pocket. Without clinical probing, such a defect at this location would be almost impossible to detect. The shape of the furcation is very unfavorable in terms of treatment; the two roots appear to fuse apically.

*Right:* Highly infiltrated granulation tissue remains attached to the tooth after extraction.

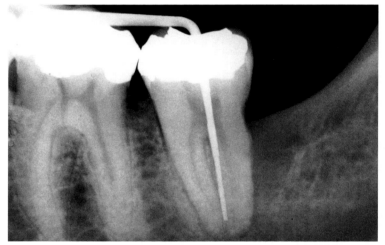
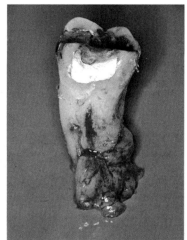

**344 Emergency situation in anterior area:
Hopeless tooth 11 – Fistula**
A fistula from the deep pocket has developed. The non-vital tooth is highly mobile and sensitive to percussion. Apical lesion is contiguous with extensive periodontal involvement. This tooth cannot be saved; it should be extracted immediately.
*Right:* The radiograph shows that a probe can be carefully inserted far beyond the apex (Endo-Perio, p. 311).

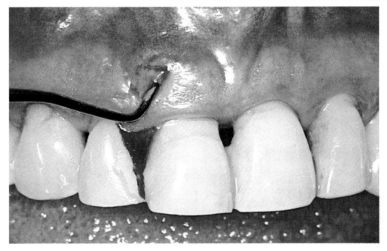
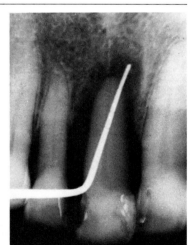

**345 Immediate extraction – Immediate temporary**
An immediate temporary is necessary for esthetics. Following extraction the root is severed and the crown is used as a temporary. A wire and acid-etched resin secure the crown to the adjacent teeth. This type of temporary can generally be maintained until periodontal therapy is completed.

*Right:* Radiographic view of the temporary replacement consisting of the patient's own tooth crown and a wire retainer.

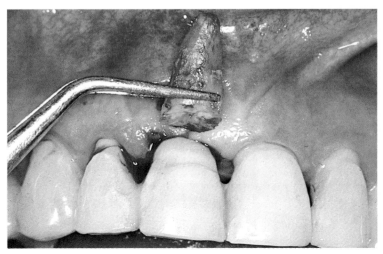
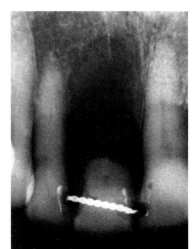

# Initial Therapy

The causes of gingivitis and periodontitis are acknowledged to be microorganisms and their metabolic products. The first goal of prevention and treatment must therefore be the creation of an oral cavity that is as free of plaque and calculus as possible. The term "initial therapy" is used to describe the various procedures that are used to achieve this goal. Thus, initial therapy is truly therapy aimed at the etiology of the disease process.

Initial therapy can be divided into two phases:

## Initial Therapy I – Hygiene

Patient motivation

Oral hygiene instruction and monitoring

Possible chemical plaque control

Supragingival plaque and calculus removal

Removal of iatrogenic irritants

Removal of naturally-occurring plaque-retentive areas

## Initial Therapy II – Pocket treatment, root planing

Subgingival plaque and calculus removal
(scaling, root planing)

Soft tissue curettage as appropriate

*Every patient* must traverse initial therapy. For gingivitis and even for mild periodontitis, initial therapy is often the only treatment necessary. Since the clinical procedures are usually simple, but time-consuming, they are delegated as much as possible to auxiliary personnel such as the dental hygienist or dental assistant. Each phase of initial therapy is performed under the dentist's direct supervision.

Functional therapy and any temporary splinting that may be necessary during initial therapy II must be performed by the dentist.

Re-evaluation of the case is performed some months subsequent to completion of initial therapy. Of special importance are symptoms of disease activity such as gingival bleeding, probing depths (residual pockets) and plaque accumulation (oral hygiene).

Post-initial therapy re-evaluation provides a check not only upon the success of treatment but also on the patient's level of cooperation in home care. A successful result after initial therapy depends in great measure upon the patient's level of motivation and the intensity of his cooperation.

# Motivation – Information

Maintenance, or restoration, of periodontal health *is* possible. However, this goal can only be achieved through a successful *cooperative* effort between dentist and patient. The patient must be interested in maintaining the health of his oral cavity, and must acknowledge the necessity for treatment. The patient must be motivated to work toward these goals. It is unfortunate that even today we still do not possess a scientifically proven method that will ensure patient motivation and interest (Sheiham 1977). Whether or not a patient can be motivated will depend on many factors including personality,

behavior patterns, intelligence, socioeconomic status, and the patient's own appraisal of his body and its general health.

The most important prerequisite for successful patient motivation is a trusting relationship between patient and dentist. An additional factor is the amount of time dedicated to patient education: *No patient can be motivated in only a few minutes!*

The recommendations presented here have their bases in practical clinical experience, and not necessarily in the scientific literature:

**346 Motivation during the initial examination**
The patient watches in a mirror as the dentist performs the Papilla Bleeding Index. The patient can hear as the PBI scores are dictated and entered into the chart (p. 37, Fig. 76).
*Right:* Upon probing, the papilla between teeth 43 and 42 bleeds (score 2).

The patient is quick to recognize diseased (bleeding) from healthy (non-bleeding) gingiva, especially in the anterior area.

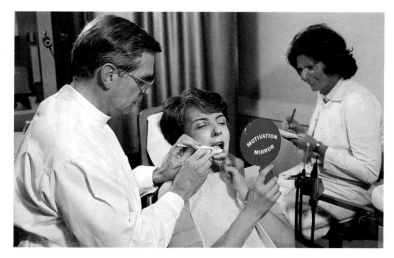
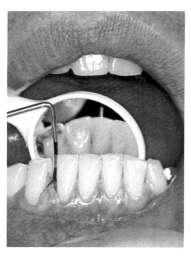

**347 Motivation with printed materials**
With the aid of modern informative brochures as well as one's own photographic materials, a dentist can effectively inform the interested patient about periodontal problems. Any discussion of the various treatment phases that are planned will be enhanced by the use of such printed material.

*Only an informed patient is a motivated patient!*

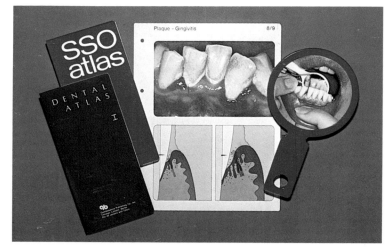

**348 Motivation with the "Plakoscope"**
The periodontal probe is used to remove a small amount of subgingival plaque, which is observed under the phase-contrast microscope. The bacterial colonization of any area of the dentition can be clearly demonstrated to the patient.

In this smear, the monitor reveals primarily filamentous organisms.

*Right:* A smear from an active pocket exhibits enormous numbers of motile spirochetes and several rods.

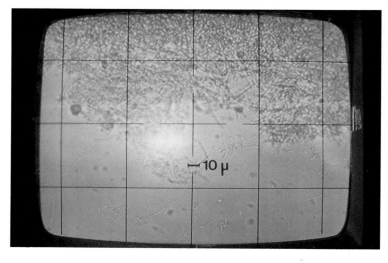
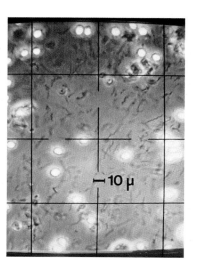

– Demonstration of bleeding gingiva during the recording of a gingivitis index
– Explanation of the symptoms of gingivitis and periodontitis using pictures and other visual aids
– Presentation of the patient's own case using the records taken during examination, especially the probing depth chart and the radiographs
– Demonstration of plaque using disclosing agents, and explanation of the microbial etiology of bleeding and inflammation ("local infectious disease").

– Presentation of the patient's "own" bacteria by means of microscope and TV monitor ("Plakoscope")

The symptom of gingival hemorrhage has achieved heightened status as a motivating factor in recent years. Using the PBI (Saxer & Mühlemann 1975, Mühlemann 1978), or the GBI (Ainamo & Bay 1975), the severity of gingival inflammation can be evaluated numerically. If the bleeding index score decreases continually during initial therapy, it will serve as a motivating factor for the patient.

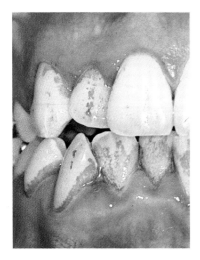
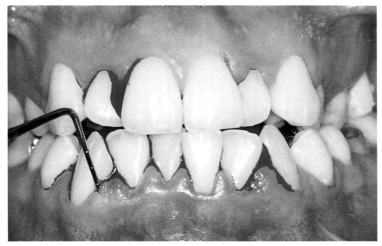

**PBI as a motivating factor**

**349   Initial finding: Moderate gingivitis**
The patient observes heavy bleeding as the PBI is recorded.

*Left:* Thereafter, a plaque-disclosing agent is used to demonstrate to the patient the cause of the bleeding he has just witnessed.
    The next step is oral hygiene instruction (OHI) and a professional cleaning of the teeth by the dentist or hygienist.

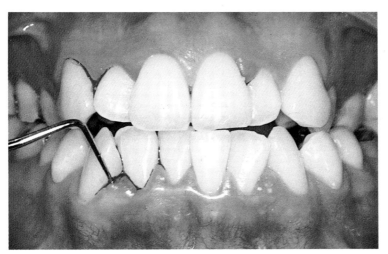

**350   Clinical situation 2 weeks later**
After prophylaxis and repeated OHI, the patient can *visualize* the improvement in his gingival health, because bleeding that occurs during PBI recording is considerably diminished.
    This can serve as motivation toward a higher level of patient cooperation.

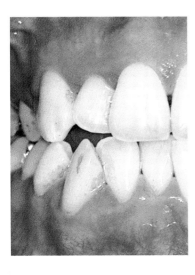
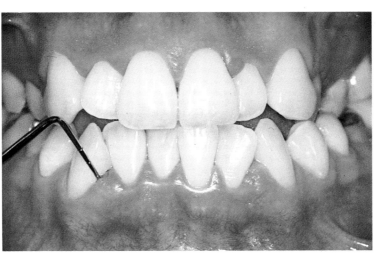

**351   Clinical situation 4 weeks later**
Bleeding has been reduced to almost nothing, and the disclosing agent reveals very little plaque accumulation. These two facts should convince the patient of the logic of the treatment.

*Left:* The dramatic reduction of plaque demonstrates the relationship: Less plaque – less gingivitis. Additional OHI is then concentrated on those tooth surfaces and interdental areas that have not been perfectly cleaned by the patient.

# Home Care by the Patient

Plaque control by the patient has been and remains a critical component of periodontal disease prevention. Furthermore, it supports therapeutic efforts and is of great significance in the maintenance of treatment successes.

Without continuing home care by the patient, all the efforts of the practitioner and the auxiliary personnel in treatment of periodontitis will achieve little success and, more importantly, any success will be of short duration. The critical aspect of patient home care is reduction of the amount of plaque at the gingival margin. The gingival massage that occurs during toothbrushing may be beneficial from a psychologic standpoint. In some special cases, home care can be enhanced by a plaque-inhibitory mouth rinse (e.g., Peridex).

Here eight issues will be discussed:

| |
|---|
| Plaque disclosing agents |
| Toothbrushes, dentifrices |
| Toothbrushing techniques |
| Interdental hygiene |
| Special cleaning aids |
| Electric toothbrushes, irrigation devices |
| Chemical plaque control (CHX) |
| Possibilities and limits of oral Hygiene |

The toothbrush is a most important tool for mechanical removal of plaque, but it can reach only the *facial, oral* and *occlusal* tooth surfaces.

This fact is important to understand because the initial lesions of gingivitis and periodontitis (as well as dental caries) usually occur in the *interproximal* areas. For this reason, the toothbrush must always be supplemented with other oral hygiene aids that can ensure cleaning of the proximal tooth surfaces.

There is no single method of oral hygiene that is right for every patient. The appropriate method and hygiene aids will be determined by the type and severity of the patient's disease, the morphologic situation (crowding, diastemata etc.), as well as the manual dexterity of the patient. The hygiene method may even need to be different for various areas within the mouth of a patient. Furthermore, during the course of periodontal therapy, the hygiene methods may have to be modified to fit the new morphologic situation (longer teeth, open interdental areas etc.).

The patient must be informed concerning the necessary frequency and duration of home care. Generally speaking, it is necessary to perform a thorough and systematic plaque removal at least one time each day (Lang et al. 1973). In the final analysis it is not the instruments, nor the technique, nor the amount of time expended that is of prime importance, it is the *result*, in terms of *freedom from plaque*. Plaque control and gingival condition must be re-evaluated at regular intervals.

# Plaque Disclosing Agents

Many times a patient will ask questions about the causes of his periodontal condition, usually when a bleeding index is being recorded.

This is an opportune time for a demonstration of microbial plaque. Using disclosing solutions, the adherent plaque on tooth surfaces and on gingiva can be selectively stained. The patient can see his own plaque in a mirror, and can watch as the dentist scrapes some off using an explorer or probe. The fact that one milligram of plaque contains up to three hundred million bacteria is always impressive to patients. This demonstrates first of all that it is necessary to remove plaque and second that it is possible to do so by means of oral hygiene procedures.

A disadvantage of plaque disclosing agents is that they tend to remain in the mouth for some time and can be an esthetic problem after an appointment. This disadvantage can be overcome through use of the Plak-Lite system. A solution that is scarcely visible under common light conditions is applied. When viewed subsequently in blue light, dental plaque fluoresces yellow.

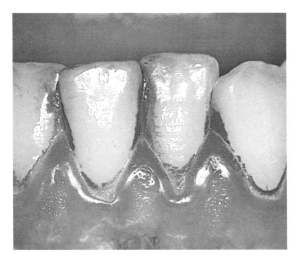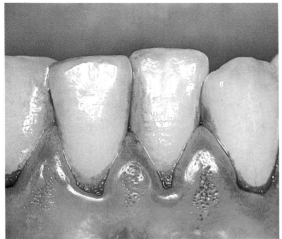

**352 Red and violet disclosing agents**
*Left:* The classic agent for plaque disclosing is erythrosin solution.

*Right:* Its disadvantage is that it is the same color as gingiva; also the plaque is not dramatically visible. The Dis-Plaque solution stains plaque violet, which makes it easier to discern from gingival tissues. Furthermore, Dis-Plaque stains older plaque a much deeper color than younger plaque.

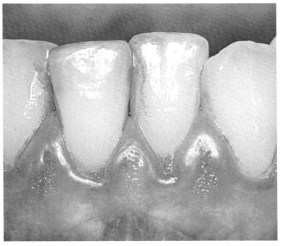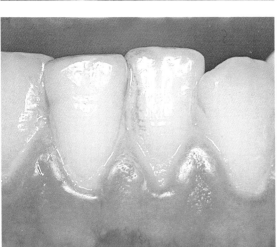

**353 Blue-green disclosing agents and Plak-Lite solution**
*Left:* Vital dyes and food coloring agents such as patent blue have also been used to advantage as plaque disclosing agents.

*Right:* The Plak-Lite solution stains plaque a yellowish color that is scarcely visible.

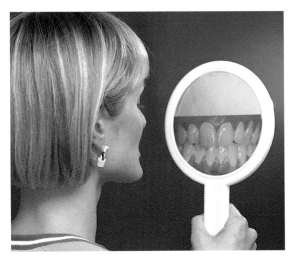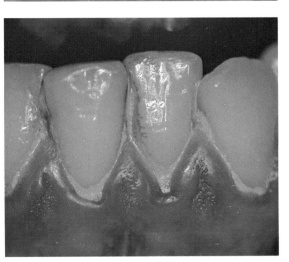

**354 Plak-Lite mirror – Fluorescing solution**
*Left:* The "filter mirror" filters out everything except the blue wavelength light, which is directed onto the teeth.

*Right:* Dental plaque stained with the Plak-Lite solution fluoresces in blue light (resonance frequencies) and can be observed in the lower portion of the mirror.

# Toothbrushes

For centuries the toothbrush in its variety of forms has served mankind for removal of plaque and food debris from *occlusal, facial* and *oral* tooth surfaces. Today the toothbrush is still the cornerstone of proper oral hygiene, but it cannot satisfactorily clean in interdental areas.

There is no "ideal" toothbrush in terms of shape, size or handle, but in the treatment of periodontal disease experience has shown that a manual toothbrush with short head and multitufted, straight, soft bristles is effective (Riethe 1988).

Hard bristles in combination with abrasive toothpastes can cause damage to both enamel and dentin, especially in the cervical area (abrasion, erosion). They can also injure the gingiva and elicit recession. Synthetic bristles with rounded ends are recommended. The *force* with which the toothbrush bristles are applied to the tooth surface should not exceed 300–400 g.

*Electric toothbrushes* (cf. p. 157)

**355  Recommended tooth-brushes (manual)**
A short head, relatively dense bristle bundles and soft to medium bristles are recommended.

- **Bristle thickness:
  0.18–0.25 mm**
- **Bristle length: 10–12 mm**

Length and diameter of the bristles determine their stiffness.

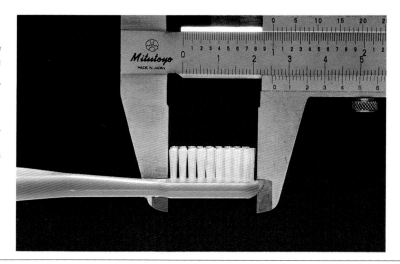

**356  Proper bristle contour – Rounded end**
Clinical view of gingiva following a single experimental brushing with a standardized, relatively heavy force (*Breitenmoser* et al. 1978). The blue acrylic block is used to standardize the photographic angulation (*Germann* 1971).

*Right:* Scanning EM shows that the bristle ends were *rounded off* during the manufacturing process, and thus do not cause gingival injury. White dot indicates bristle profile.

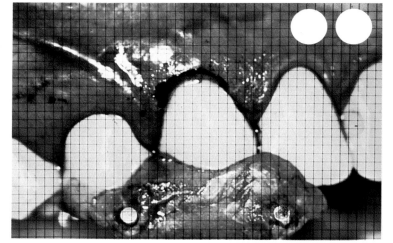

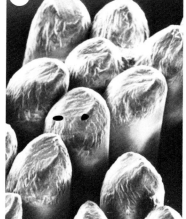

**357  Improper bristle contour – Sharp end**
Using the same standardized methods as above, the sharp bristles (triangle symbol) elicit easily visible gingival injury. The dark discoloration of the facial gingiva indicates erosion and epithelial damage. Dis-Plaque was used as disclosant.

*Right:* Sharp-ended bristle as seen in scanning electron microscope. Bristles were not rounded during fabrication.

Courtesy *W. Mörmann* and *C. Schweizer*

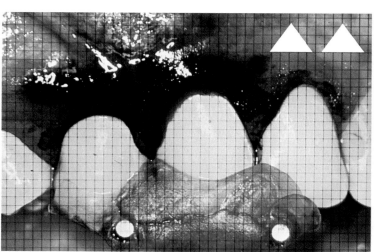

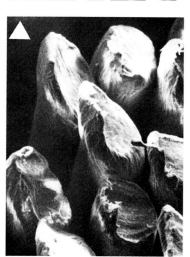

# Dentifrices

Toothpastes that contain abrasive compounds improve the mechanical cleansing of the teeth by the toothbrush. Excessively harsh abrasives, however, may also scratch the tooth surface (Riethe 1988). Some dentifrices contain various additives claimed to be beneficial for the periodontium, but such claims have yet to be fully substantiated by well controlled clinical research.

Dentifrices contain the following basic ingredients:
- *Abrasive/polishing agent:* calcium carbonate, calcium phosphate or sodium phosphate. Modern abrasives

such as silica ($SiO_2$), alumina ($Al_2O_3$) and aluminium hydroxide ($Al[OH]_3$) are very hard substances which, depending on particle size and homogeneity, can be effective for cleaning and polishing without causing excessive abrasion.
- *Binder* (e.g., carboxymethylcellulose)
- *Surfactant* (e.g., sodium N-lauroyl sarcosinate)
- *Flavoring and coloring agents*
- *Fluoride compounds* (not in all products)
- *Anti-tartar compounds*

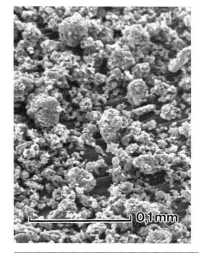

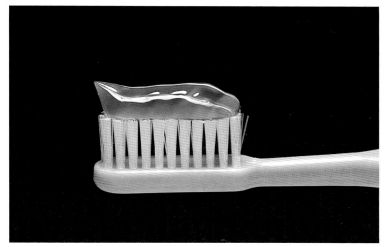

**358   Dentifrice, gel dentifrice**
The most important ingredient of any toothpaste is the abrasive.

In recent years many dentifrices have become available in gel form. These gels fulfill the requirements of a dentifrice and contain the same components as traditional pastes. Such gel-type toothpastes, however, must not be confused with "fluoride gels," which contain a considerably higher fluoride concentration.

*Left:* Sodium metaphosphate powder.

Courtesy *J.-M. Meyer*

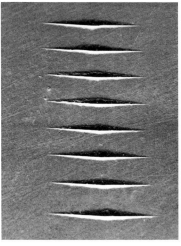

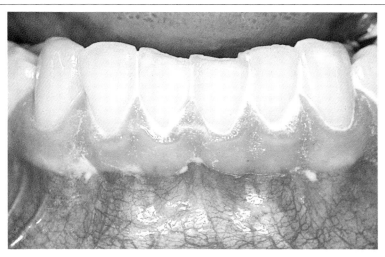

**359   Good dentifrice –**
**No enamel abrasion**
The clinical picture shows the mandibular anterior area immediately after toothbrushing.

A dentifrice must not elicit excessive tooth surface abrasion even after daily use for years.

*Left:* In experiments with various dentifrices (*Schweizer et al.* 1978), acceptable products did not cause detectable abrasion in a test system measuring effect on artificial enamel indentations subsequent to vigorous artificial brushing.

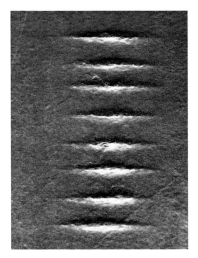

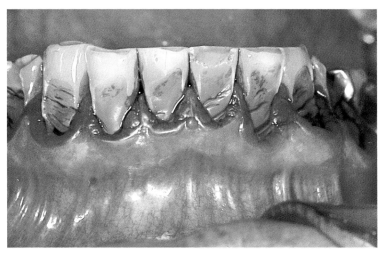

**360   Poor dentifrice – Severe enamel abrasion**
Highly abrasive dentifrices used with an improper brushing technique can lead to devastating consequences.

*Left:* Indentations in enamel in the test system (Fig. 359L) have been severely abraded after experimental brushing with a highly abrasive dentifrice.

SEMs courtesy *C. Schweizer*

# Toothbrushing Techniques

The goal of toothbrushing is plaque removal. Any method and any means that achieves this goal is acceptable, as long as neither the teeth nor the gingiva are traumatized.

The *"modified Bass technique"* (Bass 1954) has proved effective not only for patients with healthy periodontia, but especially for patients with gingivitis or periodontitis. The bristles are placed onto the tooth surface at a 45° angle and small vibratory or circular motions are made, which force the bristle tips into accessible interdental areas and into the gingival sulci. Plaque removal from these particularly vulnerable areas is thus accomplished.

The *"vertical – rotatory method"* (modified Stillman) is appropriate for periodontally healthy patients as well as for those manifesting generalized gingival recession. The bristles are moved from the gingiva toward the tooth with a simultaneous rotatory movement around the bristle long axis. Riethe (1988) recently reviewed other toothbrushing techniques.

**Modified Bass Technique**

**361  Placement of the toothbrush ...**
Toothbrush bristles positioned perpendicular to the tooth long axis will not effectively clean the interdental spaces.

*Right:* The original Bass or sulcular brushing technique is performed with toothbrushes containing only two rows of bristles (Oral-B; left).

With the more common three – and four-row bristles (center, right), the cleaning of teeth and gingival areas is improved.

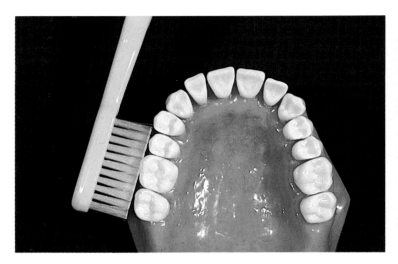
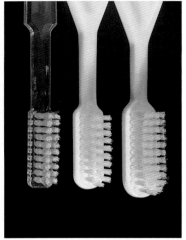

**362  ... 45° angle of the bristles ...**
When the brush is applied at a 45° angle to the teeth and then rotated toward the occlusal plane the bristles slip easily into the interdental areas and gingival sulci *without* excessive force. With the brush in this position, small rotatory or vibratory movements can effectively remove plaque.

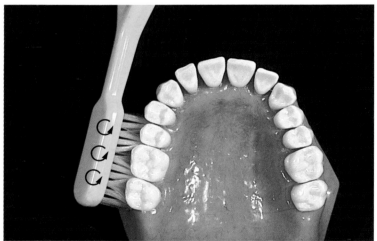

**363  ... 45° angle – Distal surface**
When viewed from the distal aspect, the position of the bristles in the Bass technique becomes obvious.

*Right:* Contact points between teeth cannot be reached by any toothbrush or through any toothbrushing technique. Therefore, an additional oral hygiene aid(s) for interdental cleaning is necessary in virtually every patient (possible exceptions: partial edentulousness, open contacts).

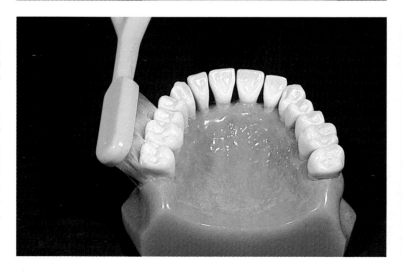
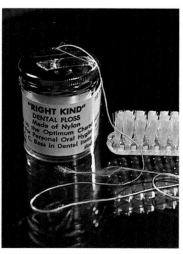

# Systematic Toothbrushing

Freedom from plaque depends upon more than just the type of toothbrush, the dentifrice and the brushing technique. The most important prerequisite for optimum plaque control is a motivated and manually dexterous patient. It is for this reason that the conventional toothbrushing methods often fail in young children, the handicapped and debilitated as well as in many elderly individuals.

Most important is a regular and *systematic* procedure by which all tooth surfaces are thoroughly cleaned.

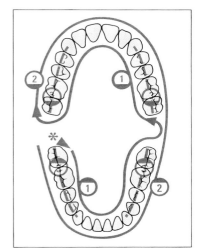

**364  Systematic toothbrushing**
This procedure has proved effective. The starting point is the lower right sextant (∗).

**1 Oral surfaces**
of mandible and maxilla, all distal surfaces of the most distal teeth in each arch
**2 Facial surfaces** of maxilla and mandible
**3 Occlusal surfaces**

**4 Interdental areas**
with special OH aids
(pp. 154–155)

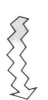

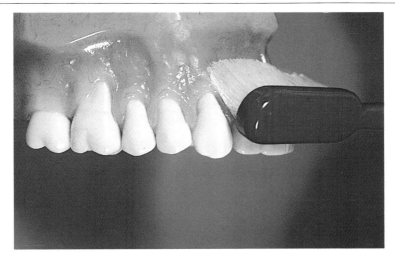

**Modified Stillman Technique
(vertical – rotatory brushing)**

**365  Initial phase of the movement – From red ...**
The soft-to-medium bristles are placed onto the attached gingiva with light pressure at a 45° angle to the tooth long axis. The bristles bend and do not injure the gingival tissue. The brush is then rotated occlusally with a slight twisting of the handle. In the original Stillman method, mild rotatory motions were recommended during this movement (see left, lateral).

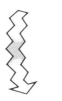

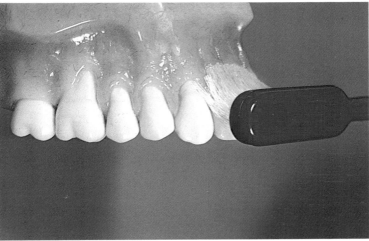

**366  [Intermediate phase]**
The toothbrush handle is now approximately parallel to the tooth surface. The bristles are still bent sharply upwards.

*Left:* The arrows symbolize the toothbrush movements of
– the *original Stillman technique:* movements from "red to white," with additional rotatory motion (left sequence)
– *modified Stillman technique:* movements from "red to white," without additional rotatory movement (right sequence).

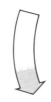
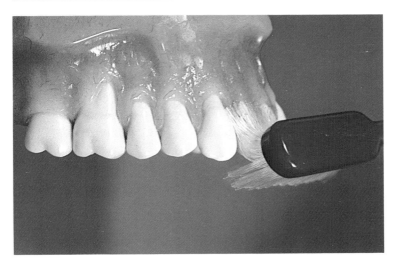

**367  ... to white – Final phase of the movement**
The toothbrush head is rotated under pressure away from the tooth, and the bristle tips effectively clean embrasure areas as well as the facial tooth surfaces. Plaque accumulations at the gingival margin are effectively removed.

This series of brush movements is repeated 5–10 times in the same area, then the brush head is moved either mesially or distally and the same series of movements is performed on another 2–3 tooth segment of the arch.

# Interdental Hygiene

Gingivitis and periodontitis are generally more severe in the interdental areas than on the facial and oral surfaces. Caries, too, is more frequent on interproximal surfaces than on facial or oral smooth surfaces. For these reasons interdental hygiene – which cannot be achieved using a toothbrush alone – is of particular importance for the periodontitis patient.

The appropriate interdental hygiene aids must be selected on the basis of each patient's individual requirements. There are many different aids available commercially; the appropriate choice depends primarily upon the morphology of the interdental areas.

In a healthy periodontium and in cases of gingivitis, mild periodontitis as well as crowded teeth, the use of *dental floss* is indicated.

If the interdental areas are open, for example after completion of periodontal therapy, *toothpicks* (e. g., stimudents) or *interdental brushes* may be appropriate for proximal plaque removal, depending upon the size of the interdental spaces.

Exposed root surfaces (grooves, furcation entrances) can only be cleaned with marginal brushes (p. 156).

**368  Interdental space size and hygiene aids**
The choice of an aid for interdental hygiene depends primarily on the size of the interdental space:

**A  Dental floss:** Indicated for narrow interdental spaces
**B  Toothpick/Stimudent:** Fine for slightly open spaces
**C  Interdental brushes:** For interdental spaces that are wide open, and for root irregularities

Each of these aids is associated with some advantages and some disadvantages.

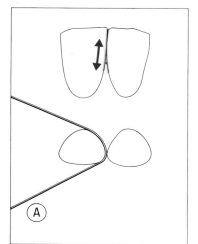
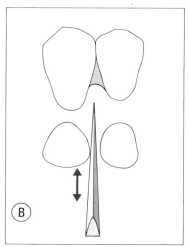
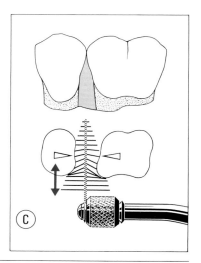

**369  Dental floss**
Unwaxed or lightly waxed floss should be recommended. Dental floss is composed of numerous individual filaments.

Floss holders may be useful for patients who lack manual dexterity.

*Right:* For special cases such as cleansing interdental areas beneath bridge pontics or bars, the following variations are available:

– **"Dental tape" (left)**
– **"Brush and Floss" (center)**
– **"Super Floss" (right)**

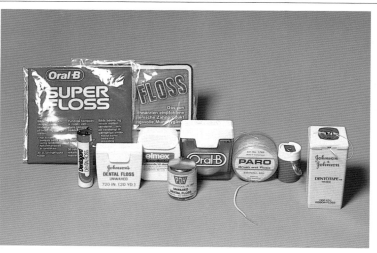
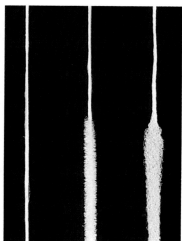

**370  Use of dental floss**
In order to avoid injury to the interdental papillae, the floss is guided with a sawing motion through the interdental contact point. Within the interdental area, the floss is first pulled against a tooth surface, then moved apically and occlusally (double arrow). The neighboring tooth surface is then cleaned identically.

Horizontal sawing motions for plaque removal are permitted with "Super Floss" or "Brush and Floss."

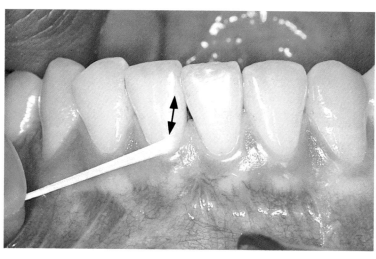

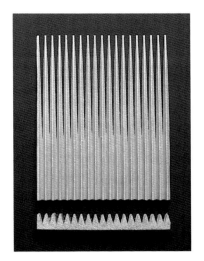

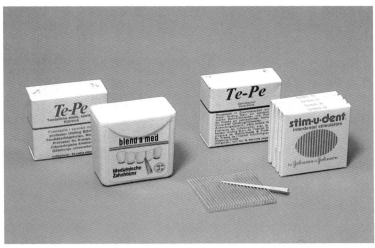

### 371 Wooden toothpicks

The ideal interdental toothpick has a triangular profile that approximates the shape of the interdental area. Different manufacturers use woods of varying hardness (balsa, birch, linden). Most commercially available wooden stimulators are effective as interdental hygiene aids if used properly.

*Left:* Wooden toothpicks with triangular profile.

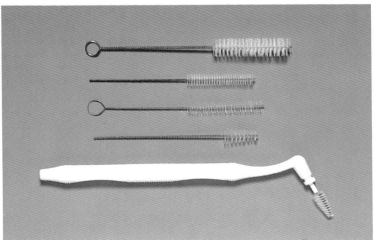

### 372 Use of wooden toothpicks

The tip is inserted into the interdental space from a slightly oblique angle as shown.

Plaque removal is accomplished by horizontal back-and-forth movements (double arrow). If the interdental space is wide, the surface of one tooth is cleaned first by applying slight pressure to one side, then the adjacent tooth is similarly cleaned.

*Remember:* The contact point itself cannot be cleaned using these wooden aids (caries!).

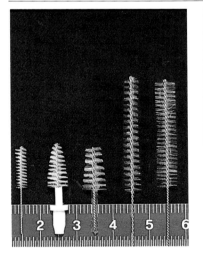

### 373 Interdental brushes

If interdental spaces are wide open, the interdental (spiral) brush is an ideal hygiene aid.

Many different varieties of interdental brushes are available, some with interchangeable heads and others with handles.

*Left:* Interdental brushes that fit a handle (brushes 1–3, from left) and longer brushes (4 and 5) can be used without a handle. A wire core that is too thick can abrade dentin and elicit pain.

### 374 Use of interdental brushes

The brush is inserted obliquely from an apical direction, as with wooden toothpicks, accommodating the morphology of the interdental papilla.

Cleaning is accomplished with back-and-forth movements (double arrow). Usually no toothpaste is used, to preclude abrasion of exposed dentin. However, if rapid calculus formation is a problem, a dentifrice with a mild abrasive may be used once per week or, in stubborn cases, daily.

## Special Cleaning Aids – Hand Instruments

In general, *two* hygiene instruments are necessary for plaque control: *One* toothbrush and *one* instrument for interdental hygiene.

It is often counterproductive to recommend half a dozen "special instruments" to the healthy patient or to the patient with gingivitis or mild periodontitis, because these will be neither regularly nor systematically employed.

On the other hand, following treatment for advanced periodontitis, the gingival margin is often irregu-

lar. Cervical areas, root irregularities and furcations may be exposed, and these are difficult to clean. In such situations, special cleaning aids may be necessary for optimum plaque removal.

In addition, patients with fixed bridgework, splinted crowns, root caps, bars, or those with removable partial dentures usually require special aids for adequate hygiene. Possibilities include interdental brushes, marginal brushes, rubber or plastic stimulators, special dental floss ("Super Floss"), floss threaders etc.

**375  Special cleaning aids**
These may be beneficial as adjuncts to the toothbrush and interdental aid for cleaning difficult-to-reach areas, plaque-retentive niches and peculiar morphologic situations:

- **Interdental/Marginal brushes** (two models)
- **Rubber and plastic stimulators**
- **Round toothpicks in a holder** (Perio-Aid)
- **Super Floss** with a stiff end for insertion
- **Threaders** for dental floss

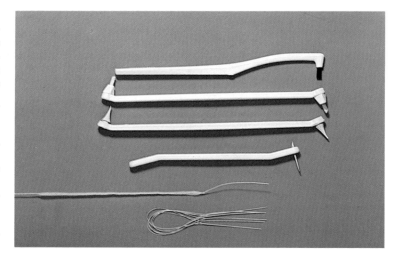

**376  Interdental/Marginal brushes**
These small brushes consist of a single bundle of bristles that may be fastened to a handle with various angulations. They are designed to reach poorly accessible sites. They are designed for plaque removal from beneath bridge pontics (photograph) or from wide open interdental areas, crown margins, root irregularities, furcation entrances, distal surfaces of the last teeth in the arch etc. Such brushes are effective if used properly.

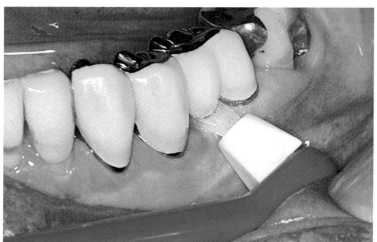

**377  "Threaders" for dental floss**
Dental floss cannot be inserted from the occlusal aspect when teeth are splinted or in the case of bar-type restorations (photograph). Floss can be effectively inserted using a "threader" (e.g., Butler), and can be used to keep the proximal surfaces of crowns, root caps etc. free of plaque.

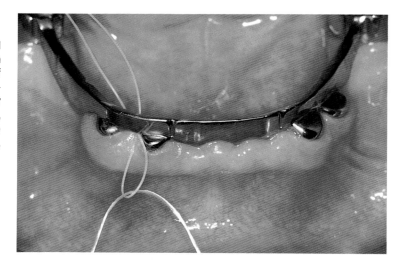

# Electric Toothbrushes

Comparative investigations have demonstrated that electric and manual toothbrushes are identical in terms of plaque removal (Niemi et al. 1986). The choice of a manual or an electric toothbrush can therefore be left to the patient. If, however, the patient chooses an electric toothbrush, its use must be demonstrated repeatedly and the patient's effectiveness in its use must be monitored.

The new "rotational" brushes (e. g., Interplak, Rota-Dent) appear to enhance plaque removal (Walsh & Glenwright 1984, Glavind & Zeuner 1986).

# Irrigators

The oral irrigator can only be considered as an *adjunct* in oral hygiene. Water sprays do not remove plaque and therefore can never replace mechanical plaque removal by means of toothbrushes and interdental hygiene aids (Hugoson 1978).

Chlorhexidine may be added in low concentrations to the irrigator fluid (Lang & Ramseier-Grossmann 1981, Aziz-Gandour & Newman 1986).

Pulsating irrigation of pockets has only a time-limited success (Mazza et al. 1981, Soh et al. 1982, Boyd et al. 1985, Greenstein 1987, Wennström et al. 1987b).

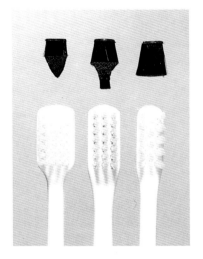
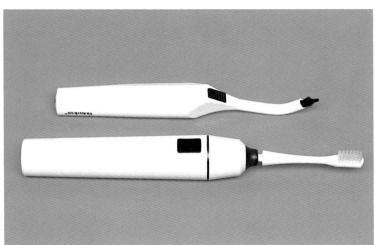

**378    Electric toothbrushes**
Two electric toothbrushes with different mechanisms.

*Above:* Rota-Dent has small rotating brushes, which are reminiscent of those used by the dentist with a professional handpiece.

*Below:* "Classic" electric toothbrush (Touch-Tronic from Water-Pik), whose head describes small ovoid movements.

*Left:* Various brush heads. Above, the Rota-Dent; below, for various electric toothbrushes.

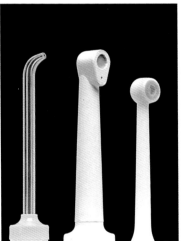
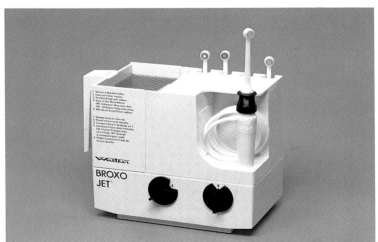

**379    Irrigators**
Broxojet has a multi-stream head. Variously colored tips permit the use a single device for the entire family.

Aromatics and disinfectant additives may be combined with the water spray (e.g., chlorhexidine, 0.05%).

*Left:* Tips for various types of irrigators, from left to right:

- **Single stream**
  (e. g., Waterpik)
- **Single or multi-stream**
  (e. g., Blend-a-Dent, Braun)
- **Multi-stream** (e. g., Broxojet)

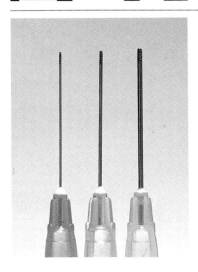
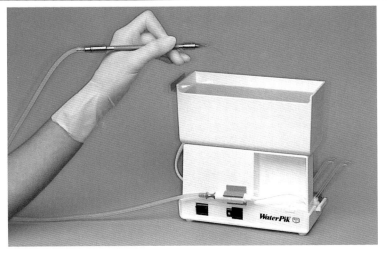

**380    Sulcus (pocket) irrigator**
Traditional irrigators have been modified for rinsing of sulci and/or periodontal pockets (WaterPik plus PeriodontoPik). These provide a pulsating flow under limited, safe pressure, to avoid injury to or activation of a pocket.

Chlorhexidine may be added in these instruments (*Soh et al.* 1982).
*Left:* Blunt tips for subgingival irrigation with different color-coded diameters (Max-i-Probe; MPL):

- **0.35 mm** (orange)
- **0.55 mm** (violet)
- **0.85 mm** (green)

# Chemical Plaque Control – Chlorhexidine (CHX)

Removal of plaque by the patient or by the dentist or hygienist using mechanical means is time-consuming and is never 100% effective.

For decades, therefore, a goal of dental research has been to discover a rinsing solution that would inhibit plaque formation. With the introduction of chlorhexidine by Davies et al. in 1956, a topical chemotherapeutic agent became available that achieved the goal of chemical plaque control. Because of its unpleasant though reversible side effects, CHX should be used for only short periods of time.

## 1. Chlorhexidine digluconate – Water soluble

Because of its cationic characteristics, chlorhexidine has a high affinity for the cell wall of microorganisms, and depending on its concentration it may be either bacteriostatic or bactericidal. It has an extended effectiveness because of anionic bonding to pellicle and salivary glycoproteins, which coat the entire oral cavity. Rinsing twice daily with 0.2% chlorhexidine solution will lead to almost total inhibition of plaque formation (Löe & Schiött 1970).

**381   Chlorhexidine (CHX) and plaque**
If all oral hygiene is ceased (day O) and only water rinsing is performed, plaque develops within only a few days (Plaque Index, PI). If rinsing is performed with CHX (0.2%), *no* plaque accumulates (red curve).

*Right:* The water-soluble neutral digluconate of CHX is frequently used as a mucosal and skin disinfectant (see chemical formula and gluconic acid).

In gel form, CHX is often used post-surgically.

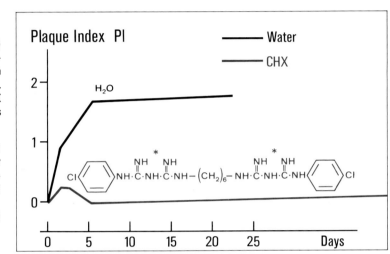

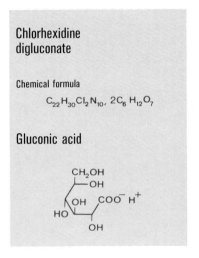

Chlorhexidine digluconate

Chemical formula
$$C_{22}H_{30}Cl_2N_{10}, 2C_6H_{12}O_7$$

Gluconic acid

**382   Staining due to CHX**
If CHX rinsing is performed for extended periods of time (weeks), the teeth (pellicle) and tongue take on a brownish discoloration.

The unesthetic staining may become so heavy in enamel fissures, on dentin and cementum etc., that it can be removed only through use of strong abrasives.

*Right:* Severe staining of the tongue following weeks of rinsing with CHX (0.2%).

*Note:* Truly effective rinsing solutions always lead to staining.

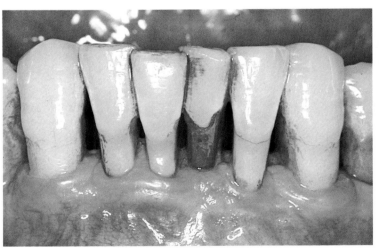

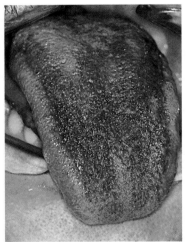

**383   High concentration – Mucosal desquamation**
Excessively high CHX concentrations may elicit epithelial desquamation. The lesions heal spontaneously and rapidly when CHX rinsing is halted. Desquamation is seldom observed with commercially available CHX oral rinses with low chlorhexidine concentrations (0.1–0.2%; e.g., Peridex).

Commercially available CHX:

– **0.12% Peridex**
– **10  % Plak-Out concentrate**
– **0.1 % Plak-Out, Chlorhexamed**
– **0.2 % Corsodyl**

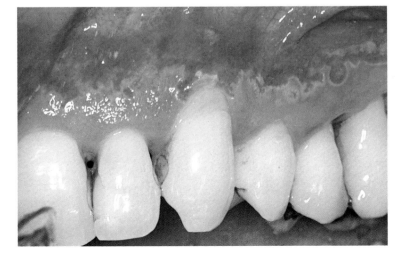

*Indications for CHX digluconate (solution):*
- disinfection of the oral cavity before dental treatment
- as an adjunct during initial therapy, especially in cases of RPP and LJP
- following periodontal surgery
- in handicapped patients (Low et al. 1989)

*Side effects of CHX digluconate:*
- staining of teeth and tongue
- taste disturbances
- mucosal desquamation
- Caution: Chlorhexidine digluconate should never be used in concentrations higher than 0.2%. If bone is exposed (extractions, flap reflection) wound healing may be disturbed (Bassetti & Kallenberger 1980).

## 2. Chlorhexidine dihydrochloride – Powder

Chlorhexidine HCl is a practically *water-insoluble* white powder of neutral pH, which is quite easy to incorporate into periodontal dressings. Tooth surfaces beneath such periodontal dressings are significantly cleaner after five days than when dressings without CHX-dihydrochloride are used (Plüss et al. 1975).

Chlorhexidine –
Dihydrochloride

Chemical formula

$$C_{22}H_{30}Cl_2N_{10},\ 2HCl$$

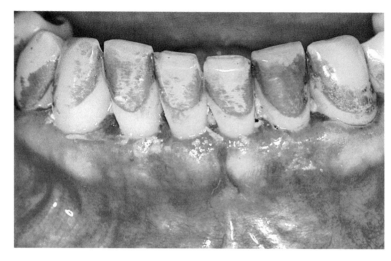

**384 Plaque inhibition beneath periodontal dressing**
Clinical picture immediately after removal of a periodontal dressing, seven days after gingivoplasty.

Chlorhexidine powder (-HCl) incorporated into the dressing almost completely inhibited plaque accumulation. The coronal portions of the teeth were not covered by the dressing, and a disclosing agent reveals gross plaque accumulation.

*Left:* Chlorhexidine dihydrochloride – Chemical formula

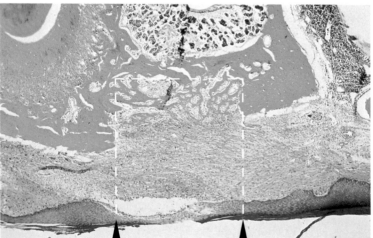

**385 Normal wound healing in a standardized mucosal wound after rinsing with Ringer's solution.**
A standardized 2 mm punch biopsy on the rat palate (dashed lines indicate wound) was rinsed twice daily with Ringer's solution for one week. Healing was without complications when evaluated clinically and histologically (Goldner, x 40).

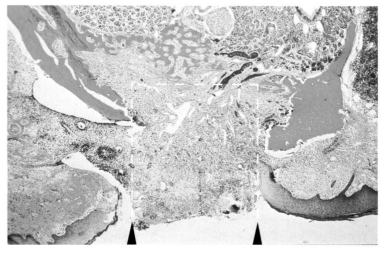

**386 Disturbed wound healing in a standardized mucosal wound after rinsing with 0.5% CHX solution**
The standardized wound in the rat palate was rinsed twice daily with a high concentration CHX digluconate solution (0.5%). Wound healing was severely impaired. Note that the wound is filled with granulation tissue and fibrin, and exhibits no re-epithelialization even after seven days (Goldner, x 40).

Histology courtesy *C. Bassetti* and *A. Kallenberger*

# Possibilities and Limits of Oral Hygiene

### Oral hygiene and prophylaxis

The influence of plaque removal by the patient has been mentioned in the literature many times (review by Lindhe et al. 1970). There exists no doubt that oral hygiene (toothbrushing, interdental hygiene) is the best preventive periodontics. In patients who form calculus, personal hygiene should be enhanced at regular intervals by professional cleaning.

Mechanical plaque control can be enhanced by short-term use of topical antiplaque rinsing solutions (chlorhexidine). Oral health can be *maintained* with optimum oral hygiene.

### Oral hygiene and gingivitis

In addition to disease prevention, optimum supragingival plaque control is also the most effective therapy for gingivitis (Löe et al. 1965). Because the patient cannot remove calcified plaque (calculus) himself, professional mechanical tooth cleaning must be performed at regular intervals.

### Oral hygiene and periodontitis

As meaningful as oral hygiene is for disease prevention, gingivitis treatment, and oral health maintenance, it is relatively ineffective, when used *alone,* for treatment of periodontitis. Even for a highly motivated and dextrous patient, there exist clear limitations: The best efforts in home care cannot reach the deep subgingival plaque. Concrements and endotoxin-containing cementum can never be removed by the patient. Moderate to severe periodontitis thus can scarcely be influenced by oral hygiene. Cercek et al. (1983) demonstrated this in a human clinical study: Patients with periodontitis were treated in three phases (Fig. 387):

A. In an initial 5-month phase, patients were instructed and motivated in the use of the *toothbrush* and dental floss. No professional tooth cleaning was performed.

B. In a second, 3-month phase, the same patients were provided with instruction for use of the *Perio-Aid* (Fig. 375), in addition to their previous oral hygiene. Patients used the rounded toothpick to clean the marginal areas as deeply as possible subgingivally.

C. Following these two hygiene phases, a professional scaling (Cavitron) was performed supra- and subgingivally using local anesthesia. Patients were then examined for 9 months.

**387 Oral hygiene versus subgingival scaling**
(*Cercek et al.* 1983)

**A** *Oral hygiene by the patient* Toothbrush and interdental hygiene aid
**B** *Oral hygiene (A); additional use of the Perio-Aid*
**C** *Professional subgingival scaling (ultrasonic instrument)*
**D** *Results after 17 months*

Patient groups by probing depth at initial examinations:

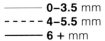

——— 0–3.5 mm
- - - - 4–5.5 mm
——— 6 + mm

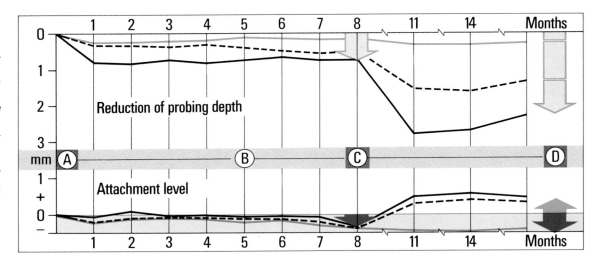

The results of this study clearly demonstrated that the oral hygiene efforts of the patients alone (first and second phases) were effective in dramatically reducing the Plaque Index (supragingival plaque) as well as the Gingival Bleeding Index. On the other hand, probing depths did *not* significantly decrease. Deeper pockets of seven and more millimeters experienced scarcely 1 mm reduction. This small reduction in probing depth was probably due to tissue shrinkage. The level of attachment did not change during the first two phases.

Only in the third phase, following professional supra- and subgingival scaling did a significant reduction of probing depths and actual attachment gain occur, especially in deeper pockets. These results demonstrate that oral hygiene *alone* cannot positively influence periodontitis.

### Oral hygiene following periodontal treatment

Home care is, however, one of the most important factors for *maintenance of the results* of successful periodontal therapy. Only with optimum plaque control by the patient, enhanced by the dentist or dental hygienist at recall appointments, can recurrence of disease be prevented (Rosling et al. 1976 b, Nyman et al. 1977, Knowles et al. 1979).

# Professional Care –
# Creating Conditions that Enhance Oral Hygiene

**Tooth cleaning**
**Supragingival scaling**
**Creation of hygiene capability**
**Gingivitis treatment**

The procedures described below are part of the *first phase of initial therapy*. Together with oral hygiene by the patient, these procedures comprise the only treatment necessary for gingivitis, and are important prerequisites in periodontitis therapy as well.

Active professional treatment should begin even as oral hygiene instruction, patient motivation and monitoring of home care are ongoing. The patient cannot be expected to improve his oral hygiene if the preconditions for optimum home care are not simultaneously created (creation of hygiene capability). Professional prophylaxis is particularly important in this regard, as well as elimination of any plaque-retentive areas that represent harbors for bacterial accumulation.

The following pages provide details concerning:

| |
|---|
| Removal of plaque, deposits, stains |
| Supragingival calculus removal |
| Removal of iatrogenic irritants (niches) |
| Reduction of naturally-occurring plaque-retentive areas (extractions, odontoplasty, elimination of crowding, etc.) |
| Subgingival plaque and calculus removal from pseudopockets and shallow gingival pockets as far as possible without anesthesia |

The various treatments performed during the first phase of initial therapy cannot be strictly separated from another, either in the presentations that follow in this book, or in the practice of dentistry. At a single appointment, for example, calculus removal, elimination of amalgam overhangs, minor odontoplasty and occlusal equilibration may all be accomplished.

The subgingival treatment of root surfaces (second phase of initial therapy) may also intersect with the first phase. In clinical situations that represent the indistinct transition from gingivitis to incipient periodontitis, i.e., when pockets are shallow, supra- and subgingival scaling often can be performed simultaneously.

On the other hand, scaling and definitive root planing in deep pockets and eventual soft tissue curettage must be relegated to the second phase of initial therapy. These procedures are often categorized as actual surgical therapy.

## Tooth Cleaning – Power-Driven Instruments ...

The removal of all stains, deposits and concrements comprises the first phase of initial therapy. It is also an important *preventive* measure in the healthy periodontium and the most significant postoperative measure following completion of periodontitis therapy. Thorough tooth cleaning is performed during each recall appointments.

The prevention/treatment/maintenance therapy trio "without end" demands the use of auxiliary personnel such as the dental hygienist or the trained dental assistant. It also demands rationalization, standardiza-

tion and work simplification as well as innovation in the development of new instruments.

Difficult-to-remove stains resulting from medicaments (e.g., chlorhexidine), tobacco, beverages and foodstuffs as well as dental plaque itself can be removed using instruments that provide a water-powder spray (e.g., Prophy-Jet). The sodium bicarbonate that is used in the water spray is abrasive for dentin and restorative materials (Atkinson et al. 1984, De Boever & Vande Velde 1985, Galloway & Pashley 1987, Iselin et al. 1989), and should only be used on enamel, with constant

**388   Powder-water spray instrument (e.g., Prophy-Jet, Cavi-Jet)**
The powdered abrasive consists primarily of sodium bicarbonate ($NaHCO_3$), which can remove tough deposits and stains when used with a water spray.

The water-powder spray requires use of a high speed evacuator, due to possibly infectious overspray and for general operatory cleanliness.

*Right:* Nozzle of the Prophy-Jet. Abrasive powder and water are mixed only after they exit the concentric nozzles.

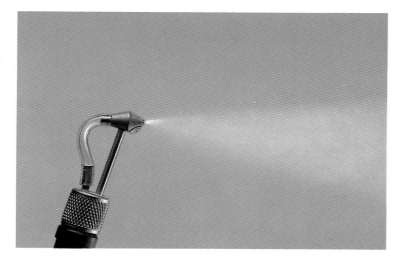
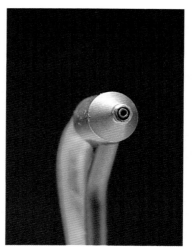

**389   Ultrasonic scaler (e.g., Cavitron, Odontoson)**
In the more modern instruments, the water coolant is directed through the instrument tip in a groove on the instrument head.

Ultrasonic scalers work at between 25,000–50,000 cycles per second (Hz, resonance frequency) with very small amplitudes.

*Right:* Three useful tips for the Cavitron (for supra- and subgingival use).

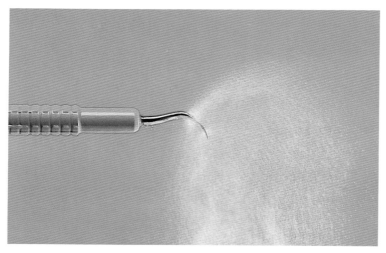
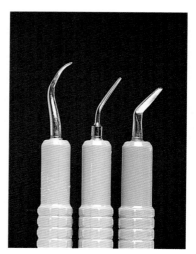

**390   Air-Scaler, "Sonic-Scaler" (Titan-S, Sonicflex)**
The new air-scalers (pictured is the Titan-S from Star Dental) have withstood the trials of laboratory investigations and clinical practice applications. These instruments have a regulatable frequency of maximum 6,000 Hz and thus are considerably slower than an ultrasonic instrument. The motion of the tip of the instrument is between 0.08–0.2 mm.

*Right:* Three tips for the Sonicflex instrument (KaVo).

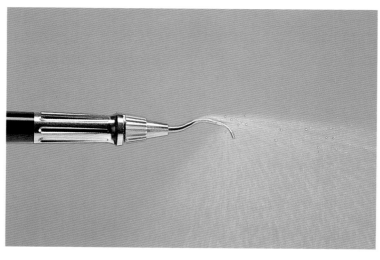
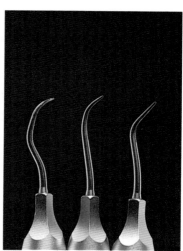

## ... and Their Use

movement of the tip. Such devices are seldom completely effective in interdental areas and gingiva may be superficially injured. The spray should never be directed into the gingival sulcus (pocket). Stains and plaque can also be removed with abrasive pastes and rubber cups or brushes. Polishing strips accomplish cleaning in interdental areas.

After removal of soft deposits, calculus becomes visible. Calculus itself is *not* a pathogen, but it is an excellent substrate for plaque accumulation and must be

completely removed. Useful are ultrasonic instruments (e.g., Cavitron), as well as several new air-scalers that attach to the dental unit (e.g., Sonicflex, Titan-S; Lie & Leknes 1985, Gellin et al. 1986, Loos et al. 1987).

Powerdriven devices may be associated with the spread infectious material.

Beyond ultrasonics and air-scalers, the most important and most precise means for removal of accretions are hand instruments (see following pages).

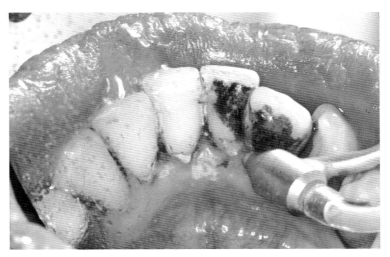

**391 Removal of soft deposits and stains with the powder-water spray device**
Tough deposits, plaque and stains from tobacco, tea, wine, or chlorhexidine, can be removed from accessible enamel surfaces using the jet. Cleaning in interdental areas, however, is insufficient. The stream should be directed onto the tooth surface at an angle of 45°. A high speed evacuator is used to retrieve the reflected solution. Do not spray directly into the sulcus (pocket)!

*Caution:* Highly abrasive on cementum, dentin and restorations.

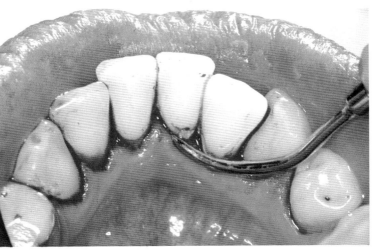

**392 Removal of hard supragingival concrements with an ultrasonic instrument**
After removal of soft debris and plaque, remaining calculus is completely removed using the ultrasonic instrument.
   In narrow, poorly accessible sites and niches, fine hand instruments must be used afterwords.

*Caution:* Overheating, cracks in enamel and porcelain.

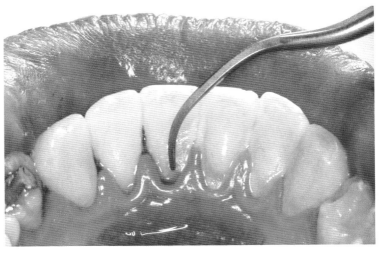

**393 Removal of hard supragingival concrements with a sonic instrument**
This instrument, which attaches to the turbine handpiece air-water orifice, permits removal of concrements in a manner similar to the ultrasonic instrument; however, the sensitivity is improved and the frequency can be regulated. Less pressure is necessary during use and rinsing is continuous. This simplifies therapy, improves visibility and permits more efficient performance.

## Tooth Cleaning – Hand Instruments, Prophy Pastes ...

Hand scalers and curettes remain the most important, indispensible instruments for periodontal therapy and prophylaxis. For the removal of soft deposits and stains, hand instruments are enhanced by the use of brushes, rubber cups and polishing strips with cleaning and polishing pastes.

The dental marketplace offers a myriad of scalers and curettes that will provide clinically adequate service if used properly. It is not the manufacturer that is critical for successful treatment, rather the shape of the instrument, especially its degree of sharpness, and above all the manual dexterity of the operator. Instruments made from high quality steel are preferable to those coated with hard metals, because they are generally more slender and can be resharpened.

Instruments for supragingival debridement include the straight *chisel,* straight and angled *scalers* and the *lingual scaler.*

On difficult-to-reach sites, in grooves and irregularities on the crown and the root, *curettes* may also be necessary for removal of supragingival accretions.

**394 Scalers**
For supragingival calculus removal and for concrements that are located only a few millimeters below the gingival margin, sharp-edged, pointed scalers in various shapes are indicated.

From left to right (color-coded):
- **Straight chisel** (white)
- **Scalers,** straight and paired L and R (blue)
- **Lingual scaler** (black)

*Right:* Working end of the chisel (45° sharpening angle!) and the lingual scaler.

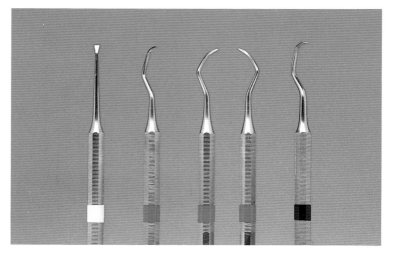
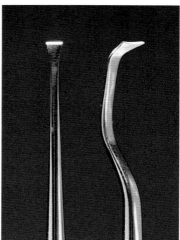

**395 Curettes**
For difficult-to-reach areas and for subgingival accretions that can be removed without anesthesia, the scaler armamentarium may be enhanced by curettes.
    From left to right:

- **Universal curettes** (yellow, 1.2 mm wide)
- **Anterior curettes** (orange)
- **Posterior curettes** (red, both ca. 0.95 mm wide)

*Right:* Working ends of a pair of broad universal curettes

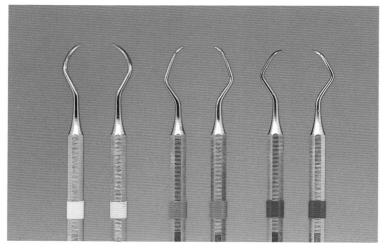
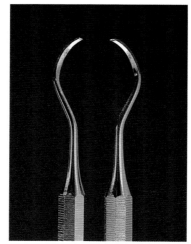

**396 Standardized prophy pastes – RDA**
Pastes are available according to abrasiveness. The standardization is achieved on the basis of dentin abrasion measured by radioactivity. All are fluoride-containing.

- **RDA  40** mild abrasion (yellow)
- **RDA 120** average abrasion (red)
- **RDA 170** moderate abrasion (green)
- **RDA 250** heavy abrasion (blue)

*Right:* Finger cups with color-coded prophy pastes.

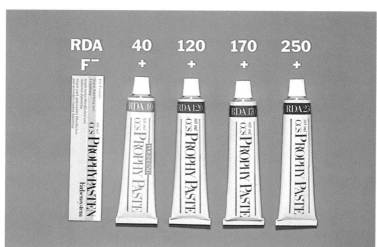
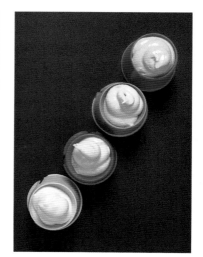

## ... and Their Use

If subgingival deposits are to be removed initially, insofar as this is possible without anesthesia, the use of curettes is obligatory. For this first phase of initial therapy the classical universal curettes are indicated. The slender *Gracey curettes,* which are sharpened on only one edge, are used almost exclusively for subgingival scaling and root planing in periodontitis patients (pp. 182–190).

If supragingival calculus is covered with thick (soft) deposits, these should be removed with brushes and coarse prophy paste before mechanical debridement.

Whenever calculus is removed, the teeth should be polished afterwards with a *rubber cup and polishing paste.* This polish of the teeth and any exposed root surfaces is performed with fluoride-containing prophy pastes which today are classified according to their dentin abrasiveness (Radioactive Dentine Abrasion = RDA).

The interdental area is finished with fine *polishing strips.* The effect of professional tooth cleaning in gingivitis is a massive reduction of supragingival plaque flora and calculus, which results in healing of the marginal gingival inflammation.

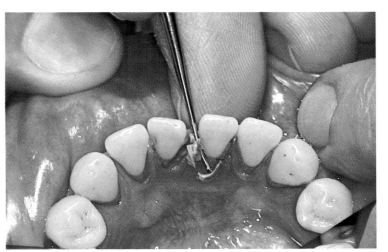

**397 Supragingival calculus removal**
The chisel is the only instrument that is used with a *pushing* motion.

It is effective for removal of gross lingual supragingival calculus in the mandibular anterior area by pushing from the facial aspect through the interdental spaces.

After the collar of calculus is removed with the chisel, straight and curved scalers are used to remove remaining deposits.

The lingual scaler (Fig. 394) smooths the narrow lingual surface of mandibular anterior teeth.

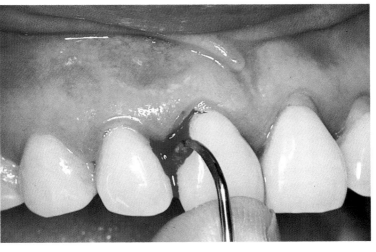

**398 Subgingival calculus removal**
The largest masses of subgingival accretions are usually located only a few mm apical to the gingival margin. These should be removed during gross debridement, using scalers and curettes as necessary.

Gingival bleeding may occur even during very careful scaling as the ulcerated pocket epithelium is injured.

*Rubber gloves should be worn during all procedures where hemorrhage may be expected (virus infection!).*

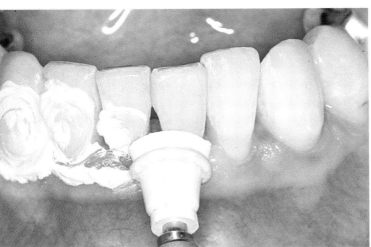

**399 Polishing with rubber cup and prophy paste**
Each time scaling is performed, the teeth must be polished, otherwise rough surfaces will enhance reaccumulation of plaque bacteria. Polishing also removes the pellicle, which is reestablished in a few hours.

Rubber cups and polishing paste are ideal for this procedure because they are kinder to the gingival margin than are rotating brushes. The rubber cup can be used carefully near shallow pockets to achieve polishing 1–2 mm beneath the gingival margin.

# Creation of Conditions that Enhance Oral Hygiene
# Removal of Iatrogenic Irritants

Concurrent with mechanical removal of plaque and calculus, all imperfect dental restorations are corrected with the goal of creating smooth supra- and subgingival tooth surfaces as well as impeccable transition areas between natural tooth structure and the margins of restorations and crowns. Only when this is done will it be possible for the patient to achieve perfect interdental hygiene: "Creation of hygiene capability."

The most important iatrogenic irritants are:

– rough, poorly contoured restorations
– overhangs of restoration margins
– open crown margins located subgingivally
– improperly contoured bridge pontics
– depressible clasps, prosthesis saddles etc., which can injure the periodontium directly.

**400  Recontouring and polishing old amalgam restorations – Instruments**
Special polishing diamonds (25 µm, Amalgashape system), finishing burs and rubber polishing wheels etc. are used in the handpiece for recontouring and re-polishing old amalgam restorations.

*Caution:* Do not overheat the restoration surface!

*Right:* Disks with varying abrasiveness are used to advantage in the proximal area. The contact point must not be destroyed.

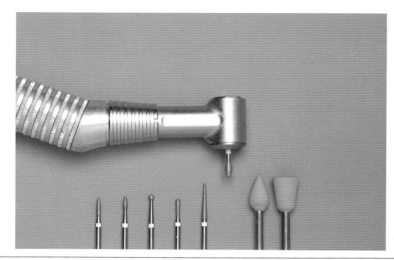
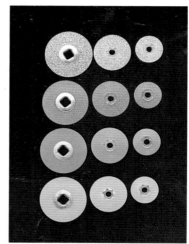

**401  Mechanical files**
Power-driven filing with water cooling is available with the EVA system. Using the thin, flexible, one-sided diamond-coated Proxoshape files, it is possible to remove overhangs and polish tooth/restoration surfaces in narrow interdental spaces (Mörmann et al. 1983).

*Right:*

– **Proxoshape files** (Intensiv Co.) diamond coating 75 µm, 40 µm (yellow), 15 µm (red)
– **EVA polishing plastic files** (Dentatus Co.)

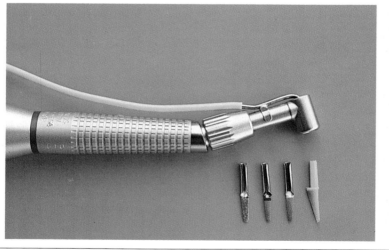
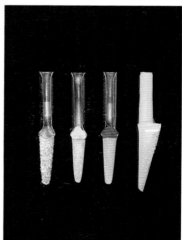

**402  Strip holders – Strips with standardized abrasiveness**
Interdental recontouring and polishing is easier with a strip holder.

– **LM holder** (above)
– **Bilciurescu holder** (below)

*Right:* Diamond-coated steel and linen strips with various standardized abrasiveness (color-coded) are indicated for corrections in the interdental area.

– **GC steel strips** (above)
– **Hawe linen strips** (below)

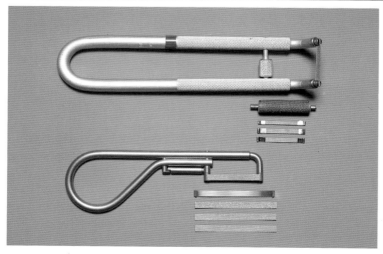
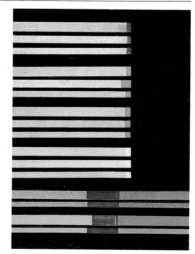

Extreme inconsistences of restoration margins (also depressible clasps etc.) can irritate the gingiva and periodontium directly (mechanically).

More important than such direct irritation, however, is the fact that even minor imperfections of dental restorative work represent plaque-retentive areas. The result at such locations is gingival inflammation and, over the long term, possibly periodontal destruction (Björn et al. 1969, 1970; Gilmore & Sheiham 1971; Renggli & Regolati 1972; Leon 1977; Lang et al. 1983; Riethe 1984; Iselin et al. 1985).

The finishing and polishing of all restoration surfaces can be performed with fine diamonds (water cooling), round burs and finishing burs and disks.

Interdental amalgam overhangs can be removed with flame-shaped diamonds and periodontal files, or with the Proxoshape files (EVA system; Mörmann et al. 1983). *Old* restorations with overhangs *should be replaced* because recurrent caries is common.

Metal and plastic strips, either hand-held or in an appropriate holder, are also useful in the marginal/proximal regions for smoothing of restoration margins.

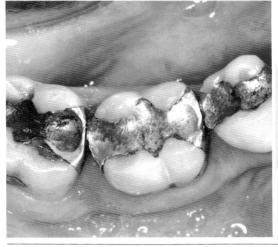 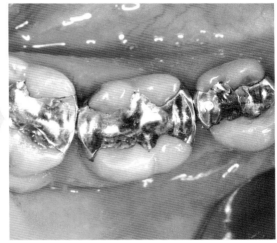

**403 Old amalgam restorations before and after recontouring**
*Left:* The rough, discolored surface of old restorations enhances plaque accumulation. Smoothing and polishing of such restorations will reduce the magnitude of microorganisms in the oral cavity. Care must be taken not to disturb functional contacts in centric and lateral occlusion during the smoothing and polishing of occlusal surfaces.

*Right:* Contoured and polished old amalgam restorations.

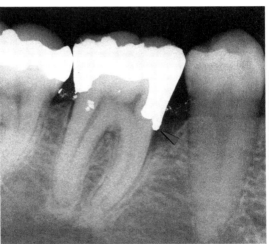 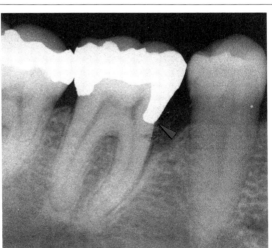

**404 Amalgam overhang before and after removal**
*Left:* Tooth 46 exhibits a pronounced marginal overhang on the mesial aspect (massive plaque accumulation, arrow). A deep bony pocket is also located near this iatrogenic niche.

*Right:* The proximal overhang was removed and the restoration was polished. The margin is now perfect, discouraging any further plaque accumulation.

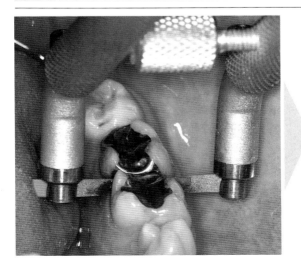 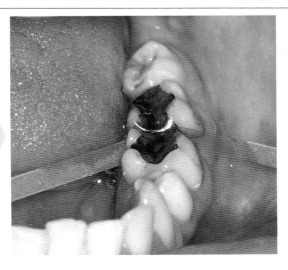

**405 Smoothing the proximal restoration surface with strips**
*Left:* LM strip holder with diamond-coated steel strip during smoothing of the distal surface of tooth 36. The contact area is protected.

*Right:* The interdental surface of the restoration is finally polished using fine, very mildly abrasive linen strips, which can also be used in the contact area.

*Goal:* Smooth proximal surfaces make possible perfect interdental hygiene with dental floss.

## Removal of Iatrogenic Irritants – Overhanging Crown Margins

The open margins of full cast crowns that extend below the gingival margin represent particularly massive iatrogenic irritants that can lead to destruction of periodontal tissues. It is commonly accepted that subgingival margins represent potential plaque-retentive areas that can foster caries and periodontal involvement (Hammer & Hotz 1979), but there is no proof that a subgingival margin is caries-prophylactic. Compromises should only be tolerated for esthetic reasons in the anterior area.

The removal of a subgingival and/or open crown margin during initial therapy is generally only a temporary measure. Thereafter the old crowns or bridges serve as fixed temporary restorations. Following completion of periodontal therapy, such faulty restorations are usually replaced.

Removal of overhanging crown margins is accomplished using diamond burs. An attendant problem is the incorporation of gold fillings into the gingival tissues (p. 170). Severely open or overhanging crown margins may be removed through use of a finishing bur or a round bur supragingivally (Fig. 406).

**406  Subgingival overhanging crown margins**
This often observed iatrogenic irritant can be detected clinically using a fine pointed explorer. Plaque accumulates beneath the open margin, and gingivitis often persists for years.

Such massive crown margin overhangs may be removed with a diamond *supragingivally,* or a round bur may be used to remove the entire crown margin, as depicted here.

*Right:* The radiograph clearly reveals that the crown margin is overhanging interproximally (arrows).

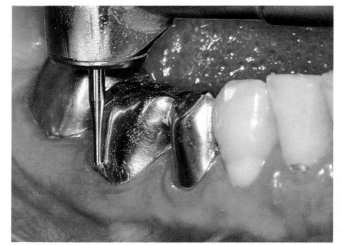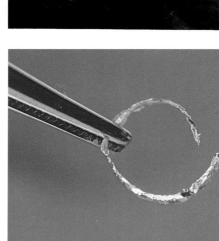

**407  Overhanging crown margin removed**
Caries is often encountered following radical removal of an overhanging subgingival crown margin. Before initial therapy, this carious process could not be diagnosed either radiographically or clinically.

*Right:* The crown margin, removed in one piece!

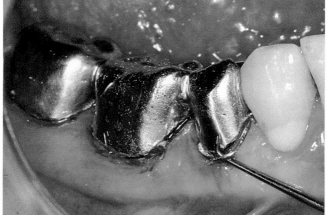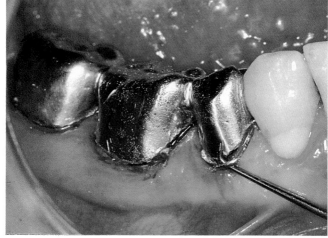

**408  Crown margins now supragingival**
The old crowns serve nicely as "temporaries" following treatment of the cervical caries. Interdental hygiene can now be accomplished using Stimudents.

These crowns will be replaced following completion of periodontal therapy.

*Right:* The radiograph depicts the removal of the major overhangs (metal residue in tissue; compare p. 170).

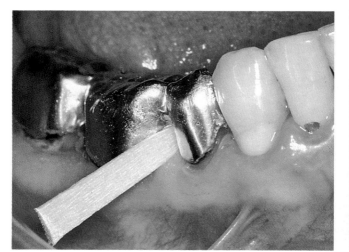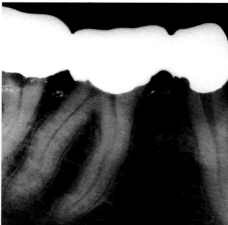

# Correction of Iatrogenic Irritants – Bridge Pontics

Pontics in the *anterior area* should lightly contact the attached gingiva at a point or along a line (pp. 358–359). A pontic should never extend onto the mobile oral mucosa. There must be no pressure exerted upon the marginal gingiva of the adjacent abutment teeth. In *posterior areas,* where esthetics is not a consideration, it is often beneficial to leave ca. 2 mm of space beneath pontics to facilitate use of hygiene aids in the removal of plaque *under* the pontic.

A facetted pontic makes it easier to use interdental brushes, Stimudents or Super Floss to clean abutment teeth, because of the guidance that is absent when the pontic is far removed from the gingiva or when a bar-like pontic is used.

Improperly constructed bridge pontics may be corrected on an emergency basis using flame-shaped diamonds. The undersurface of pontics treated in this manner can be polished almost to laboratory smoothness using Proxoshape files (15 µm abrasiveness).

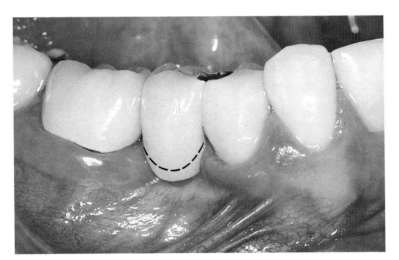

**409   Improper bridge pontic form**
This pontic is too long and its saddle shape contacts both attached gingiva and mobile oral mucosa on the facial aspect. It is also too wide, contacts the mesial abutment over a broad expanse, encroaches on the mesial gingival papillae and precludes any interdental hygiene.
   The planned shortening and contouring is indicated by the dashed line.

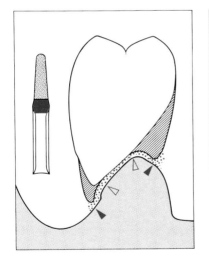

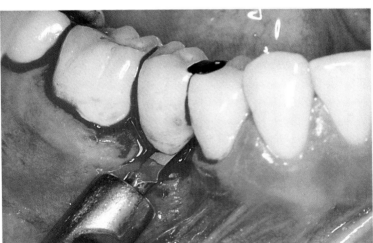

**410   Correction of the pontic**
Use flame-shaped diamonds to shorten and recontour the improper pontic, especially at its mesial and distal aspects. Local anesthesia may be required. Proxoshape files are used to smooth the undersurface of the pontic.

*Left:* Massive plaque-retention area beneath the concave, saddle-shaped pontic (solid red arrow).
   Contouring renders the pontic's undersurface flat to convex, plaque retention is reduced (empty arrow) and improved cleaning is made possible.

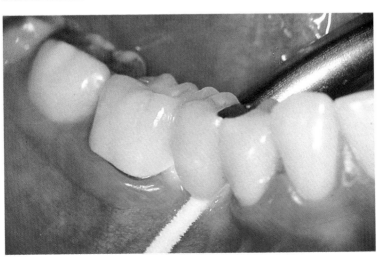

**411   Pontic area accessible for hygiene**
After the soft tissues heal, optimum hygiene is possible in the interdental areas and under the pontic using Super Floss or Brush and Floss.
   The yellowish fiber-optic light used from the lingual aspect reveals healthy keratinized gingiva.

## Removal of Iatrogenic Irritants – Metal Pigmentation

The cervical extent of fixed restorations, from a simple amalgam to extensive bridgework should be located supragingivally whenever possible, and should exhibit optimum closure at the margins. Correction of inadequate fixed restorations can be difficult, and does not always lead to the desired result.

In addition, attempting to correct subgingival inadequacies in fixed restorations is almost always accompanied by gingival trauma. Metal dust or fine particles of metal may become sequestered within the soft tissue, usually without any clinical sequelae.

Silver amalgam lodged in soft tissue often presents as a clinical "tattoo" that is esthetically undesirable. A foreign body reaction can be observed histologically. Amalgam particles may be phagocytosed by connective tissue cells, decomposed and transported within the tissue, leading to expansion of the clinical tattoo.

|  |  |
|---|---|
| **Amalgam** | **Gold** |

**412　Metal pigmentation viewed radiographically**
*Left:* Amalgam residues can enter the gingival tissues during removal of overhangs; these are visible in the radiograph. Some particles are expelled from the tissue. It is not always possible to remove all metal fragments, even by means of curettage of the sulcus/pocket wall.

*Right:* Gold residue and gold dust after recontouring a poor crown margin.

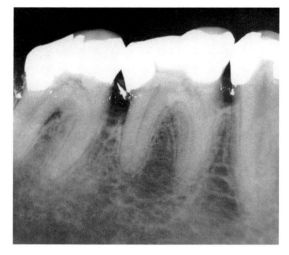 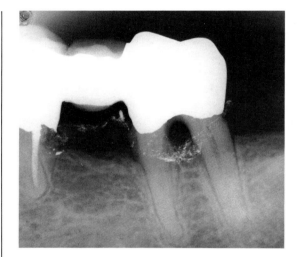

**413　Reaction of gingival tissue**
*Left:* Two amalgam particles surrounded by an infiltrate of multinucleated foreign body giant cells (Masson, x 250).

*Right:* Gold particle in the gingiva without any visible reaction of the tissue (H & E, x 250).

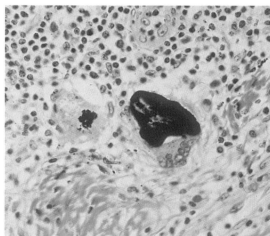 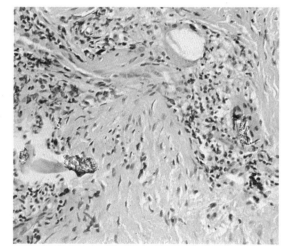

**414　Phagocytosis – Foreign body reaction**
*Left:* Amalgam can be degraded within connective tissue, whereupon fibroblasts phagocytose the amalgam dust (Masson, x 1,000).

*Right:* A large gold particle (✳) was lost from the tissue during sectioning for histologic examination. Multinucleated foreign body giant cells surround the area (H & E, x 1,000).

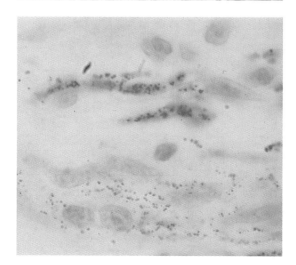 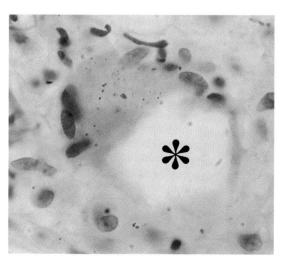

# Removal of Natural Plaque-Retentive Areas – Extraction

If *hopeless* teeth are not extracted on an emergency basis, the extractions should be performed during the hygiene phase of initial therapy. The deep and usually active periodontal pockets surrounding such teeth represent enormous bacterial reservoirs. These endanger the interdental septa of adjacent teeth and therefore the periodontal support of these teeth may continue to be compromised. Grassi et al. (1987 b) demonstrated that after extraction of a tooth the pocket associated with the adjacent tooth was reduced, but the attachment level did not change. Before extraction of a hopeless tooth, any restorations in the adjacent teeth should be polished. Immediately after extraction, the interproximal crown and root surfaces of the adjacent teeth can be cleaned and polished.

Excess gingival tissue or periodontal pockets in the proximal areas of the remaining teeth can be eliminated by means of a wedge excision followed by root planing and suture closure (cf. pp. 253–257). Temporary replacement of an extracted tooth in the posterior segment may not be necessary immediately.

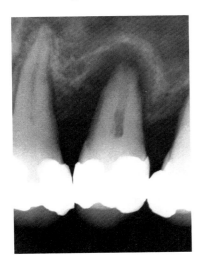
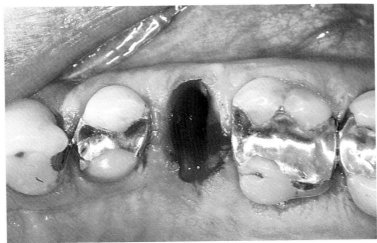

**415 Elimination of a plaque-retentive area through extraction**
A hopeless tooth with defects extending to the apex was extracted to preclude compromising the osseous support of the adjacent teeth.

*Left:* The radiograph reveals that tooth 25 has no remaining osseous support. The advanced attachment loss on this tooth appears to have damaged the periodontal support of its adjacent teeth (24, 26).

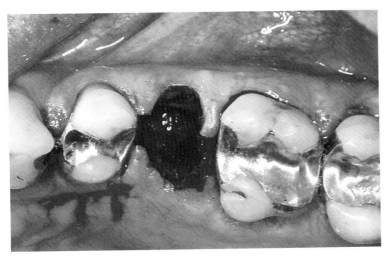

**416 Gingival excision and scaling of adjacent teeth**
Inflamed gingival and pocket tissues around adjacent teeth are excised as a wedge. The interproximal surfaces of these teeth can now be cleaned and smoothed under direct vision.

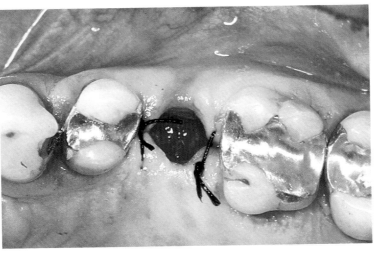

**417 Suture placement**
Individual sutures partially close the extraction wound mesially and distally, and also serve to adapt the tissues to the remaining teeth.

# Removal of Natural Plaque-Retentive Areas
## Odontoplasty of Grooves, Ridges, Irregularities ...

The natural morphology of a tooth manifests grooves, irregularities, depressions etc. on both the crown and the root. In a healthy dentition, these can usually be cleaned adequately with the toothbrush and interdental hygiene aids. However, morphologic anomalies that represent plaque-retentive areas may be found at the cervical aspect of some roots. Frequently encountered are *narrow grooves* that extend apically from the lingual pit of an incisor far down the root surface (Fig. 419).

Furthermore, fused roots of multirooted teeth may exhibit an irregular profile, with large grooves that may extend deeply into the subjacent dentin. Following initial periodontal pocket formation, such grooves are exposed and become plaque-retentive areas that are difficult to ascertain clinically. They may assume an etiologic role in localized, progressive destruction of periodontal supporting structures.

To a certain degree, such niches can be opened by means of mild odontoplasty and rendered more accessible for cleaning.

**418 Diamonds for odontoplasty – Perio-Set**
This set consists of slender, conical and flame-shaped diamonds for subgingival debridement, contouring (odontoplasty) and final polishing of ground tooth or root surfaces.

*Right:* Flame-shaped Perio-Set diamonds in three degrees of abrasiveness and two shaft lengths (SEM):

- **Perio-Set** (Intensiv Co.)
  75 µm (blue),
  40 µm (yellow),
  15 µm (red)

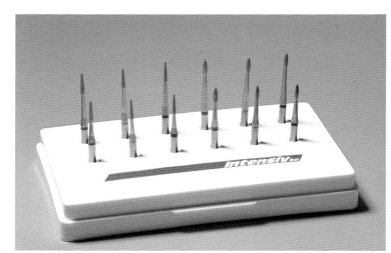
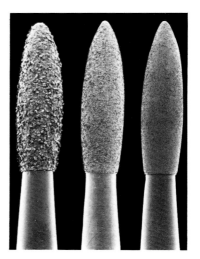

**419 Recontouring a depression on tooth 22**
Apical to the lingual pit amalgam on this lateral incisor, a fine groove that could be detected clinically with an explorer extended 5 mm apically into the periodontal pocket.

The groove was so narrow that its depth could not be probed with either a scaler or a curette. An odontoplastic modification was indicated, which included widening, rounding and polishing with a 15 µm diamond.

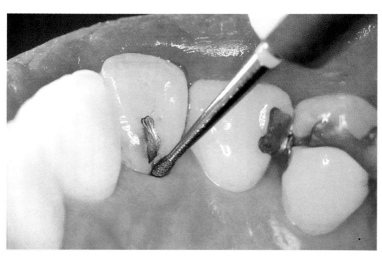

**420 Tooth 22 after odontoplasty**
The narrow groove was opened up using diamond burs. The depth of the groove can now be reached with fine hand instruments (e.g., an 0.8 mm wide curette), making adequate professional debridement possible.
After odontoplasty tooth surfaces should be repeatedly treated with topical fluoride.

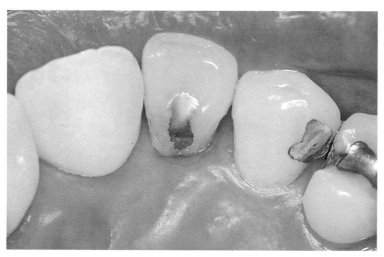

## ... and Furcations

Furcations can pose a clinical problem after even minor loss of periodontal supporting structure, because the entrance to a furcation may be located immediately apical to the crestal bone margin, e.g., in mandibular molars. When such a furcation is exposed, it becomes a plaque-retentive area that is virtually impossible to reach with any hygiene aid. The enamel pearls and enamel projections frequently located at the furcation entrance just apical to the CEJ represent potential weak links in the plaque control chain.

During the combined clinical and radiographic examination of each individual tooth, such anomalies must be discerned. In most cases they can be corrected easily by means of minor odontoplasty, making the plaque-retentive areas accessible for hygiene. Teeth that have undergone odontoplasty should be carefully polished (15 µm diamond, rubber cups and polishing paste if accessible). Finally the areas should be treated with topical fluoride. It is not uncommon for a patient to experience sensitivity of the cervical area for some time following odontoplasty.

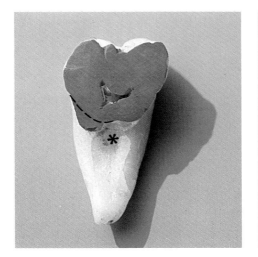
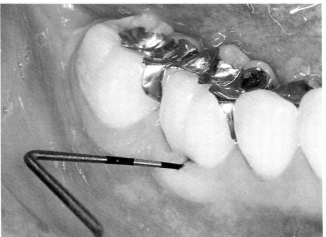

**421 Furcation (Class F1) as a plaque-retentive area**
This mandibular molar furcation can be probed 3 mm horizontally from the buccal aspect. A cavernous hollow is located behind the overhang (dashed line). Without odontoplasty this kind of plaque-retentive area is impossible to reach for cleaning.

*Left:* For demonstration of this situation, a similar mandibular molar was sectioned through the furcation area. The interradicular "cave" (*) and the planned odonto-plastic procedure are shown.

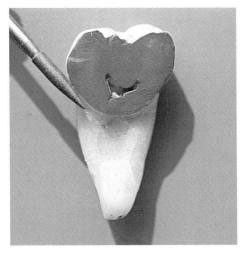
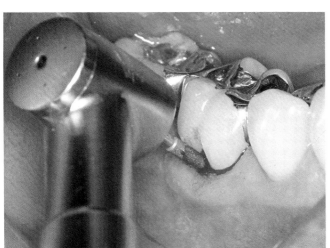

**422 Odontoplasty of the furcation entrance**
Using coarse diamond burs, the overhanging enamel is removed and the entrance to the furcation area opened. It is now accessible for professional plaque control (scaling).

*Left:* Polishing the treated furcation entrance using the 15 µm diamond.

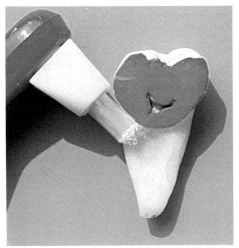
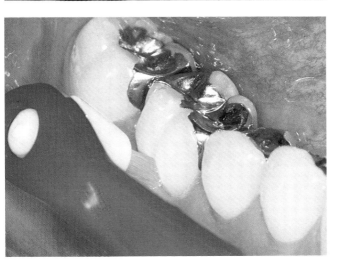

**423 Hygiene with the marginal/interdental brush**
The furcation entrance can now be cleaned easily by the patient using, for example, the marginal/inter-dental brush (Lactona no. 27).
At each recall appointment, this area must be carefully reevaluated.

*Left:* This section through the tooth shows how the small brush has access to the furcation entrance.

# Reduction of Plaque-Retentive Areas Caused by Crowding – Odontoplasty

Crowding of teeth is one of the few tooth positional anomalies that can be of significance indirectly in the etiology of gingivitis and periodontitis. This has less to do with functional occlusal factors than with the accumulation of plaque that occurs around crowded teeth, coupled with the fact that the patient has difficulty keeping the area clean.

Extensive orthodontic treatment including selective extractions is often refused by adults due to the cost in time, effort and money.

Careful *odontoplasty* of crowded teeth is an alternative to orthodontic treatment, albeit a limited alternative. Such recontouring also may enhance the esthetic situation. The corrections are performed *only in enamel* using fine diamonds.

Tooth surfaces must subsequently be smoothed, polished and treated with topical fluoride.

**424  Crowding**
There is severe gingivitis, and a disclosing agent reveals heavy plaque accumulation on tooth surfaces that cannot be reached by the normal self-cleansing mechanisms, e.g., lip and tongue contact. This clinical situation can be improved by careful morphologic grinding.

*Right:* View of the mandibular anterior teeth from the incisal. As a result of the crowding, the facially displaced tooth 31 is not touched by the tongue.

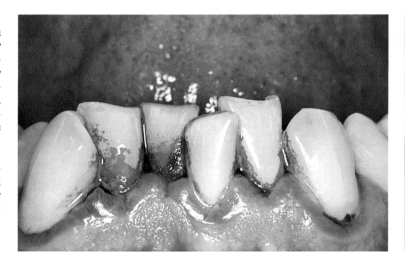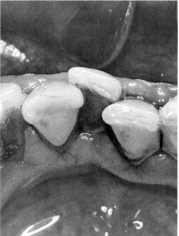

**425  Odontoplasty**
The incisal edges were first evened somewhat for esthetic reasons, but incisal contacts were left intact (red). The labial tooth surfaces were then selectively recontoured, as indicated by the black markings, to eliminate the plaque-retentive area as much as possible.

The interdental spaces were filed using abrasive strips to permit the use of dental floss.

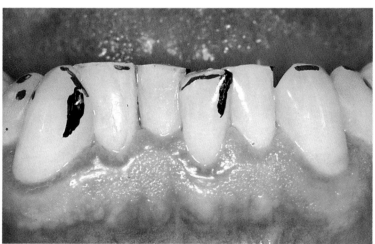

**426  After grinding and initial therapy**
The plaque-retentive areas are less dramatic as indicated by the disclosing agent, which reveals only minor plaque accumulations. Interdental hygiene by means of dental floss is now possible for the patient.

Initial therapy and optimum home care have eliminated inflammation for the most part.

*Right:* The situation has also been improved on the lingual aspect. However, a mild marginal inflammation persists in this area.

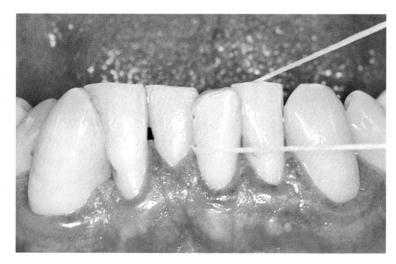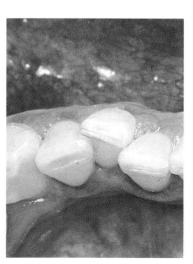

# Gingivitis Treatment

## Operative procedure

Gingivitis therapy is a component of the first phase of initial therapy. It consists of patient motivation, information, oral hygiene and monitoring, as well as *plaque and calculus removal*. These are time consuming; they will be demonstrated in the mandibular anterior area.

The 30-year-old female patient exhibits a moderate, plaque-induced gingivitis. There is *no* attachment loss, but pseudopockets to 4 mm are noted. The patient has never received comprehensive oral hygiene instruction. OHI is therefore provided simultaneously with professional tooth cleaning procedures.

---

*Initial findings* (values for the mandibular anterior area)

| | | | |
|---|---|---|---|
| HI: | 28% | GI-S: | 69% |
| TM: | 0–1 (Severity of TM cf. Fig. 307) | | |

See Figs. for clinical picture and radiographic findings.

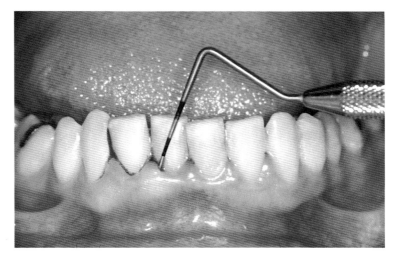

**427  Initial findings –
Moderate gingivitis**
The gingivae are swollen by edema, especially in the papillary area. Profuse hemorrhage occurs immediately after gentle probing particularly in interdental areas. The patient's generally mediocre oral hygiene is enhanced in the mandibular anterior area by mild crowding, which favors plaque accumulation. The width of attached gingiva is normal.

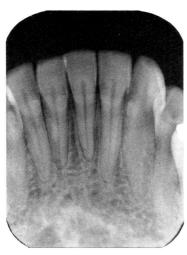

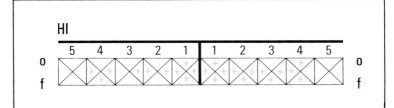

**428  Bleeding Index (GI-S)
and Hygiene Index (HI)**

**GI-S:** On 22 of the 32 measured sites (mesial, facial, distal, oral) bleeding occurs after gentle periodontal probing (69% gingivitis; see Indices, pp. 35–40).

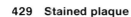

**HI:** On 23 of the 32 examined tooth surfaces (teeth 34–44) plaque is detected (28% hygiene).

*Left:* Radiographic findings. Despite the gingivitis, which has persisted for many years, there is no radiographic bone loss.

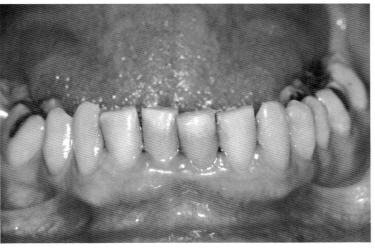

**429  Stained plaque**
On almost all teeth there are more or less pronounced plaque accumulations (see HI in Fig. 428: 72% plaque corresponds to HI of 28%).

**Plaque and calculus removal; mandibular anterior area – Procedure observed from the oral aspect**

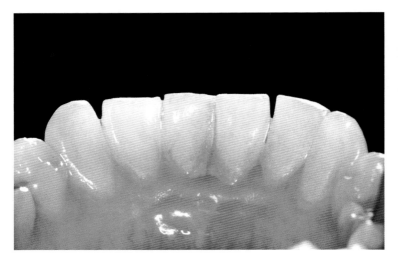

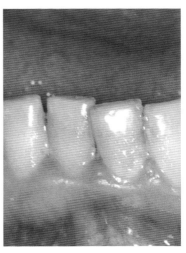

### 430 Initial condition

A plaque-induced gingivitis with supragingival calculus is shown from the *oral* aspect.

Oral hygiene instruction including toothbrush and dental floss is provided.

*Right:* The gingivitis is equally pronounced on the facial aspect.

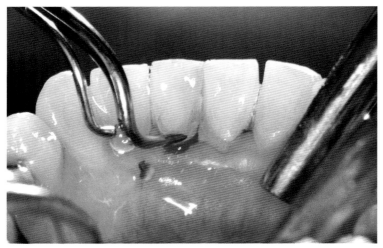

### 431 Debridement using the ultrasonic scaler

For rapid removal of soft and hard supragingival deposits, but especially for calculus, ultrasonic and sonic scalers are excellent. Even when hemorrhage is severe, the washed-field technique provides continuously good visibility.

Ultrasonic and sonic scalers may also be inserted a few millimeters into the pocket/pseudopocket.

*Caution:* Aerosols are created (Viral infections: HIV, hepatitis!).

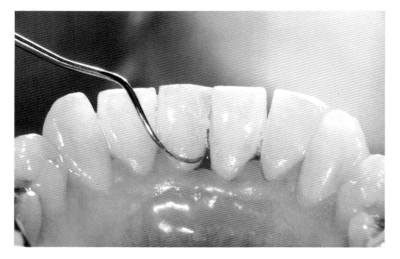

### 432 Checking with a pointed explorer

The smoothness of the tooth and root surfaces is checked with a very fine cowhorn or shepherd's crook explorer. Pictured is the CH3 from Hu-Friedy.

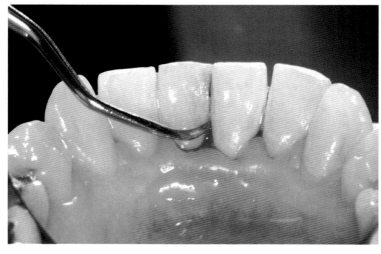

### 433 Scaling – Tooth cleaning supragingivally using hand instruments

After use of power scalers it is imperative that hand instruments (scalers/curettes) be systematically employed for fine debridement.

The relatively gross ultrasonic instruments routinely leave behind islands of soft and hard deposits, especially in interdental areas. Residual calculus must be removed with scalers/curettes (tactile sense!). Plaque is removed with rubber cups and paste (cf. Fig. 436).

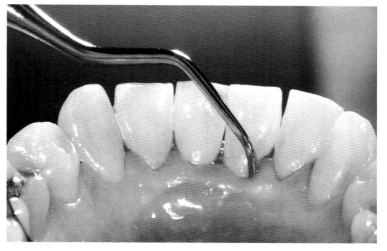

**434    Subgingival cleaning with universal curettes**
Even in gingivitis therapy, fine curettes are used. Their rounded ends injure gingiva only slightly even when they are used subgingivally in pseudopockets.

The working stroke of this anterior curette may be vertical, diagonal or horizontal to the long axis of the tooth.

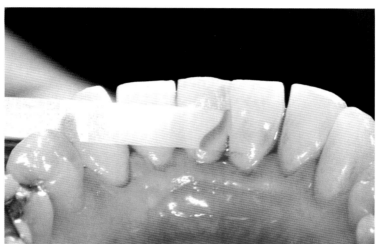

**435    Plaque removal in the interdental area – Strip with mild abrasiveness**
Following mechanical therapy of the oral and facial tooth surfaces, the proximal surfaces and the contact areas are cleaned with strips incorporating fine abrasive.

For polishing, dental tape or smooth, uncoated strips may be used with a fluoride-containing prophy paste.

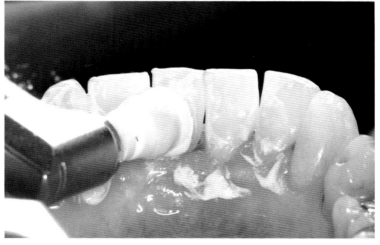

**436    Polishing the teeth**
Using the "*R*ubber *C*up and *P*aste" method (RCP), the tooth surfaces are treated with rubber cups and prophy paste. It may be necessary to polish first with an abrasive paste (e.g., RDA 120), and finally with a polishing paste (RDA 40; cf. p. 164, Fig. 396).

Whenever possible soft deposits (plaque) should be removed by means of RCP, because repeated mechanical scaling (e.g., at recall appointments) may elicit slight recession (attachment loss) even in healthy patients.

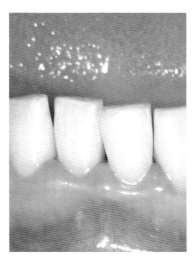
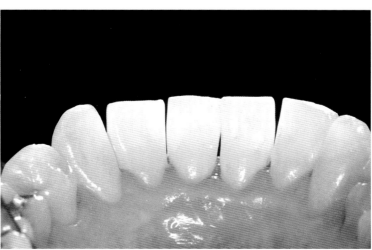

**437    Mandibular anterior area immediately after treatment**
Plaque and calculus have been removed. The time for these procedures was ca. 20 min. Even with very careful mechanical treatment of the tooth surfaces, minute trauma to the gingiva cannot be avoided.

*Left:* View from the facial immediately following plaque and calculus removal.

*All of these procedures (which constitute gingivitis therapy) may be performed by the dentist or by the dental hygienist.*

# Gingivitis Treatment

## Summary

In this 30-year-old female patient, restorations were placed from time to time over many years. At these infrequent dental appointments, however, oral hygiene instruction was never provided. The patient reported that a very brief calculus removal was performed at such appointments.

During gingivitis therapy in all sextants by the dental hygienist, the patient was readily motivated. She learned the demonstrated plaque control methods using toothbrush and dental floss without any difficulty.

The Hygiene Index for the entire dentition increased quickly to 88%, and virtually no bleeding occurred upon sulcus probing (GI-S: 9%, Fig. 439).

The patient's continued excellent cooperation was to be expected; thus, 1–2 short term follow-up appointments were scheduled. Subsequently, a recall interval of ca. 6 months should be sufficient to maintain the successful treatment result.

**438  Initial condition – Mandibular anterior area**
Inflamed and slightly swollen gingiva, pseudopockets, bleeding on probing.

Generalized marginal plaque accumulation is barely visible (HI only 28%).

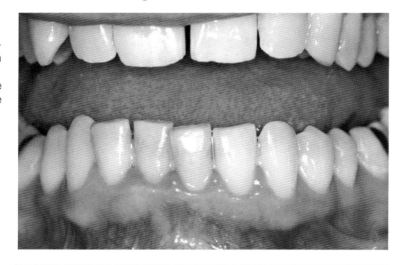

**439  Bleeding Index (GI-S) before initiation of therapy**
Over two-thirds of all marginal and interdental areas bleed after probing (GI-S: 69%).

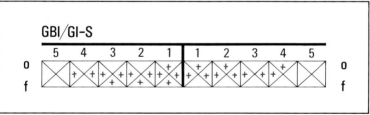

Before

**Bleeding Index (GI-S) after treatment**
The number of bleeding sites was reduced from 69% to 9% by means of the local therapy. In the depicted region, there are only three sites that exhibit mild, point bleeding upon probing.

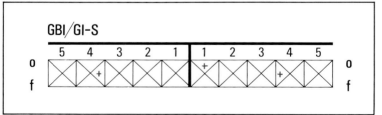

After

**440  After 6 months**
Gingivitis has been eliminated. The gingiva exhibits normal form, color and contour. It is coral pink, keratinized and lightly stippled.

Plaque is virtually absent. The patient uses the modified Bass technique for toothbrushing and cleans interdental areas with dental floss.

She understands the etiology of gingivitis; thus, she can prevent recurrence.

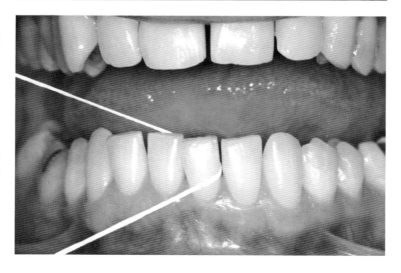

# Initial Therapy II – Conservative Therapy

## Subgingival Scaling – Root Planing
## Gingival Curettage

The second phase of initial therapy includes closed debridement of periodontal pockets. This treatment is also referred to as *conservative* therapy, in contrast to periodontal surgery (p. 207). It is non-surgical therapy.

The following procedures comprise this therapy:

| |
|---|
| Cleaning the root surfaces of plaque and calculus |
| Removing endotoxin-containing cementum layers (?) |
| Root planing |
| Possible soft tissue curettage |

## Definitions

Nomenclature for these procedures is not internationally uniform. The following definitions are presented for clarity in this *Atlas* (AAP 1986 a, b).

### Subgingival plaque and calculus removal (scaling)

Removal of adherent and non-adherent plaque as well as calcified plaque (calculus) from the gingival or bony pocket and from the root surface.

### Cleaning the root surfaces

Removal of endotoxin-containing cementum once the root surfaces have been cleaned. This procedure cannot be sharply delineated from subgingival calculus removal and root planing.

### Root planing

Smoothing the root surface using curettes and possibly also polishing diamonds. This procedure is also not a distinct entity vis-à-vis subgingival scaling or cleaning root surfaces.

### Gingival curettage

Removal of the pocket epithelium and infiltrated subepithelial connective tissue. This procedure borders on surgical therapy.

### Closed curettage – Conservative therapy

All of the above-defined procedures are carried out without reflecting the gingivae, i. e., without direct vision into the pocket or onto the root surface.

### Open curettage – Surgical therapy

Following a marginal incision or an internal gingivectomy (see ENAP, Open Curettage and Modified Widman Procedure, pp. 217–230), the gingiva is reflected to such an extent that scaling and root planing can be performed with direct vision.

The differences between these Phase II procedures and *supragingival* plaque and calculus removal (Initial Therapy I) are not sharply defined, because during supragingival tooth cleaning procedures the scalers, ultrasonic instruments, air-scaler and curettes often enter the subgingival area insofar as this is possible without anesthesia.

## Conservative, Non-Surgical Therapy – Goals of Treatment

The goal of conservative, non-surgical therapy is the elimination of the microorganisms responsible for periodontal destruction, from the pocket and surrounding tissue. The creation of a clean tooth and a clean, biologically compatible root surface that is as smooth as possible, and the possible removal of diseased or infected tissues are essential to therapy (Frank 1980, Saglie et al. 1982, Allenspach-Petrzilka & Guggenheim 1983, O'Leary 1986, Adriaens et al. 1988).

### Indications
Conservative procedures *without* surgery are indicated for mild to moderate periodontitis (pockets $\leq$ 6 mm). At re-evaluation several months later, the dentist can decide if local surgery is needed.

### Contraindications
None, although patients with severe systemic diseases require special attention (patients taking anticoagulants or those who require antibiotic coverage; see p. 314).

**441    Principles of conservative pocket therapy**
This stained (H & E, x 20) histologic section through a periodontal pocket will be used to illustrate root planing and soft tissue curettage.

Soft tissue curettage (**2**) is *never* used alone. True "causal" therapy includes the thorough cleaning of the root surfaces (**1**). Curettage always elicits a transient bacteremia.

**1. Root planing**
The unilaterally sharp Gracey curette (**1**) removes plaque, calculus, endotoxin-containing cementum and sometimes dentin from the tooth surface. The arrow indicates the direction toward which the curette tip is pulled.

**2. Gingival curettage**
A Gracey curette sharpened on its other edge (**2**) is used to remove pocket epithelium and remaining (apical) junctional epithelium, as well as the infiltrated connective tissue (destroyed collagenous matrix) that is sharply demarcated from the intact, healthy tissue.

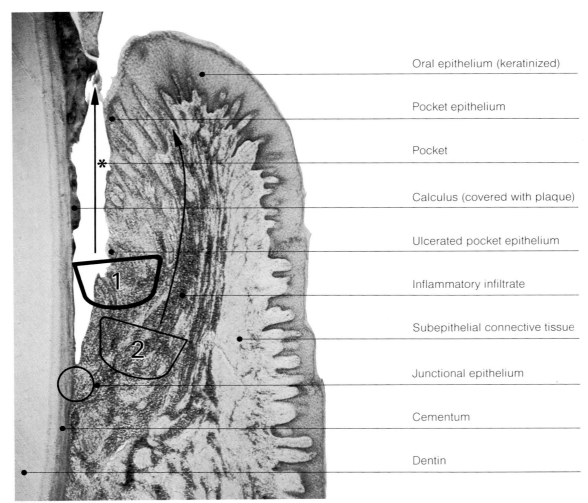

Oral epithelium (keratinized)

Pocket epithelium

Pocket

Calculus (covered with plaque)

Ulcerated pocket epithelium

Inflammatory infiltrate

Subepithelial connective tissue

Junctional epithelium

Cementum

Dentin

### Advantages
Closed treatment of the periodontal pocket is, in principle, a simple operation. It causes less trauma and hemorrhage than a surgical procedure. Gingival shrinkage during the healing phase is less than after invasive surgery. This may be important for esthetics.

The conservative procedure is associated with long-term maintenance of attachment level with regular recall (p. 209, Michigan studies, Knowles et al. 1979). Single-rooted teeth respond particularly well to the conservative, closed procedure (Badersten 1984; Badersten et al. 1984 a, b).

### Disadvantages
Subgingival scaling is one of the most technically difficult treatment modalities because it is performed without direct vision. It is therefore not surprising that such scaling procedures do not achieve all root surfaces or that treated surfaces are not always completely free of residual plaque and calculus (Waerhaug 1978, Thornton & Garnick 1982, Rateitschak-Plüss 1985, Eaton et al. 1985, Nordland et al. 1987, Lie et al. 1987). Closed pocket treatment is especially difficult in deep and narrow pockets, in furcation areas and where root irregularities exist. The danger of recurrence and reinfection of residual pockets exists in these areas.

# Root Planing – With or without Gingival Curettage

Absolute cleanliness of the root surface is the most critical goal in pocket therapy. All substances must be removed from the root surface including plaque, calculus and endotoxin. These toxins (lipopolysaccharide, from gram-negative bacteria) are found in the superficial layers of cementum, and can inhibit attachment of epithelium and regenerated connective tissue to the root surface. For this reason, the root surface must be planed and smoothed until only healthy (hard) cementum or dentin remains. Once the root surface is treated, the "peeling out" of the pocket epithelium and infiltrated connective tissue can be accomplished. This procedure is currently the topic of some controversy. If the curettes used for root planing are sharp on both edges, some soft tissue curettage will be accomplished inadvertently while the hard tooth structure is being planed.

The goals of these procedures are the elimination of pocket infection and healing of the periodontal lesion. Some shrinkage of the tissue will occur, producing longer appearing teeth.

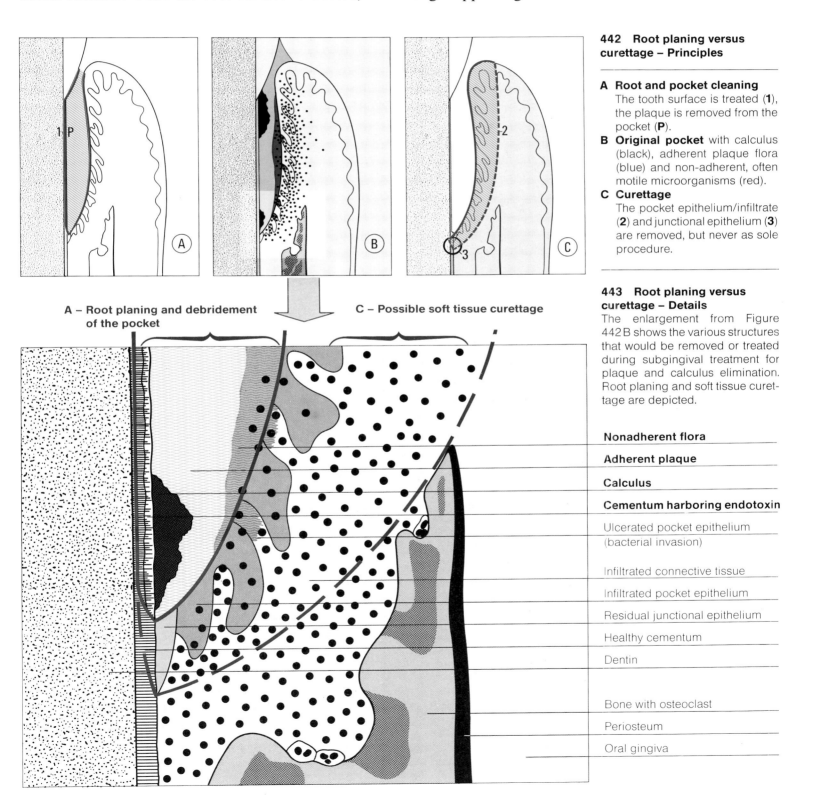

**442  Root planing versus curettage – Principles**

**A  Root and pocket cleaning**
The tooth surface is treated (**1**), the plaque is removed from the pocket (**P**).

**B  Original pocket** with calculus (black), adherent plaque flora (blue) and non-adherent, often motile microorganisms (red).

**C  Curettage**
The pocket epithelium/infiltrate (**2**) and junctional epithelium (**3**) are removed, but never as sole procedure.

**443  Root planing versus curettage – Details**
The enlargement from Figure 442B shows the various structures that would be removed or treated during subgingival treatment for plaque and calculus elimination. Root planing and soft tissue curettage are depicted.

A – Root planing and debridement of the pocket

C – Possible soft tissue curettage

Nonadherent flora

Adherent plaque

Calculus

Cementum harboring endotoxin

Ulcerated pocket epithelium (bacterial invasion)

Infiltrated connective tissue

Infiltrated pocket epithelium

Residual junctional epithelium

Healthy cementum

Dentin

Bone with osteoclast

Periosteum

Oral gingiva

# Instruments for Scaling and Root Planing ...

For the removal of large accumulations of subgingival calculus, *hoes* and *curettes* are the instruments of choice. For plaque removal, root planing and soft tissue curettage, curettes are indicated exclusively; hoes are inappropriate for this purpose.

The dental marketplace offers innumerable instruments of various designs and varying quality. Every dental school and every dental practitioner have favorites. This *Atlas* makes no recommendations as to brand names, but it is important that the assortment of curettes selected must be able to reach all root surfaces.

In practice, the instrument should be used with its working tip an angle of 80° to the root surface. All instruments must be sharpened before each use (except hoes with carbide tips).

Note that the common universal curettes are sharp on both sides of the working end, while the special Gracey curettes are sharpened on only one side of the blade. Graceys are used more often for cleaning root surfaces (root planing) than for soft tissue curettage.

### 444　Hoes
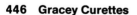

#### – TC 210–213 (Ash Co.)

These hoes have carbide steel tips and are useful for removal of hard subgingival accretions even in deep pockets. These instruments can cause deep scratches and are therefore not indicated for root planing. Four shapes are available.

*Right:* Shank and working tip of hoes 212 and 213; (green-black) for use primarily on facial and oral root surfaces.

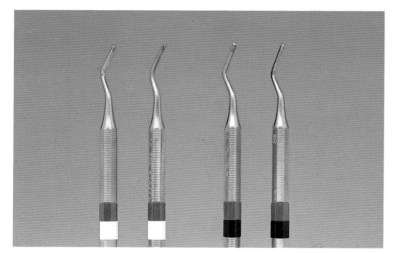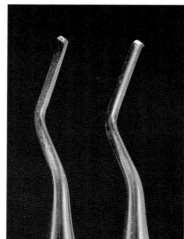

### 445　Curettes
(Deppeler Co.)

#### – Universal curette ZI 15
(yellow)
#### – Anterior curette GX 4
(orange)
#### – Posterior curette M 23 A
(red)

ZI 15 is used for the first gross debridement. GX 4 is indicated for incisors, canines and sometimes premolars; M 23 A, premolars and molars.

*Right:* Shank and working ends of the double-ended posterior curette (M 23 A).

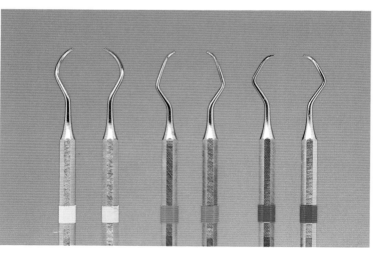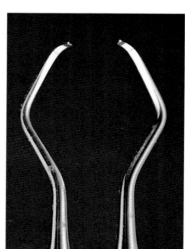

### 446　Gracey Curettes

A complete set consists of 14 instruments with different bends of the shanks, or seven *pairs* of double-ended instruments (cf. Fig. 453).

The following double-ended instruments, with color-coded handles, are sufficient (cf. pp. 186–190).

#### – Gracey 5/6 (yellow)
#### – Gracey 7/8 (grey)
#### – Gracey 11/12 (brown)
#### – Gracey 13/14 (blue)

*Right:* Shank and working end of the paired Gracey curettes 13/14 (Deppeler Co.).

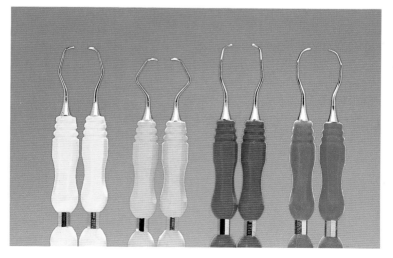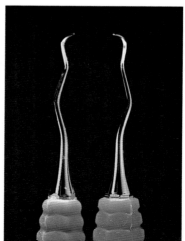

# ... and Their Use

Closed subgingival scaling can only be a successful procedure if it is performed systematically, generally by quadrants or sextants, and using local anesthesia. The operator must be aware of the probing depths and attachment loss on all root surfaces of each tooth to be treated.

The procedure can be performed *"tooth by tooth"* or *"instrument by instrument."* Here, the degree of precision demanded by the procedure is pitted against a rational approach. It is more rational, time-effective and easier to treat all tooth surfaces in a dental segment with one instrument, and then switch to the next instrument. However, when probing depths vary greatly from one tooth to another, and when teeth exhibit root fusions, furcation involvement, or other anatomic peculiarities, it often makes more sense to treat completely all surfaces of one tooth, even though it requires several instrument changes. This is the only way to insure that every root surface is appropriately addressed, treated, and not "forgotten."

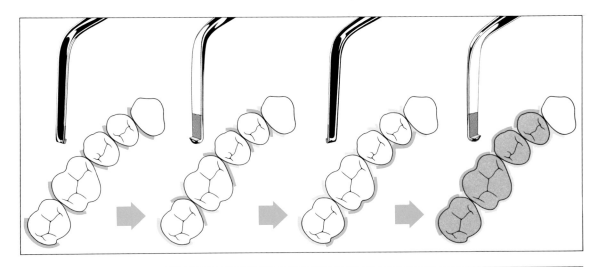

**Systematic procedure**

**447 Tooth surface by tooth surface – Hoe instrument**
The operator holds a double-ended hoe scaler (Ash TC 210–211) and treats all distal surfaces of teeth in the maxillary right sextant.

He then turns the instrument over and treats all mesial surfaces of the same teeth.

The same procedure is performed on buccal and palatal surfaces using the TC 212–213 hoe.

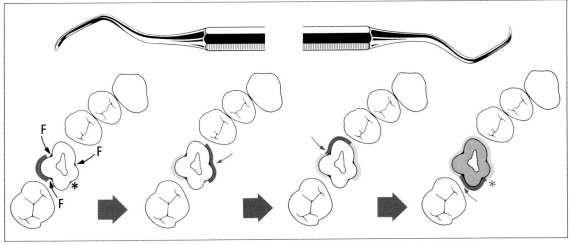

**448 Tooth by tooth – Posterior universal curette**
In the example depicted, a molar (16) with a palatal depression and incipient furcation involvement is to be completely treated.

Using one side of a double-ended posterior curette (M 23 A), the distobuccal aspect of the tooth is treated first, then the mesiopalatal. With the other end of the instrument, the mesiobuccal and finally the distopalatal root segments are treated. Note the depression (∗) and the furcation entrances (**F**).

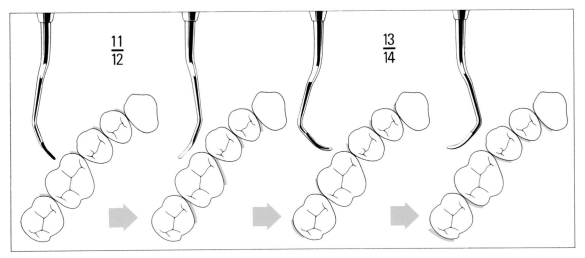

**449 Tooth surface by tooth surface – Garcey curettes**
The approach when using Gracey curettes is different, because they are sharp on only one side, as compared to universal curettes, which have two sharp edges. Furthermore, the working end of the Gracey is offset 70° to the shank.

The double-ended (paired) instruments are used as depicted here to treat the mesial surfaces of the premolars and molars (no. 11/12) and the distal surfaces of these same teeth (no. 13/14).

Buccal and palatal surfaces are then treated with the no. 7/8 curette.

# Gracey Curettes – Areas of Use

### Complete set

For closed subgingival scaling and root planing, special instruments are indicated that are adaptable to the most varied root shapes. As early as the 1930s a practitioner named C. H. Gracey, together with an instrument maker by the name of Hugo Friedman (Hu-Friedy!) conceptualized his first set of instruments which "... *gives every dentist the possibility to treat even the deepest and least accessible periodontal pockets simply and without traumatic stretching of the gingiva; the possi-*

*bility to remove completely all subgingival calculus and to clean and plane every root surface perfectly, which will in turn make possible subsequent tissue adaptation and re-attachment."*

Numerous modifications of the instruments lead finally to the Gracey curettes of today.

The use of these instruments has been described in detail (Pattison & Pattison 1979, Hellwege 1987) and will be depicted here.

**Anterior teeth to the premolars**

Figures 450–456 demonstrate the systematic use of all Gracey curettes in quadrant 2 (maxillary left).

**450  Gracey (GRA) 1/2 – Incisors, canines**
The primary area of use for this paired instrument is the *facial* root surfaces of incisors and canines.

*Right:* **GRA 1/2**
Medium length shank, mild angulation

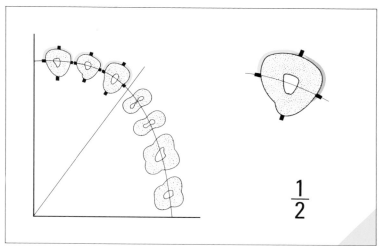 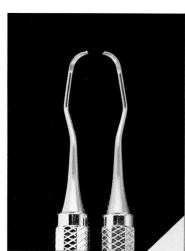

**451  Gracey 3/4 – Incisors, canines**
Primary use is the same as with GRA 1/2, but because of the more severe angulation, the 3/4 is particularly indicated for *palatal* and *lingual* surfaces.

*Right:* **GRA 3/4**
Short shank, sharper angulation.

The cutting edge of these paired instruments is the "outer" edge, along the *convex* curvature of the working tip (only one edge of the blade is sharp).

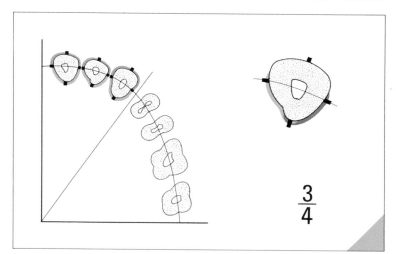 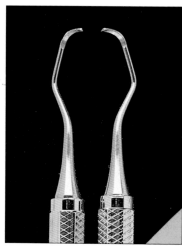

**452  Gracey 5/6 * – Anterior teeth and premolars**
The area of use corresponds for the most part to that of an anterior universal curette (e.g., GX 4, Fig. 445).

Additionally this Gracey curette with its long straight shank can be used in virtually all areas of the dentition where deep pockets exist.

*Right:* **GRA 5/6**
Long shank, slight angulation.

---

\* The four double-ended instruments marked with an asterisk comprise the reduced Gracey set (cf. Figs. 446 and 458–474).

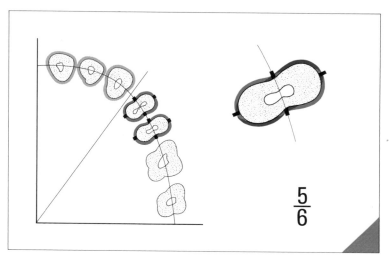 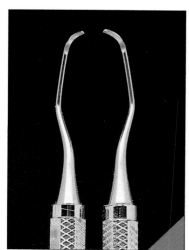

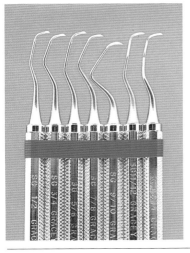

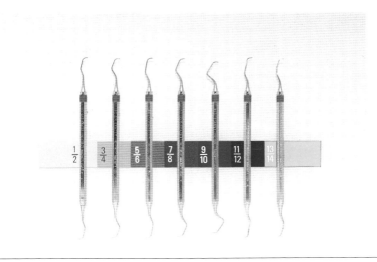

### 453  Complete Gracey curette set
(Original Hu-Friedy Co.)

| GRA | 1/2 | yellow |
|-----|------|--------|
| GRA | 3/4 | orange |
| GRA | 5/6* | red |
| GRA | 7/8* | magenta |
| GRA | 9/10 | purple |
| GRA | 11/12* | violet |
| GRA | 13/14* | blue |

(Color-coding valid for this double page)

*Left:* The seven different working ends of the complete Gracey set.

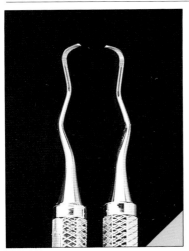

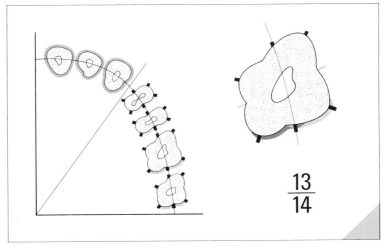

$$\frac{13}{14}$$

### Posterior area

### 454  Gracey 13/14*
**Molars (and some premolars) – distal**
First, for example, all *distal surfaces* are cleaned, from the facial (buccal) aspect and then from the oral (palatal) aspect. The *line angles* are indicated by short bars. This is the transition from one tooth (root) surface to another, where the use of individual instruments changes.

*Left:* **GRA 13/14***
Triple-bend shaft.

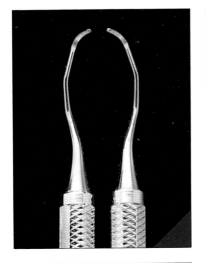

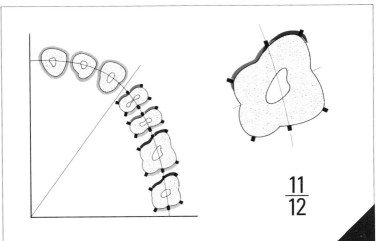

$$\frac{11}{12}$$

### 455  Gracey 11/12*
**Molar (and some premolars) – mesial**
This instrument, with its sharp convex cutting edge, is indicated for treatment of all *mesial surfaces* from the facial (buccal) aspect, and the other end for mesial surfaces from the oral (palatal) aspect.

Like the GRA 13/14, the GRA 11/12 is particularly well suited for multirooted premolars as well as in furcations and depressions.

*Left:* **GRA 11/12***
Longer shaft with several shallow angulations.

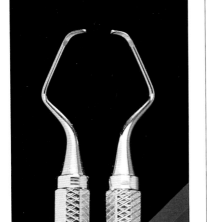

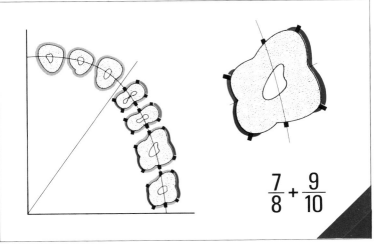

$$\frac{7}{8} + \frac{9}{10}$$

### 456  Gracey 7/8* and 9/10
**Molars (and some premolars) — Facial and oral surfaces**
Due to the rather severe angulation of the longer shaft, both instruments, in addition to their primary indication on facial and oral surfaces in the posterior area, are also useful in deep depressions and furcations. In addition this angulation permits not only axial but also oblique and horizontal strokes parallel to the gingival margin.

*Left:* **GRA 7/8***
Medium length, severely angulated shaft.

# Scaling Technique with Gracey Curettes – Systematic Clinical Procedure

### Reduced, minimum set

An introduction to the scaling technique using Gracey curettes is simplified by limiting the choice to four double-ended instruments. Color-coded handles simplify their assignment to certain tooth surfaces. The reduced instrument set is adequate for the treatment of mild to moderate periodontitis, and for recall patients.

In addition to an adequate armamentarium, certain prerequisites must be fulfilled in order to optimally perform the technically difficult scaling procedures (Wolf 1987 b).

*Prerequisites for optimum scaling technique:*

– Position of the patient and the operator
– Operatory lighting
– Sharp instruments, selecting proper cutting edge
– Secure stroke (modified pen grasp) and finger rest
– Precise knowledge of all probing depths
– Systematic procedure
– Exploratory and working strokes
– Monitoring roughness

### 457 Scaling technique

Even though the entire subgingival scaling procedure is performed blind, an excellent view of the field of operation is of prime importance. Proper lighting and a trained assistant are essential.

Conservative pocket treatment is associated with considerable hemorrhage, which demands rubber gloves and other barrier techniques by the operator.

The position of the patient's head should be adapted to the ideal posture of the operator. Exceptions to this rule need only be made for the handicapped, pregnant etc.

The operator holds the instrument in a modified pen grasp: The middle finger is in contact with the first bend of the instrument shank, which serves to stabilize the instrument.

### Basic armamentarium:

– Anesthesia
– Mirror, cotton forceps, sharp explorer
– Periodontal probe
– Minimum Gracey set (No. 5/6, 7/8, 11/12, 13/14)
– Scalers, universal curettes
– Perio-Set diamonds (Fig. 418)
– Rinsing solution, NaCl 0.9%
– Sterile sharpening stone

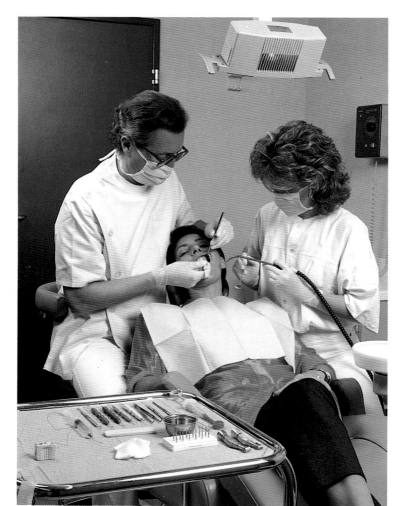

**Checklist – Scaling technique**

● Operatory light

● Protective eyewear
● Mask

● Surgical gloves

● Position of operator and patient's head

● Instrument grip (modified pen grasp)
● Rest position (fulcrum)

● Armamentarium with sharpening stone

*Pages 187–190 depict systematic scaling using the minimum set in the upper left quadrant.*

### 458 Areas of use for the Gracey curettes – Minimum set

– **Gracey 5/6** (yellow)
Incisors and canines
– **Gracey 7/8** (grey)
Molars and premolars, *buccal* and *oral*
– **Gracey 11/12** (brown)
Molars and premolars, *mesial,* furcations
– **Gracey 13/14** (blue)
Molars and premolars, *distal,* furcations

*Right:* Minimum Gracey set with color-coded handles ("Col-grips," Deppeler Co.).

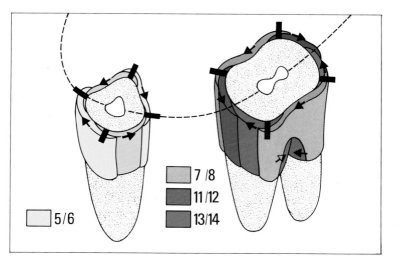

7 /8
11 /12
13/14
5/6

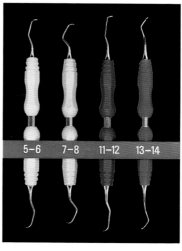

5–6   7–8   11–12   13–14

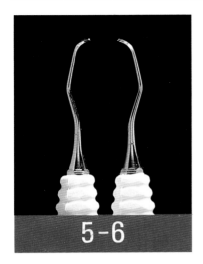

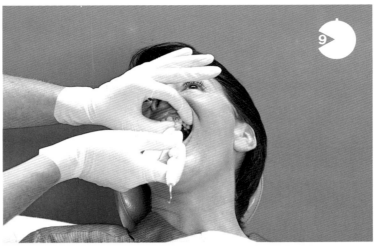

## 5–6

▶ **Anterior region – Facial**

**459   Scaling on distobuccal surfaces – Tooth 22**
*Patient's head:* Reclined position, head inclined to the right

*Dentist:* 9 o'clock position
*Rest position:* Intraoral, indirect upon the thumb of the left hand
*Vision of the operator:* Direct

*Left:* No. 5/6 working ends

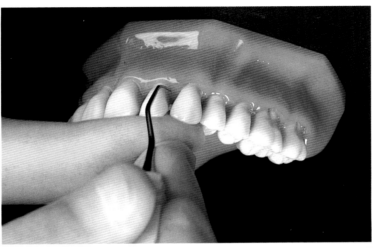

**460   Model situation**
This indirect, intraoral rest position permits the fulcrum point of the working hand to be placed nearest to the root surface being treated.

*Left:* The cutting edge of the instrument cleans all *distobuccal* root surfaces, then the *mesiobuccal* surfaces are treated with the other blade of the double-ended Gracey 5/6 curette. Instrument changes are made at the indicated markings. In these regions the working areas of both blades should overlap.

▶ **Anterior region – Palatal**

**461   Scaling on distopalatal surfaces – Tooth 22**
*Patient's head:* Extended to the right and dorsally

*Dentist:* 11 o'clock position
*Rest position:* Intraoral, directly on tooth 21
*Vision:* Indirect (mirror)

*Left:* Parallel, 3–4 mm working strokes from the palatal toward the interdental area. The facial tooth surface has already been cleaned.

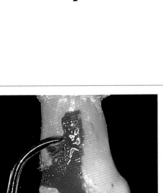

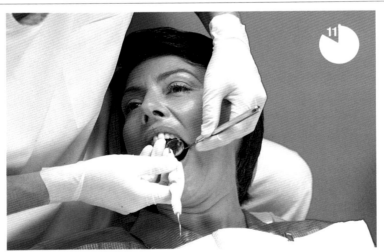

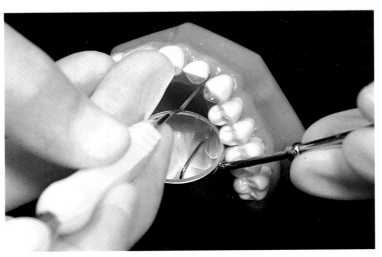

**462   Model situation**
The mouth mirror permits indirect vision and ensures proper lighting of the working field.
    Observe the modified pen grasp.

*Left:* Mesiopalatal and distopalatal root surfaces are approached using alternate ends of the 5/6 Gracey curette.

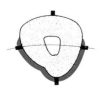
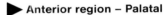
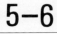

## 13-14

▶ **Posterior segment — Distal**

**463   Scaling on distal surfaces from the buccal — Tooth 26**
*Patient's head:* Inclined far to the right

*Dentist:* 10 o'clock position
*Rest position:* Intraoral, directly upon the neighboring tooth
*Vision:* Direct; mirror retracts cheek.
*Right:* The cutting edge is on the longer, convex surface of the working tip (No. 13/14).

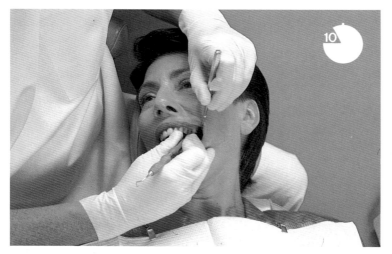
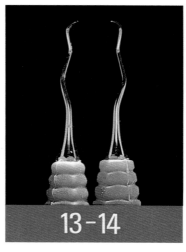
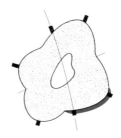

**464   Model situation**
The rest position is with the ring finger on tooth 25 very near the working area of tooth 26. The shank portion immediately adjacent to the curette blade must be parallel to this tooth surface.

*Right:* Section through tooth 26. Contact points and the four line angles are depicted. From the buccal approach, No. 13/14 is indicated for the distal surface from the disto-buccal line angle to the contact area.

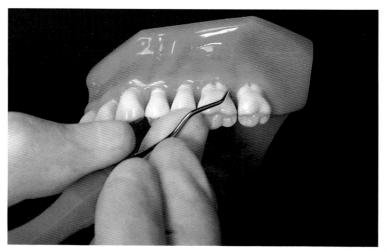

▶ **Posterior segment — Distal**

**465   Scaling on distal surfaces from the palatal — Tooth 26**
*Patient's head:* Inclined to the left

*Dentist:* 9 o'clock position
*Rest position:* Intraoral, indirect on the back of the first finger of the left hand. This finger also serves to guide the instrument and apply pressure to it.
*Vision:* Direct

*Right:* The palatal root is treated from the palatal toward the contact area and the distal furcation.

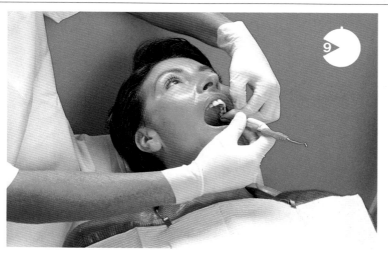
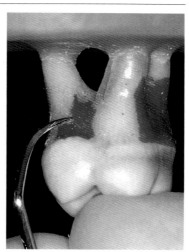

**466   Model situation**
The first finger of the left hand serves two functions when scaling in this area:
- fulcrum for the working hand
- guidance and lateral pressure for the curette

*Right:* Beginning on the palatal surface, the No. 13/14 curette scales the distal surface of tooth 26 from the line angle, across and into the furcation region, then under the contact area.

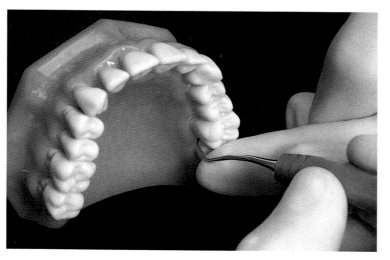
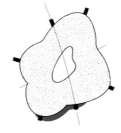

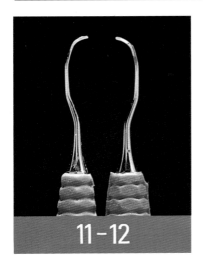

11-12

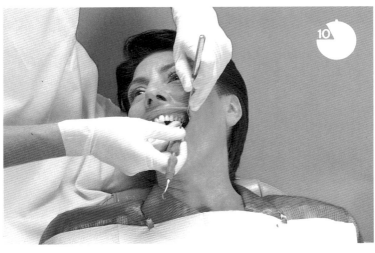

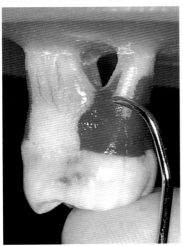

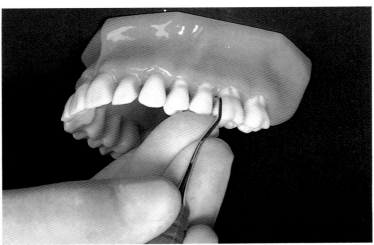

## 11-12

▶ Posterior segment — Mesial

### 467  Scaling on mesial surfaces from the buccal – Tooth 26
*Patient's head:* Inclined slightly to the right

*Dentist:* 10 o'clock position
*Rest position:* Intraoral, directly on the adjacent tooth
*Vision:* Direct

*Left:* The two working ends of the double-ended No. 11/12 curette

### 468  Model situation
The ring finger establishes a fulcrum for the working hand as near as possible to the mesial surface of tooth 26. The working strokes for subgingival scaling are initiated by a rotating movement of the *forearm* around the fulcrum point.

*Left:* Section through tooth 26. No. 11/12 is used from the buccal approach to scale the mesial surfaces from the mesiobuccal line angle, under the contact area, toward the palatal, including the mesial furcation.

▶ Posterior segment — Mesial

### 469  Scaling on mesial surfaces from the palatal – Tooth 26
*Patient's head:* To the left and back

*Dentist:* 8 o'clock position
*Rest position:* Extraoral on the mandible, or intraoral on the opposing arch. Guidance and additional support through the thumb of the left hand.
*Vision:* Direct

*Left:* Entrance to mesial furcation only via palatal.

### 470  Model situation
The left thumb guides and stabilizes the curette. Only light pressure is necessary for scaling the root surface if the instrument is properly sharpened.

*Left:* Section through tooth 26. The working area for curette No. 11/12 is from the palatal approach.

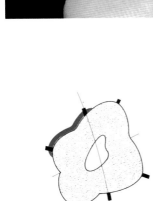

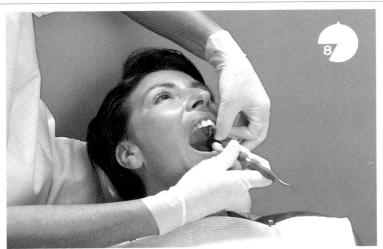

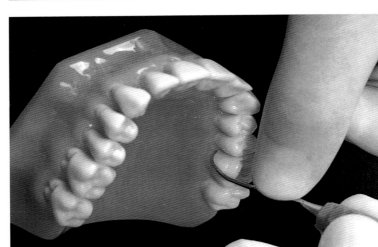

## 7–8

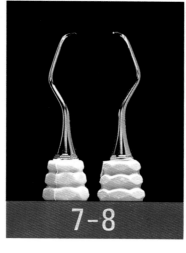
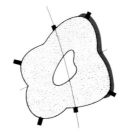

7-8

### ▶ Posterior area – Buccal

#### 471 Scaling the buccal surfaces – Tooth 26
*Patient's head:* Tilted slightly toward the operator

*Dentist:* 10 o'clock position
*Rest position:* Intraoral, directly on the adjacent tooth
*Vision:* Direct.

*Right:* Working ends of No. 7/8 curette. Medium shank length, severely angulated.

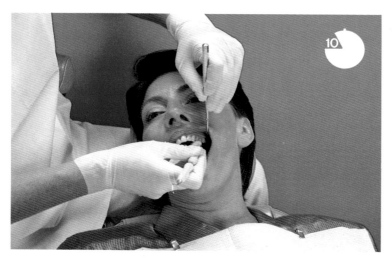

#### 472 Model situation
In addition to axial strokes, the buccal molar surfaces are often treated using oblique or horizontal strokes. The modified pen grasp is obvious, with the middle finger in the first curve of the instrument shank.

*Right:* The indentation represents the entrance to the buccal furcation.
Note: Mesial and distal sections of exposed roots near the furcation are treated using the No. 11/12 (mesial) and No. 13/14 (distal).

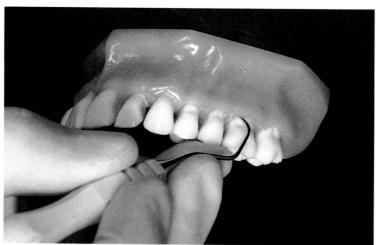

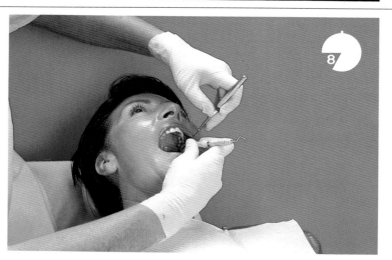

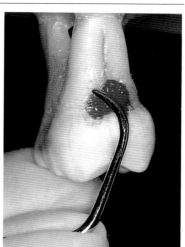

### ▶ Posterior area – Palatal

#### 473 Scaling the palatal surfaces – Tooth 26
*Patient's head:* Tilted toward the left away from the operator

*Dentist:* 8 o'clock position
*Rest position:* Intraoral, directly upon the occlusal surfaces
*Vision:* Direct

*Right:* The palatal root sections of teeth 26 and 27 are basically round in shape, however shallow grooves do occur and these may present difficulties during scaling.

#### 474 Model situation
Rest position directly on the occlusal surface of tooth 26.

*Right:* Gracey 7/8 curette is used to scale the palatal surface from the distopalatal to mesiopalatal line angles. In this area there are no furcations, but often grooves.

*After scaling this final (palatal) posterior tooth surface, systematic treatment of the upper left quadrant is complete. The pockets are then rinsed and any bleeding is staunched.*

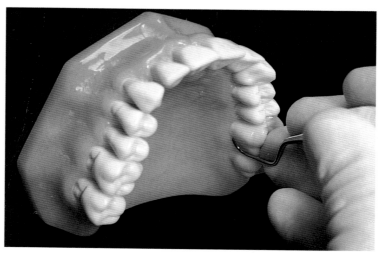

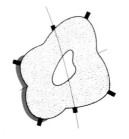

# Instrument Sharpening

The common instrument that serves both conservative as well as surgical periodontitis therapy is the curette. It is used for scaling, subgingival scaling, root planing and curettage. Knowledge of its characteristics and maintenance of its function are therefore of great significance. Instruments that have become dull must be re-sharpened; no degree of manual dexterity or force can compensate for the disadvantage of a dull instrument. Dull instruments lack "bite," calculus is burnished rather than removed.

Systematic sharpening of curettes may be accomplished before, during or after patient treatment. Especially the small slender curettes quickly become dull during scaling in a quadrant because of contact with metal restorations or enamel. Such instruments must be *resharpened* during the treatment appointment, using a sterile, mildly abrasive sharpening stone (Fig. 479).

Instruments that have lost their proper shape or which were improperly sharpened must be recontoured using more abrasive sharpening stones.

Instruments whose tips become thin may break.

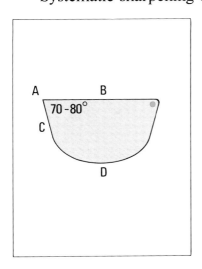

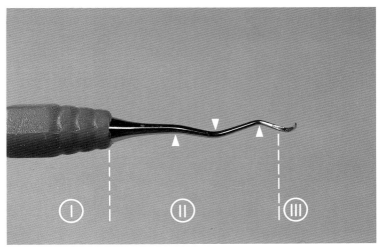

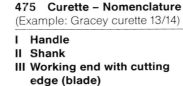

**475   Curette – Nomenclature**
(Example: Gracey curette 13/14)

**I   Handle**
**II   Shank**
**III  Working end with cutting edge (blade)**

*Left:* Section through the working end

**A   Cutting edge**
Only one edge of a Gracey curette is sharpened.
**B   Face**
**C   Sides**
**D   Back**

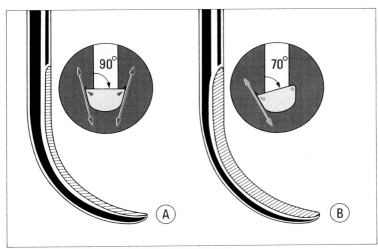

**476   Difference between universal (A) and Gracey curettes (B)**

1   The face (B in Fig. 475) of the working end forms a 90° (universal) or 70° (Gracey) angle to the shank when the terminal portion of the shank is perpendicular to the floor.

2   Both edges of the universal curette are sharpened; but only the "lower" edge of the Gracey.

3   Only in Gracey curettes is the working end arched over the surface as well as over the edge.

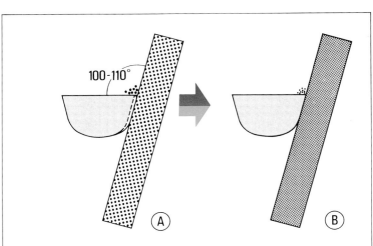

**477   Principles of sharpening**

A   Totally dull or improperly sharpened instruments must be reshaped through use of a coarse sharpening stone on the sides. Heavy loss of metal must be expected.

B   Dull but properly shaped instruments need only be resharpened. For this purpose only mildly abrasive stones should be used (see next page).

# Sharpening Stones

### Silicium carbide – Aluminum oxide

Sharpening stones are available in various shapes, colors, compositions and abrasiveness. The most commonly used abrasive materials in such stones are the artificially produced *silicium carbide* (SiC, trade name Carborundum) as well as *aluminum oxide* ($Al_2O_3$).

Relatively coarse carborundum and colored India stones are manufactured with the mineral abrasive powder (SiC, $Al_2O_3$) in a ceramic matrix. These stones are indicated for reshaping of dull or misshapen instru-

ments, but they create deep grooves in the edge and quickly reduce the instrument tip size.

The naturally occurring, mildly abrasive Arkansas stones ($Al_2O_3$) vary in color and crystalline size. They can be sterilized for resharpening of curettes during the treatment appointment. A few drops of acid-free mineral oil prevent excessive heating of the instrument tip, and metal particles cannot penetrate the "oil stone." Nevertheless some experts recommend that oil *not* be used on sharpening stones.

**478   Sharpening stones – Materials**

**C  "Carborundum"**
SiC, silicium carbide; artificial, coarse grained, highly abrasive

**I  "India"**
$Al_2O_3$, aluminum oxide, artificial, coarse grained, abrasive

**A  "Arkansas"**
$Al_2O_3$, aluminum oxide, natural, average-to-fine grained, mildly abrasive

*Right:* Acid-free mineral oil (SSO, Hu-Friedy) for the Arkansas stone.

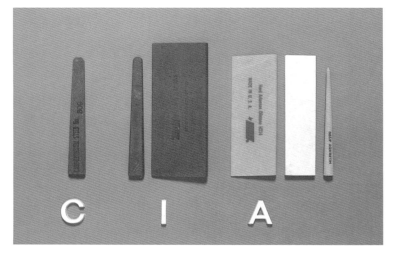

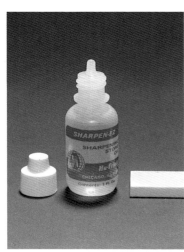

**479   Resharpening**
Fine curettes for subgingival scaling (pictured: GRA 5/6) become dull after 20–30 working strokes. They must be sharpened repeatedly during the procedure. The natural fine-grained Arkansas stones are indicated for this purpose (pictured: No. 4 from Hu-Friedy).

For sharpening, the curette is held in the left hand with its face parallel to the floor. The right hand guides the sharpening stone at the appropriate angle.

*Right:* Proper relationship between stone and Gracey curette.

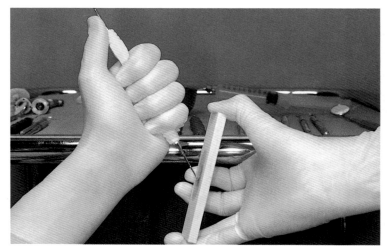

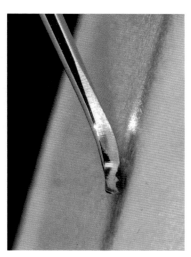

**480   Tests for sharpness: Light reflection test and scratch test**
Dull cutting edges on scalers and curettes are rounded. They reflect incident light when "rolled," sharp edges do not. This reflection test is more certain and cleaner than the antiquated, unhygienic "fingernail test" or the scratch test.

*Right:* Scratch test on an acrylic rod (PTS, Hu-Friedy). Sharp instruments cut into the acrylic and create spurs. *Remember:* The final test is the desired "bite" of an instrument on the tooth surface.

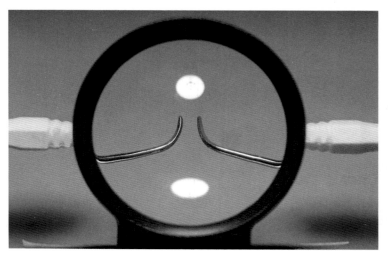

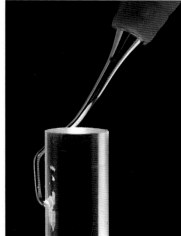

# Subgingival Scaling and Root Planing
# Closed Curettage

## Operative procedure

Closed subgingival scaling is performed without direct vision. Depending upon the extent of attachment loss and upon root morphology, the time required to thoroughly treat a *single* tooth ranges from three to ten minutes. In the following case, *closed* scaling was indicated in the maxillary right quadrant because the pockets were not very deep. The localized deep defect on tooth 14 might better have been treated with an open procedure.

This 43-year-old female presented with mild adult periodontitis (AP) and one advanced defect on the mesial of 14. The patient was readily motivated but had received no oral hygiene instruction to date.

*Initial findings:*

HYG: 58%          PBI: 2.1          TM: 0–1

See Figures 481–483 for the clinical picture, probing depths, gingival contour and radiographic survey.

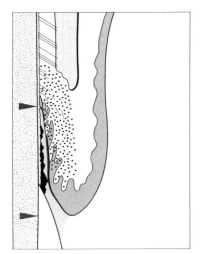

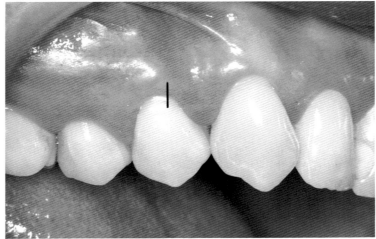

**481   Initial condition –**
**Before creation of hygienic relationships**
The gingivae are mildly edematous but only slightly reddened. The gingiva appears "glassy" and exhibits no stippling. Bleeding occurs after gentle probing.

*Left:* The schematic depicts the facial surface of tooth 14. The root surface harbors calculus, adherent plaque (blue) and some non-adherent, primarily gram-negative plaque (red). The gingival connective tissue exhibits an inflammatory infiltrate.

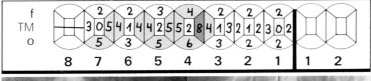

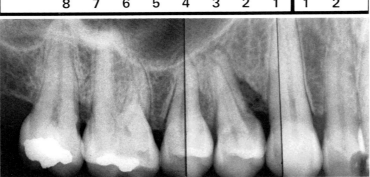

**482   Probing depths, tooth mobility (TM)**
Attachment loss (AL) is clearly visible between 17 and 16, 15 and 14, and especially pronounced on the mesial of 14. With the exception of 14, there is very little AL on facial surfaces. Pockets to 6 mm are measured on the oral aspect.

**Radiographic survey**
X-ray corroborates the probing depths. Tooth 14 appears to possess two roots (fused?). It will be difficult to treat this area by closed scaling.

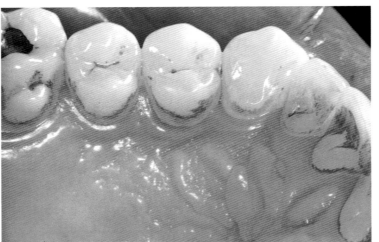

**483   Initial condition from the oral aspect**
The teeth exhibit a brown staining. The patient is a tea drinker and heavy smoker.

The gingivae exhibit thickened and rolled borders, without particularly pronounced inflammation.

Upon probing a great deal of subgingival calculus is discovered; the root surfaces are rough. Especially around the deep pockets on tooth 15 and tooth 14, bleeding occurs on the palatal aspect and especially interproximally.

## Scaling and root planing

### 484 Anesthesia

Two weeks after plaque and calculus removal and OHI, the gingiva is less red and swollen.

The subgingival scaling, root planing and curettage of the bony pockets are performed using block anesthesia administered into the vestibulum. Palatal injections are also given, as well as intrapapillary anesthesia.

*Right:* Facial surface of tooth 14. *Subgingival* accretions and plaque remain after gross debridement.

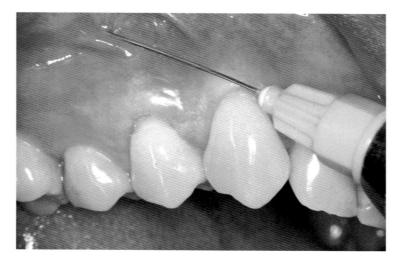
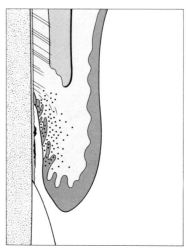

### 485 Probing the depth of the pocket

Before the mechanical treatment of the root surfaces, the base of the pocket is ascertained around the entire tooth, under anesthesia. Pocket topography is usually very irregular, as in this case. Frequently only one or several aspects of a root surface exhibit pronounced attachment loss.

*Right:* The radiograph shows that with a force ca. 25 g the probe tip penetrates almost to the bone.

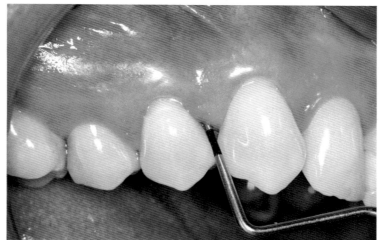
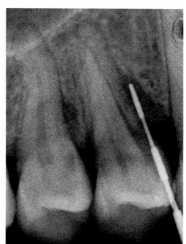

## Hoes

### 486 Hoe – Entering stroke

The hoe scaler with its carbide tip (Ash Lustra 211) is inserted into the pocket on the mesial surface of tooth 14, parallel to the tooth long axis, as deeply as possible. These instruments are indicated for gross subgingival calculus removal, but not for root planing.

*Right:* The radiograph clearly reveals that the relatively gross instrument does not get to the bottom of the pocket.

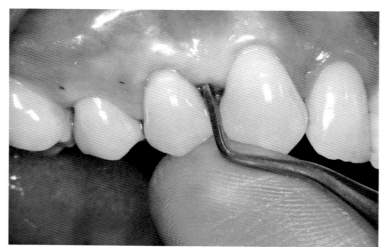
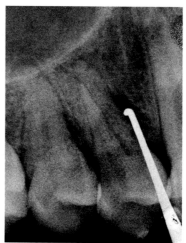

### 487 Hoe – Working stroke

The hoe requires considerable space and is generally used with a stroke from apical toward coronal, parallel to the tooth long axis.

The sharp edge of the carbide-tipped hoe may leave deep grooves in the tooth. For this reason they are not indicated for actual root planing. Many practitioners eschew carbide-tipped hoe scalers entirely for this reason.

*Right:* Schematic depiction of the hoe in action. Working stroke from apical toward coronal.

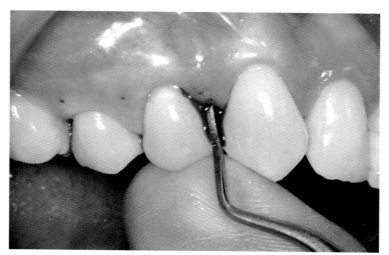
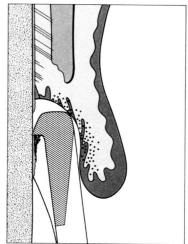

### Curettes

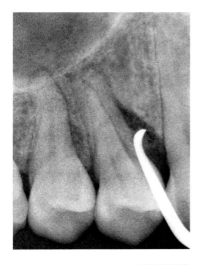
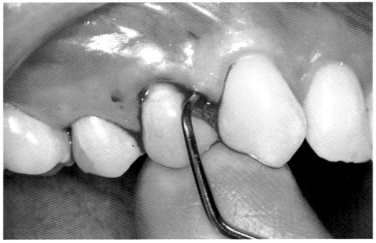

**488   Universal curette, mesio-buccal**

The sharpened posterior universal curette (M 23 A, Deppeler) is inserted to the base of the pocket.

Short working strokes are performed with light pressure axially and diagonally from apical toward coronal.

*Left:* The radiograph depicts the size relationships between the tooth/pocket and the curette blade.

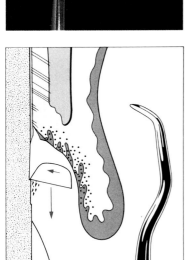
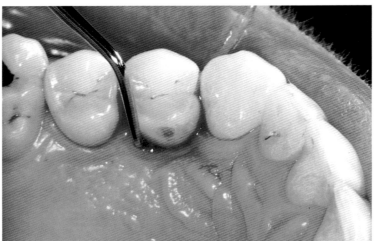

**489   Universal curette, disto-palatal**

The same curette blade used on the mesiobuccal root surface (cf. Fig. 488) also performs root cleaning and planing on distopalatal surfaces.

*Left:* Depressions, "figure 8" root cross section, furcation entrances etc. must be cleaned using a fine sense of touch. The morphology of the roots rather than the probing depth determines the limitations of closed subgingival scaling!

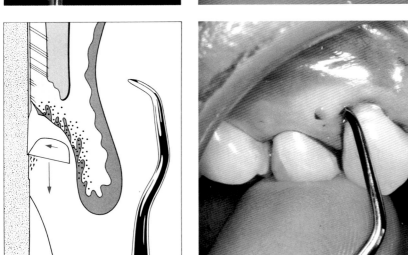

**490   Universal curette, disto-buccal**

After planing the mesiobuccal and distopalatal root surfaces, the paired, double-ended instrument is *reversed* and the distobuccal surface is planed, as above.

*Left:* The angle of attack of the curette blade upon the root surface during the working stroke should be approximately 80°.

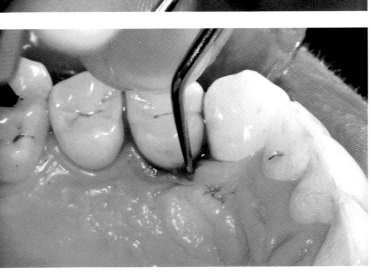

**491   Universal curette, mesio-palatal**

Finally, using the same curette blade as in Figure 490, the mesio-palatal root surface is cleaned and planed.

The association of a particular tooth surface with a particular curette results from the shape of the root surface and the bend at the working end of the curette.

Nevertheless, these curette-tooth surface associations are not "etched in stone" according to the depictions above; the determining factor is the possibility to apply the curette blade at an angle of 80°.

**492 Soft tissue curettage, supporting the tissue**

Intentional gingival curettage is no longer a component of modern periodontal therapy. There exists no proof that this measure improves the healing of a pocket. In fact, the tissue shrinkage seems to be somewhat more severe than after root planing alone.

*Right:* The gingiva must be supported by a finger. This will prevent tearing the tissue.
 Today rubber gloves are mandatory!

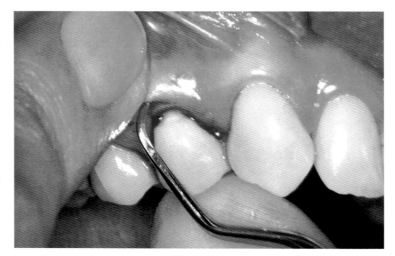
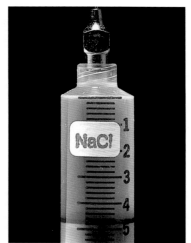

**493 Pocket rinsing**

Following mechanical therapy the pocket is rinsed with physiologic saline or Ringer's solution in order to remove all residues of plaque, loose calculus, and pieces of cementum or dentin dislodged during cleaning and root planing.

*Right:* Physiologic saline (0.9%) in disposable syringes with blunt tips.

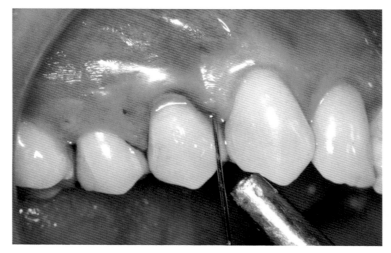

**494 Cleaning the field of operation**

Gingiva and teeth are sprayed off. Spraying, rinsing as well as constant evacuation during the entire treatment procedure provides the operator, who is working blind in conservative (closed) pocket therapy, with a clean and clear field of operation.

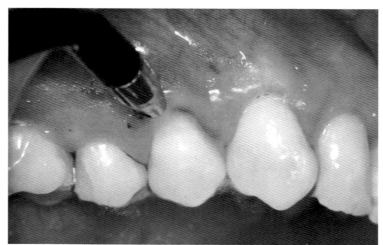

**495 Checking the root surface – Adaptation**

Using a pointed "cowhorn" explorer (CH 3, Hu-Friedy), the root surface is checked for smoothness; surfaces that feel rough (calculus, grooves) must be re-treated.

*Right:* Adaptation of the tissue. In the case of open wounds, the gingiva should be adapted using a periodontal pack. If papillae have been released, simple interdental sutures are indicated.
 The coagulum should be as small as possible (cf. Fig. 528).

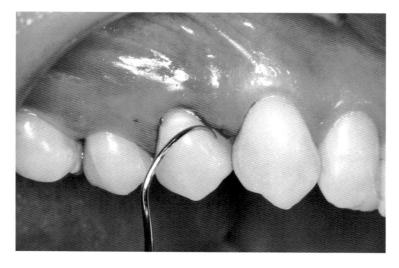
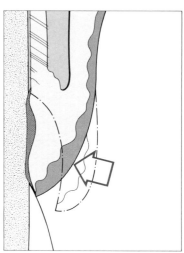

# Subgingival Scaling and Root Planing
## Closed Curettage

### Summary

The 43-year-old patient demonstrated excellent co-operation from the very beginning. The Hygiene Index improved considerably even after supragingival pre-treatment, and there was a reduction in the bleeding tendency.

Following subgingival scaling and root planing the shallow pockets in the depicted quadrant were reduced to physiologic levels. The especially deep pocket on the mesial aspect of tooth 14, with a deep infrabony furcation defect was reduced to 4 mm (see radiograph, Figs. 482, 485).

Both the relatively high degree of tissue shrinkage and the gain of attachment led to a significant reduction of probing depths. The quality of periodontal regeneration in the depth of the previously existing pockets cannot be judged clinically (Periodontal Healing, pp. 136–137).

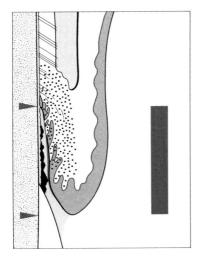

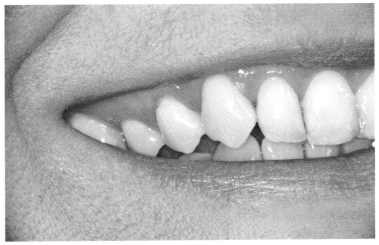

**496   Initial findings – Before treatment**
Gingivitis, generalized mild periodontitis (AP) with localized deep defect on 14. The gingiva bleeds copiously after probing, especially in papillary regions.

The patient had never been adequately oriented with regard to personal oral hygiene.

*Left:* Pocket on the buccal aspect on tooth 14, filled with plaque and calculus (red bar = probing depth).

Pocket epithelium, infiltrated subepithelial connective tissue.

**Before**

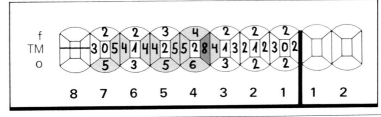

| | 2 | 2 | 3 | 4 | 2 | 2 | 2 | | |
|---|---|---|---|---|---|---|---|---|---|
| f TM o | 3 0 5 | 4 1 4 | 4 2 5 | 5 2 8 | 4 1 3 | 2 1 2 | 3 0 2 | | |
| | 5 | 3 | 5 | 6 | 3 | 2 | 2 | | |
| | 8 | 7 | 6 | 5 | 4 | 3 | 2 | 1 | 1 2 |

**497   Probing depths, initial findings**
The localized defect on the mesial aspect of tooth 14 is evident (root fusion? furcation?).

Interdental probings of 5 mm. On the palatal aspect of teeth 17 and 15 deeper pockets are detected.

**After**

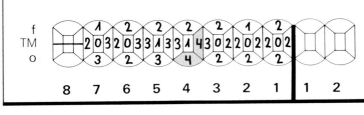

| | 1 | 2 | 2 | 2 | 2 | 1 | 2 | | |
|---|---|---|---|---|---|---|---|---|---|
| f TM o | 2 0 3 | 2 0 3 | 3 1 3 | 3 1 4 | 3 0 2 | 2 0 2 | 2 0 2 | | |
| | 3 | 2 | 3 | 4 | 2 | 2 | 2 | | |
| | 8 | 7 | 6 | 5 | 4 | 3 | 2 | 1 | 1 2 |

**Probing depths 6 months after scaling and root planing**
Dramatically reduced probing depths between 1 and 4 mm. Even the deep bony pocket near tooth 14 has been reduced (shrinkage, attachment gain).

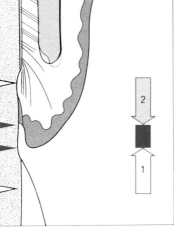

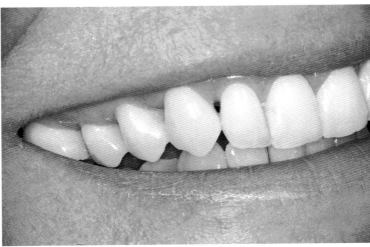

**498   Final results 6 months after scaling and root planing**
The gingiva exhibits healthy, though yet somewhat thickened structure. Especially near the deep infrabony pocket mesial to 14, some shrinkage of the papilla is observed.

The type of regeneration that occurred in the depth of the pocket cannot be ascertained clinically.

*Left:* The former active pocket was greatly reduced (red bar = inactive "residual" pocket).

**1** = shrinkage
**2** = attachment gain

# Treatment of Mild Furcation Involvement (Class F1)
# Scaling, Root Planing

Class F1 furcation involvements can be successfully treated conservatively by means of scaling and planing the furcation entrance (Ramfjord & Ash 1979). In some cases a minor odontoplasty is also indicated. The depression at the entrance to the furcation must not remain as a plaque-retentive area. Full coverage crowns, as depicted by the case below, must be contoured so that natural crown and root form is duplicated. The furcation entrance is an "endangered area"; crown margins in this area should not be located subgingivally.

Following the clinical procedures, the gingiva must be well adapted onto the root surface in order to provide optimum conditions for healing, especially if odontoplasty has been performed in the furcation area. Tissue adaptation can be accomplished with a periodontal dressing or with tissue adhesive (cyanoacrylates, e.g., Histoacryl).

**499   Root planing and curettage of a mild furcation involvement (F1)**
During supragingival debridement the open crown margin is corrected as much as possible. During curettage the crown margin is definitively smoothed and polished, and the buccal furcation is widened slightly coronally by means of odontoplasty.

*Right:* This radiograph was taken *before* revision of the overhanging crown margins (arrows, mesial and furcation area).

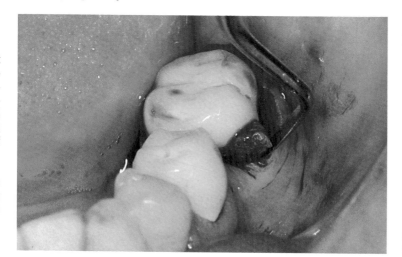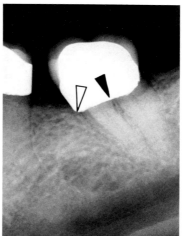

**500   Adaptation of the gingiva using tissue adhesive**
Following odontoplasty and scaling the gingiva must be adapted closely into the furcation that has been altered via odontoplasty. The tissues are pressed against the tooth, then sealed to place using cyanoacrylate. The adhesive must *not* be permitted to flow between the tooth and gingiva; this would render attachment impossible and could elicit a severe foreign body reaction.

*Right:* The tissue adhesive can be readily applied using a plastic instrument.

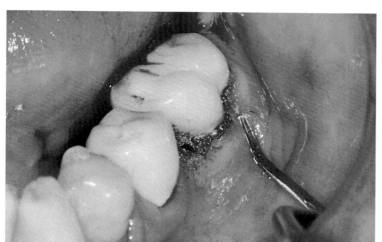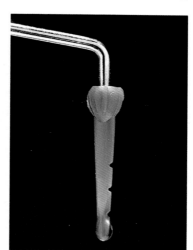

**501   Six weeks after conservative therapy**
The pocket is almost completely healed via shrinkage and regeneration. The crown margin is supragingival and follows the contour of the root surface depression in the furcation area.

Special hygiene aids (e.g., Lactona no. 27 marginal/interdental brush) must be used in this area to enhance the toothbrush (Bass technique).

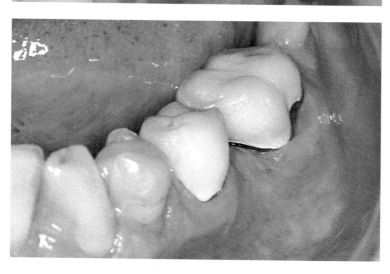

# Treatment of Moderate Furcation Involvement (Class F 2) Odontoplasty and Root Planing

By the time furcation invasion has advanced to the F 2 stage (horizontally probable 3 mm or more, but not through-and-through), the involvement is in a narrow area where the roots converge. Even the finest curette cannot gain entrance to such an area, making debridement and root planing in the furcation region impossible. If the tooth must be maintained in terms of the total treatment plan, the problem may be better solved by means of odontoplasty. Using coarse diamonds initially (75–40 µm), the furcation is widened to such an extent that narrow curettes can gain entrance. A final polishing using 15 µm diamonds is then performed.

Such class F 2 furcation revisions are easier to perform with direct vision, e.g., following reflection of the gingiva. If an odontoplastically treated furcation remains exposed after treatment, there exists a danger of caries development and dentin hypersensitivity. Optimum hygiene is critical. The furcation entrance must be checked at each recall, professionally cleaned and fluoridated topically.

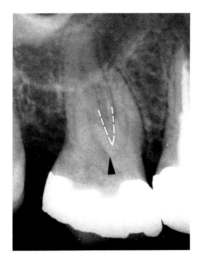

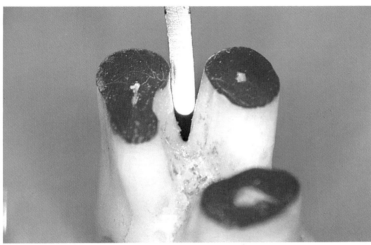

**502   Narrow buccal furcation entrance**
Even a fine curette, only 0.9 mm wide, cannot effectively reach the involved furcation.

*Left:* The radiograph reveals the closely spaced buccal roots (arrow). However, the severity of the furcation involvement (periodontal pocket, plaque, calculus) cannot be ascertained radiographically, especially in 3-rooted maxillary molars.

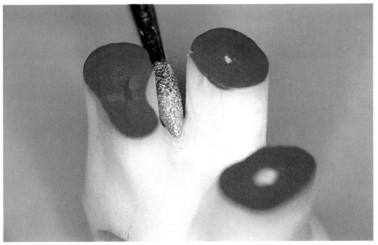

**503   "Furcation-plasty"**
If access is good, the procedure can be performed "closed" but it is easier to do after reflecting a small flap. Using flame-diamonds (Perio-Set, coarse 75 µm and medium 40 µm), the involved furcation can be opened just enough so that a fine curette can enter for debridement and root planing.

Furcations that have been treated via odontoplasty are particularly susceptible to caries! Once opened, they must be polished with the finest diamond bur (15 µm, Fig. 418) and treated with topical fluoride.

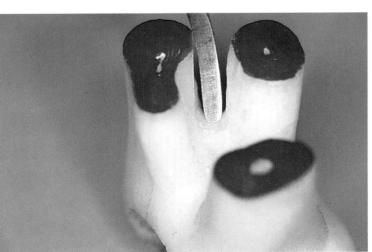

**504   Hygiene made possible**
Debridement and root planing with fine curettes can now be performed during the course of periodontal therapy as well as at each recall appointment after therapy is completed.

In such cases, cervical sensitivity may be particularly troublesome and persistent. The patient should be warned of this possibility *before* performing the odontoplasty. The area must be treated with topical fluoride to enhance remineralization, prevent plaque accumulation and reduce sensitivity. Special dentifrices may be recommended.

# Open Scaling and Root Planing

Complete planing of a root surface is extremely difficult during *closed treatment (without direct vision)* because root surfaces exhibit such a wide variety of irregularities, depressions and grooves. Good results can only be achieved with a systematic procedure, a fine tactile sense, a talented operator and the expenditure of considerable time.

The *open approach (with direct vision),* on the other hand, simplifies considerably the task of perfect debridement and root planing. Marginal incisions are made facially and orally, and the gingivae reflected minimally.

This procedure exposes the root surfaces, which can be planed with direct vision (p. 210, Fig. 530). Wound margins are then repositioned and adapted around the teeth by means of interdental sutures. Gingival shrinkage and postoperative bone resorption will be more pronounced than after closed treatment, but less than after radical flap procedures.

When the incision for open curettage is an internal gingivectomy (inverse bevel), it is very similar to the ENAP and modified Widman techniques (pp. 217, 225).

**505 "Open curettage"**
A marginal incision is made and the gingiva reflected. Pocket epithelium and granulation tissue are removed and the papillae are thinned internally to enhance subsequent adaptation. The root surfaces are cleaned and planed with direct vision.

*Right:* Using extracted teeth it has been demonstrated that in deep pockets only the coronal 5 mm of the root surface can be effectively treated by *closed* scaling (*Waerhaug* 1978).

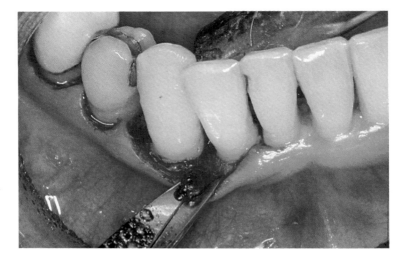
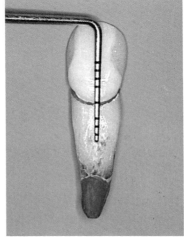

**506 Adaptation of the gingiva**
Following open treatment the papillae must be readapted and repositioned, then sutured to place. Sutures should be placed using atraumatic straight or curved needles and thin suture material (3–0 to 5–0).

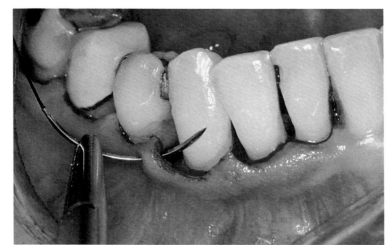

**507 Wound closure after open treatment**
After a marginal incision with minimal reflection it is not always possible to completely close the interdental space, and small interdental soft tissue craters may persist after healing. With intensive interdental hygiene (e.g., Butler no. 614 interdental brush) and frequent recall such craters will close with time. It may be necessary to subsequently perform a minor papilloplasty to improve gingival contour. Electrosurgery is often used for such minor revisions.

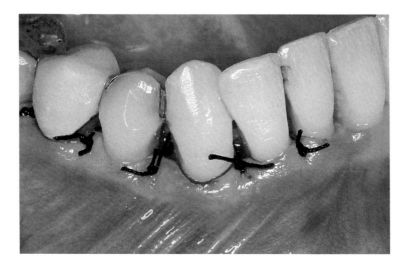

# Root Planing  –  Correction of Undercontoured Crown Margin

Plaque-retentive areas due to overhangs and over-bulked crown margins are usually corrected during the first appointment for initial therapy.

In the esthetically important anterior region, correction of a crown margin without injury to the gingival margin can often only be accomplished by reflecting the soft tissue. In order to avoid replacing a restoration that has clinically unacceptable marginal relationships, the dentist may attempt to recontour the restoration or the tooth itself by grinding with direct vision, as shown in the clinical example below. Gingival tissue is reflected mini-

mally, if necessary with an intrasulcular incision. The procedure is the same regardless of whether the crown is overcontoured or undercontoured. Ground surfaces of tooth and restoration must be smoothed and polished with fine diamonds. Some shrinkage of the tissue will *always* occur, even when procedures are performed carefully and atraumatically.

If there is a gap between the restoration margin and the margin of the prepared tooth ("open margin"), no amount of grinding will adequately correct the situation. In such cases, the crown must be replaced.

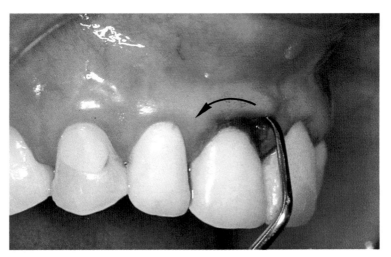

**508   Scaling in the area of a jacket crown**
On the labial aspect of the two incisor jacket crowns, the gingivae are inflamed and swollen. Root planing was attempted, but it quickly became evident that the margin of the jacket crown on tooth 11 was undercontoured, creating a plaque-retentive area.

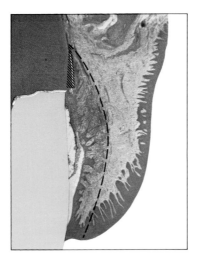 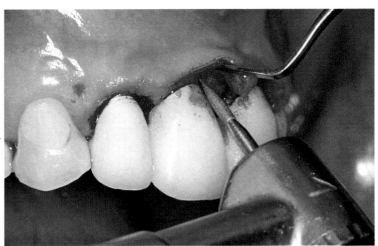

**509   Correction of the marginal inadequacy**
Reflecting the gingiva revealed a discrepancy between the crown margin and tooth structure. Coarse (75 μm, then 40 μm) diamonds were used with direct vision to reduce the tooth structure until it met the crown margin.

*Left:* In the histologic section the odontoplasty (hatched area) and the soft tissue curettage are indicated. A tiny cement line remains between the jacket crown (blue) and the preparation.

Courtesy of *N. P. Lang*

**510   Two years later**
Despite the crown margin that is still located somewhat subgingivally (an esthetic compromise), the gingiva is well adapted and inflammation-free two years after treatment. The probing depth is 2 mm.

# What does "Root Planing" Really Mean?

Root planing, i.e., the definitive treatment of the root surface, is the most important component of periodontal therapy. Following subgingival plaque and calculus removal and elimination of cementum layers that are saturated with endotoxin, the root surface must be planed and smoothed.

The rationale for this procedure is the assumption that a smooth root surface will be less plaque-retentive and that therefore the danger of reinfection and recurrence of disease should be less. Some have also espoused the theory that reattachment of either epithelial or (ideally) connective tissue would be more likely on a smooth root surface than on a rough one. Other factors, such as root treatment with citric acid, could also enhance regeneration of a new attachment, and many clinical studies are currently underway to evaluate this possibility.

The photographs below demonstrate clearly that the term "planing and smoothing" is, indeed, relative, regardless of whether it is performed with curettes or with the finest rotating diamonds (Schwarz et al. 1984).

**511 Dentin planing with curettes**
Using a standardized method (250 gm pressure, 10 strokes downward) for evaluating conventional mechanical root planing, parallel grooves with an average depth of 2 μm were created.

*Right:* **Factory-new curette (CUR)**
The curette tip is shown at high magnification (above). Note the irregularities and spurs of metal, which can never be completely eliminated.

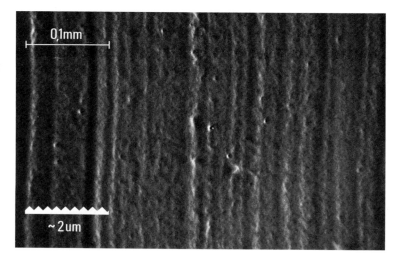
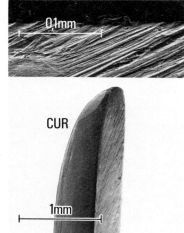

**512 Dentin planing with a 15 μm diamond**
Compared to the curettes, the diamond leaves scratches that are a bit deeper and less regular. This standardized test employed 60 gm pressure and 10 passes with the flame-shaped diamond rotating at 6000 rpm.

*Right:* **Diamond for root planing (D 15)**
The magnification (above) reveals the fine surface structure of the 15 μm diamond (cf. Fig. 418, right).

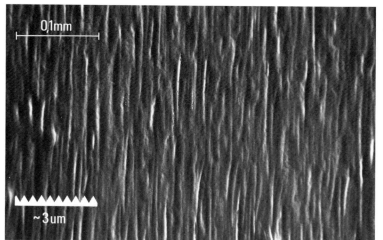
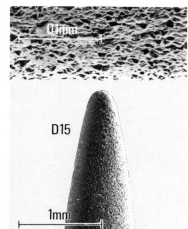

**513 Dentin roughening by a 75 μm diamond**
The coarse 75 μm diamond, commonly used for tooth preparation, leaves deep grooves and irregularities in the dentin. Scratches are as deep as 15 μm. The test conditions were the same as for the 15 μm diamond.

*Right:* **Diamond for tooth preparation (D 75)**
A normal flame diamond may be employed for odontoplasty, before final polish. It is *not* acceptable for root planing.

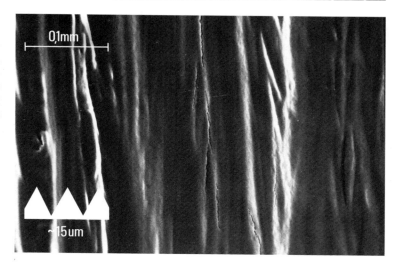
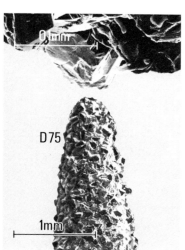

# Initial Therapy – Possibilities and Limits

Initial therapy (Phase I: Plaque control, supragingival debridement; Phase II: Subgingival scaling, root planing, possible curettage) is considered to be the most important component of complete periodontal treatment. In the truest sense it is "causal therapy," because its goal is the elimination of etiologic factors.

Complementing initial therapy is periodontal surgery, which permits root cleaning with direct vision and is therefore also "causal therapy." In addition, surgery can eliminate or reduce the symptoms and some of the consequences of periodontal disease.

## Gingivitis

In cases of *gingivitis,* initial therapy is usually the *only* treatment necessary. An exception is fibrous gingival overgrowth, which may persist even after inflammation is eliminated.

Overgrowth may occur in cases of severe gingivitis, in patients who are mouth breathers, and with certain systemic medications that cause hyperplasia as a side effect (e.g., phenytoin, p. 58; nifedipine, p. 59; cyclosporine-A, p. 60).

In these situations, initial therapy must be complemented by gingivectomy/gingivoplasty.

## Mild periodontitis

Initial therapy alone may bring satisfactory results in cases of *mild periodontitis,* especially on single-rooted teeth (Badersten 1984; Badersten et al. 1984a, b).

## Moderate and severe periodontitis

There are certain limits to the success that can be achieved by initial therapy alone in cases of *moderate and severe periodontitis.* It has been demonstrated unequivocally that nonsurgical removal of subgingival plaque and calculus becomes increasingly more difficult with increasing pocket depth (Waerhaug 1978). It is impossible to completely plane root irregularities, grooves, furcations and fusions; removal of diseased cementum and smoothing of the root surface can be accomplished imperfectly at best without direct vision. The result of this is a lack of new attachment (regeneration) postoperatively. Remaining pockets can become re-infected despite the patient's conscientiousness in home care.

For all these reasons it is imperative to re-evaluate the case ca. 8 weeks after initial therapy to determine whether surgical intervention is required or whether the patient should be retreated during a recall visit, for example by repeated subgingival scaling and root planing.

**514 Pocket depth reduction and gain of attachment after various treatment methods in 4–6 mm pockets (Knowles et al. 1979)**

——— Root planing and curettage
——— Modified Widman procedure
– – – – Surgical pocket elimination

Compare also Figure 527: Pocket reduction and attachment gain in deeper pockets.

## The Michigan long-term study

Ramfjord and his coworkers performed an 8-year longitudinal study to evaluate the long-term effects of three treatment modalities (Knowles et al. 1979, 1981):

1. Root planing and curettage
2. Modified Widman procedure
3. Surgical pocket elimination
   (flaps, ostectomy, apical repositioning)

The results of this landmark study revealed that with pocket depths of 4–6 mm all three treatment modalities gave similar results (Fig. 514), although *closed* treatment led to slightly less reduction in pocket depth than the two surgical techniques. On the other hand, *attachment gain* after closed curettage was similar to the results obtained with modified Widman surgery, and somewhat more when compared to radical pocket elimination (ostectomy).

In cases of advanced periodontitis with probing depths of 7–12 mm, the modified Widman technique was superior to closed therapy in terms of both pocket elimination and attachment gain (p. 209).

**Initial therapy I**

### 515 Severe, plaque-elicited gingivitis

Before treatment, the clinical picture was one of severe inflammation, especially in the maxillary anterior region, with pronounced edematous enlargement of interdental papillae. The PBI score was 3.8.

Inflammation in the mandibular area was less severe (PBI 3.0).

No attachment loss was detected in either area.

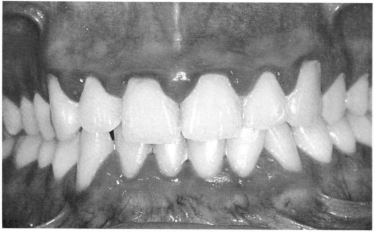

Before

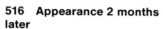

Gingivitis

### 516 Appearance 2 months later

Severe gingivitis has been completely eliminated *(Restitutio ad integrum)*. The patient's level of motivation and dexterity using the Bass technique and dental floss rendered any further treatment unnecessary. In cases such as this, a recall interval of six months is adequate.

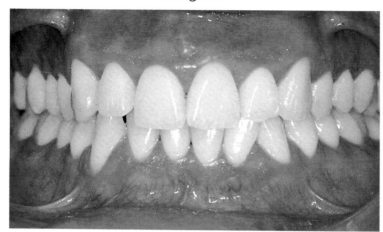

After

**Initial therapy I and II**

### 517 Generalized moderate periodontitis with pronounced gingivitis

In addition to the severe manifestations of gingivitis in papillary and marginal areas (PBI 3–4) probing depths to 6 mm were detected (attachment loss).

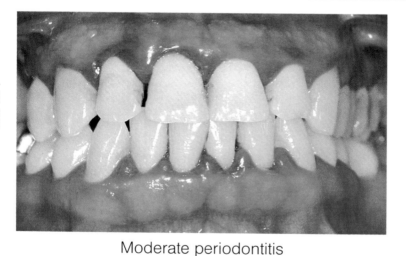

Before

Moderate periodontitis

### 518 Appearance 2 months later

The inflammation has been reduced (PBI 1.8). Probing depths were generally half of the original values. The gingivae have shrunk, and exhibit irregular fibrous thickening.

A subsequent surgical procedure was indicated to improve gingival contour.

Replacement of defective anterior restorations would considerably simplify interdental hygiene.

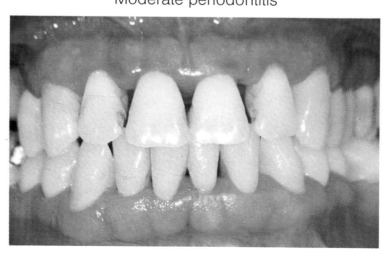

After

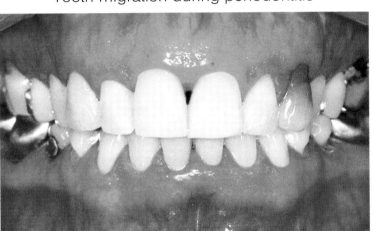

Before

Tooth migration during periodontitis

After

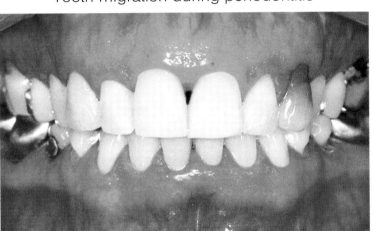

**Initial therapy I and II**

**519   Moderate periodontitis – Diastema caused by the drifting of teeth**
The patient reported (dental history, old photographs) that the diastema between teeth 11 and 21 had developed over the course of two years.

Drifting of the maxillary anterior teeth could be due to the severe gingival inflammation and the localized deep periodontal pockets, as well as functional forces from premature contacts, overbite and a shift during intercuspation.

**520   Appearance 9 years later**
The only treatment provided for this patient was initial therapy, occlusal adjustment in centric occlusion and protrusive excursion, and slight shortening of tooth 21. The gingival inflammation remained under control despite the patient's less than optimum motivation and cooperation with home care. The diastema closed *spontaneously* six months after initial therapy, without any orthodontic measures.

Tooth 23 became dark after endodontic treatment for pulpitis.

Courtesy of *M. Leu*

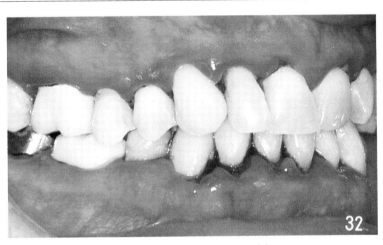

Before

Advanced periodontitis

After

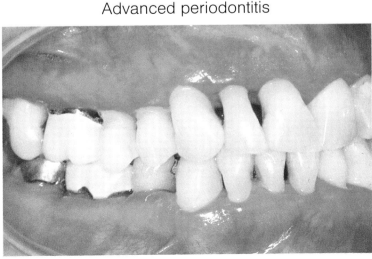

**Initial therapy I and II**

**521 Advanced periodontitis**
Pronounced marginal inflammation, hemorrhage at the lightest touch (PBI 4). Probing depths of up to 10 mm were detected. Some pockets exhibited symptoms of activity (pus).

The margins of posterior full crowns are at least 2 mm apical to the gingival margin.

**522   Appearance 3 months later**
Inflammation is absent for the most part. Gingival tone has returned after tissue shrinkage that resulted in irregular contour. Crown margins are now supragingival. However, some deep pockets (cratering) persist, some with signs of active disease.

Reevaluation of this case clearly demonstrates that without surgical intervention the deep active pockets cannot be expected to disappear. Surgical correction of the gingival contour is also indicated.

**Initial therapy I and II**

### 523 Acute stage of ulcerative periodontitis (ANUG/P)

The gingivae are severely inflamed (PBI 3–4) and exhibit pronounced ulceration in interdental areas. Gingival contour is "inverted" (reverse architecture) as a result of attachment loss associated with osseous interdental cratering.

The probing depths (4–5 mm) appear relatively slight; this is common in ANUG/P because the necrotic process attacks interdental papillae.

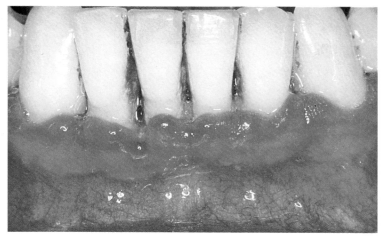

Before

ANUG/P

### 524 Appearance 6 months later

The *acute* phase was completely eliminated by initial therapy. A surgical procedure is required in the mandibular anterior region, especially between 42 and 41, to create morphology that the patient can keep clean. If the results achieved are to be maintained, a short-term recall interval (3 months) is necessary. In patients with this type of ulcerative periodontitis, the establishment of proper and above all long-term effective home care is often a difficult process that involves changing life habits.

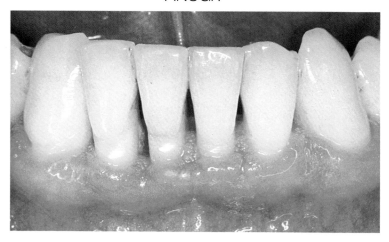

After

**Initial therapy I**

### 525 Trauma or Stillman's cleft? – Secondary inflammation

Calculus is visible in the gingival cleft on tooth 21. Use of erythrosin disclosing solution also revealed a small accumulation of microbial plaque. This patient practiced oral hygiene vigorously but incorrectly using a horizontal scrubbing technique with a hard bristle toothbrush. Thus the etiology of this cleft could involve both plaque-elicited inflammation and trauma from toothbrushing.

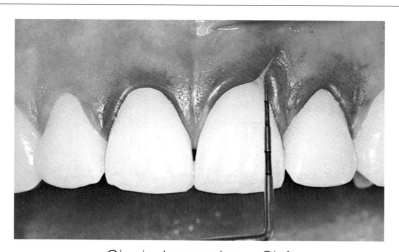

Before

Gingival recession – Cleft

### 526 Appearance 3 months later

The cleft closed spontaneously solely as a result of repeated careful cleaning of the tooth surface in the area of the cleft, and "freshening up" of the edges of the soft tissue. The patient's brushing technique was changed to modified Stillman (vertical rotatory). Sulcus depth at the location of the former cleft is completely normal!

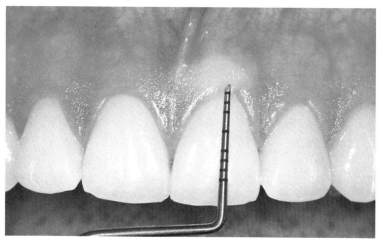

After

# Periodontal Surgery
# Corrective Phase

Periodontal surgical therapy is only *one component* of complete periodontal treatment. If surgery is necessary, it is usually performed as a second phase of therapy. The patient must have first demonstrated appropriate motivation and home care. The first phase of initial therapy, professional supragingival tooth cleaning, must be complete. It is also preferable to perform subgingival scaling before any surgical intervention. When initial therapy is this comprehensive, surgery must be performed less often and less radically. In addition, surgical procedures are associated with less hemorrhage, and the morphologic results are better; tissue loss is also reduced.

When all periodontal treatment is completed, a regular recall interval must be established (maintenance phase). If this is not done, *every* periodontal surgical procedure will eventually fail (Rosling et al. 1976 b, Nyman et al. 1977, Westfelt et al. 1983).

The art and science of periodontal surgical therapy will be presented as follows:

| |
|---|
| Purposes and goals of periodontal surgery |
| Indications for and methods of periodontal surgery |
| Re-evaluation after initial therapy is complete |
| Preparation for a periodontal surgical procedure |
| Various standard surgical techniques |

## Purposes and goals of surgical therapy

1. Root cleaning and smoothing (planing) with direct vision
2. Reduction or elimination of plaque-retentive areas that promote infection, especially periodontal pockets
3. Elimination of inflammation and pocket activity
4. Enhancing the regeneration of periodontal tissues
5. Creation of physiologic morphology of the marginal periodontium and the mucogingival border

Periodontal surgery, its goals and purposes, can only be considered in conjunction with complete periodontal treatment. For example, initial therapy and surgery are two entities with identical goals, but which use different methods (closed root planing versus root planing with direct vision) to achieve those goals. Furthermore, initial therapy may be the only therapy required for mild periodontitis, whereas in severe cases it may represent only a preparatory presurgical phase.

### Root cleaning with direct vision

The root surface is exposed to clinical view either by reflecting mucoperiosteal flaps or by simple gingivectomy. The root surface, including its depressions, irregularities and the furcation area, is then debrided of plaque and calculus insofar as this was not accomplished completely during initial therapy. Endotoxin-containing cementum is planed away and the root surface is smoothed. These measures make possible the healing and regeneration of periodontal structures.

*Reduction or elimination of plaque-retentive areas*

The most important retentive areas for microbial flora are periodontal pockets. Additional niches include open furcations, root depressions, anomalies of tooth position and iatrogenic irritants such as poor margins on restorations and crowns.

Pockets with persistent signs of activity may be treated by various flap procedures or via gingivectomy.

Furcations can be treated by odontoplasty and rendered accessible for oral hygiene; alternatively, root resection may be performed to eliminate the furcation problem entirely.

*Elimination of inflammation and pocket activity*

The primary goal of periodontal surgery does not always include total elimination of the pocket itself, but elimination of any signs of pocket *activity* (infection) such as exudate, hemorrhage or suppuration. The goal is to halt the progression of the disease process. Elimination of inflammation *always* leads to tissue shrinkage, reduction of probing depths, and exposure of the cervical area.

*Enhancing regeneration of periodontal tissues*

The result of all periodontal surgery should be healing and regeneration (Periodontal Healing, pp. 136–137). Early results with "guided tissue regeneration" are promising and may make it possible to avoid resective surgery.

*Creation of physiologic morphology of the marginal periodontium and the mucogingival border*

A physiologic contour of the marginal periodontium can be achieved by means of gingivectomy/gingivoplasty, flap surgery with internal gingivectomy and (infrequently) minor osteoplasty.

Mucogingival surgery may be employed to enhance the width of attached gingiva or to correct unphysiologic frenum attachments that extend into the marginal gingiva. Such procedures can stop further gingival recession.

## Indication for and methods of periodontal surgery

The choice of a periodontal surgical technique depends on the type and severity of the periodontal disease, as well as on the pathomorphologic situation at the site to be operated.

The specific techniques for treating periodontitis surgically possess some similarities. The goals are virtually identical (see above).

Common standard surgical methods include:

- **ENAP procedure, open curettage** (p. 217)
- **Partial flap reflection (modified Widman/Ramfjord technique)** (p. 221)
- **Full flap reflection with variable flap repositioning** (p. 231)
- **Combined and special operations** (p. 241)
- **Gingivectomy/gingivoplasty** (p. 273)
- **Mucogingival surgery** (p. 289)

– *Open curettage and ENAP procedure*

These are very similar interventions that preserve tissue. Both permit root cleaning/planing with direct vision following minimal reflection of the gingiva, especially in the interdental area. They are especially indicated in the anterior area (esthetics).

– *Modified Widman procedure* (Ramfjord technique, partially reflected flaps)

The modified Widman operation is the most universally applicable periodontal surgical modality. It is indicated in mild to moderate periodontitis. Its principles are valid for all flap procedures.

– *Fully reflected flaps (with or without vertical incisions)*

This technique is indicated in severe periodontitis with irregular bone loss and for advanced furcation involvement. Fully reflected flaps simplify osteoplasty, ostectomy, implants in osseous defects, and attempts at periodontal regeneration.

– *Special periodontal surgical procedures*

These include wedge excisions, implants of various materials into osseous defects, treatment of isolated furcation involvement, and extraction of hopeless teeth with simultaneous revision of the periodontal supporting tissues of the adjacent teeth.

– *Gingivectomy/Gingivoplasty* (GV/GP)

Indications for GV/GP are limited to gingival enlargement/overgrowth, shallow suprabony pockets, local contouring. The GV/GP is *contraindicated* for treatment of infrabony pockets and osseous thickening, and when attached gingiva is narrow or absent.

– *Mucogingival surgery*

Indicated only for advanced and progressing gingival recession.

## Re-evaluation and surgical planning after initial therapy

Two to three months after initial therapy, maximum periodontal tissue consolidation and regeneration should have occurred. At this time, probing depths, attachment loss, gingival inflammation and plaque accumulation (home care!) are re-evaluated. Only now can definitive planning of necessary surgery be done. The chances for success in terms of attachment gain and pocket elimination are assessed. Decisions are made regarding which surgical technique to use in particular segments (sextant or quadrant), and what teeth must be extracted. Surgery should only be considered if the hygiene (HI) is at least 80% and gingival bleeding on probing is essentially absent.

Another critical factor is the *general systemic health* of the patient, e. g., diabetes, hematologic disorders, hypertension, hemorrhagic diathesis, focal infection or elderly persons with a history of poor healing. Patients undergoing radiation therapy and those on anticoagulant medication should not be treated surgically without prior consultation with the physician.

## Preparations for a periodontal surgical procedure

Surgery is usually performed per sextant, less often per quadrant. The patient should always be left postsurgically with one side functional for chewing.

The preparations for periodontal surgery are similar to those for routine small oral surgical procedures, and include the usual rubber gloves, mouth mask, operatory disinfection and instrument sterilization.

It is prudent for the dentist and his auxiliary personnel to be immunized against hepatitis-B, since the danger of infection is quite high in dental practice. The risk of AIDS transfer must also be considered.

Finally, the entire dental practice team should be well schooled in how to handle emergency situations (Schijatschky 1979).

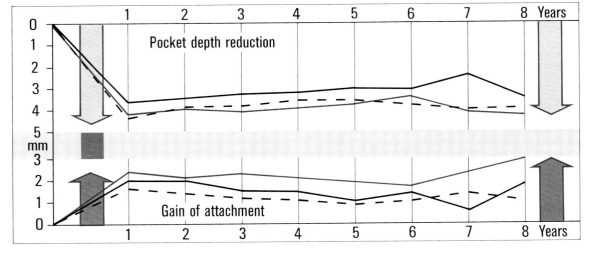

**527  Pocket depth reduction and attachment gain following various treatment methods for 7–12 mm pockets (Knowles et al. 1979)**

———— Modified Widman procedure

———— Root planing and curettage

– – – – Surgical pocket elimination

Compare also Fig. 514; same study with pockets of 4–6 mm.

*Premedication* is not necessary in healthy patients with good oral hygiene. It is advisable, however, to have the patient rinse thoroughly (30 sec) with chlorhexidine solution (Peridex) immediately before the surgery begins. This elicits a reduction in the quantity of microorganisms in the oral cavity for several hours. *Antibiotic coverage* may be required (e. g., endocarditis). Systemic medication may be indicated as supportive therapy in distinct types of periodontal disease (e.g., RPP, LJP; see Medicaments, p. 314).

## Surgical techniques described in this atlas

In the following pages, the most important basic periodontal surgical methods are first described *comparatively,* then *"in principle"* and finally in *a practical case.*

Indications and contraindications as well as advantages and disadvantages of each surgical technique are discussed.

# Comparison of Therapeutic Methods

## Advantages and disadvantages of conservative (closed) and surgical (open) pocket therapy

The goal of "causal" therapy for periodontitis is removal of disease-causing microorganisms from tooth and root surfaces as well as from the pocket. Various pathways lead toward this goal:

### A Subgingival scaling, root planing
*Advantages:* Relatively simple and free of hemorrhage in *mild* cases, with minimal tissue shrinkage.

*Disadvantages:* Technically difficult; no direct vision.

### B Gingival curettage
This is *never* the sole therapy; it is only performed in combination with scaling and root planing.

*Advantages:* Removal of pocket epithelium and infiltrated connective tissue (granulation tissue).

*Disadvantages:* More pronounced tissue shrinkage.

| | Scaling | Gingival curettage | ENAP (open curettage) |
|---|---|---|---|
| **Treatment method** | | | |
| Gingival margin | | | |
| **Preoperative situation**<br>– Incisions<br>– Excised tissues<br>– Logos of main instruments | | | |
| ◀ MGL – Mucogingival line | | | |
| **Cross-section of approach and incision** | | | |
| **Postoperative situation** | | | |
| Former gingival margin | | | |
| – Tissue reflection<br>– Tissue adaptation<br>– Coagulum | | | |
| ◁ Original MGL | | | |

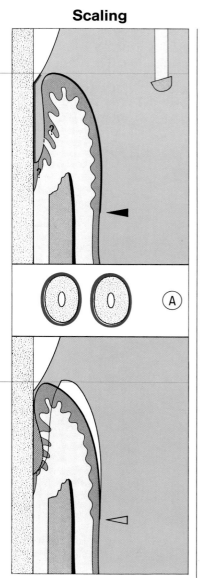

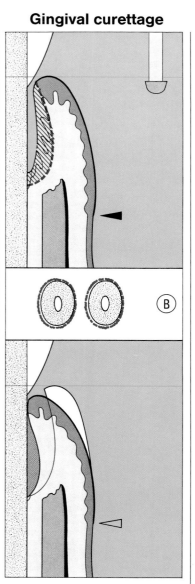

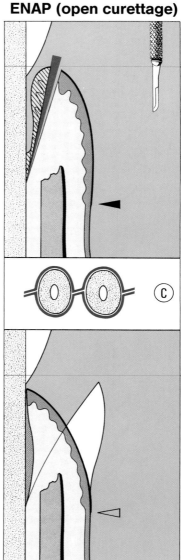

**Characterization of the methods of therapy (right)**
– Instrumentation

**528 Subgingival scaling, root planing (A)**
Removal of plaque and concrements from the root surface. Removal of endotoxin-containing cementum (dentin) layers. Removal of the pocket epithelium is *not* attempted.

The Gracey curettes, sharpened on only one side of the blade, are indicated for this procedure.

**529 Gingival curettage (B)**
"Peeling out" of the pocket epithelium.

This measure must be combined in every instance with the scaling procedure, shown at left.

The universal curettes, sharpened on both edges, are indicated for this gingival curettage.

**530 ENAP, open curettage (C)**
Excision of the pocket epithelium with a small, slender scalpel. Slight reflection of the gingiva, especially in papillary areas. Scaling and root planing. Adaptation of the papillae by means of interdental sutures.

For the incisions, very slender scalpels (e.g., Beaver) are indicated.

## C ENAP, open curettage

*Advantages:* Root planing is performed with limited direct vision. Removal of pocket epithelium, especially interdentally. Gingival shrinkage is minimal.

*Disadvantages:* Limited view of the aveolar bone.

## D Modified Widman flap procedure (MWF)

*Advantages:* Direct vision. Removal of pocket epithelium and portions of the connective tissue.

*Disadvantages:* Tissue loss; more severe shrinkage.

## E Flap operations

*Advantages:* Expansive view. Access to furcations. Possible to reposition the flaps.

*Disadvantages:* Tissue loss; severe shrinkage.

## F Gingivectomy

*Advantages:* Radical pocket elimination; gingival contouring; direct vision.

*Disadvantages:* Massive tissue loss; only possible in attached gingiva.

| **MWF (modified Widman)** | **Flap procedures** | **GV (Gingivectomy)** | |
|---|---|---|---|

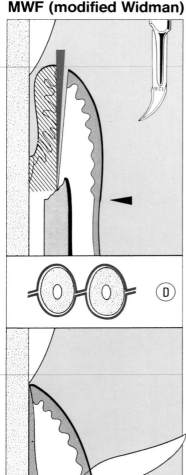
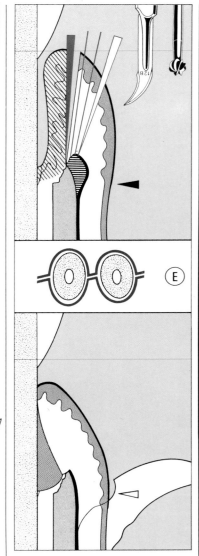
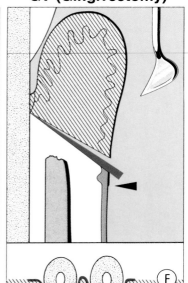
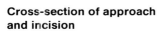

**Treatment method**

Gingival margin

**Preoperative situation**
– Incisions
– Excised tissues
– Logos of main instruments

◀ MGL – Mucogingival line

**Cross-section of approach and incision**

**Postoperative situation**

Former gingival margin

– Tissue reflection
– Tissue adaptation
– Coagulum

◁ Original MGL

**531  Modified Widman flap (D)**
Arcuate, minimum inverse bevel incision to the alveolar crest. Reflection of the partially mobilized flap, wherever possible not beyond the mucogingival line. Scaling and root planing. Flap adaptation by means of interdental sutures.

For the first incision, the double-edged 12 B scalpel is suited best.

**532  Flap procedures (E)**
The incision (inverse bevel) is made at varying distances from the gingival margin. A fully mobilized mucoperiosteal flap is reflected to reveal the root surface, furcation areas and the alveolar crest. Then roots are scaled and planed.

Osteoplasty and furcation treatment etc. are possible. Interdental sutures. Repositioning of flap, if necessary at a different location.

Incision: 12 B scalpel.

**533  Gingivectomy (F)**
Excision of gingiva (GV) and / or gingival recontouring (GP). The MGL should not be touched.

Scaling and root planing.

Healing (epithelialization) of the GV/GP wound occurs by secondary intention beneath a periodontal dressing.

Excision and recontouring using gingivectomy and papilla knives or the electrosurgical loop.

**Characterization of the methods of therapy (left)**
– Instrumentation

# Anesthesia

### Nerve block anesthesia

Only in the mandibular posterior segments is true nerve block anesthesia used for periodontal surgery (inferior alveolar block).

### Terminal anesthesia

Terminal anesthesia may be used in addition to nerve block in the mandible. An advantage of this procedure is that it provides a degree of vasoconstriction for the field of operation and provides the surgeon better vision because of reduced hemorrhage.

### Direct infiltration

Injection of anesthetic solution directly into interdental papillae, for example prior to a gingivectomy, can enhance the anesthetic effect and provide tissue ischemia.

### Vasoconstrictors

Most anesthetic solutions contain 0.5–1 mg% epinephrine. If there is a contraindication for epinephrine in a particular patient, it may be substituted by an alternative vasoconstrictor (e.g., vasopressin).

**534 Surface anesthesia**
A topical anesthetic is used at the site of injection to reduce the discomfort of needle penetration.
  Reducing the pain of an injection can contribute greatly to the patient's psychic well-being during the entire operation.
  *Procaine-free* topical agents reduce the chance of an allergic reaction.

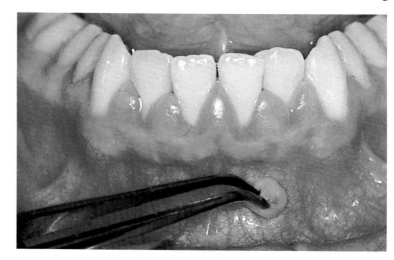

**535 Terminal anesthesia in the vestibular fold**
On the facial surface, anesthetic solution is injected near the periosteum in the loose submucosal connective tissue.

*Right:* Schematic depiction of the injections into the facial vestibulum and lingually at the border between the attached and mobile mucosa.
  On the *palate,* anesthetic solution should be infiltrated 5–10 mm from the gingival margin.

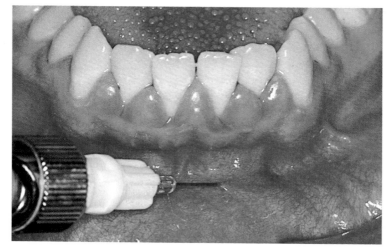
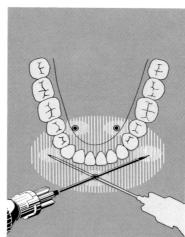

**536 Infiltration into interdental papillae**
Immediately before surgery the dentist may choose to inject directly into the papillae. In addition to increasing the anesthetic effect, this procedure will also greatly reduce hemorrhage.

*Caution:* Direct infiltration should *never* be attempted into severely inflamed tissue.

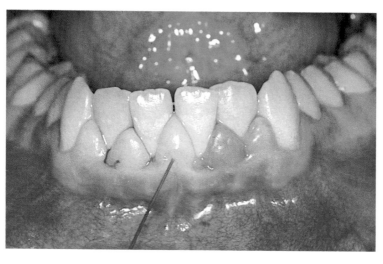

# Flap Procedures

During the comparison of the various therapeutic methods (pp. 210–211) and the listing of their advantages and disadvantages, it became clear that flap procedures are the most universal and the most frequently employed periodontal surgical procedures. If one considers all of the various forms and variations of flap procedures, only gingivectomy/gingivoplasty and mucogingival surgery can be differentiated from them. In all flap procedures, the reflection of soft tissue is always nothing more than a method for gaining visual access to deeper periodontal structures, which can then be treated with direct vision (see Indications, below).

In order to ensure adequate vascular supply and regeneration, the full thickness (mucoperiosteal) flap is almost always used. The entire soft tissue complex (gingiva, mucosa, periosteum) is separated and reflected from the root and alveolar bone surfaces. Less often, "split thickness" flaps are reflected in which the mucosa and connective tissue are separated from the subjacent periosteum. An example of the split flap may be found in mucogingival surgery.

The modified Widman flap procedure (Ramfjord technique) and the ENAP procedure are the most often selected, particularly for patients manifesting mild to moderate periodontitis.

### General indications

Flap procedures are indicated in cases of periodontitis with active pockets 5–6 mm deep or greater that do not respond satisfactorily to initial therapy.

### Special indications

- Infrabony pockets
- Implants and osseous transplant into infrabony pockets
- Pronounced thickening of the marginal bone
- Hemisection of a tooth, or root resection
- Tooth extraction with immediate periodontal treatment of remaining adjacent periodontal structures
- Crown lengthening procedures to expose restoration margins

### Contraindications
- Pronounced gingival enlargement/overgrowth, which is handled more efficiently by means of GV/GP
- Combined minor procedures to facilitate placement of, for example, class V restorations

### Advantages

Flap procedures have the following advantages over closed root planing/curettage or GV/GP:

- Pocket epithelium is removed by the inverse bevel incision
- Optimum subgingival scaling and root planing to the base of the pocket can be performed with direct vision
- At the end of the surgery, the flaps can be replaced at the original location, or repositioned apically, coronally or laterally
- The interdental bone or infrabony defects can be covered by the flaps
- No open wound persists postoperatively

### Disadvantages
- When flaps are repositioned apically, the cervical areas of the teeth are often exposed, long and sensitive, due also to shrinkage of the tissues

# Instruments for Flap Procedures ...

In general, the instruments used for periodontal flap procedures are the same as those employed for other oral surgical procedures. These include scalpels, elevators and needle holders. The instruments should be as fine as possible, to promote sensitive handling of the delicate tissues.

The various instruments depicted and described below have proved useful in practice. Many other types and manufacturers are available that will yield satisfactory results if used correctly.

If the flap procedure is to be combined with a gingivectomy/gingivoplasty, the gingivectomy knives described later in this text may also be required (gingivectomy knife, papilla knife; p. 274). The flap surgery "kit" also contains various forceps, explorers, periodontal probes, surgical scissors and clamps, and most importantly curettes for scaling and root planing. In addition, bone burs or bone files (osteoplasty) as well as fissure burs or diamond stones may be required for hemisection or root resection.

### 537 Scalpel blades
From left to right:

- **11**  (Martin)
- **12 B** (Bard-Parker)
- **15**  (Martin)
- **15 C** (Bard-Parker)

To insure sharpness, only disposable blades are utilized, providing a minimum of tissue trauma and enhanced healing.

Only fine and delicate scalpels are indicated for periodontal surgery, where precision is demanded and access often limited.

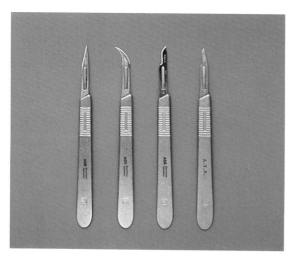
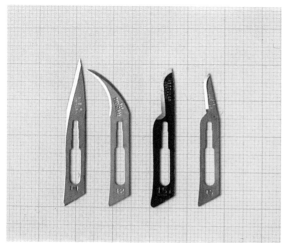

### 538 Elevators

- **6 mm** (FK 300; Aesculap; *white*)
- **5 mm** (VT 24, 22, 23; Deppeler; *red*)
- **4 mm** (VT 27; Deppeler; *yellow*)
- **2.5 mm** (Special manufacture; Zabona; *blue*)

Small, narrow elevators (2–6 mm wide) are used to mobilize and reflect the flaps.

Larger instruments may also be used during root planing or osseous recontouring to deflect the flaps from the field of operation and improve visibility.

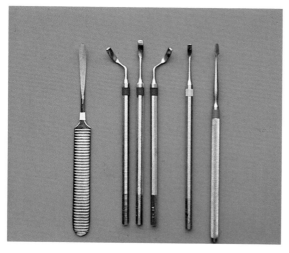
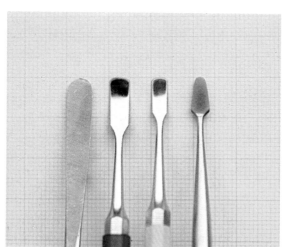

### 539 Needle holder – Elasticity of the closure (in gm)

- **"Mathieu"** (Aesculap; 1500 gm)
- **"Boyton"** (Hu-Friedy; 1200 gm)
- **"Castroviejo"** (Aesculap; 500 gm)
- **"Gillis"** (Dufner; without closure, with scissors)

Needle holders must fulfill opposing demands: They must hold the needle securely, while allowing the surgeon to release the locking mechanism easily.

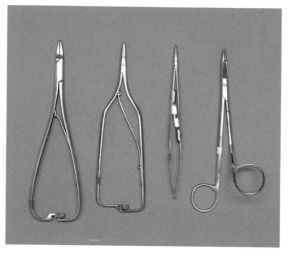
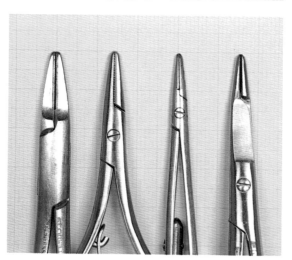

## ... and Their Use

The use of periodontal surgical instruments is depicted in the clinical photographs below. Only the most important steps for flap design and reflection, as well as for repositioning the flap are shown. First is the primary incision, here with the 12 B scalpel. It takes the form of an arcuate, inverse bevel incision with subsequent flap reflection using the narrow, rounded elevator. The flap is finally repositioned and stabilized by means of interrupted interdental sutures.

The instruments depicted below are for flap reflection and repositioning.

The most important instruments for any periodontal surgical procedure, however, are the *curettes* (as well as scalers, ultrasonic instruments, air-scaler, polishing diamonds). As has been emphasized repeatedly, mechanical root cleaning, smoothing and planing are the most important aspects of any periodontal surgical procedure. Reflection of a flap is actually nothing more than a means to this end.

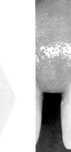
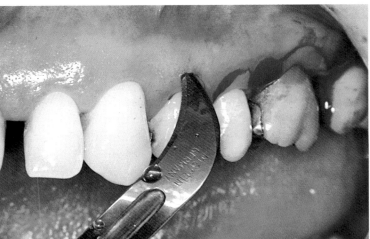

**540   Scalloped inverse bevel incision**
The first incision made during a modified Widman operation (Ramfjord technique) is a scalloped inverse bevel incision.

This type of incision can, of course, also be employed during creation of a fully reflected flap.

The preferred instrument for this procedure is the 12B scalpel, which is sharp on both edges of its sickle-shaped blade.

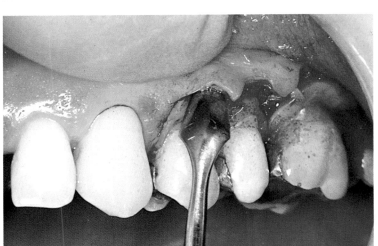

**541   Flap reflection**
In the region of tooth 24, a small elevator is used to raise a concise tissue flap, following the scalloped line of incision.

Narrow elevators can follow the scalloped incision better than wide elevators, thus preventing tissue trauma.

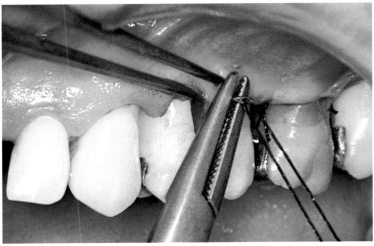

**542   Flap fixation with interrupted sutures**
Fine needle holders and fine needles are required for atraumatic periodontal surgery. Thin papillae and mucosal flaps can easily be torn by thick needles and large needle holders that are clumsy and difficult to open.

"Atraumatic" needles and suture combinations are recommended (needle without "eye").

# Needles, Sutures and Suture Knots

Adaptation of periodontal flaps may be accomplished using a variety of suture materials available in varying thicknesses with curved or straight needles. The needles are also available in various sizes, degrees of curvature, and cross-sectional profiles. Needles may have an "eye," or may have the suture incorporated into the blunt end of the needle ("atraumatic" needles).

Periodontal surgeons normally use interrupted sutures but may occasionally employ continuous or mattress sutures. Although there are numerous "surgeon's knots" known, a few will serve adequately in the majority of periodontal surgery situations. The most important considerations in flap repositioning are close adaptation to the alveolar bone and around the teeth, and complete coverage of the interdental area.

**543 Needles and sutures**
The needle, suture material and needle holder should be synchronized to each other. Atraumatic suturing requires a pointed needle, which cuts as it penetrates.

The suture material should be supple and should permit knots that hold well. The type of suture material (catgut, nylon, silk) determines the type of knot used.

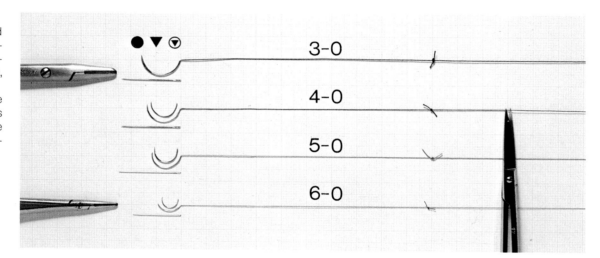

**544 The "2–1" surgeon's knot**
A double and a single loop are used together in a simple surgeon's knot.

The first double loop prevents any loosening of the suture tension while the second (single) loop is being added.

*Right:* The "2–1" knot pulled tight. This simple knot is used primarily with braided suture, whether synthetic or natural (silk).

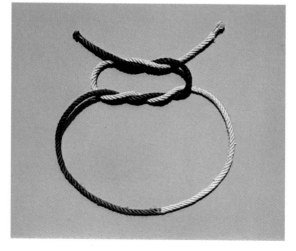
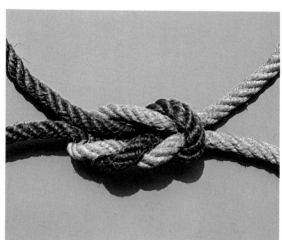

**545 The "2–2" double surgeon's knot**
Knots placed in catgut or in monofilament synthetic suture loosen easily. When these materials are used, it is wise to employ two double loops when tying sutures.

*Right:* The "2–2" knot pulled tight. *Caution:* Large knots such as the 2–2 surgeon's knot may lead to formation of aphthous ulcers on the vestibular mucosa due to irritation. If the patient is particularly susceptible to such ulcer formation, suture knots should be covered with a soft periodontal dressing (e.g., Coe-Pak, Barricaid).

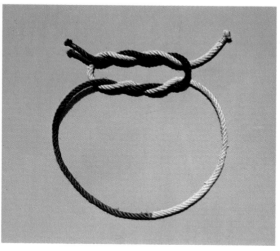
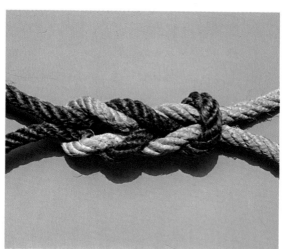

# ENAP – Excisional New Attachment Procedure
# Papillary Flaps – "Open Curettage"

Already in the 1970s the tissue-conservative treatment concepts that are propagated widely today for the treatment of periodontitis were being examined. The so-called ENAP procedure was developed during this period in the U.S. Naval Dental Corps (Yukna et al. 1976, Yukna 1976, Fedi 1985).

### Indications
– Localized, mild to moderate periodontitis, especially interdentally in the anterior region (tissue-conservative!)

### Contraindication
– Advanced periodontitis with deeper infrabony pockets, or osseous thickening whose treatment requires excellent vision during the operation

### Advantages
– Minimum tissue loss
– Can be performed with minimum attached gingiva
– Good healing potential

### Disadvantages
– In comparison to limited vision larger flaps
– Not applicable when pockets are deep or irregular

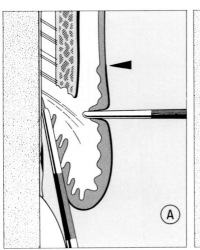
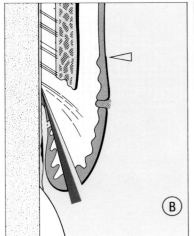
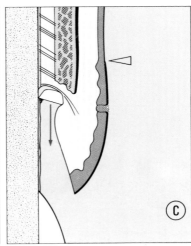

**546   Principles of the ENAP**

**A  Measurement/Marking**
Probing the suprabony pockets and marking the base of the pocket on the oral epithelium of the gingiva by means of a bleeding point. The mucogingival line is identified by arrows.

**B  Incision**
Conservative incision to excise pocket epithelium. "Sharp" curettage with a fine scalpel.

**C  Root cleaning/Planing**
After removal of the pocket epithelium, root cleaning and planing with direct vision.

## Principles of the operation

The *original method* was described as follows: The clinical pocket is measured with a periodontal probe, which is then used to mark the probing depth on the facial aspect by a superficial penetration (bleeding point).

Next a conservative intrasulcular incision is made in the direction of the base of the pocket, extending from the gingival or papillary margin.

The same incision is made on the oral aspect. The excised pocket epithelium is removed and the root surfaces are cleaned, smoothed and planed with curettes. The tissues are adapted tightly interdentally and to the tooth surfaces by means of interdental interrupted sutures and with a periodontal dressing if indicated.

# ENAP

## Operative procedure

This 45-year-old female presented the relatively rare combination of gingival recession (no pockets) on the facial surface and an interdental localized periodontitis.

For esthetic reasons, this patient stated that she did not want the periodontal therapy to lead to additional exposure of the necks of her maxillary anterior teeth.

For this reason, the conservative ENAP was performed almost exclusively in the *interdental areas.* Presurgical therapy consisted solely of professional tooth cleaning. The vertical-rotatory brushing method (modified Stillman) was demonstrated.

It is possible that closed subgingival scaling might have also been effective; however, distal to teeth 23 and 24, 6 mm pockets were present.

*Findings after initial therapy:*
HYG: 80%     PBI: 0.8     TM: 1
See accompanying Figures for clinical picture, gingival contour, probing depths and radiographic survey.

### 547 Appearance after tooth cleaning

A cursory inspection reveals gingivae that appear for the most part healthy. The rather pronounced facial recessions are of note. Pockets are present only interdentally.

Of primary concern is the healing of the pathologically deepened interdental pockets.

An attempt to cover the esthetically unpleasant recessions in the anterior area should be considered only if it is the patient's particular desire (cf. Mucogingival Surgery, p. 289).

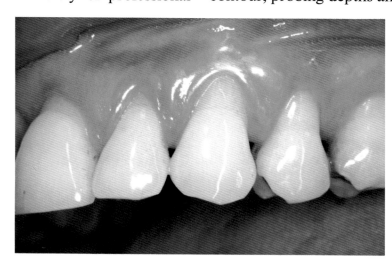

### 548 Probing depths and tooth mobility (TM)

As in cases of classic gingival recession, no periodontal pockets are present on the facial aspect (probing depths: 2 mm).

Interdentally, on the other hand, probing depths up to 6 mm were recorded.

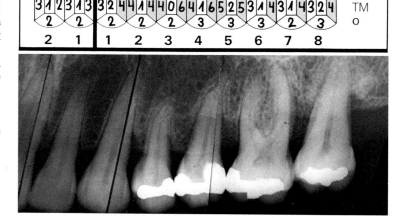

### Radiographic survey

Interdental horizontal bone loss is obvious (suprabony pockets).

### 549 Marking the base of the pockets

Using the CP 12 periodontal probe (Hu-Friedy) the probing depths are measured and marked on the facial surface of the gingiva.

*Right:* After measuring the probing depths mesial from 23, the depth of the pocket at this location is marked.

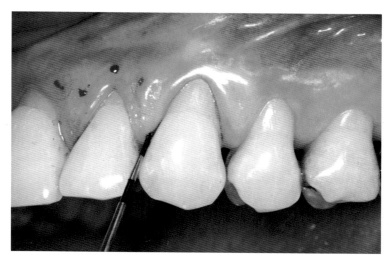
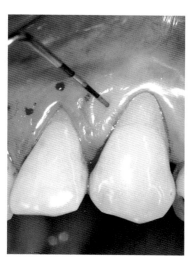

---

*In this series the ENAP-procedure is shown on tooth 23, mesial surface.*

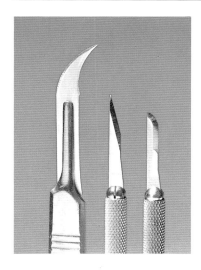

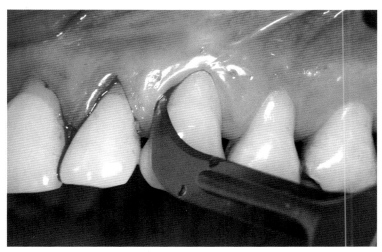

### 550  Incision
In this special case the incision is made only in the papillary region in order to protect the facial margin of the gingiva, where no pockets exist.

Using the double-edged no. 12B scalpel or the even narrower Beaver knives (from ophthalmic surgery), the incision is made, an extremely conservative internal gingivectomy (inverse bevel, Fig. 546B).

*Left:* Scalpels for the marginal (intrasulcular) ENAP incision.

– **No. 12B** (Bard-Parker)
– **No. 6500/6700** (Beaver)

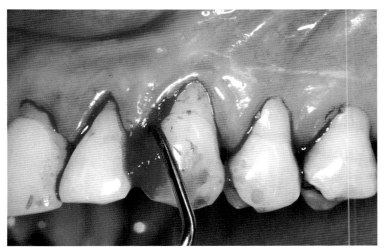

### 551 Removal of pocket epithelium
By removing the excised pocket tissue with a universal curette, a small gingival flap in the region of the papilla remains. This simplifies access for cleaning the root surfaces. In the marginal/facial area, where no pockets are present, the gingiva is not reflected.

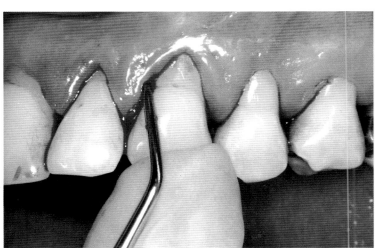

### 552 Root planing
All root surfaces on all teeth that are included in the surgical area (e.g., a localized pocket or a sextant/quadrant) are now systematically cleaned and then planed with curettes (cf. Subgingival Scaling – Root Planing; Closed Curettage, p. 179).

Only areas with pockets are treated; areas exhibiting normal sulcus depths are not touched (here, e.g., the facial surfaces).

The photograph depicts root cleaning on only the mesial surface of 23.

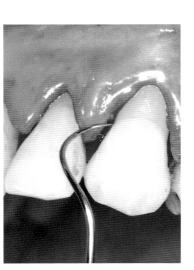

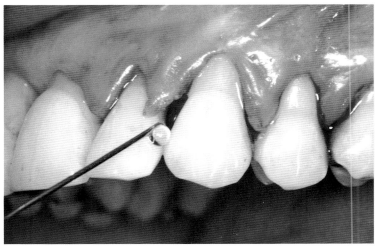

### 553 Rinsing the pocket
During cleaning and smoothing of the root surface, the surgical field is rinsed often with Ringer's solution.

Left: Checking the root surface with a pointed explorer. All root surfaces are checked repeatedly with a fine pointed explorer (e.g., CH 3, Hu-Friedy). In addition to visual control, this is the only possibility for ensuring the smoothness, i. e., cleanliness of the root surfaces.

**ENAP – Wound healing**

### 554 Repositioning and adaptation of the papillae using interrupted sutures

After applying pressure with moist gauze, to stop bleeding and ensure only the thinnest coagulum between the flap and the tooth surface, the interdental spaces are closed by approximating the papillae.

In comparison to the initial situation (Fig. 547), it is clear that the removal of the pocket epithelium and granulation tissue resulted in somewhat opened interdental spaces (cf. Fig. 557).

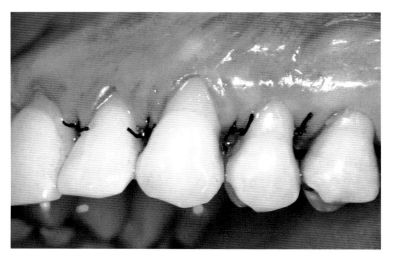

0

### 555 Periodontal dressing

In order to enhance undisturbed healing by primary intention, the original ENAP method prescribed use of a eugenol-free dressing in addition to the tight suture closure. If no dressing is placed, the patient should clean the operated area carefully on the very next day.

0

### 556 Ten days postoperatively

Dressing and sutures have been removed. During this first phase of healing, the patient rinsed with a 0.12% chlorhexidine solution (Peridex). The surgical area appears clean.

Oral hygiene can now be carefully reinstituted. Interdental hygiene (e.g., with Super Floss or toothpicks) is of particular importance.

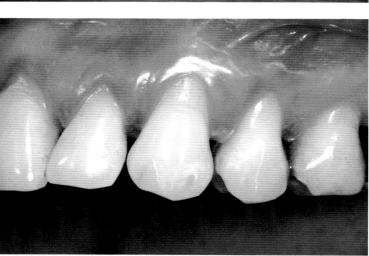

10 days

### 557 Three months postoperatively

The probing depths have been reduced to 2 mm, even in proximal areas. The *facial* recessions have not become more severe.

In the region of the papillae some shrinkage has occurred.

---

*As of this writing, there exist no proven (traditional) therapeutic modalities – from closed root planing to fully reflected flaps – that are not attended by some degree of gingival shrinkage!*

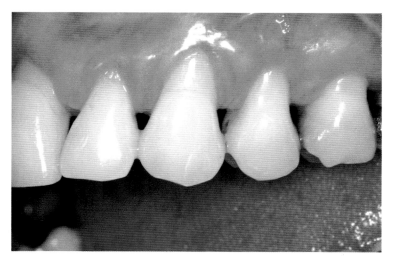

3 months

## Partially Reflected Mucoperiosteal Flaps
## Modified Widman Procedure (Ramfjord Technique)

Of all the available periodontal surgical procedures, the versatile "modified Widman flap" (MWF) procedure is probably the most often employed. It provides favorable long term results. Ramfjord and Nissle (1974) and Ramfjord (1977) modified and improved the original technique of Widman (1918) by means of defined incisions, conservative flap reflection and an atraumatic approach. The goal of the procedure is "healing" of the periodontal pocket with minimum loss of tissue, and not pocket elimination *per se*. Because the alveolar process is only minimally exposed, postoperative pain or swelling almost never occur. Similar techniques are used in the "ENAP" operation and in "open curettage."

The most important component of the Ramfjord technique is complete removal of subgingival plaque and calculus as well as smoothing and planing of the root surface with direct vision. No ostectomy is performed. On the contrary, with elimination of all pathogenic irritation and healing of the pocket, actual new bone formation may be expected in infrabony pockets. Corrective osteoplasty may be performed to improve the facial or palatal (lingual) bony architecture, and can be very important in obtaining complete closure over interdental bony defects when repositioning the flaps.

### Indications

– The MWF is indicated for the treatment of all types of periodontitis, and provides excellent results with probing depths up to ca. 6 mm.

– Advantageous use of MWF will depend upon the pathomorphologic situation on individual teeth and at various periodontal sites. The Ramfjord technique can be combined with more extensive fully mobilized flaps as well as special operations such as wedge excisions, root resections, tooth hemisections, implants and less frequently also with gingivectomy/gingivoplasty (see Combined Procedures, p. 241).

### Contraindications

There are hardly any contraindications for the Modified Widman procedure:

– If attached gingiva is absent or is very thin and narrow, the Ramfjord technique is difficult to perform properly because the scalloped inverse bevel incision is practically impossible. In such situations it may be necessary to utilize the classic intrasulcular incision.

– The MWF technique will be contraindicated if osteoplasty or ostectomy are planned in the case of very deep defects with *irregular* bone loss on facial and oral aspects, and if the marginal crest of bone is very bulbous.

### Advantages

– Root cleaning with direct vision
– Protective of tissues, reparative
– Healing by primary intention
– Lack of pain or complications postoperatively

### Disadvantages

– See contraindications

# Principles of the Ramfjord Technique

- Scalloped inverse bevel incision, along the long axis of the root, down to the alveolar crest; *no* vertical incisions
- Reflection of a mucoperiosteal flap within the attached gingiva, but only to the crest of the alveolar bone
- Intrasulcular incision
- Horizontal incision (especially interdental)
- Root planing with direct vision; removal of granulation tissue from osseous defects

- Tight adaptation of the flaps and coverage of interdental septa by means of interrupted interdental sutures

In the Ramfjord technique the first incision serves to sharply demarcate the pocket epithelium and subjacent infiltrated tissue from the adjacent healthy tissue and to pre-form "new papillae." The marginal gingiva is simultaneously thinned.

An elevator then is used to mobilize and reflect the flap, but only far enough to expose the crest of the alveolar bone.

**558 First incision – Scalloping inverse bevel**
This incision determines the shape of the flap and is performed facially and orally using the 12 B scalpel. It is an inverse bevel incision, extending to the alveolar crest. The distance of the incision from the gingival margin will vary according to the width of the interdental spaces that must be covered, between 0.5–2 mm. The incision may become intrasulcular in interdental areas.

*Right:* The initial inverse bevel incision is depicted schematically (red).

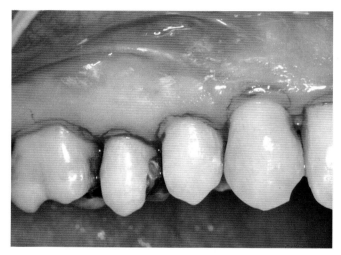 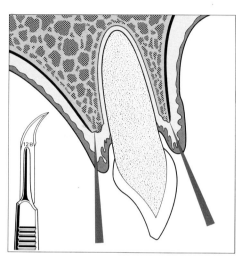

**559 Flap reflection**
A small elevator is used to reflect a full thickness yet only partially mobilized mucoperiosteal flap, as atraumatically as possible. The flap is reflected for one reason only: To permit direct visualization of the root surface and the alveolar crest.

*Right:* The schematic shows clearly that the facial flap is *not* reflected beyond the mucogingival line (black arrow): Conservative flap reflection.

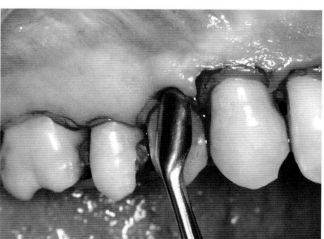 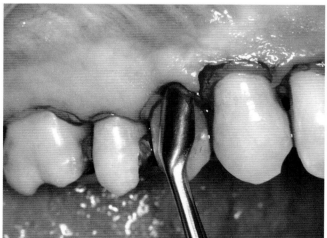 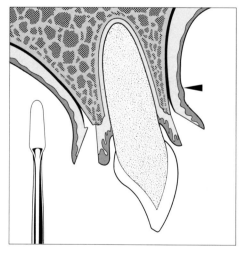

**560 Second incision – Intrasulcular**
This incision is a purely intrasulcular incision that is carried around each tooth, between the hard tooth structure and the gingiva, beyond the base of the pocket and extending to the apical end of the junctional epithelium.

The 12 B scalpel is also indicated for this second incision.

*Right:* Schematic depiction of the second, intrasulcular incision (red).

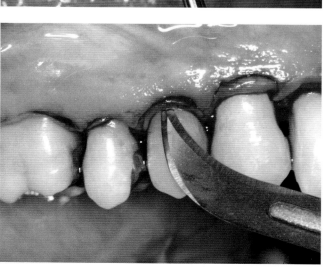 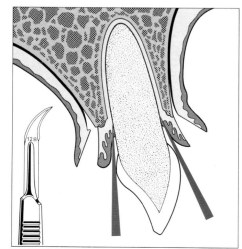

A second incision is made intrasulcularly around the tooth to the depth of the pocket; this frees pocket epithelium and connective tissue from the root surface. In many cases these two incisions will be sufficient to permit removal of the delineated pocket and granulation tissue using a curette.

Ramfjord suggests a third, horizontal, incision to ensure sharp and atraumatic removal of diseased pocket tissue.

The most important component of the Ramfjord procedure now follows: Systematic scaling and planing of the root surfaces using fine curettes, with *direct vision.*

Supportive alveolar bone is *not* removed, but minimum osteoplasty to facilitate flap closure may be performed as necessary.

Finally, the flaps are repositioned. Because of the shape of the flaps created by the initial scalloped incision, tight and complete coverage of the interdental bone is possible. This enhances healing by *primary intention.* Adherence to these principles is routinely associated with excellent long-term results in terms of maintenance or even true gain in periodontal attachment (Knowles et al. 1979; Fig. 527).

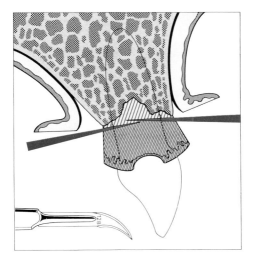
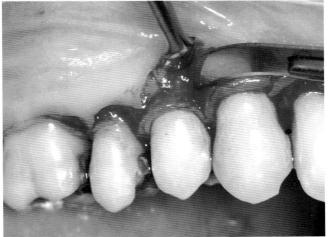

### 561  Third incision – Horizontal
The horizontal incision is carried along the alveolar crest from the facial to the oral aspect, or the reverse, thus separating the supracrestal pocket tissue from its supporting subjacent tissues, especially in the interdental area.

*Left:* The schematic clearly depicts the bony pocket, especially the interdental osseous crater. The horizontal incision does not approach the base of the pocket (note red spears and the profile of the bony architecture apical to it).

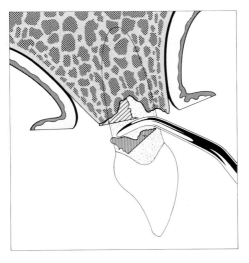
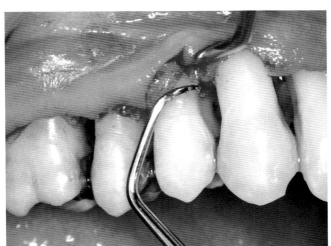

### 562  Root planing with direct vision
Fine curettes are used in the depth of interdental craters to remove remnants of pocket epithelium and granulation tissue. Systematic root planing is performed with direct vision and repeated rinsing.

*Left:* Schematic depiction of the removal of granulation tissue, and root cleaning with a universal curette.

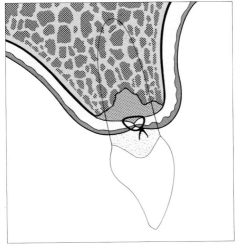
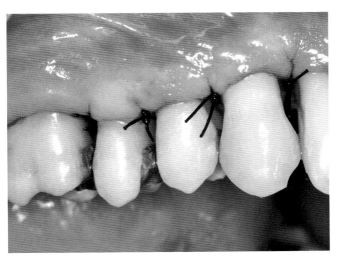

### 563  Tight coverage of interdental defects
The facial and oral flaps are tightly adapted over the bone and teeth by means of interrupted interdental sutures. Because "new papillae" were created by the initial scalloping incision, it is possible to cover interdental defects (e.g., infrabony defects).

*Left:* The schematic shows clearly the coverage of the interdental area. In molar regions, this is not always possible (healing occurs via granulation tissue, by secondary intention).

# Principles of the Ramfjord Technique (MWF) – Occlusal View

The surgical principles of the Ramfjord technique described above clinically will be depicted here from the occlusal. The anatomy of flap design and flap repositioning can be appreciated particularly well when viewed from the occlusal aspect.

The initial incision is scalloped, somewhat removed from the free gingival margin buccally and palatally, creating "new papillae" for subsequent closure of interdental defects.

In the premolar and molar regions the incision may become a pure intrasulcular incision interdentally to provide adequate tissue for complete closure of the interdental space. The primary incision can terminate distally as a wedge excision, permitting treatment for any pockets or furcation involvements at this site (Wedge Excision, p. 248).

The scalloped margin of the flap provides tight closure of the curetted interdental areas as well as coverage for any implant material that may have been used in 2-wall osseous defects.

**564　Initial incision**
The first incision is a scalloped inverse bevel incision (internal gingivectomy) in the maxillary posterior segment (cf. Fig. 558).

The inverse bevel incision continues into a wedge excision distal to the last tooth in the arch (p. 248).

The second (intrasulcular) and third (horizontal) incisions are not depicted here.

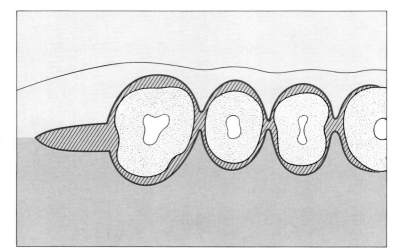

**565　Flap reflection**
After reflecting mucoperiosteal flaps, the excised soft tissues are removed, the osseous defects are carefully curetted, and all root surfaces are cleaned and carefully planed with direct vision.

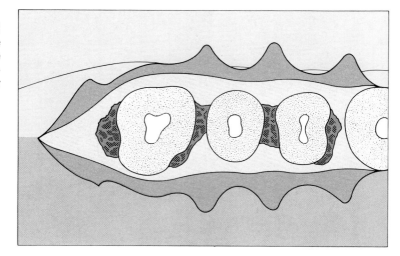

**566　Adaptation of flaps, suturing**
Complete coverage of the interdental bone is accomplished by fixation of the papilla tips using interrupted sutures. If enough tissue is available, the facial and oral papilla tips can actually be repositioned side-by-side before fixation.

If there is insufficient tissue to cover the interdental area, crater-like soft tissue defects may persist. Such defects generally fill in with time. If plaque control is too difficult in such areas, a corrective gingivoplasty may be performed.

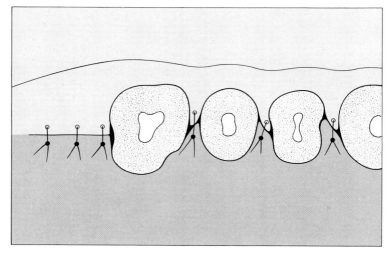

# Modified Widman Procedure
# Partially Reflected Mucoperiosteal Flap

### Operative procedure

The systematic procedure for conservative flap reflection according to the principles of the Ramfjord technique will be depicted in the maxillary right sextant. The 42-year-old female presents a mild to moderate, slowly progressing periodontitis (AP). Initial therapy is complete. Patient cooperation was "only average." In other sextants that are not depicted here, smaller surgical interventions were planned.

*Findings after initial therapy:*
HYG: 70%     PBI: 1.1     TM: 0–2
See accompanying Figures for the clinical picture, probing depths, gingival contour and radiographic survey.

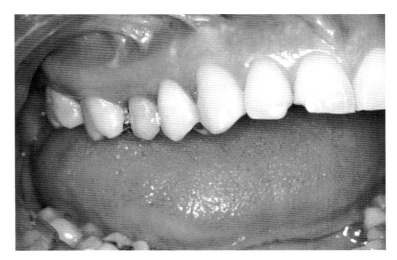

**567  After initial therapy**
The gingivae are inflamed despite initial therapy. Mild hemorrhage occurs upon probing of the pockets. The patient's oral hygiene must be checked repeatedly and OHI provided even after the planned surgical procedures are completed.

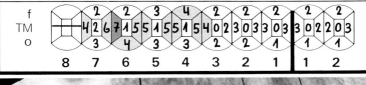

| f | | | 2 | 2 | 3 | 4 | 2 | 2 | 2 | | 2 | 2 |
| TM | | | 4 2 6 | 7 1 5 | 5 1 5 | 5 1 5 | 4 0 2 | 3 0 3 | 3 0 3 | | 3 0 2 | 2 0 3 |
| o | | | 3 | 4 | 3 | 3 | 2 | 2 | 1 | | 1 | 1 |
| | 8 | 7 | 6 | 5 | 4 | 3 | 2 | 1 | | 1 | 2 |

**568  Probing depths following initial therapy**
Interdental probing depths up to 7 mm persist after initial therapy.

**Radiographic survey**
Mild to moderate attachment loss is observed in the premolar region. Between teeth 17 and 16 the interdental septum has resorbed down to the midpoint of the root.

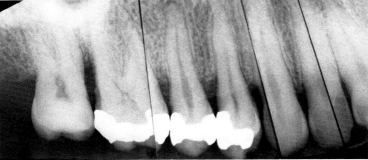

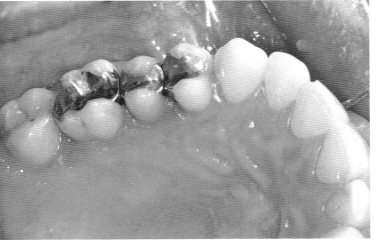

**569  Occlusopalatal view**
Mild inflammation is also obvious from the oral aspect in the sextant between 13 and 17, especially in the interdental area. Near the deep pocket around 17 and 16, signs of pocket activity (exudate) persist despite initial therapy.

**570 Planning the surgery**
The planned initial scalloping incision and the extent of the flap to be reflected are indicated.

---

*Solid line:* Initial incision.

*Hatched area:* Planned mobilization. The flaps are not reflected beyond the mucogingival line (dashed line and arrow).

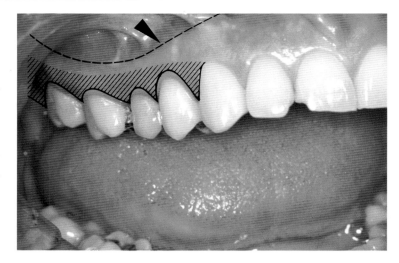

**First incision**

**571 Scalloping primary incision**
The initial scalloping incision is inverse bevel (internal gingivectomy). If teeth are crowded this incision may become a purely intrasulcular one in interdental areas, to ensure sufficient tissue for the "new" papillae.

*Right:* The incision targets toward the marginal crest of the alveolar bone (12B scalpel).

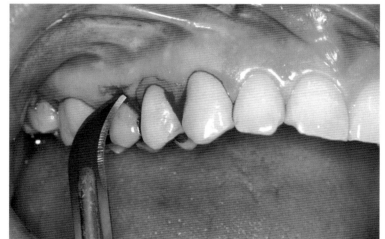
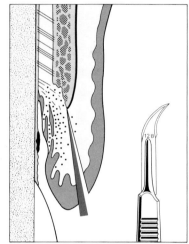

**572 Primary incision complete – Facial view**
Because the partially reflected flaps will be replaced at the original location, vertical incisions are unnecessary.

The inverse bevel incision is depicted here as it terminates near the canine as a pure intrasulcular incision; this provides sufficient mesial release of the flap (no pocket exists on the facial surface of the canine).

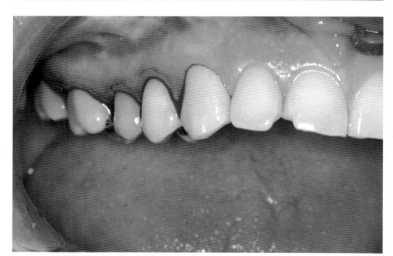

**573 Scalloped primary incision – Palatal view**
The incision is performed identically on the oral surface. In order to ensure that the rather resilient palatal flaps can be readapted to the tooth and bone surfaces, the primary incision should not be made too far removed from the height of the gingival margin. The incision targets toward the marginal crest of the alveolar bone (12B scalpel).

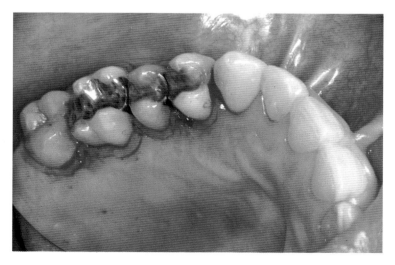

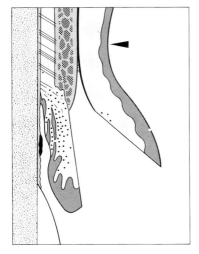

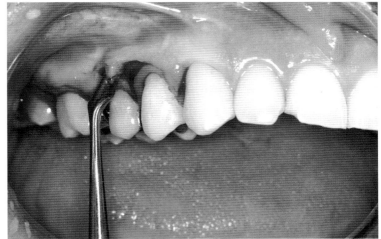

**574 Partial reflection of the facial gingival flap**
Using a small elevator, the gingiva is reflected just far enough to reveal the course of the alveolar margin.

*Left:* Because the flaps are *not* reflected beyond the mucogingival line (black arrow) into the mobile mucosa, they cannot be repositioned apically or coronally during closure and suturing.

### Second incision

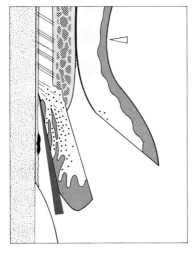

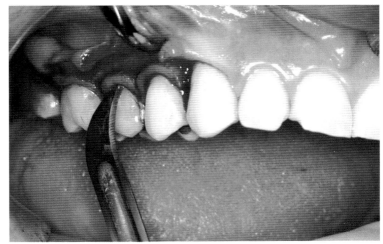

**575 Intrasulcular incision**
Using once again the 12 B scalpel the second, intrasulcular incision is made. These two incisions are often sufficient to permit removal of the delineated pocket tissues using curettes. If difficulty is encountered the third, horizontal incision must be performed (Fig. 576).

*Left:* The second incision is made between the tooth and the gingiva and extends somewhat beyond the base of the pocket.

### Third incision

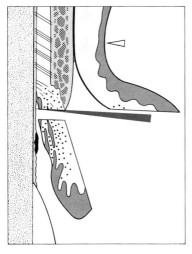

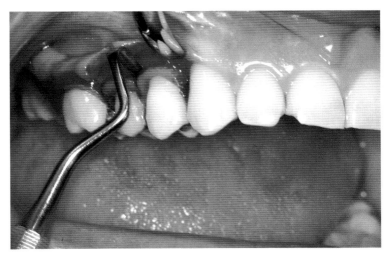

**576 Horizontal incision**
Using a papilla knife or a fine scalpel, a third (horizontal) incision is made.

*Left:* This final incision frees completely and sharply the tissues to be removed. Not clear in the schematic is that this third incision is primarily *interdental* (cf. Fig. 561).

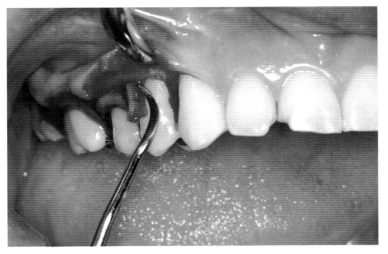

**577 Removal of the delineated pocket tissues**
The tissues that are delineated and freed up by the three incisions can be easily removed using curettes. Granulation tissue is also removed and this provides a clear view of the root surfaces. The absolute removal of *all* infiltrated tissue *per se* is *not* necessary for complication-free healing.

### 578 Root cleaning and root planing using curettes

After removal of the pocket soft tissues, and curettage of the bony pocket and craters, the root surfaces are cleaned and planed using fine universal or Gracey curettes. Extensive removal of cementum, even into the dentin, as was formerly advocated, is no longer recommended today. Any endotoxins usually occupy only the superficial cementum portion.

*Right:* Schematic depiction of root surface cleaning with universal curette (M23A).

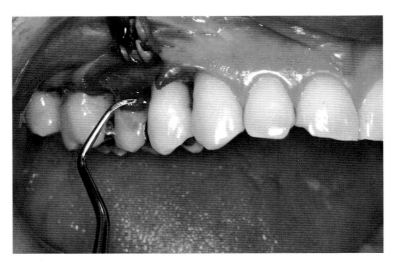
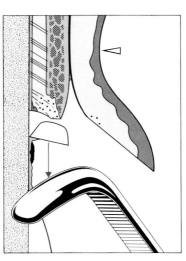

### 579 Root cleaning and planing with fine diamond

Cleaning the root surfaces (calculus removal) can also be performed with diamonds (Perio-Set, 40 µm), and root planing with 15 µm diamond stones. Low rpm and constant rinsing with Ringer's solution must always accompany the use of rotating diamonds.

The diamonds of the Perio-Set (Fig. 418) should not be considered as replacements for curettes, but enhancements! Diamonds are indicated for use in grooves, depressions, and furcation areas; less for smooth surfaces.

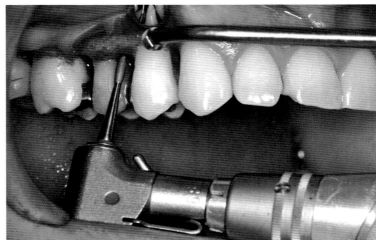

### 580 Flap adaptation using interrupted sutures

The close approximation of the flaps upon bone and tooth surfaces is a prerequisite for optimum healing. Fixation of the flaps is accomplished by means of interdental interrupted sutures. The scalloping form of the initial incision usually permits tight closure in the interdental spaces. The facial and oral papillae should touch each other or even overlap somewhat side-by-side.

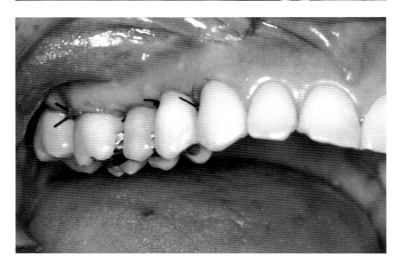

### 581 Flap adaptation, palatal

The scalloping primary incision on the oral aspect should permit closure of the interdental spaces and coverage of curetted interdental craters (right). In addition to suture closure, a periodontal dressing (e.g., Coe-Pak) may be placed. The patient is instructed to rinse with chlorhexidine (e.g., Peridex) daily until sutures are removed.

*Right:* The interdental crater that persists following curettage and root cleaning is especially pronounced between 17 and 16.

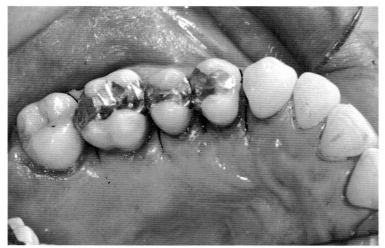
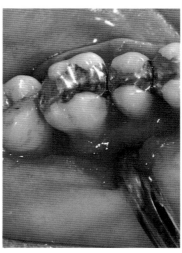

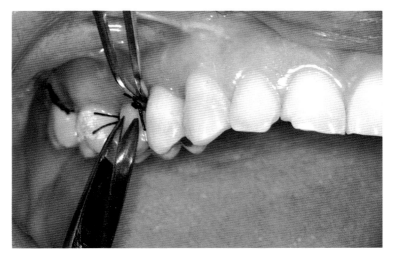

### Wound healing

#### 582 Suture removal – Carefully!

Eight days following surgery, sutures are carefully removed. By this time the wound margins have adhered to each other and the healing process is well underway; however, careless handling of the sutures could nevertheless disturb the delicate attachments between and among the flaps, the osseous surface and the tooth/root. This might defeat the entire purpose of the operation: Complete healing.

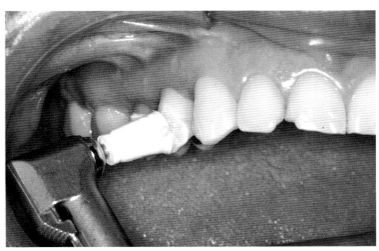

#### 583 Tooth cleaning

Following suture removal the surfaces of the teeth are thoroughly cleaned with a soft rubber cup and a mildly abrasive prophy paste (or dentifrice).

Since wound healing is not yet complete (regeneration, new junctional epithelium) care must be exercised that no paste is forced into the sulcus.

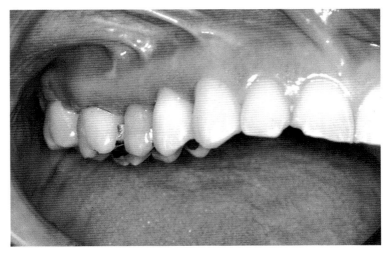

#### 584 Following suture removal and tooth cleaning

At this stage the patient should reinitiate home care, but carefully! For the next few days, until more vigorous toothbrushing can be practiced, it is recommended that chlorhexidine rinsing be continued. The field of operation should be professionally cleaned by the dental hygienist during subsequent appointments for the surgical treatment of other areas of the dentition.

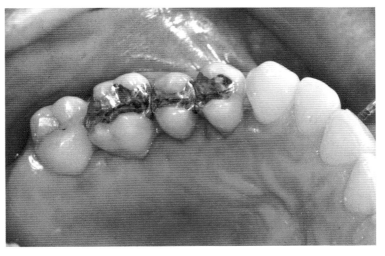

#### 585 Occlusopalatal view following suture removal and tooth cleaning

Oral hygiene is particularly critical in the palatal region.

Despite all efforts to close the interdental spaces immediately after surgery, a small gingival crater persists between teeth 17 and 16. Such depressions can usually be eliminated by routine oral hygiene procedures (interdental brushes). Sometimes a minor gingivoplasty via electrosurgery must be performed to even out the area.

# Modified Widman Procedure
# Partially Reflected Mucoperiosteal Flap

## Summary

The 42-year-old patient with mild to moderate adult periodontitis exhibited deficient oral hygiene at the first examination. Even after initial therapy, mild gingival inflammation was in evidence. Between molars 16 and 17 signs of mild pocket activity (exudate) persisted.

Probing depths returned to physiologic levels subsequent to the surgical procedure. Even the deep defect between 16 and 17 exhibited a probing depth of only 4 mm. These excellent results can also be attributed to the great improvements by the patient in home care. Because of the shrinkage, mainly in the interdental region, special emphasis should be placed on interdental hygiene.

The initial recall is set at three months; if patient cooperation continues, subsequent recalls may be at 4–6 month intervals.

**586 Before surgery**
Despite initial therapy mild gingival inflammation persists (PBI 1.1); application of finger pressure between 16 and 17 elicits release of minimal exudate. The treatment of choice is *surgical*, with direct vision.

*Right:* An untreated pocket (facial surface of 14). The probing depth is marked in red (bar and arrows).

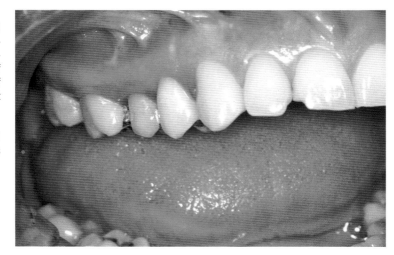
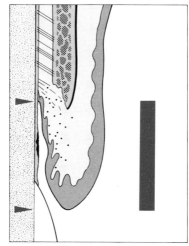

**587 Pocket probings and TM following initial therapy – Before surgery**
Following initial therapy which consisted of closed supra- and subgingival scaling without anesthesia, pockets of 4–7 mm persist, especially interdentally.

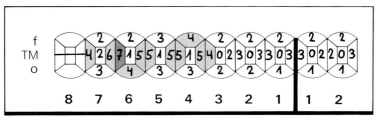

Before

**Pocket probings and TM six months after surgery**
At the recall examination six months after the surgical procedure, no probing depths beyond the 4 mm level are detected.

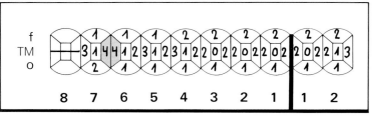

After

**588 Six months postoperative**
Even after the careful and conservative operation involving partial mobilization of flaps, the teeth appear slightly "elongated" and the interdental spaces are more open. Recommendations for interdental hygiene are determined by the anatomic situation.

*Right:* A slightly deepened sulcus persists (red bar). The former probing depth has been reduced through shrinkage (**1**) as well as periodontal regeneration (**2**).

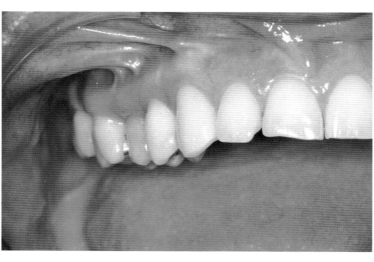
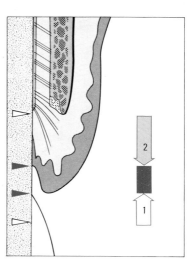

# Fully Reflected Mucoperiosteal Flaps

Flaps that are reflected beyond the mucogingival border into the region of the mobile oral mucosa in vestibular and lingual regions are termed fully reflected mucoperiosteal flaps. Full thickness flaps are differentiated from split-thickness flaps. The former are used primarily in the treatment of periodontitis, while the latter are employed for mucogingival surgical procedures.

A fully reflected mucoperiosteal flap permits a broad overview of the surgical field and simplifies the important decision as to whether or not the alveolar bone should be recontoured, or whether teeth should be extracted, or whether individual roots should be resected or whether implants should be placed in osseous defects. The reflection of full thickness mucoperiosteal flaps may require that vertical incisions be made (Fig. 589). These can make it possible to reposition flaps (e. g., apical).

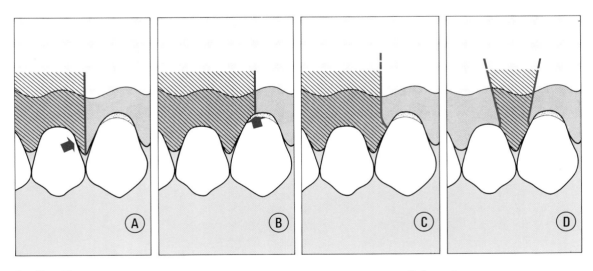

**589  Vertical releasing incisions**

*Unfavorable incisions ?*
**A  Interdental:** Necrosis, shrinkage of the papilla tip
**B  Midfacial:** Recession; shrinkage may be desirable in the case of periodontal pockets on the facial surface

*Favorable incisions?*
**C  Paramedian:** Best compromise, minimal shrinkage
**D  Triangular flap:** Two diverging paramedian incisions = minimum fully mobilized flap for localized interdental defects

## Indications
- Pronounced, irregular bone loss on various teeth that will be treated simultaneously
- Necessary osteoplasty to correct deep pockets or thickened bony margins. *Tooth-supporting bone must never be sacrificed.* Bone must be conserved!
- Hemisections of teeth or resection of individual roots
- Implants into infrabony pockets

## Contraindications
- Fully mobilized flaps are contraindicated anywhere that partial flap reflection (e. g., modified Widman procedure) will suffice.

## Advantages
- Excellent direct vision; good access to all root surfaces in furcations, depressions etc.
- Possible flap repositioning (apical, lateral, coronal)

## Disadvantages
- Postoperative edema, pain
- Superficial resorption of exposed bone (attachment loss, bone loss)
- Exposed tooth necks (esthetics, hypersensitivity, caries)

## Osseous Surgery?
## Instruments/Materials ...

In the treatment of periodontitis today, osseous surgery maintains only minimum importance. A basic premise is that *no* tooth-supporting bone should be removed; the total elimination or "evening out" of osseous defects by means of ostectomy is regarded today as necessary in only rare instances. The target is rather that by means of curettage of the bony pockets and cleaning/planing of the adjacent root surfaces, new bone formation and filling of the osseous defect should occur, especially in 2- and 3-wall infrabony pockets.

A question that has not yet been definitively answered is whether or not, or to what degree, the filling of osseous defects by autologous or alloplastic material actually enhances formation of new bone (pp. 245 & 259).

The removal of bone in the course of a periodontal surgical procedure must be only in the form of *osteoplasty*. This permits better *adaptation* of the mucoperiosteal flap and healing that results in gingival morphology favoring optimum *oral hygiene*.

**590 Round burs – Bone bur**
At left, three different sizes of normal round burs; at right the smallest bone bur with internal cooling.

- **Round bur** nos. 014, 018, 023
- **Bone bur** with internal cooling no. 473 RS/040 (Jota Co.)

Bone should be approached only at low rpm and with constant sterile cooling solution. Even with a mild warming above 50°C, necrosis of osteocytes can occur.

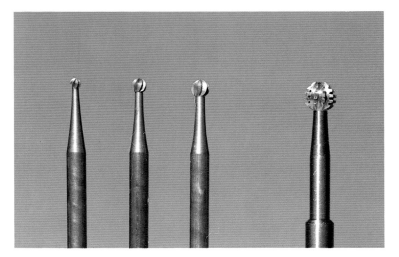

**591 Rongeurs**
This special bone-cutting forceps with its round (left) and pointed working ends is indicated for removal of sharp or protruding bony margins, e.g., the alveolar margin following tooth extraction.

- **Luer-Friedmann** FO 409 (red, Aesculap)
- **Cleveland** 5S (yellow, Hu-Friedy)

The rongeur forceps is indicated only seldom for actual periodontal osseous surgery, e.g., for recontouring of the alveolar bone, because it is a rather gross instrument.

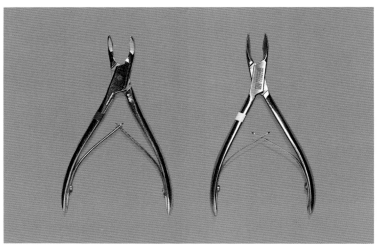

**592 Alloplastic implant material**
Implant materials in the form of calcium phosphates are available in various particle sizes:

- **Coarse tricalcium phosphate (TCP, left)**
  Resorbable TCP (Ceros 82)
- **Average hydroxyapatite (HA, center)**
  HA, non-resorbable (Periograf)
- **Fine-grained HA (right)**
  Experimental HA, slowly resorbable (Bio-Oss)

Particle size of ca. 0.2–0.5 mm is recommended.

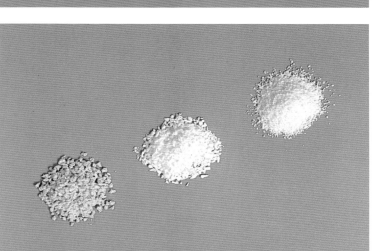

## ... and Their Use

Tooth-supporting bone may be removed for reasons unrelated to the periodontal therapy, e.g., crown lengthening procedures for restorative dentistry (pp. 236–237).

Round burs or special bone burs are best indicated for *recontouring* of bone. Rotating sterile instruments should only be used under cooling with Ringer's solution; this in combination with low rpm serves to avoid heat damage to the bone (max. 50 °C for osteocytes!).

For the removal of sharp bony margins after tooth extraction, bone forceps ("rongeurs") are indicated.

Two different crystalline forms of calcium phosphate are available for the *filling* of osseous defects with alloplastic material: Resorbable tricalcium phosphate and non-resorbable hydroxyapatite. This procedure remains controversial. Both of these materials are available commercially in various porosities and particle sizes (p. 259).

**Osseous surgery – Examples**

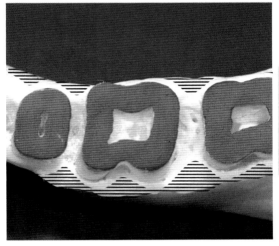
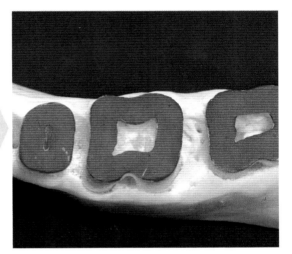

### 593 Osteoplasty of a thickened alveolar process
*Left:* The irregular and thickened alveolar process resulting from periodontal destruction inhibits proper adaptation of the soft tissue flap into the interdental and furcation areas subsequent to periodontal surgery. If left untreated, this would render oral hygiene very difficult. The hatched areas indicate the planned osteoplastic recontouring of the alveolar process.

*Right:* Appearance following conservative osteoplasty.

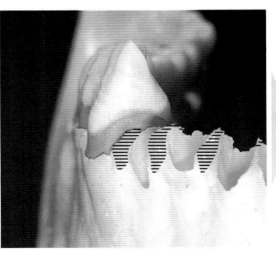
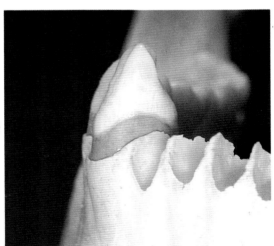

### 594 Recontouring a sharp alveolar margin subsequent to tooth extraction
*Left:* Following extraction during a periodontal flap procedure (cf. p. 255, Fig. 665), sharp bony edges should be eliminated, as well as undercut areas of the edentulous alveolar process, in order to protect the soft tissue flap from perforation (preprosthetic surgery). The actual *height* of the alveolar process should never be reduced.

*Right:* Situation following careful reduction of the facial bony margins using the rongeur forceps.

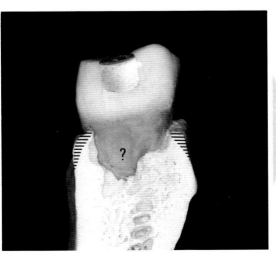
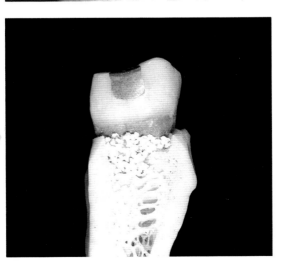

### 595 Fill a pocket with an implant material?
*Left:* Interdental bony crater, 2-wall osseous defect. After thorough curettage and root planing, one can expect some new bone formation. It remains questionable whether this can be enhanced by an implant.

Facial and oral thickened bone should be carefully remodeled, to improve adaptation of soft tissue flaps (hatched area).

*Right:* Osseous crater filled with alloplastic material. Implant material must be mixed with blood.

# Mucoperiosteal Flap without Vertical Incisions
# Osteoplasty – Flap Repositioning

In this young patient, only 21-years-old, advanced periodontitis was diagnosed, with varying degrees of severity throughout the arch. Following initial therapy a flap procedure was performed. Incisions were made according to the principles of the Ramfjord technique. However, the labial flap was subsequently fully reflected beyond the mucogingival line in order to gain access for osteoplasty of the bulbous margin of the alveolar crest.

Following the osseous correction, the flap was repositioned at its approximate original location.

*Diagnosis:* Moderate progressive periodontitis (RPP?) with a localized deep lesion on the mesial of 26. The patient's preoperative home care was only average.

*Findings before surgery:*
HYG: 78%     PBI: 1.4     TM: 1–2

The clinical picture, gingival contour, probing depths and radiographic survey are shown in the Figures below.

**596  After initial therapy**
In the upper left quadrant, active pockets to 8 mm remain after initial therapy (see charting).

The soft tissue and possibly also the bone are thickened, especially on the facial aspect lateral to the interdental craters (arrows), although this is not readily visible in the photograph.

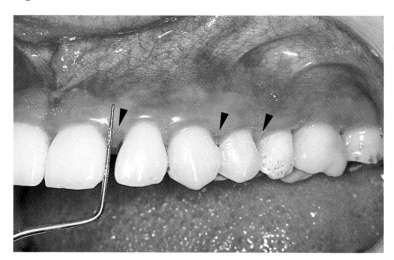

**597  Probing depths and tooth mobility (TM) after initial therapy**
Interproximal periodontal pockets are severe. Bone loss is not uniform throughout the segment.

**Radiographic view**
The radiographs reveal a crater-like bony defect on the mesial of tooth 26.

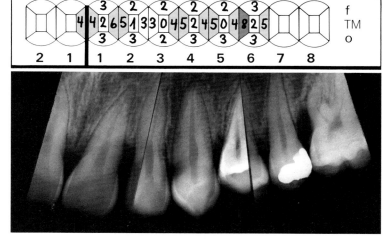

**598  Initial incision**
When mucoperiosteal flaps are extensively reflected, the principles of the modified Widman technique should also be followed. The scalloped form provides "papillae" (facial and oral) that can be used subsequently to completely cover interdental defects.

Because the surgery was intended to correct the bulbous, thickened buccal bone, the buccal flap had to be reflected apically beyond the mucogingival line.

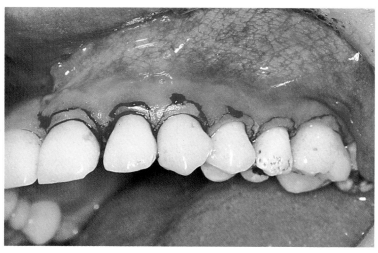

*Case:* A 59-year-old patient desired an esthetically acceptable reconstruction for her severely abraded, often filled, "stubby" anterior teeth. Periodontal pockets (mild AP) were present before initial therapy.

The surgical procedure is conveniently divided into individual steps, as depicted below:
- Pre-preparation of abutments, with a marginal step
- Full reflection of facial and oral mucoperiosteal flaps
- Ostectomy around the tooth at a *constant distance* from the marginal step
- Osteoplasty to facilitate flap adaptation
- Scaling of the exposed roots to remove cementum
- Apical repositioning of the facial flap and the oral flap, which was shortened by gingivectomy
- Placing of interrupted sutures
- Tooth preparation with a circular step at new gingival margin
- Seating the trimmed and adapted temporaries

Crown lengthening by means of gingivectomy alone is depicted on p. 286.

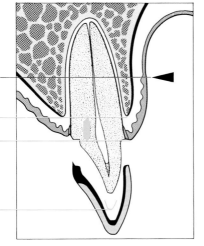

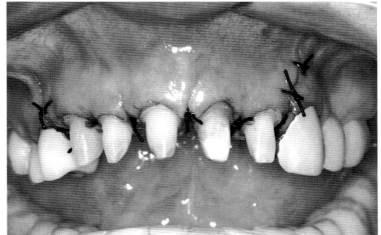

**606  Apical flap repositioning – Definitive preparation of the lengthened abutment teeth**
The facial flap is apically repositioned and sutured to the oral flap. The preparation margins of the abutment teeth are then carefully adjusted down to the "new gingival margin."

*Left:* In the schematic, beginning apically blue lines indicate the new position of the mucogingival line (arrow), the new alveolar border and the gingival margin, as well as the incisal edge of the porcelain-fused-to-metal crown.

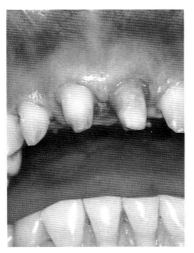

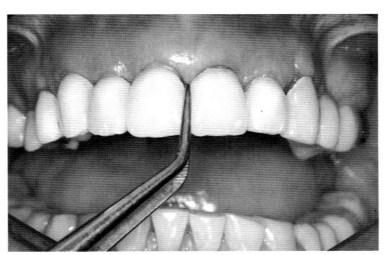

**607  Temporary crown – Postoperative care 7 days later**
The acrylic crown fabricated in the laboratory was seated on the prepared abutment immediately after the surgery.

Seven days later the sutures and the temporary crown were removed. The unsightly temporary was recontoured to approximate the form of the natural teeth, the tight interdental spaces were opened somewhat to make oral hygiene easier (Super Floss).

*Left:* After suture removal, 7 days postoperative. Gingival healing has proceeded normally.

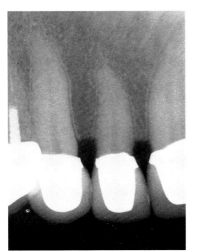

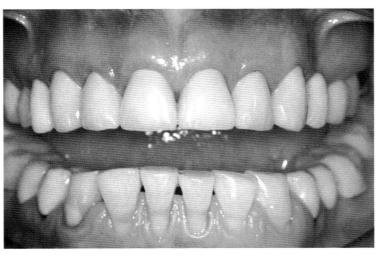

**608  Six months postoperative – Definitive reconstruction**
The definitive porcelain-fused-to-metal crowns were seated 3 months postoperatively. The old bridge 23–26 was also remade, at the patient's request.

Despite wide interdental spaces, anatomically normal interdental gingival papillae regenerated spontaneously during the period when the temporary crowns were in place.

*Left:* The radiograph reveals the wide interdental septa.

# Mucoperiosteal Flap with Vertical Incisions
## Osteoplasty – Apical Repositioning

The apically repositioned flap is employed only seldom in the treatment of periodontitis today. It is indicated only in cases with very deep pockets on the facial aspect. The technique for this procedure will be demonstrated in a 34-year-old patient with advanced periodontitis in the mandibular anterior region. Full reflection of the mucoperiosteal flaps was necessary to gain visual access into the extremely deep defects, and vertical releasing incisions were required because the planned surgery included apical repositioning of the flaps.

Clinically visible inflammation was almost completely eliminated by initial therapy, but the hyperplastic gingivae did not shrink appreciably. Several deep pockets continued to exhibit signs of activity.

*Findings after initial therapy:*
HYG: 80%     PBI: 1.3     TM: 2–3!

The clinical picture, gingival contour, probing depths and radiographic survey are depicted in the Figures below.

**609   After initial therapy**
Probing depths were not significantly reduced by initial therapy, which included subgingival scaling. Pockets to 9 mm persisted, as indicated by the Michigan-O probe. The *activity* (inflammation) of the pockets was nevertheless reduced, though not completely eliminated.

*Right:* Section through the interdental space between 41 and 42. The base of the osseous pocket (probe tip) is located apical to the mucogingival line (black arrow).

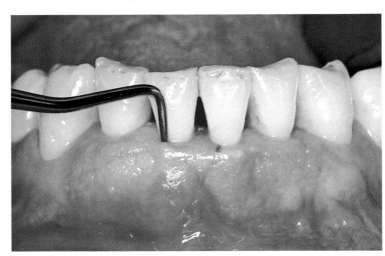
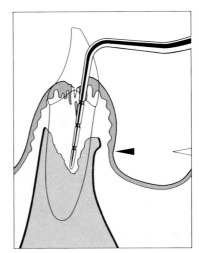

**610   Probing depths and tooth mobility (TM) after initial therapy**

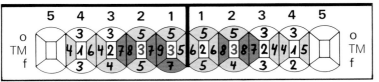

| | 5 | 4 | 3 | 2 | 1 | 1 | 2 | 3 | 4 | 5 | |
|---|---|---|---|---|---|---|---|---|---|---|---|
| O | | 3 | 3 | 5 | 5 | 5 | 5 | 3 | 3 | | O |
| TM | 4 1 | 6 4 | 2 7 | 8 3 | 7 9 3 5 | 6 2 6 | 8 3 8 | 7 2 | 4 4 | 1 5 | TM |
| f | | 3 | 4 | 5 | 7 | 5 | 4 | 3 | 2 | | f |

**Radiographic survey**
Less than half the root length of the mandibular incisors remains anchored in the bone. The exceptionally deep defect between 41 and 42 is not clearly revealed in the radiograph (Figs. 612, 613).

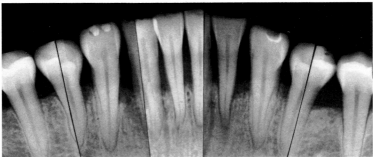

**611   Surgical planning**

1 Scalloped, inverse bevel incision
2 Vertical incisions bilaterally
3 Crevicular incision
4 Full flap reflection

The primary incision (inverse bevel) is performed relatively liberally because the pockets on the facial surfaces are very deep and because there is sufficient width of attached gingiva.

The bilateral vertical incisions permit apical flap repositioning.

*Right:* First incision in the interdental area toward the alveolar crest.

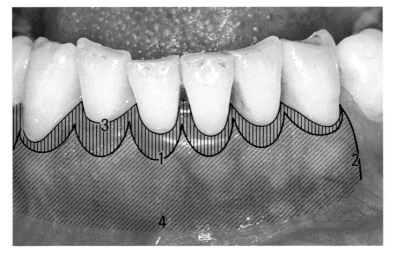
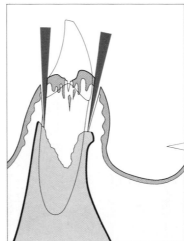

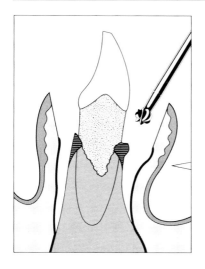

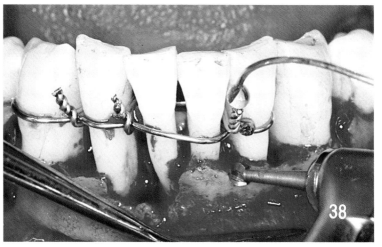

### 612 Osteoplasty
A round bur with saline irrigation is used to reduce the bulbous, sharp bony edges (osteoplasty). *Tooth-supporting bone is not removed.*

The anterior teeth were so mobile that it was necessary to fabricate a crude temporary wire splint during the surgery.

*Left:* The extensive flap reflection beyond the mucogingival line (empty arrow) is shown. The planned osteoplasty is indicated (hatched).

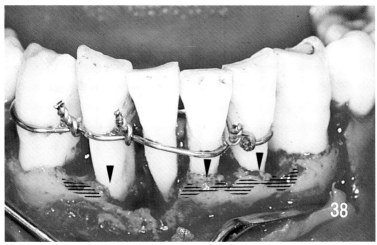

### 613 After osteoplasty
The horizontal lines indicate areas where bone was removed. Note that *no* osseous reduction was performed on tooth-supporting bone near the cervix (arrows). This case demonstrates that even when reverse architecture is present due to advanced disease, removal of bone is still performed most sparingly.

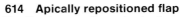

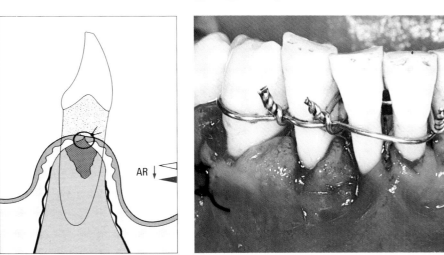

### 614 Apically repositioned flap
The flap is repositioned apically so that the interdental craters, now filled with coagulum, can be tightly covered with gingival tissue when sutured.

The wire splint serves a dual purpose since it will also help retain the periodontal dressing.

*Left:* Root surfaces are exposed as a result of the liberal inverse bevel incision (Fig. 611) and because of the apical repositioning (AR) of the flaps.

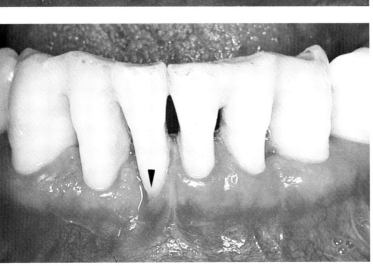

### 615 Six weeks postoperatively
The teeth appear considerably longer in comparison to the pre-operative clinical view. Tooth 41 exhibits no attached gingiva at all (black arrow). A minor, localized Edlan procedure is planned for this area.

The extremely mobile anterior teeth were splinted in two groups of three teeth each (43–42–41 and 31–32–33) using a composite resin (acid-etch technique, p. 349).

# Osteoplasty – Apical Repositioning of Flap

## Summary

In a 34-year-old patient, initial therapy eliminated most of the gingival inflammation. Selective occlusal equilibration was performed due to a parafunctional habit and increasing tooth mobility.

Pocket-free conditions were achieved by means of a relatively radical surgical procedure involving fully reflected flaps, osteoplasty and apical repositioning of the mucoperiosteal flaps.

Several months later a minor surgical procedure (modified Edlan-Mejchar) was performed to create some attached tissue in the region of tooth 41.

The long term prognosis in such a case is good only if the patient maintains excellent oral hygiene, especially in interdental areas.

This large and complex therapeutic endeavor was justified by the fact that loss of these teeth would reconcile the patient to an expansive 6- to 8-unit fixed bridge or a removable partial denture.

**616    After initial therapy**
Findings before flap surgery:
- "short" teeth
- minimum visible inflammation
- very deep pockets (to 9 mm, red in diagram)
- interdental osseous cratering

*Right:* Relationship between severe inderdental attachment loss and a relatively normal height of the gingival margin (red bar = probing depth).

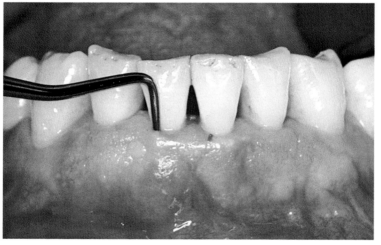
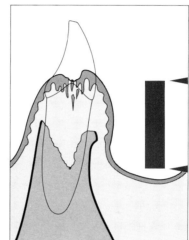

**617    Probing depths and tooth mobility (TM) after initial therapy**

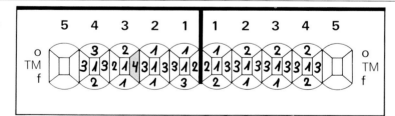

Before

**12 months postoperative**
The tooth mobility (TM) values represent the two splinted units (3 teeth each).

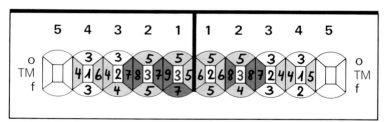

After

**618    Clinical picture one year later**
The former pockets have been eliminated; however, the teeth appear elongated and the cervical areas remain sensitive. A minor vestibular extension procedure ("Edlan") stabilized the mucosa near 41.

*Right:* The residual probing depth is depicted (red bar).

1  Apical repositioning and shrinkage
2  Bone regeneration; new attachment

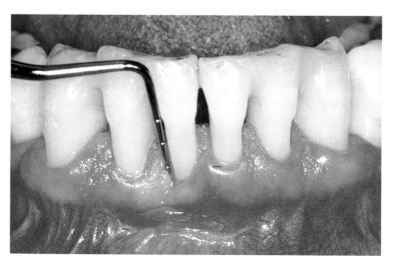
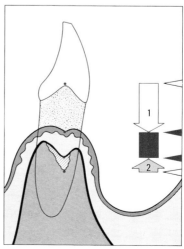

# Flap Surgery in a Combined Procedure

Advanced periodontitis is rarely distributed evenly throughout the dental arch. Inflammation, attachment loss and probing depths must therefore be evaluated for each individual tooth ("single tooth diagnosis"). It is not exceptional to find in one patient an area of localized gingivitis, elsewhere severe periodontal destruction, as well as areas of localized gingival recession.

Depending upon the localization of attachment loss, the treatment plan may include initial therapy and patient home care as the only treatment necessary in certain areas, while conservative surgical interventions such as the modified Widman procedure, "ENAP," gingivoplasty or gingivectomy may be necessary in other areas. In still other segments of the dentition it may be necessary to reflect expansive mucoperiosteal flaps in order to perform osteoplasty, root resection, hemisection, or intraosseous implants.

Similarly, it is possible for two *different* surgical procedures to be indicated in the *same* operative area. Because a palatal flap cannot be repositioned apically due to its lack of elasticity, it is not unusual for a surgical appointment to combine a gingivectomy (*palatal*) and a flap procedure (*buccal*). Yet another possibility is the performance of a flap procedure and gingivectomy on the same surface of the same tooth.

These frequently encountered combination techniques are described and depicted below:

| | | |
|---|---|---|
| **Fully reflected flap** ← → | **Partially reflected flap (Widman)** | (p. 234) |
| **Flap** ← → | **GV/GP** | (p. 242) |
| **Flap** ← → | **Infrabony implants** | (pp. 243, 259) |
| **Flap** ← → | **Wedge excisions** | (pp. 248, 262) |
| **Flap** ← → | **Tooth extractions** | (p. 253) |
| **Flap** ← → | **Hemisections, root resections** | (p. 265) |

Combining a periodontal flap procedure with removal of an impacted third molar is not recommended, because of the danger of infection in the extraction wound. It is also unwise to perform surgery for periodontitis (flaps, GV/GP) at the same time as mucogingival surgery for recession. In such cases, the periodontitis is generally treated first. Only when the initial surgical site has completely healed should the mucogingival problem be approached surgically.

# Combined Surgical Technique – Schematic Presentation
# Flap (buccal) – GV and Flap (palatal)

A frequently indicated periodontal surgical technique involves a buccal flap and a palatal gingivectomy with subsequent flap reflection. Gingivectomy is often performed on the palate because of the difficulty of repositioning the highly resilient tissue. Furthermore, it is often technically difficult to reflect a flap on the lingual aspect of the mandibular posterior region.

The reflection of a palatal flap *after* gingivectomy is indicated when deep pockets are present interproximally and palatally. This procedure permits root planing with direct vision on palatal and interproximal tooth surfaces. It also makes possible adequate coverage of interdental defects with soft tissue. The palatal gingivectomy wound, which is usually not very expansive, must be covered with a periodontal dressing and permitted to re-epithelialize.

This procedure is depicted diagramatically below for the maxillary premolar region.

**619   Incision/Gingivectomy**

**Buccal: Flap**
A horizontal inverse bevel incision is made to create the flap, according to the Ramfjord principles.

**Palatal: Gingivectomy**
A standard gingivectomy incision eliminates to a great degree the palatal pocket.

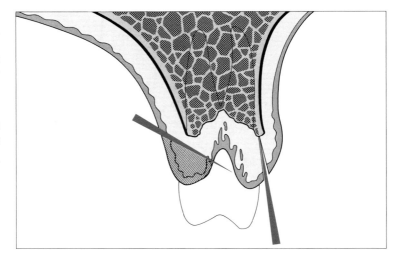

**620   Reflection of buccal and palatal flaps – Root planing**
After removal of the tissue excised via GV, a crevicular incision is made on the palate and a flap is reflected; thus, the flap is not covered with epithelium. The root surface and osseous contour are now exposed so that debridement, root planing and any indicated osteoplasty (hatched area) can be accomplished with direct vision from both buccal and palatal aspects.

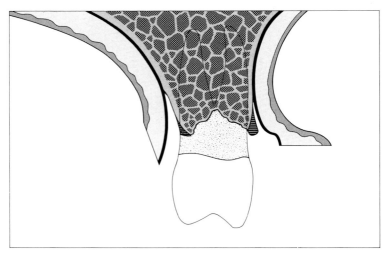

**621   Flap adaptation – Wound care**
Interrupted sutures serve to closely adapt the buccal and palatal flaps to the bone and tooth surfaces. Every effort should be made to completely cover interdental craters. This can only be accomplished by sliding the buccal flap into and through the interdental area, which causes the mucogingival line to be displaced coronally. Thus the mucobuccal fold becomes shallower.

The gingivectomy wound on the palatal surface must always be covered with a dressing.

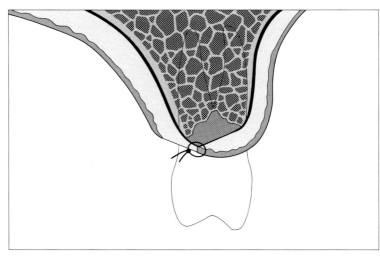

# Combined Surgical Technique
# Flap (buccal) – GV and Flap (palatal) – Alloplastic Intraosseous Implant

## Operative procedure

In the case presented here various periodontal surgical procedures were combined. The primary goal of the surgery was to attempt to enhance bone regeneration in the 8 mm pocket mesial to the left central incisor by placement of an alloplastic implant (resorbable β-tricalcium phosphate, TCP). This was an esthetic as well as a functional measure.

The patient was a 27-year-old female manifesting generalized mild to moderate periodontitis. The 8 mm pocket on the mesial of 21 persisted after initial therapy.

---

*Findings before surgery:*
HYG: 85%     PBI: 1.8
TM:  average of 1, but grade 3 on tooth 21.
Clinical picture, gingival contour, probing depths and radiographic survey are depicted in the Figures below.

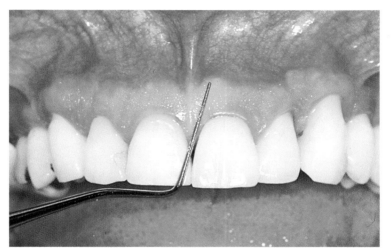

**622   After initial therapy**
The gingivae are essentially free of clinical signs of inflammation following initial therapy, but several active pockets persist. The deepest, an 8 mm 2- to 3- wall infrabony defect, is mesial to tooth 21.
   The pocket extent is indicated with the Michigan probe.

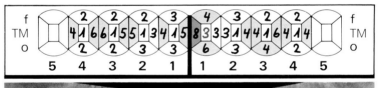

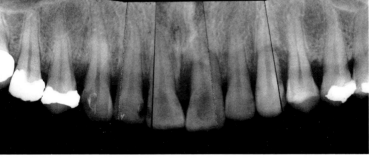

**623   Probing depths and tooth mobility (TM) after initial therapy**
The highly mobile tooth 21 must be approached surgically.

**Radiographic survey**
The relatively "soft" radiograph does not provide an entirely clear picture of the deep defect mesial to tooth 21 (cf. Initial findings, Fig. 637).

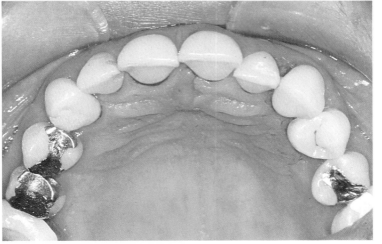

**624   Occlusal view after initial therapy**
Despite initial therapy, mild gingivitis persists. The relatively steep anterior palatal vault permits gingivectomy without creation of an expansive wound surface.

**Palatal procedure**

### 645 Palatal gingivectomy
The first step is a gingivectomy (oblique incision; p. 273) without contacting bone.

Use of a Kirkland knife with a *double-angled* shank makes access easy and overcomes any technical problems.

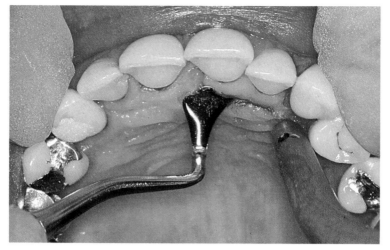
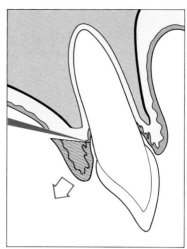

### 626 Mobilization of the palatal flap
Following the gingivectomy, a crevicular incision (not shown) is made using the scalpel (e. g., no. 12B).

The flap is reflected with the aid of an elevator, and direct access is gained to the root surfaces, alveolar bone crest and the osseous craters.

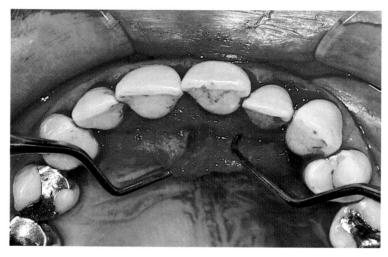

**Labial procedure**

### 627 Labial flap
The mucoperiosteal flap on the labial aspect is created by means of a modified horizontal incision: Around the central incisors a scalloped inverse bevel is used because of the infrabony pockets, while a crevicular incision is sufficient around the other teeth where no deep pockets are present.

*Right:* The inverse bevel incision for flap elevation has been made. The depicted intrasulcular incision is the second step.

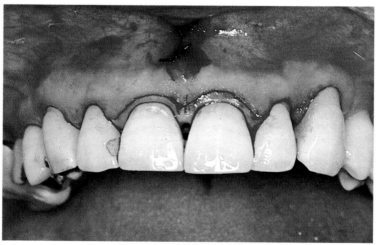
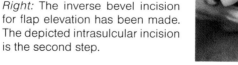

### 628 Root planing
The deep osseous crater mesial to 21 has filled with blood following thorough but careful debridement and root planing.

Regeneration of new bone in the depth of this crater may be anticipated, without the use of an implant of any kind.

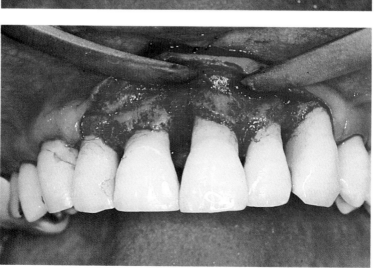

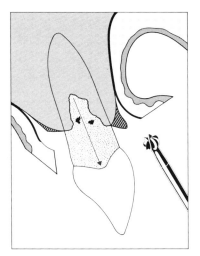

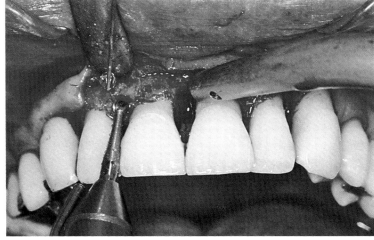

**629 Osteoplasty**
The bulbous bony margin between 11 and 12 is carefully recontoured without reducing the *height* of the supporting alveolar bone.

*Left:* The anticipated osteoplasty is indicated. After recontouring of the bone, definitive planing of the root surfaces (red arrow) is performed.

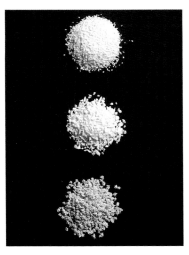

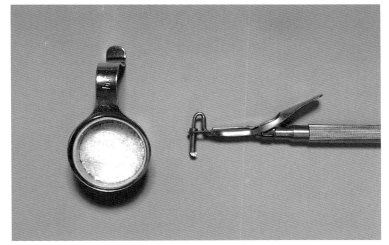

**630 Alloplastic implant material – TCP (β-tricalcium phosphate)**
The relatively fine-grained material is mixed with sterile saline to form a thick paste. Using a small sterile amalgam carrier (F-10-11, Hu-Friedy) it can conveniently be placed into the osseous defect, where it must be mixed with blood.

*Left:* Alloplastic implant materials with various particle sizes and porosities (cf. p. 259):

| | | |
|---|---|---|
| above | **0.2–0.5 mm** | fine |
| center | **0.6–1.4 mm** | medium |
| below | **1.5–2.8 mm** | coarse |

**TCP – Tricalcium phosphate**

- Ceros 82
- Synthograft
- Others

**HA – Hydroxyapatite**

- Allotropat 50
- Alveograf
- Bio-Oss
- Calcitite
- Ceros 80
- Interpore 200
- Osprovit
- Periograf
- Others

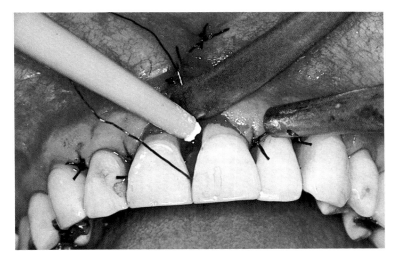

**631 Filling the bony defect with TCP**
The buccal and palatal flaps have already been adapted and sutured, except in the area of 21 where the suture has been placed but not yet tied. Note that a frenotomy was also performed.

The implant material is forced into the pocket where it must become well mixed with blood. *Immediately* after placement, the remaining flaps are adapted and securely sutured.

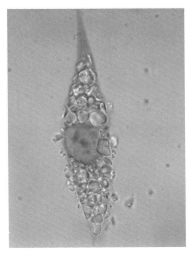

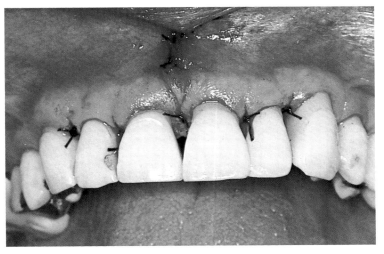

**632 Tight flap adaptation**
To preclude loss of the implanted material, flaps must be closely adapted and completely closed over the interdental defect.

*Left:* This cultured fibroblast has phagocytosed extremely fine TCP particles (experimental material, not indicated for periodontal implant at this fine particle size).

The glassy round spheres in the cell cytoplasm are fine TCP particles (carbol fuchsin, x 1000).

This experiment demonstrates the biocompatibility of TCP.

**Wound healing**

**633 Periodontal dressing**
In order to guarantee undisturbed wound healing, the operative site is protected from mechanical trauma by placement of a well-adapted periodontal dressing. Coe-Pak rolled in chlorhexidine-HCl was employed in this case.

*Right:* The blood coagulum (red) with TCP particles (blue) fills the infrabony defect completely. The suture location (arrow) is protected by the dressing (light blue).

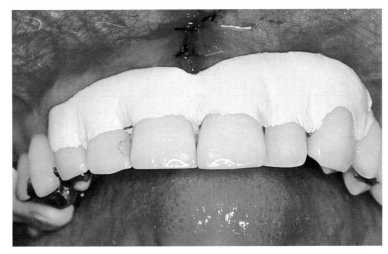 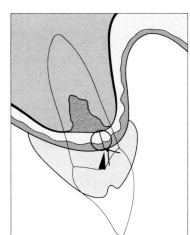

**634 Two weeks postoperative**
After dressing removal, whitish patches consisting of desquamated epithelial cells are visible.
    Sutures are removed and the area is cleansed gently but thoroughly using hydrogen peroxide (3%) on cotton pellets. The tooth surfaces are polished with rubber cups and dentifrice.
*Caution:* Paste must not be rotated into the sulcus because healing of the periodontal tissues is not yet complete!

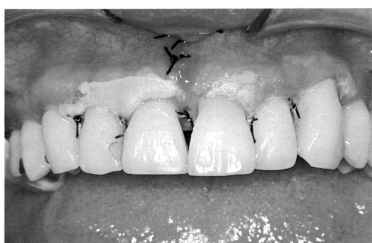

**635 Clinical view after suture removal and cleansing**
Gingival shrinkage has occurred mesial to 21.

*Right:* New bone begins to develop from the crater walls (hatched area). The TCP particles (blue) are partially resorbed.

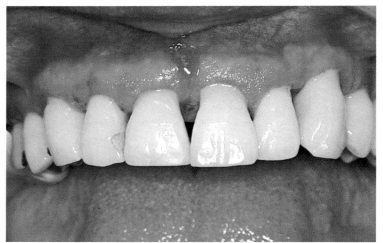 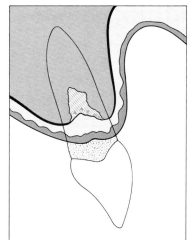

**636 Six weeks postoperative**
The palatal view reveals persistent slight gingival erythema. The patient must be encouraged to improve home care in this area.

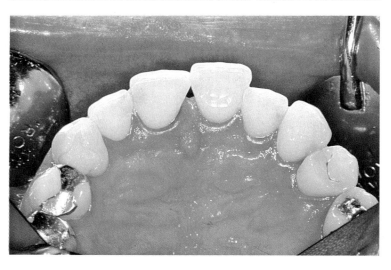

# Combined Surgical Technique – Intraosseous Implant

## Summary

The young female patient responded positively to initial therapy and demonstrated a high level of motivation before the surgical intervention. Despite this, some active pockets persisted, especially in the interdental areas (cratering).

The combined surgical procedure successfully eliminated all periodontal pockets. Only the treatment of the maxillary anterior teeth was presented here.

The 8 mm pocket mesial to 21 was reduced to 3 mm, due primarily to a significant amount of gingival shrinkage. It is possible that some osseous regeneration occurred in the depth of the pocket, but whether or not the tricalcium phosphate implant accelerated or increased bone regeneration cannot be determined (Scott-Metsger et al. 1982, Strub et al. 1979; see also Transplants and Implants in Bony Pockets, p. 259).

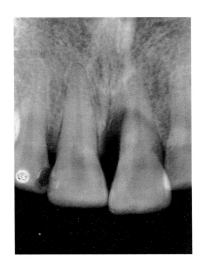

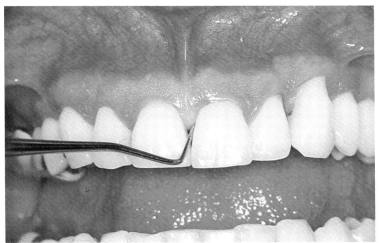

**637 After initial therapy**
The gingival contour is satisfactory after initial therapy. A deep infrabony pocket (8 mm) is present on the mesial of the left central incisor.

*Left:* The radiograph reveals a 2- to 3-wall defect on the mesial aspect of tooth 21.

Before
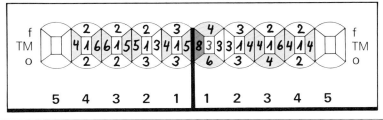

**638 Probing depths and tooth mobility (TM) after initial therapy**

After
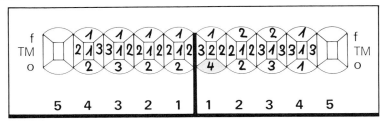

**Probing depths and tooth mobility (TM) one year after surgery**

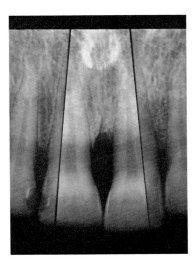

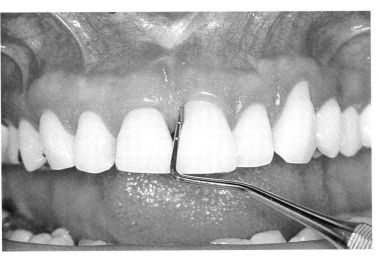

**639 One year postoperative**
The combined surgical procedure led to a reduction of pocket depth from 8 to 3 mm. This reduction could be accounted for by gingival shrinkage and possibly some osseous regeneration.

*Left:* The radiograph reveals what appears to be some filling of the osseous defect mesial to 21 (cf. Preoperative radiograph, Fig. 637).

# Wedge Excision

## Surgical principles

Periodontal pockets distal to the last tooth in an arch, as well as pockets on lone standing teeth (p. 252), are often difficult to eliminate surgically. The best solution in such cases is often the wedge excision. This procedure is generally successful only if it can be performed within the region of the attached gingiva.

The danger of recurrence is particularly high in the mandible distal to the second molar, i.e., in the region of mobile mucosa at the periphery of the retromolar pad. If surgery in this area is unavoidable, care must be taken to avoid the lingual nerve, which often assumes a more superior position. For this reason repeated root planing is preferable to surgical intervention in many cases.

Wedge excisions are often combined with flap procedures in the same sextant or quadrant (p. 262).

Three various possibilities for surgical pocket elimination distal to end-standing teeth are depicted diagrammatically in the Figures below.

**640 "Classic" distal wedge excision**
The triangular-shaped wedge excision is generally used for pocket elimination distal to the last tooth in an arch. The initial incisions (red, left) delineate the wedge. These two incisions converge at the base of the pocket.

*Right:* The second incisions serve to undermine (arrow) and thin the buccal and lingual tissue flaps overlying the alveolar ridge. Repositioning the flaps with sutures essentially eliminates the distal pocket.

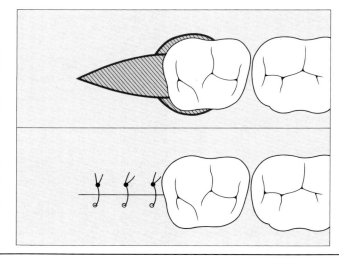
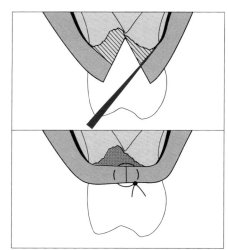

**641 Modified incision**
If the elimination of a pocket distal to the last tooth in the arch is performed as one phase of a more extensive flap procedure in the region, a *modified* wedge excision may be employed.

The modified technique considerably simplifies the reflection of facial and oral flaps, and direct vision of the root surface and bone is improved. The procedure is depicted in the clinical situation that follows (p. 249).

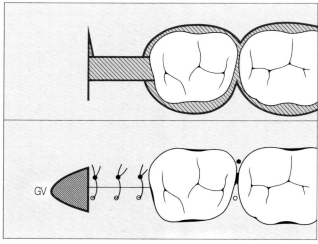
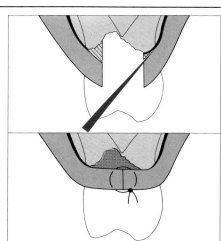

**642 Wedge excision according to Chaikin (1977) – Facial incision**
After making a curved incision from the buccal around the distal of the tooth (see schematic), a lingual pedicle flap is reflected. Subjacent tissue is excised down to bone, and root planing is performed.

The tip of the half-moon shaped flap is shortened somewhat, then sutured to the primary incision site. The slight tension placed on the flap by this suturing method serves to adapt the flap well around the distal aspect of the tooth (small arrows).

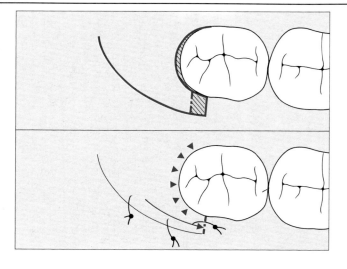
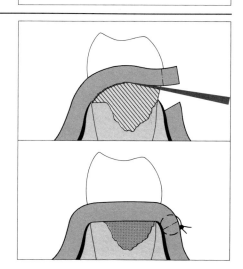

## Wedge Excision – Most Distal Tooth

### Operative procedure

In a 38-year-old female mild inflammation and an active 7 mm pocket persist distal to 26 following initial therapy. The treatment plan calls for elimination of the pocket by means of a modified wedge technique (Fig. 641).

The operation is feasible because there is sufficient attached gingiva distal to the tooth. The distal furcation is involved slightly (Class F1).

No surgery is indicated for the remainder of the dentition, but repeated scaling will be performed. The composite restorations in 24 and 25 should be replaced after conclusion of the periodontal therapy.

*Findings after initial therapy:*
    HYG: 60%        PBI: 2.2        TM: 0–1
Clinical findings and radiographic survey are depicted in the Figures below.

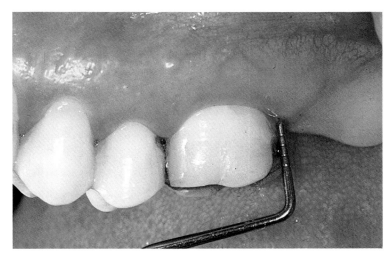

**643    Active distal pocket**
An active 7 mm pocket distal to 26 persists after initial therapy. The distal furcation could be probed 2 mm horizontally using the Nabers-2 probe, indicating a Class F1 furcation involvement.

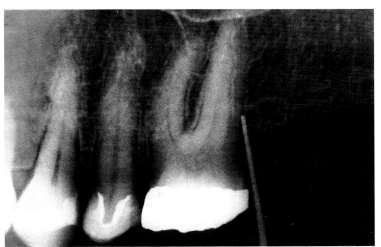

**644    Radiograph with probe in situ**
The Williams probe encountered no resistance from the inflamed tissue, and penetrated to the alveolar bone.

The markings on this probe are at 1, 2, 3, 5, 7, 8, 9 and 10 mm. The thickness of alveolar soft tissues in relation to the clinical situation (Fig. 643) can be appreciated in this view.

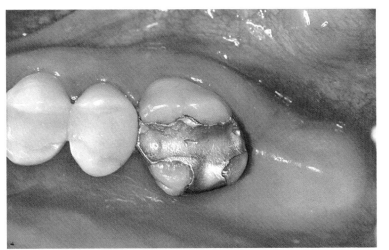

**645    Occlusal view of 26**
Sufficient attached gingiva is present distal to 26. This makes the operation much simpler and virtually excludes any risk of recurrence.

The old amalgam restoration should be recontoured and polished before surgery.

**646 Surgical plan – Incisions**

1 Half-moon shaped inverse bevel incision from the midbuccal to the midpalatal aspect of 26, then a corresponding pure intrasulcular incision
2 Wedge-shaped parallel incisions carried ca. 10 mm distally
3 Perpendicular incision at the distal extent of the parallel incisions
4 Undermining incisions for flap formation and reflection (oblique hatching; cf. Fig. 649 R).
5 Contouring gingivectomy to eliminate redundant tissue

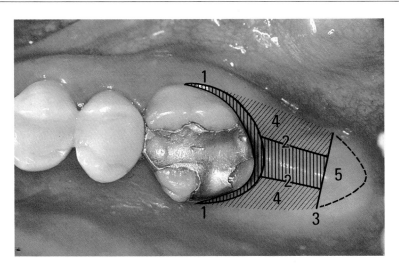

**647 Incisions**
Clinical view after performing the incision depicted above. The old amalgam was recontoured and polished before surgery.

*Right:* The schematic depicts the wedge excision in orofacial section (incision no. 2; Fig. 646).

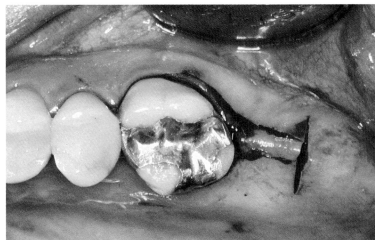
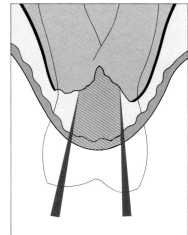

**648 Removal of the wedge**
A lingual scaler may be used to advantage for freeing the tissue wedge from subjacent bone.

*Right:* Wedge removed; lingual scaler (Fig. 394).

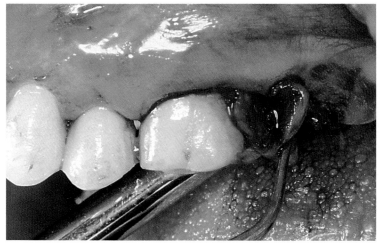
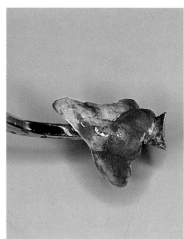

**649 Flap reflection – Root planing**
The undermining incisions parallel to the gingival surface create flaps of uniform thickness (2–3 mm) both facially and orally (see schematic; incision no. 4, Fig. 646).

*Right:* Undermining incision (red spear). The exposed root surface is thoroughly planed (thin red arrow), especially in the furcation area.

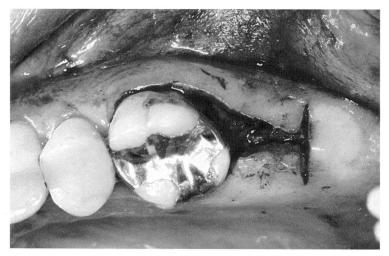
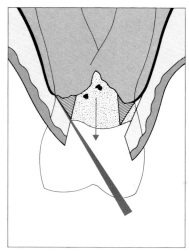

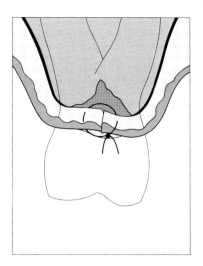

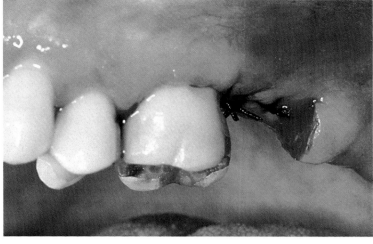

### 650 Suturing the thinned flaps

The technique of wedge excision with modified incisions permits particularly effective flap adaptation and secure closure of the defect.

At the distal end of the operative site redundant tissue remains in the tuberosity area.

*Left:* Sutured flaps, coagulum in the osseous crater.

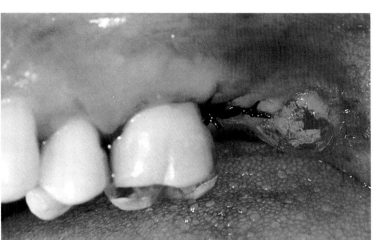

### 651 Gingivectomy of redundant tissue

The excess tissue distal to the molar may be removed by means of electrosurgery or scalpel. The goal is to recontour the tuberosity. This small open wound is left to epithelialize without any periodontal dressing; the patient may experience some discomfort initially.

Alternatively, the wound may be covered with a cyanoacrylate tissue adhesive.

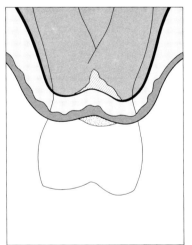

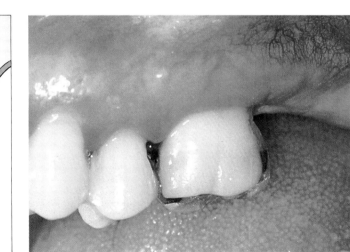

### 652 Two months postoperative

Pocket depth has been reduced by about 4 mm (note restoration margin and gingival contour). The sulcus can be probed to a depth of 3 mm, and there are no signs of disease activity.

*Left:* The schematic shows that some degree of osseous regeneration may be expected in the defect. The slight depression in the gingiva distal to the molar (furcation) must be given special attention by the patient during home care procedures.

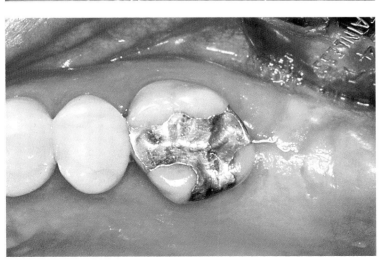

### 653 Occlusal view – Four months postoperative

At the first recall appointment an inflamed papilla was noted facially between 25 and 26. Treatment included plaque removal, root planing, patient motivation and re-instruction. Gingival inflammation was eliminated within a few days.

The posterior composite restorations must be replaced with metal or ceramic.

# Wedge Excisions – Lone-Standing Tooth

The surgical elimination or reduction of pockets on lone-standing teeth requires a special technique that is similar to that used for wedge excisions on the most distal tooth in an arch.

A 55-year-old female, whose case is depicted below, presented with advanced periodontitis. In the mandible, all hopeless teeth and an old bridge were removed. On the three remaining teeth (47, 43; 33), the probing depths after subgingival scaling were 7 mm mesially and distal-

ly, but only 2 mm facially and orally. The treatment plan included surgical elimination of the mesial and distal pockets by means of wedge excisions.

Following healing, an Edlan vestibuloplasty was performed on teeth 43 an 33 to enhance the narrow band of attached tissue, for definitive prosthetic treatment (removable prostheses over telescope crowns).

The modified wedge procedure is demonstrated below on tooth 43.

**654 Mesial and distal wedges**
The pointed gingivectomy knife is used to make mesial and distal incisions outlining the wedge to be excised.

The wedges must be large enough to permit direct vision of the exposed root and the bony margins.

After removal of the tissue wedges, undermining incisions are made to create thin, even flaps (p. 250, Fig. 649).

*Right:* Schematic representation of the initial incision and the osteoplasty (hatched area).

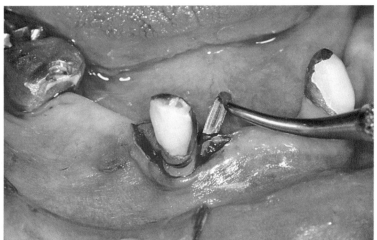

**655 Osteoplasty**
Following root planing, the sharp bony edges are smoothed, but *no supporting bone is removed* (see schematic above, Fig. 654 R).

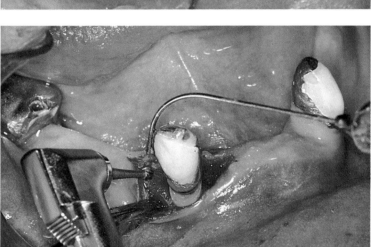

**656 Flap adaptation and wound closure**
The triangular wounds mesial and distal to tooth 43 are closed using interrupted sutures, without creating tension. Wound closure can be enhanced by application of a tissue adhesive (cyanoacrylate).

*Right:* The definitive telescoping reconstruction was completed 6 months after surgery. The margin of the primary abutment lies supragingivally. This abutment is too long (lever effect!).

The scar from the Edlan procedure is visible at the lower border.

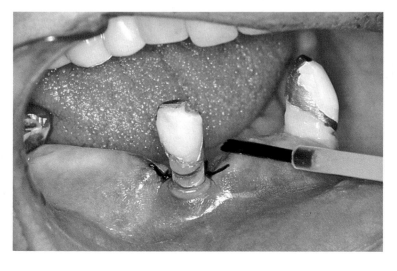
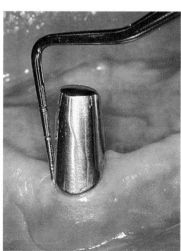

# Combined Surgical Technique
# Flap – Extraction – Revision of Adjacent Periodontal Structures

## Operative procedure

In the treatment of advanced periodontal diseases, teeth with poor prognoses often must be extracted. Following initial therapy, this may be accomplished during a flap procedure, at which time the periodontal supporting structure of the adjacent maintainable teeth can be treated *simultaneously*. This procedure is demonstrated here in the maxilla of a 45-year-old female. The treatment plan was radical because of the patient's desire for a long-term prosthetic solution. Seven teeth were extracted (17, 15, 14, 12, 11; 21, 25); five were treated periodontally and maintained as abutments (16, 13; 22, 23, 24).

---

*Findings before initial therapy:*
   HYG: 53%                          PBI: 2.2
   TM: 3 (hopeless teeth);   2 (maintainable teeth)
   The clinical picture, gingival contour, probing depths and radiographic survey are depicted in the Figures below.

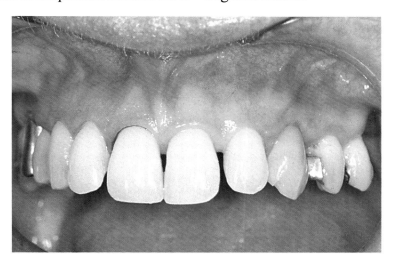

**657  Before initial therapy**
The severity of the periodontal destruction cannot be totally appreciated from the clinical presentation. Probing depths of up to 10 mm were recorded.
   Consideration of the medical history and clinical findings led to the diagnosis: Advanced adult periodontitis (AP), which had traversed acute exacerbations in recent years. Note that the attachment loss is very irregular.

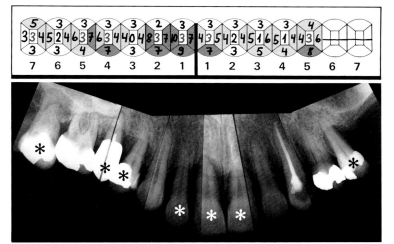

**658  Initial findings:**

**Probing depths and tooth mobility (TM)**
Several teeth were highly mobile and some of the periodontal pockets very deep.

**Radiographic findings**
Teeth destined for extraction due to the severity of periodontal destruction are marked (✳) on this film and in the clinical photographs below.

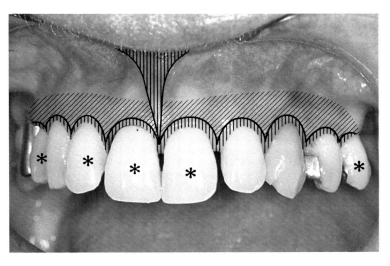

**659  Surgical plan**

---

**1** Scalloping horizontal inverse bevel incisions on buccal and palatal aspects (solid line)
**2** Flap reflection. The zone of reflection is relatively narrow (oblique hatch)
**3** Extractions. The asterisks indicate teeth destined for extraction
**4** Frenotomy of the high labial frenum attachment (hatched area)

---

**660 Flap reflection**
Following a horizontal scalloped inverse bevel incision, the buccal and oral mucoperiosteal flaps are elevated, revealing the alveolar bone.

Subsequently a purely marginal incision is made so that the tissue to be excised is easier to remove from the teeth to be maintained (and those to be extracted).

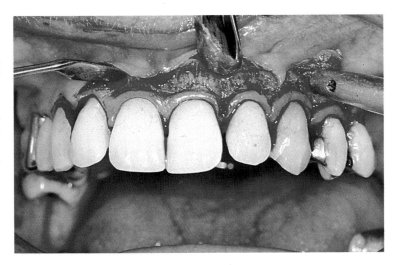

**661 Extractions**
The hopeless anterior teeth (12, 11; 21) are removed.

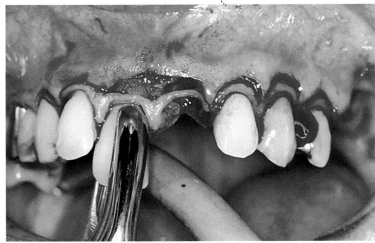

**662 Palatal surfaces of the extracted teeth**
It is clear how little of the roots of these teeth was still anchored in bone (dashed line indicates remaining periodontal ligament).

*Right:* The radiograph of the initial condition with periodontal probes in place reveals the minimum osseous support for the extracted teeth.

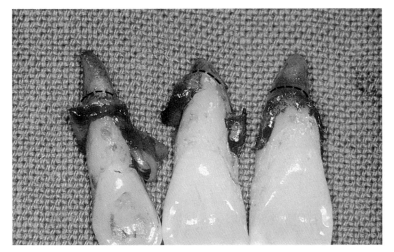
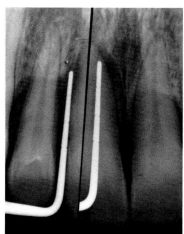

**663 Thinning the flap**
The pocket epithelium and loose granulation tissue that were not completely removed by the initial incision are excised from the internal surface of the flap using a small, curved scissors.

This gives the flap a uniform thickness throughout, enhancing repositioning and adaptation.

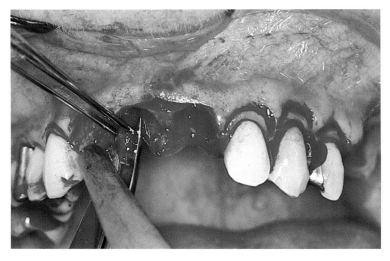

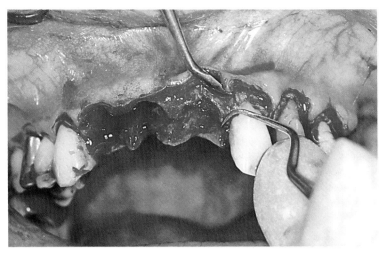

**664   Debridement and root planing**
The root surfaces of teeth destined for maintenance (abutment teeth) are systematically cleaned and planed under direct vision. Once again, this is the most important step in any periodontal surgical procedure.

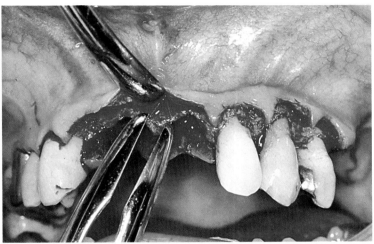

**665   Correcting bony marginal contour**
Sharp bony edges are removed using rongeurs or bone burs to preclude damage to the tissue of the repositioned flaps.

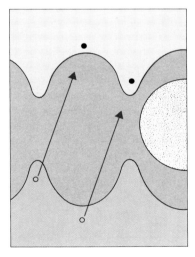

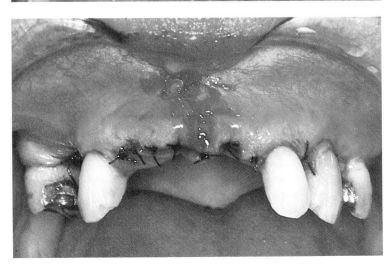

**666   Flap adaptation**
Flaps are first adapted closely to the remaining teeth.

*Left:* The extraction wounds can then be almost completely closed if the papilla tips of one flap are sutured into the depression between the papilla tips of the other flap (see diagram: Buccal flap = light blue; palatal flap = darker blue). Complete closure ensures healing by primary intention.

Schematic modified from Krüger 1977

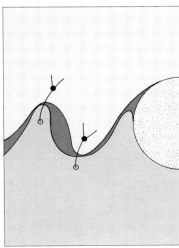

**667   Surgical procedure complete**
In addition to the extractions and the periodontal treatment, a frenotomy was performed.
    The flaps have been closed tightly over the alveolar process. A temporary denture, prepared in advance, can be seated.

*Left:* The staggered replacement of the well-adapted papilla tips of each flap cover the blood-filled alveoli tightly.

**Wound healing – Prosthetic treatment**

**668 Suture removal 10 days postoperatively**
Plaque and stains are carefully removed using rubber cup and dentifrice.

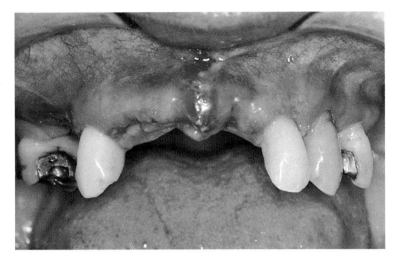

**669 Relined temporary denture**
Depending upon the severity of the periodontal destruction, an extended healing and consolidation phase of 6 ± 3 months follows between the periodontal surgery and definitive prosthetic treatment.

*Right:* The temporary denture will be worn for an extended period of time; it must be tooth-born, with clasps that hold each tooth bodily. It is often necessary to reline the temporary denture during the healing period (Reconstruction, p. 355, Fig. 930).

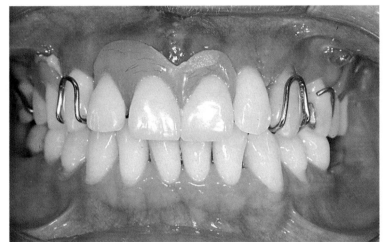
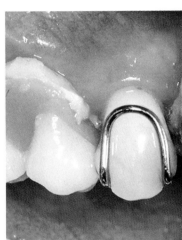

**670 Four weeks postoperative**
The recall interval is established at this point, based on the patient's degree of motivation and the clinical re-evaluation.

The light brown stains are from chlorhexidine, which the patient used as a mouthwash for several weeks after the surgery.

The definitive restoration, using a telescope construction, was performed ca. 9 months later (p. 361, Figs. 944–946).

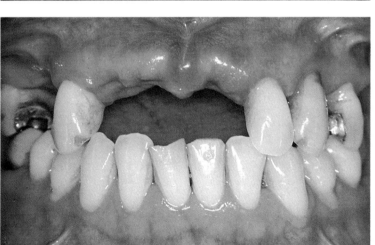

**671 Telescoping definitive reconstruction**
A purely tooth-born 11-unit, removable bridge was fabricated and seated upon the five remaining periodontally treated maxillary teeth. During speaking and laughing the patient's lip covered the necks of the teeth, which made it permissible to place the telescoping crown margins supragingivally (no esthetic compromise necessary).

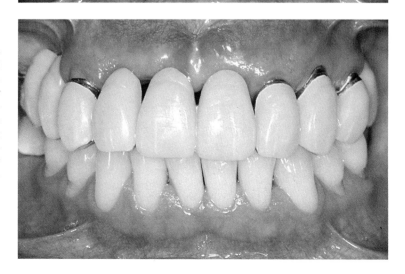

# Extraction with Revision

## Summary

In this 45-year-old patient with relatively advanced adult periodontitis (AP), a somewhat more radical surgical approach was made in the *maxilla,* in accordance with the patient's wishes.

Following the first phase of initial therapy on all teeth (supragingival scaling, creation of hygienic relationships), subgingival scaling was performed on the teeth that were to be maintained.

Several weeks later, seven teeth were extracted (17, 15, 14, 12, 11; 21, 25) and the definitive periodontal surgical revision of the five remaining abutment teeth was simultaneously performed (16, 13; 22, 23, 24). Immediately following the surgery, a tooth-born removable temporary denture was seated.

After an extended (9 mo) healing and consolidation phase, the definitive removable telescoping bridge was seated. Telescoping bridges permit optimum hygiene, and can be modified later if necessary.

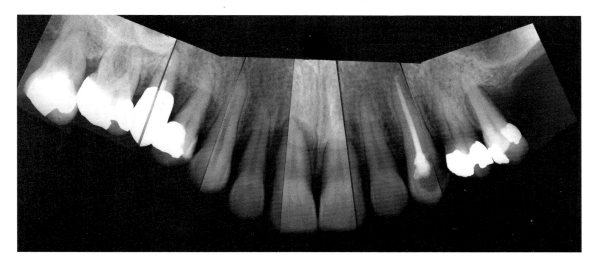

**672 Radiographic survey**
Several teeth are hopeless, others could be maintained with a great investment of therapeutic effort. The relatively radical planning included extraction of the following teeth:

· 7 · 5 4 · 2 1 | 1 · · · 5 · · ·

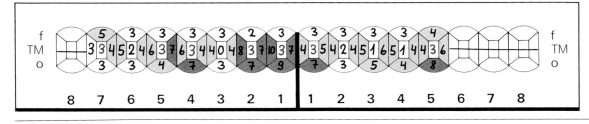

**673 Initial probing depths and tooth mobility (TM)**
Deep pockets and highly mobile teeth characterize the clinical situation.

Before

After

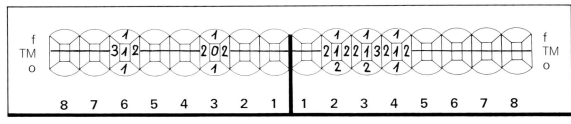

**Post-treatment probing depths and tooth mobility (TM)**
Before beginning definitive prosthetics, physiologic probing depths exist around abutment teeth.

**674 Final radiographs**
Ten months after periodontal surgery, all 5 remaining maxillary teeth bear telescope crowns:

· · 6 · · 3 · · | · 2 3 4 · · · ·

The long-term prognosis is good if the patient is diligent in home care and with regular maintenance.

On a 4-6-month recall the bridge has remained functional for over 8 years without recurrence of periodontal symptoms.

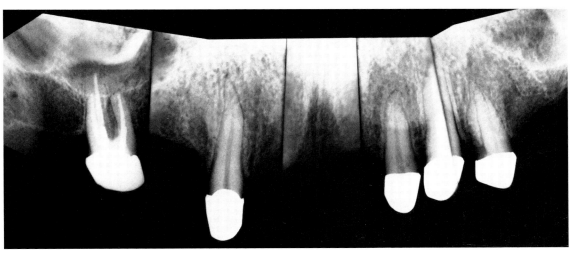

# Surgical Removal of Impacted Third Molar Prevention of a Pocket Distal to Second Molar

Impacted third molars are often associated with a periodontal pocket on the distal of the second molar. Removal of such third molars should therefore be performed early on. The extraction must be as atraumatic as possible, to protect the periodontal structures of the adjacent second molar. Sectioning the third molar prior to removal is often indicated. This operation is often associated with loss of attachment on the second permanent molar (Quee et al. 1985).

The postoperative results are generally better in young individuals than older persons, who often manifest a persistent active pocket distal to the second molar. In young persons, third molar root formation may not be complete and the osseous structure is not so compact. For all these reasons, third molar extraction should be done as early as possible to preclude persistent active periodontal pocketing distal to the second molar (Eichenberger 1979, Osborne et al. 1982).

**675   Third molar extraction later in life**
Nine months after the surgical extraction of the wisdom tooth in this "older" (45 yr) patient, no osseous regeneration is detectable distal to the second molar, despite repeated debridement and planing of the root surface.

An active pocket of 12 mm can be probed (arrow).

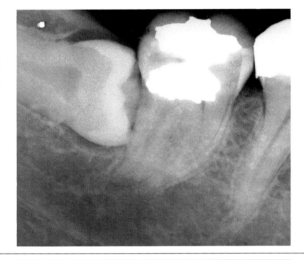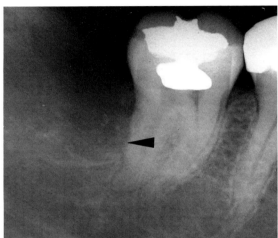

**676   Atraumatic third molar extraction – Skull preparation**
Injury to the mandibular canal can occur during surgical removal of third molars. Wire demonstrates mandibular canal. When such teeth are removed the supporting structures of the adjacent second molar must be preserved.

The distal root of the second molar must be thoroughly cleaned and planed to remove endotoxin-containing cementum, enhance healing, and preclude recurrence of periodontal pocketing.

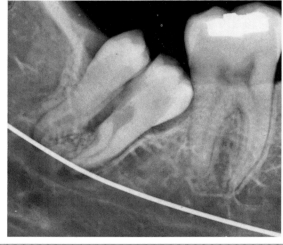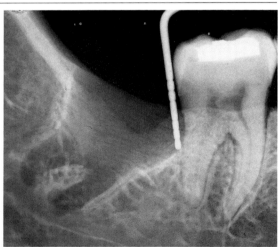

**677   Timely third molar extraction**
In this 24-year-old female, osseous regeneration within 6 months has almost completely filled the defect created by surgical removal of the horizontally impacted third molar. Probing the distal aspect of the second molar reveals only a 3 mm sulcus (arrow).

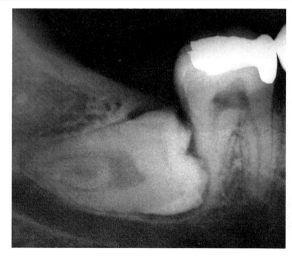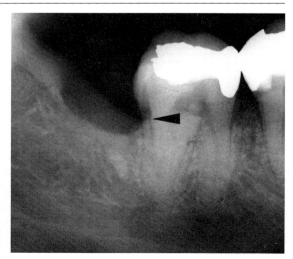

# Transplants and Implants in Infrabony Pockets

*Transplantation* signifies surgical transfer of a *living* tissue or organ to a different site or to a different individual. The tissue must maintain its vitality in the transplant bed of the new location.

The term *implantation* implies surgical insertion of a *nonvital* tissue or material. In discussing osseous replacement techniques, both old and new terminology for transplant and implant materials are still used (see Table).

| Old nomenclature | New nomenclature | Origin of the material | Type of material |
|---|---|---|---|
| autologous ⟶ | autologous | – Same individual | **Bone** |
| homologous { ⟶ | isologous (syngeneic) | – Monozygotic twin or inbred strain | **Bone** |
| ⟶ | allogeneic | – Same species (no genetic "matching") | **Bone bank Lyophilized bone and cartilage** |
| heterologous ⟶ | xenogeneic | – Different species | **Bone (fetal) Collagen** |
| alloplastic ⟶ | alloplastic | – Inorganic, "foreign body" material (e.g., ceramic, metal etc.) | **Calcium phosphates** – **HA – Hydroxyapatite** *(nonresorbable)* – **TCP – Tricalcium phosphate** *(resorbable)* |
| Combined techniques | Combined techniques | see above | e.g., autologous bone and alloplastic materials |

**678 Nomenclature, origin and type of transplant and implant materials for filling osseous defects**

Generally speaking the most successful implants are of autologous bone.

All other implant materials yield but questionable results.

The many and varied types of alloplastic materials currently available may serve to stabilize the blood coagulum and reduce shrinkage. Whether these implants actually stimulate new bone formation in addition to their role as a space holder is questionable.

---

*New bone formation does not mean that new periodontal attachment with simultaneous formation of new cementum and periodontal ligament fibers has necessarily occurred!*

The benefit of transplants and implants in periodontal osseous surgery remains a topic of discussion and controversy. The literature contains numerous references to new bone formation in periodontal pockets after transplantation or implantation. However, similar results have been reported following thorough root planing and curettage in infrabony pockets after reflecting flaps for access. A tight postoperative suture closure coupled with perfect plaque control would appear to be more important prerequisites for osseous regeneration than the filling of bony pockets with "some material."

*Autologous* bone is the most promising material in terms of enhancement of new bone formation. The source for such bone may be the alveolar process, for example between two tooth roots or from an edentulous area (see Operative Procedure, p. 262).

Bone spicules gathered on a filter during osteoplasty may also be used as a transplant material.

Cancellous bone from the hip, though a successful transplant material, does not represent a realistic solution to the problem of periodontal pockets because of the costs in time, discomfort and money (Schallhorn et al. 1970, 1972). The general surgical effort and risk for the patient far outweigh the potential gain, i.e., the filling in of periodontal bony defects.

# Instruments for Removal of Autologous Bone ...

Allogenic, xenogenic and alloplastic materials have the advantage that they can be stored in the dental office (see Combined Surgical Techniques, p. 243).

Autologous bone, on the other hand, must be obtained fresh during the surgical procedure. Various instruments are available for this purpose. For example, a filter inserted distal to the evacuation tip during osteoplasty can trap particles of bone for subsequent use in infrabony pockets (Robinson 1969, Dayoub 1981).

Additional instruments for harvesting autologous bone include trephine drills. These are available in various sizes for use manually or in the contraangle handpiece.

Fine fissure burs or Lindemann drills can also be used to gather bone from the edentulous ridge, from exostoses etc., which may necessitate a second surgical site.

**679  Bone filter in-line in the surgical evacuation tip**
This sterilizable filter system can be dismantled for cleaning, and is available from Gelman Sciences, Inc.
The grid size of the filter is
ca. 0.25 x 0.25 mm (Dayoub 1981).

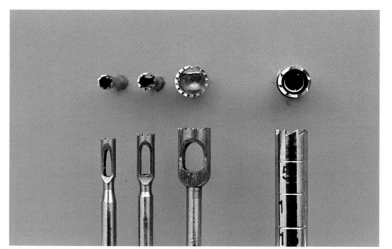
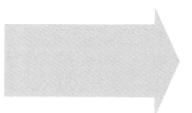

**680  Trephine drills**

*Left:* Three trephine drills for use in the handpiece (Jota, Inc.)

| Outside diameter: | **2.3 mm** |
| | **2.8 mm** |
| | **5.0 mm** |

*Right:* Working end of the manual trephine drill (see below), with dispensing attachment.

| Outside diameter: | **5.0 mm** |

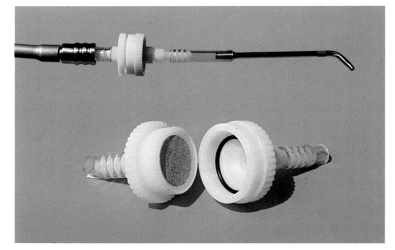

**681  Hand trephine**
This trephine is engraved every one-quarter inch or 5 mm so that the surgeon can always ascertain how deep the tip has penetrated (Maurice Bovard, Inc.).

Reducing the solid core of bone removed with the trephine to small chips can be difficult. Possibilities include squashing with a forceps or cutting with a scissors or scalpel.

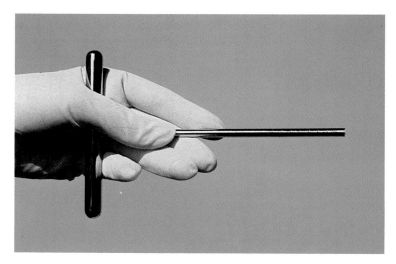

# ... and Their Use

In order to obtain autologous bone with a trephine, the periodontal surgical site usually must be extended beyond normal limits. Extending the flaps may expose an adjacent edentulous area as a site for harvesting autologous bone for transplantation.

It may be necessary to raise mucoperiosteal flaps in another area of the mouth in order to gain access to an appropriate site for the harvest of autologous bone. The transplant should include spongy or – less desirable –cortical bone. Before transferring autologous bone to the periodontal defect, it must be split into tiny chips that do not exceed 1 mm³. The rongeurs or scissors can accomplish this.

Extension of the surgical site or creation of a second site can be avoided if osteoplasty is planned for the primary site. If this is the case, a sterile filter system can be used to collect autologous bone for transplantation.

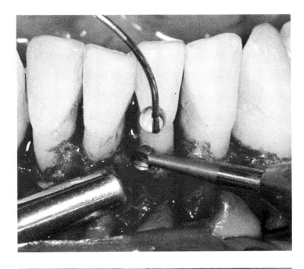
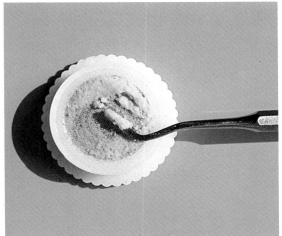

**682 Harvesting bone**
*Left:* Considerable amounts of osseous substance can be collected on a sterile filter in the evacuation system when a round bur is used for osteoplasty with copious irrigation using sterile saline.

*Right:* Bone chips in the filter. This material becomes mixed with blood when placed into a debrided defect *("osseous coagulum")*. Two- and 3-wall infrabony defects are easily filled with osseous coagulum.

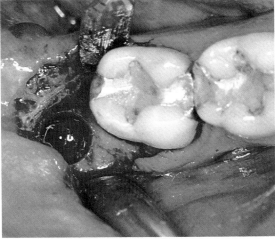
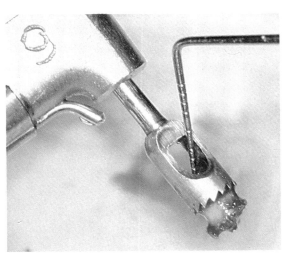

**683 Harvesting autologous bone with a handpiece-mounted trephine drill**
*Left:* The retromolar area has been the site for collection of autologous bone, using a 5 mm trephine drill mounted in the contraangle handpiece. Constant irrigation with sterile saline is mandatory during such procedures. The core of bone must be freed using the drill or an elevator.

*Right:* The durable Williams probe is used to dislodge the bone, which is reduced to chips in saline solution before implantation.

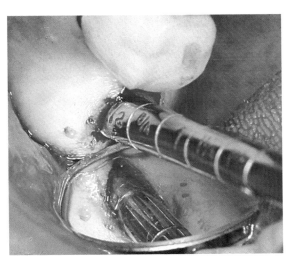
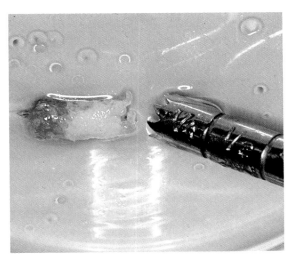

**684 Harvesting autologous bone with the manual trephine drill**
*Left:* Access in the oral cavity is difficult with this relatively gross instrument. It is indicated almost exclusively for harvesting bone from the edentulous ridge, especially in the tuberosity region. A sagittal incision through the mucosa is made to permit entry.

*Right:* Adherent soft tissue should be removed from the osseous material before transplantation, and the bone must be reduced to small chips.

# Autologous Bone Transplantation

### Operative procedure

A 30-year-old female wished to have the space in her upper left quadrant closed by means of a fixed bridge. Because the mandible was fully dentulous, it was prudent to maintain the lone-standing maxillary second molar (27) as an abutment, but a 7 mm infrabony pocket could be probed on the mesial aspect of this tooth. The examination led the practitioner to suspect a multi-walled defect.

The treatment plan called for filling this defect with autologous bone. The edentulous area between 24 and 27 was available as a site for harvesting the transplant material; however, because of the proximity of the maxillary sinus, this is a "dangerous" donor site.

*Findings after initial therapy:*
 HYG: 82%    PBI: 1,2
 TM: Grade 2 for tooth 27, grade 1 for 23 and 24.
 The clinical picture and radiograph are presented in the figures below.

**685    After initial therapy**
The persistent 7 mm infrabony pocket mesial to the second molar is depicted clinically with a Goldman probe *in situ.*

A 5 mm gingival pocket was present on the distal surface of 24.

*Right:* The deep pocket mesial to tooth 27 is depicted in the radiograph even more clearly than in the clinical view.

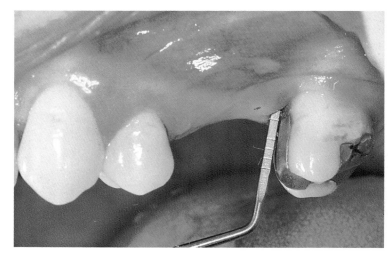 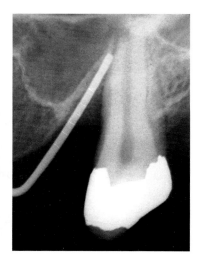

**686    Incisions**
Facial and oral flap reflection is necessary in order to perform periodontal treatment on 24 and 27 with simultaneous harvest of autologous bone. The primary incison courses parallel to the alveolar crest in the edentulous area between the two teeth. As the incision approaches the teeth, it becomes a sulcular incison on both facial and oral aspects.

Distal to 27, the incision ends as a modified wedge procedure (cf. Fig. 647).

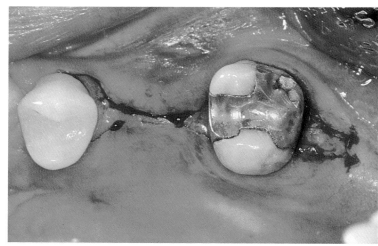

**687    Surgical field exposed**
Following root planing and debridement of the infrabony pocket, the 3-wall defect mesial to 27 and two of the three donor sites are visible.

Instead of a single large (5 mm) explant, three small (2.8 mm) pieces were taken, without altering the contour of the alveolar ridge. The 3 pieces of bone were further reduced in size before transfer to the defect.

*Right:* Radiographic view of the trephine drill during bone removal.

*Caution:* Maxillary sinus!

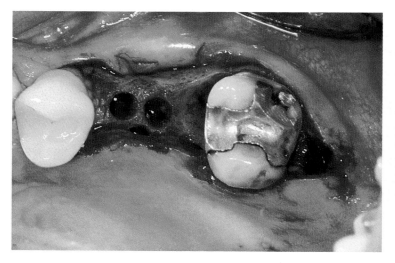 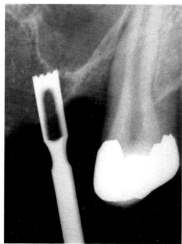

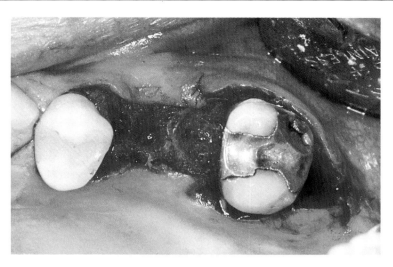

**688    After transplantation of the bone**
Bony chips with a maximum size of 1 mm$^3$ are tightly wedged into the 3-wall defect.
   The crater is completely filled, and blood clots fill the donor sites. Such sites reossify quickly, similar to a minor extraction site.

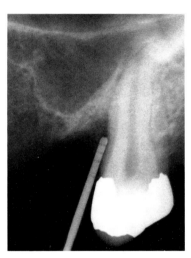

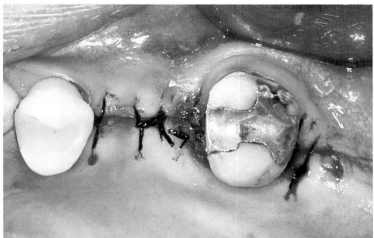

**689    Tight closure of the surgical site**
Healing of the site can only occur optimally if the flap closure is complete and secure.
   The surgical site should be protected from mechanical trauma by a periodontal dressing or, as in this case, with a tissue adhesive (Histoacryl).

*Left:* Radiographic check of the osseous fill. Compare the initial radiograph (Fig. 685 R).

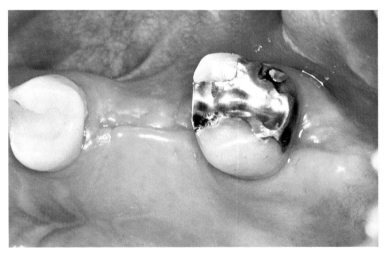

**690    Three months postoperative**
Healing proceeded without complication. Fabrication of the fixed bridge can begin in a few more months, after complete consolidation of the site.

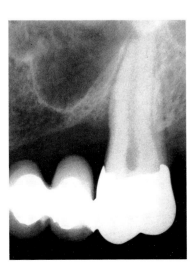

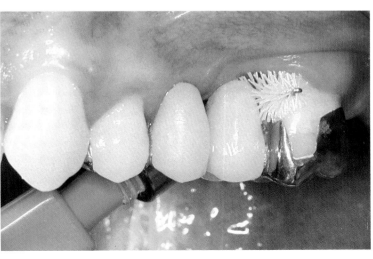

**691    Seven months postoperative – Seating the bridge**
The 4-unit bridge is first seated temporarily. The bridge abutments were prepared for three-quarter crowns, with all margins located supragingivally. Interdental hygiene is easy, using spiral brushes. The periodontal pocket mesial of 27 has been eliminated via apical positioning of the gingiva and possible osseous regeneration.

*Left:* The radiograph reveals that the previous osseous crater has filled with newly regenerated bone.

# Bone Regeneration without Transplantation

It is not universally accepted, nor has it been unequivocally proven, that osseous regeneration in periodontal pockets can be initiated, enhanced or accelerated by means of transplants or implants.

However, it has been demonstrated that significant osseous regeneration may occur spontaneously in the absence of any sort of "filling" in a bony defect. Prerequisites for such regeneration include perfect root planing, curettage and long term postoperative plaque control (Polson & Heijl 1978).

The radiographs below depict this type of spontaneous osseous regeneration, which occurred over a 6-month period in a 35-year-old male.

However, osseous regeneration is *no* guarantee that new cementum and new periodontal ligament have formed (p. 136). In many cases only a *long junctional epithelium* ensues, extending apically beyond the newly formed bone, even to the depth of the original pocket. Despite this, new bone formation may be viewed as a therapeutic success since the osseous defect is reduced in size and tooth mobility is often reduced.

**692   9 mm infrabony pocket**
The pocket distal to tooth 46 was debrided and root planed with direct vision (flap procedure).

*Right:* The schematic representation of the radiograph depicts the level of the CEJ (red line), the level of the original bony margin (black line) and the expanse of the osseous defect.

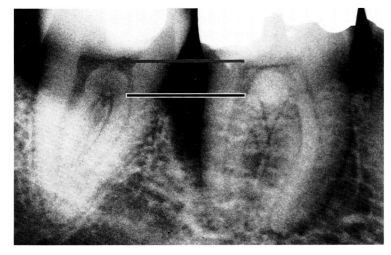 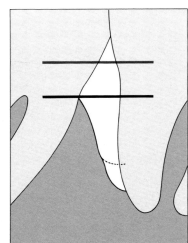

**693   Beginning osseous regeneration**
Several weeks after the surgery the defect appears to be 1/3 filled.

*Right:* In the schematic the initial osseous formation is shown in red.

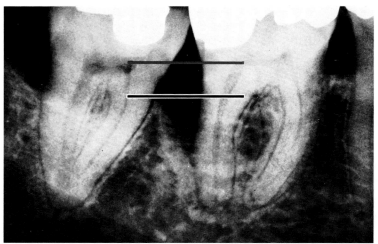 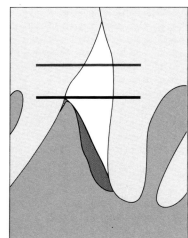

**694   Bone regeneration 6 months postoperatively**
The original vertical defect has almost completely filled in. The clinical probing depth is 3 mm.

The osseous regeneration observed in the radiograph, however, cannot be taken as a qualitative indication of the degree of true new attachment.

*Right:* The schematic depicts the extent of new bone formation (red).

Courtesy G. Cimasoni

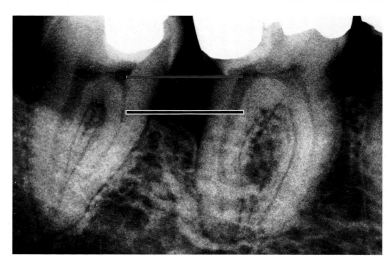 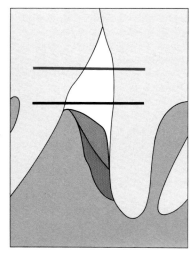

# Surgical Treatment of the Furcation

The various degrees of severity of furcation involvement in multirooted teeth were described and portrayed in preceding chapters ("Diseases of the Periodontium," pp. 80–81; "Charting – Diagnosis – Prognosis," pp. 118–119). Furcation involvements of classes F1 to F3 are based on horizontal probing. The treatment of class F1 and F2 furcation involvement was discussed in "Initial Therapy, Phase II" (pp. 198–199), but it is appropriate at this point to return to a discussion of basic treatment planning for furcation involvement, in the broader scope of comprehensive dental care (see Fig. 695).

The goal is not to save individual multirooted teeth "at all costs," rather it is to ascertain the potential *value* of heroic measures in terms of comprehensive patient care (Ramfjord & Ash 1979; Mutschelknauss & Von der Ohe 1982, 1983; Lindhe 1983; Löst 1985; Saadoun 1985; Brägger & Lang 1988; Kocher & Plagmann 1988).

In the future, effective techniques for true regeneration of lost tissues are expected to greatly enhance more traditional therapeutic methods, especially in the case of strategic abutment teeth.

| Furcation diagnosis | F 1 | F 2 | F 3 |
|---|---|---|---|
| **A Complete dention** | ● | ● | ●/▲ |
| **B Partial edentulousness** | ● | ●/▲ | ▲ |
| **C Prosthetic abutments** Strategically important tooth | ● | ▲ | ▲ |
| **D "Palliative therapy"** For patients with inadequate oral hygiene | ● | ● | ●/ ex |

**695 Choice of therapy for furcation involvement**

● *Retain the tooth,* usually with all roots intact. Therapy targeted toward healing, whether conservative or surgical methods employed. Special oral hygiene measures.

▲ *Radical procedures:* Hemisection, root resection and root amputation, "tunneling", (extraction).
Maintenance of strategically important teeth or roots requiring radical procedures usually need endodontic treatment.

## Indications for various treatment techniques

In cases of *class F1 furcation involvement* and shallow pocketing, therapy consisting of subgingival scaling, root planing and curettage (cf. p. 198) is usually successful, sometimes in conjunction with a furcation-plasty (odontoplasty). Treatment may also be combined with a gingivectomy or a modified Widman flap, depending on comprehensive findings and the overall treatment plan.

In the case of *class F2 furcation involvement,* surgical revision after flap reflection is usually indicated in order to reveal the morphology of the furcation entrance and to permit scaling and root planing with direct vision. A corrective odontoplasty at the cervix of the crown (cf. p. 199) can minimize the plaque-retentive area represented by the furcation entrance.

In the case of *class F3 furcation involvement,* the prognosis is relatively poor for the untreated tooth, especially in advanced cases; without excellent cooperation by the patient, these teeth are often hopeless. Simple extraction is often indicated. If the tooth is indispensible either for *chewing function* or as an *abutment,* several treatment possibilities are available (see "Radical Procedure," Fig. 695), but the prognosis remains questionable.

## Hemisection in the Mandible – Reconstruction

In this 45-year-old female, the furcation of tooth 46 was involved in a through-and-through manner (class F3), and the radiograph revealed a massive periapical radiolucency. The treatment plan included hemisection of the tooth and extraction of the mesial root for both periodontal *and* endodontic reasons. This procedure was chosen in order to preclude a free-end saddle situation against the existing dentition of the maxillary arch.

The hemisection was performed after reflecting a conservative flap. A temporary bridge was required during the healing and consolidation phase to prevent drifting of the remaining root. Definitive restorative therapy was accomplished 7 months after the periodontal surgery. The patient exercised excellent home care.

*Findings before surgery:*
HYG: 92%     PBI: 1.3     TM: 1

The clinical picture and radiographs are depicted in the Figures below.

**696  Molar 46 with class F3 furcation involvement**
The crown of 46 is severely broken down, and the furcation involvement is through-and-through (class F3).

*Right:* The radiograph reveals an expansive radiolucency at the apical area of the mesial root of 46. Primarily for endodontic reasons, hemisection of the tooth and extraction of the mesial root are indicated. The root canal of the retained distal root must be treated endodontically *before* the hemisection procedure.

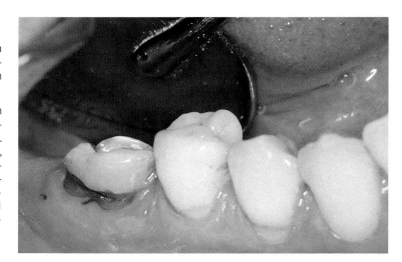
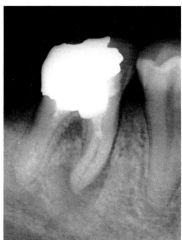

**697  Flap reflection and hemisection**
The crown is halved using diamond and carbide burs (pictured is a diamond cylinder that is somewhat too thick).

*Right:* On this a model of the molar, the line of hemisection is shown to be toward the mesial root. This prevents any damage to the distal root, which will be retained; however, this precautionary measure often leads to a detectable overhang (plaque retention) in the furcation region. This must be removed during tooth preparation.

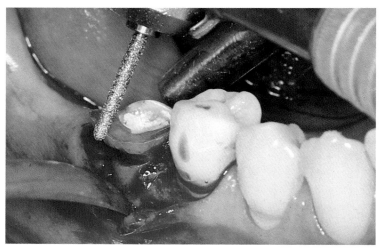
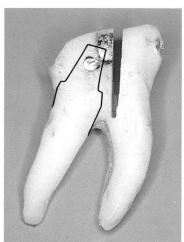

**698  After extraction of the mesial root**
All sharp edges of the remaining portion of the tooth should be smoothed before terminating the procedure. This may be considered as "initial tooth preparation."

*Right:* In the radiograph the distal root of 46 appears similar to a single-rooted premolar.

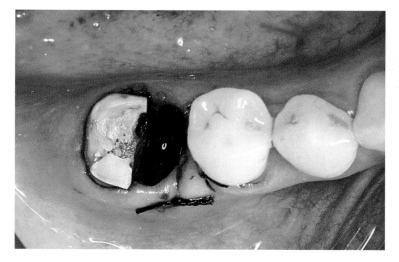
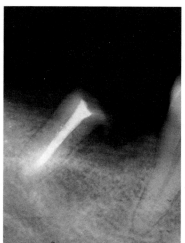

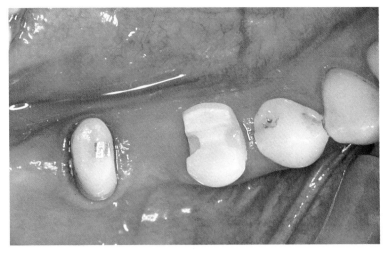

**699   Six months after hemisection**

After primary healing of the extraction wound, the distal portion of 46 was prepared to receive a full cast crown using a screw-type post and a composite resin build-up. The mesial abutment, tooth 45, was prepared for a three-quarter crown.

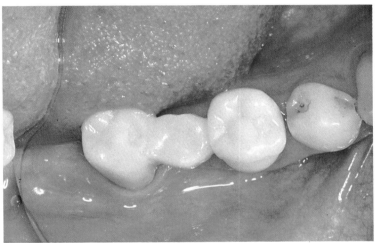

**700   Temporary resin bridge**

The temporary bridge should be seated as soon as possible because lone-standing roots of hemisected teeth tend to drift. The shape and occlusal form of the temporary bridge should anticipate that of the planned definitive restoration.

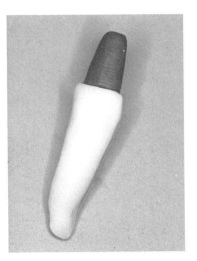

**701   Seven months after hemisection – Definitive bridge in situ**

Teeth were definitively prepared 6 months after the hemisection, and the definitive bridge was constructed. The bridge extends from the premolar to the distal root of the first molar.

*Left:* This model demonstrates the premolar-like form of a prepared distal molar root.

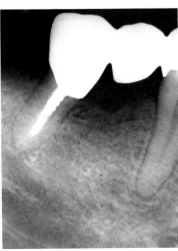

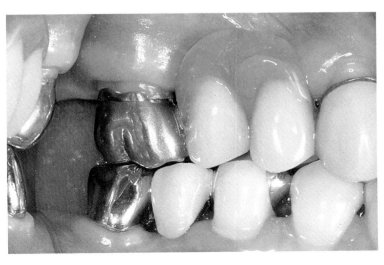

**702   Final documentation – Prognosis**

Cemented bridge. The teardrop-shaped pontic lightly contacts the ridge. The interdental spaces are contoured so that hygiene can be accomplished with spiral brushes.

The maxillary antagonist is a removable partial denture over telescope crowns.

*Left:* The radiograph shows the cemented bridge with the single-rooted molar 46 as its distal abutment. To date, this bridge has been in function for 8 years.

# Root Resection in the Maxilla – Reconstruction

Depending on the degree of trifurcation involvement, it may be necessary to resect one or two roots from three-rooted maxillary molars.

The case presented here is a 39-year-old female, who presented with severe mobility and class F3 furcation involvement of both maxillary left molars. Tooth 27 was hopelessly involved, and was extracted. Both buccal roots and the buccal portion of the crown of 26 were resected. After healing of the surgical site, the remaining palatal root of 26 and the two premolars (24, 25) were prepared for full coverage restorations. The two premolar crowns were soldered to serve as a firm anchor for the palatal root of 26, which remained highly mobile (permanent splint).

---

*Findings after initial therapy:*
    HYG: 78%        PBI: 2
    TM: 3 for teeth 26 and 27
    The clinical view and radiographs are shown in the figures below.

**703  Initial clinical situation**
Interproximal probing depths of 7 mm were detected around teeth 26 and 27. Both molars exhibited class F3 (through-and-through) involvement of the trifurcation.

Both teeth were highly mobile (TM = 3). The premolars 24 and 25 display old, unsatisfactory reconstructions.

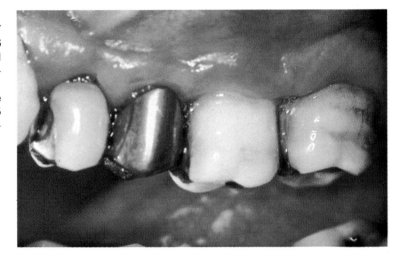

**704  Radiographic view**
The furcation involvements (all class F3) are obvious, as is the especially pronounced loss of support on the buccal roots of the molars.

The enormous palatal root of 26 is clearly visible.

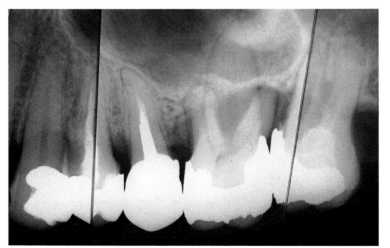

Before

**705  Periodontal surgery**
After initial therapy, the first molar (26) was treated endodontically, but it was found that none of the three roots of the second molar (27) could be maintained. Reflection of a mucoperiosteal flap revealed the wide open furcations; 27 was extracted and both buccal roots of 26 were resected.
Only the palatal root of the first molar could be maintained as participant in a cast splint reconstruction.

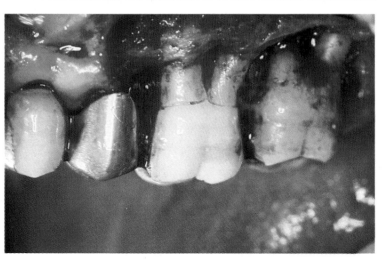

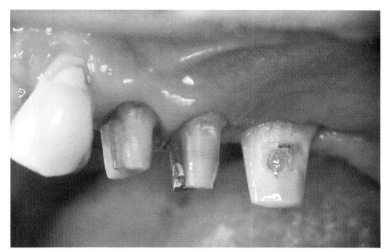

**706    Six weeks after root resection**
Teeth 24, 25 and the palatal portion of 26 have been prepared to receive temporary full coverage restorations. The buccal surface of 26 reveals the former pulp chamber, now filled with AH-26.
For the definitive reconstruction, this palatal root will receive a post and core.

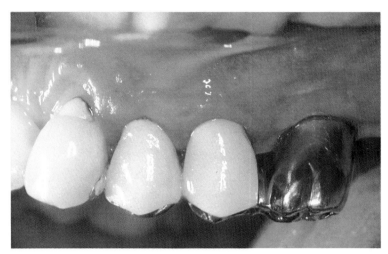

**707    Definitive reconstruction**
Eight months postsurgically, the teeth were definitively prepared and the palatal root of 26 received a post. Cast gold crowns with porcelain facings (24, 25) were fabricated. The two premolar crowns were soldered and the molar crown was incorporated into an intracoronal precision attachment; this splinting was done to enhance patient comfort, as the palatal root of 26 remained highly mobile and was palatally positioned. The interdental areas were left wide open to facilitate hygiene.

After

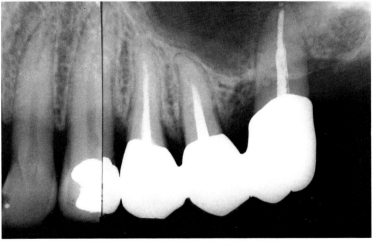

**708    Radiographic view 8 months after surgery**
The three-unit splint consists of two soldered crowns and a precision attachment from the molar, the latter necessitated by the tipped, palatal position of 26.

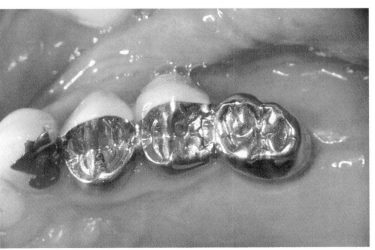

**709    Occlusal view 6 years later**
Despite the palatal position of the remaining root of 26, it was possible to achieve harmonious dental arch form. The intracoronal precision attachment effects a stable splinting of 26 to the soldered crowns on 24 and 25.
The long-term prognosis for this segment of the dental arch remains good.

Today – as this second edition of the *Atlas* is completed – this reconstruction remains in the mouth after 10 years without complications.

# Root Resection in the Maxilla – No Reconstruction

An alternative method for treating a class F3 furcation in a maxillary molar involves resection of one root with maintenance of the entire crown. An advantage of this approach is that it eliminates the inaccessible plaque-retentive area. This procedure can be employed only if the furcation between the two remaining roots is not involved.

The case presented below is a 54-year-old male with good oral hygiene. The last remaining maxillary right molar had a class F3 involvement connecting the buccal and distal furcations. The furcation between the palatal

and mesiobuccal roots was not involved. Resection of the distobuccal root was indicated, with concomitant recontouring of the tooth crown via odontoplasty, to facilitate home care.

---

*Findings after initial therapy:*
  HYG: 83%
  PBI:    1.1
  TM:     0–1

The clinical situation and radiographs are depicted in the figures below.

**710 Probing prior to root resection**
Vertical probing depth of 5–6 mm is noted between the buccal roots of the first molar.

*Right:* The radiograph reveals considerable bone loss, arousing suspicion of furcation involvement. Careful horizontal probing detected a through-and-through (class F3) involvement between the distobuccal and palatal roots.

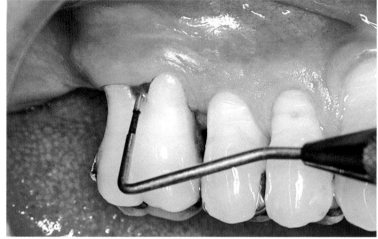
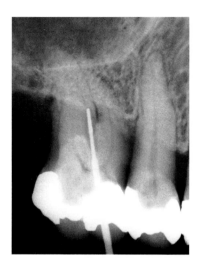

**711 Separation of the distobuccal root, and odontoplasty**
Prior to root resection, the tooth was treated endodontically and the coronal portion of the distobuccal root canal was filled with amalgam.

*Right:* Lines on this extracted tooth depict the resection area and the degree of odontoplastic recontouring.

Because the resection site is located supragingivally, root extraction can be accomplished without reflecting a mucoperiosteal flap.

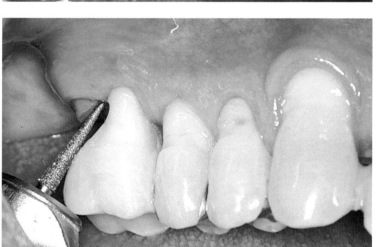
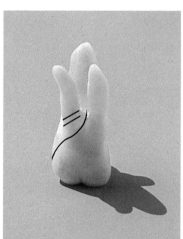

**712 Extraction of the distobuccal root using an elevator**
The odontoplasty is performed and the site is completely smoothed and polished before extracting the distal root. This prevents the introduction of amalgam dust or debris into the extraction site.

The distal surfaces of both mesial and palatal roots were thoroughly cleaned and planed.

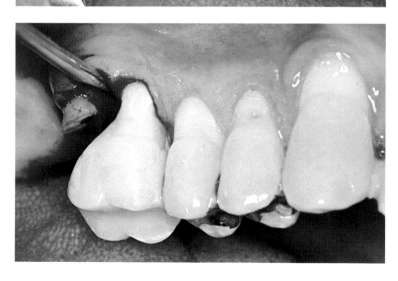

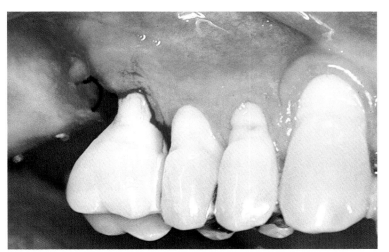

**713 Suture closure**
The thin buccal osseous plates are depressed toward the open alveolus. After thorough planing and smoothing of the resection site and the remaining tooth roots, sutures are placed to close the extraction site and adapt the gingiva around the tooth.

Before

After

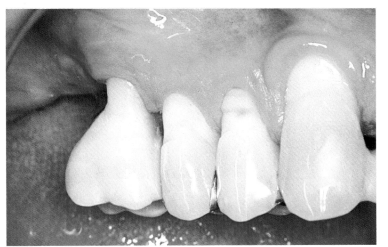

**714 Six weeks postoperative**
The tooth is retained without any type of splint or reconstruction.

The occlusal surface of the tooth is essentially unchanged, but makes contact with its antagonist *only* in centric occlusion. The tooth should not serve any guidance function during lateral or protrusive mandibular excursions.

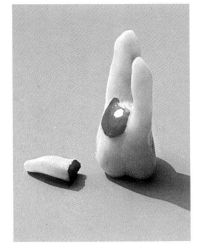

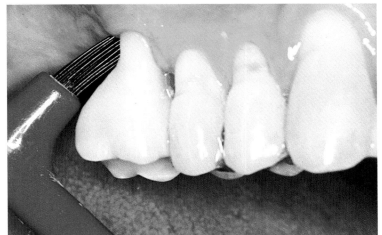

**715 Hygiene for the resection site**
The patient must be made aware of the particular home care technique demanded by the new tooth form. Marginal/interdental brushes are indicated (e.g., Jordan or Lactona no. 27). The resection site receives regular topical applications of fluoride.

*Left:* The model demonstrates the recontoured resection site (red) and the root canal closure (amalgam).

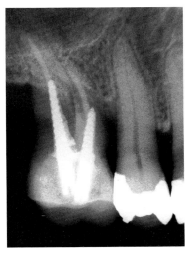

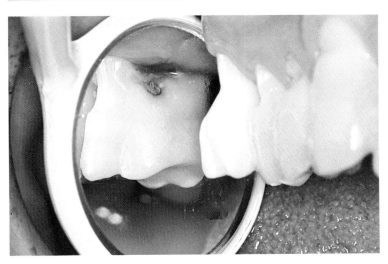

**716 Findings after 6 weeks**
The entrance to the pulp chamber of the former distobuccal root canal was filled with amalgam. The gingiva is mildly inflamed because the patient's home care in the area is not yet optimum.

*Left:* The radiograph reveals the metal posts used in the endodontic treatment; these obscure the amalgam closure of the root canal.

*Three years later, a porcelain-fused-to-metal crown had to be incorporated due to the fractured distobuccal cusp.*

# "Hemisection" (Tri-section) in the Maxilla – Maintenance of All Roots with F3 Furcation Involvement

In cases with severe furcation involvement (class F3, subclass C; cf. pp. 81, 118), a decision concerning which root(s) to extract and which to maintain can often be made only after *complete separation* of the tooth. This permits probing each individual root around its entire circumference and determining mobility.

A 45-year-old female desired to maintain tooth 16 after the hopeless tooth 17 had been extracted, in order to avoid a free-end saddle situation.

After removal of the defective bridge between 16 and 14 and separation of the roots of 16 it became obvious that all of the roots were equally mobile, with only 2–3 mm of remaining attachment. *All* roots were treated endodontically and periodontally, with enlargement of the interradicular area. This heroic treatment included a temporary acrylic bridge. Thanks to the patient's excellent oral hygiene, it was possible 6 months later to seat the definitive reconstruction, which has remained in function and health for the last 6 years.

**717 Severe furcation involvement (F3) – Situation following removal of bridge**
The two Nabers probes demonstrate on tooth 16 the horizontal through-and-through involvement from distal and palatal toward mesial (mesiopalatal). Hopeless tooth 17 has already been extracted.

*Right:* Initial situation before extraction of 17. The etiologic factors of this disease picture become clear: Massive open crown margin, periodontal pockets and furcation involvement, incomplete root canal filling (combined endo-perio problem, cf. p. 311).

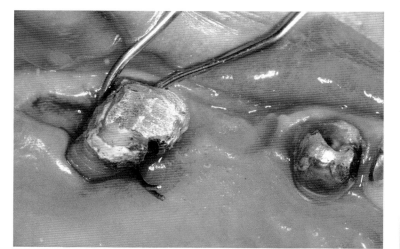
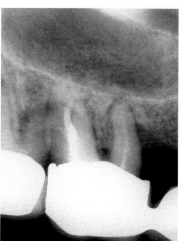

**718 "Hemisection" of molar 16 – Temporary and definitive reconstruction**
Using a temporary bridge that could be easily corrected, adapted, reshaped etc., a "waiting period" was observed in order to see if the patient could maintain all three roots of tooth 16 plaque free. Only after 6 months was the definitive reconstruction seated, and then only temporarily at first.

*Right:* Occlusal view of the 3 molar roots.

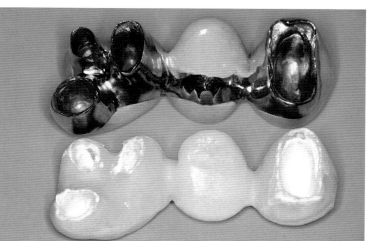
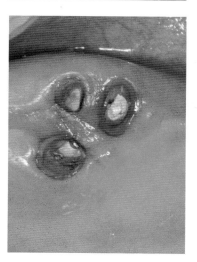

**719 Definitive reconstruction – Oral hygiene**
Premolar 14 and pontic 15 exhibit normal crown form and occlusal surfaces; the castings for coverage of the roots of 16 were fabricated with minimal undercut areas.

The furcation entrances of the crown are easily accessible for cleaning with Super Floss or interdental brushes.

*Right:* The brightly illuminated distal furcation is seen in mirror photography. All crown margins are supragingival.

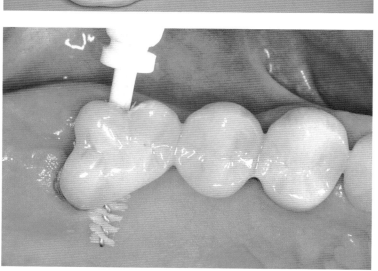
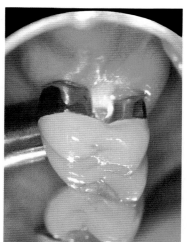

# Gingivectomy (GV) and Gingivoplasty (GP)

The *gingivectomy* (GV) used to be a frequently performed operation; however, it has lost most of its significance as a procedure in the treatment of periodontitis today. The goal of the operation is elimination of gingival pockets by resection of gingival tissue. This is in sharp contrast to the primary goal of modern periodontal therapy, which is *healing* of diseased periodontal structures.

The GV, even today, does maintain its value for exposing crown and cavity margins, for crown lengthening procedures etc.

The *gingivoplasty* (GP) also remains useful, for example for reducing gingival hyperplasias, and for creation of physiologic gingival contour.

GV and GP are almost always performed simultaneously. Either operation may also be combined with flap procedures (p. 241, "Combined Procedures").

## Indications

- Gingival enlargement or overgrowth (caused by medicaments or hormonally)
- Idiopathic fibrosis
- Suprabony pockets in areas with limited access
- Minor corrective procedures

Suprabony pockets are best treated conservatively by scaling and root planing or by means of the modified Widman procedure.

## Contraindications

- Narrow or absent attached gingiva
- Infrabony pockets
- Thickening of marginal alveolar bone

## Advantages

- Technically simple; good visual access
- Complete pocket elimination
- Predictable morphologic result

## Disadvantages

- Very limited indication
- Gross wound; postoperative pain
- Healing is by secondary intent (ca. 0.5 mm re-epithelialization per day)
- Danger of exposing bone
- Sacrifice of attached gingiva
- Exposes cervical area of tooth (sensitivity, esthetics, caries)
- Phonetic and esthetic problems in anterior areas

## Principles of the operative procedure

- Continuous incision at 45° angle toward the base of the pocket
- Sharp dissection of tissues in the interdental areas
- Smoothing of the incision edge
- Scaling and root planing
- Contouring of the gingival surface (GP)
- Wound coverage (periodontal dressing; tissue adhesive)

# Instruments for Gingivectomy/Gingivoplasty ...

Virtually every dental manufacturer offers instruments that fulfill the requirements of a gingivectomy procedure. The original GV/GP instruments are decades old (e.g., Kirkland knives), and continue to be modified and improved. The main function of the instrument is to provide the operator with the ability to perform an uncomplicated, rapid and clean procedure. This will be determined primarily by the size, shape and angulation of the working tip, and also by the handle, which should be comfortable.

Generally speaking, a GV/GP procedure requires a gingivectomy knife and a papilla knife, each of which may be singly or doubly angled. For superficial recontouring of the gingiva (GP) as well as for minor operations such as exposing crown and cavity margins, electrosurgery may be chosen over knives.

Forceps for measurement and marking the pocket fundus are not obligatory. Such measurements and markings can be performed with the periodontal probe.

### 720   Pocket marking forceps
The paired pocket marking forceps (Deppler; L & R) is used exclusively in the GV/GP procedure for indicating the location of the base of the pocket. Pocket depths can also be marked using a fine periodontal probe.

*Right:* Working end of marking forceps. The straight arm is inserted to the bottom of the pocket, then the forceps is closed. The point thus penetrates the surface of the gingiva and creates a bleeding point corresponding to the base of the pocket.

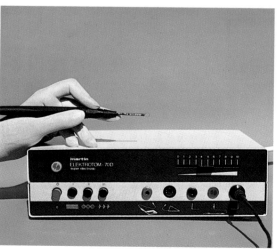

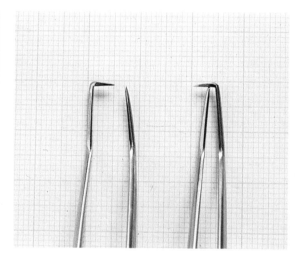

### 721   Gingivectomy knives
(Deppeler Co.)

- **GV knife** (Kirkland; GX 7 L & R), single bend
- **Papilla knife** (Orban; Zl 14 L & R), single bend
- **Universal knife** (Zl 19), single bend

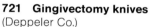

These knives are also available with two bends, and as double-ended instruments.

*Right:* Working ends of the gingivectomy knifes.

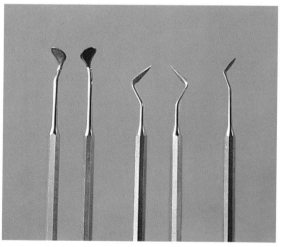
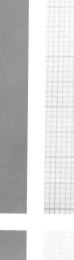

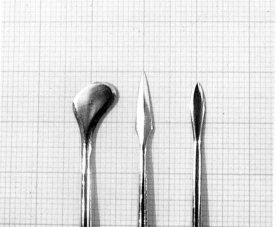

### 722   Electrosurgery – Device and tips
(Martin, Ellman)
Electrosurgery finds its primary function in the gingivoplasty procedure, where it is useful for contouring soft tissue, for papillectomy, for smoothing out abrupt tissue edges, and for exposing the margins of restorations. Electrosurgery is not recommended for expansive gingivoplasty because of the possibility of injury to the tooth root, periosteum, bone or the tooth pulp.

*Right:* The three most important tips for the electrotome.

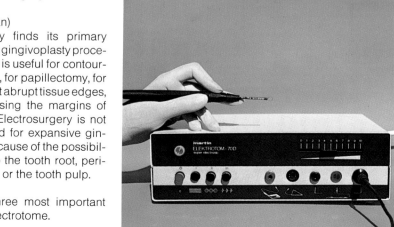

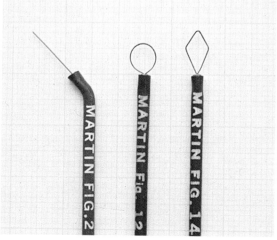

## ... and Their Use

*More important than design and manufacturer is the sharpness of the instruments.* Gingivectomy knives must be sharpened using an Arkansas stone with oil before each operation. This requirement can only be avoided through use of instruments with disposable blades.

For contouring the gingival surface (GP), fine electrosurgical tips are indicated. Electrosurgery is also indicated for minor procedures such as exposing the margin of a tooth preparation before taking an impression, or before seating a restoration. Because electrosurgery exerts a certain hemostatic effect, it may be used to advantage for excision of highly vascular, edematous soft tissues.

The typical use of some gingivectomy instruments is depicted below. A complete clinical procedure will be provided later to illustrate their detailed use.

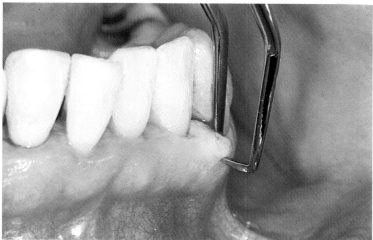

**723 Marking the pocket depths**
The straight arm of the forceps is guided into the buccal pocket on tooth 33, much as a periodontal probe would be. When the base of the pocket is encountered, the forceps is closed, causing the horizontal tip to mark the depth of this 4 mm pocket.

By repeating this procedure at each tooth surface, a series of bleeding points is created, which are used subsequently as a guide for the line of incision.

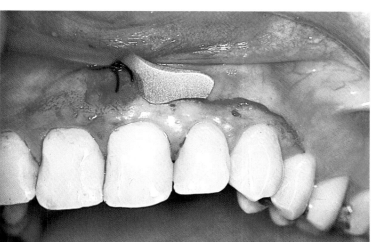

**724 GV/GP using the Kirkland knife**
The blade is positioned at a 45° angle to the tooth long axis and a continous incision is made. Here, the single-bend Kirkland knife is used in the anterior area.

For a gingivectomy on the less accessible palatal or lingual areas, a double-angled instrument is often useful.

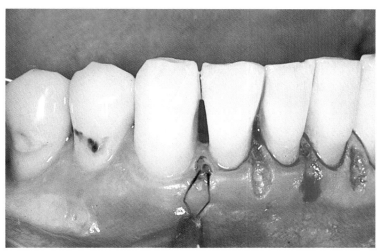

**725 Gingivoplasty using the electrosurgical loop**
The small rhomboid electrode is used to reduce the bulbous marginal gingival contour while creating physiologic morphology. The excision should be definitive, because a portion of the wound will fill with granulation tissue during healing. The alveolar bone must not be exposed or touched.

# Periodontal Dressing and Tissue Adhesives

In almost every case, the open gingivectomy wound must be covered with a dressing, more for patient comfort than for acceleration of wound healing. A dressing can significantly reduce postoperative pain during the first few days. The periodontal dressing is generally left in situ for 7–10 days. A second dressing may be indicated if healing is inadequate.

Only eugenol-free dressings are recommended. Coe-Pak, for example, is a 2-component dressing composed of zinc oxide and fatty acids, while Peripac comes ready-to-use from the container and has a gypsum base.

A periodontal dressing can prevent colonization of the wound surface by plaque microorganisms if a disinfectant, e. g., chlorhexidine powder, is added (Plüss et al. 1975).

Minor injuries such as those created by an electrosurgical procedure to expose the margin of a crown or restoration can be covered with a cyanoacrylate tissue adhesive (see Figs. below).

### 726 Eugenol-free dressings

**– Peripac (left)**

A ready-to-use dressing composed of gypsum and acrylic. It sets quickly upon contact with saliva. If a Peripac dressing is in contact with the mobile oral mucosa, pressure ulcers can form.

**– Coe-Pak (right)**

A two-component dressing composed of zinc oxide and fatty acids. Coe-Pak remains somewhat pliable even after the setting reaction is complete; no irritating edges are created.

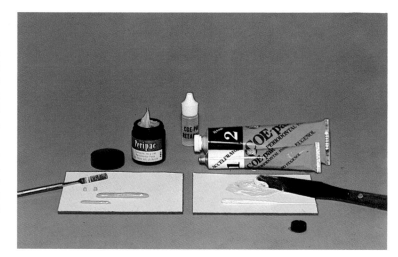

### 727 Chlorhexidine powder (CHX)

Periodontal dressings can be rolled in the water-insoluble CHX-HCl powder immediately before placement over a wound. This will serve to reduce plaque formation beneath the dressing. Wound healing progresses without inhibition (pp. 159 and 316).

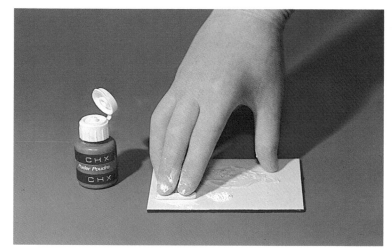

### 728 Tissue adhesives (cyanoacrylates)

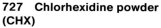

– **Histoacryl** (B. Braun, above)
– **Bucrylate** (Ethicon, below)

For minor GV/GP wounds, tissue adhesive may be used in place of a periodontal dressing. Adhesives may also be used instead of sutures for stabilization of repositioned flaps or free gingival grafts, and for covering the palatal donor site.

Adhesives are applied by means of plastic cannulae, brushes or tubes.

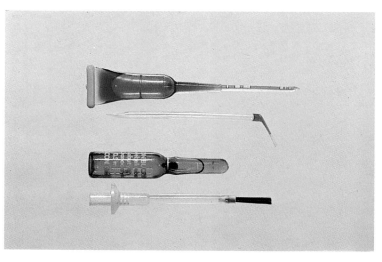

# Gingivectomy/Gingivoplasty

## Operative procedure

The systematic procedure for a GV/GP operation is depicted below in the case of an 18-year-old male who exhibited severe hyperplastic gingivitis without any history of phenytoin medication. Abundant plaque accumulation, maxillary anterior crowding, malocclusion and mouth breathing were all factors in the etiology of this condition.

Orthodontic therapy was recommended, but not accepted at that time by the parents or the patient; initial therapy therefore included minimal occlusal equilibration by means of selective grinding.

*Initial findings:* HYG: 0%    PBI: 3.5    TM: 0–1
*Findings after initial therapy:*
HYG: 75%    PBI: 1.5

The clinical picture, gingival contour, probing depths and radiographs are presented in the figures below.

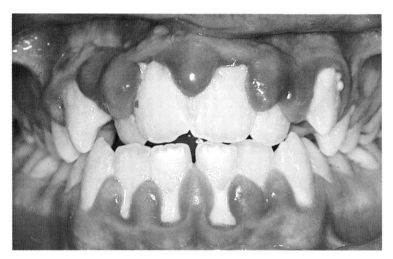

**729  Clinical picture before initial therapy**
Extreme gingival hyperplasia with pseudopockets to 6 mm. Heavy plaque accumulation, especially in anterior area; mouth breathing, malocclusion.

The situation prevented effective home care. The patient stated that the gingival problems had already begun during puberty.

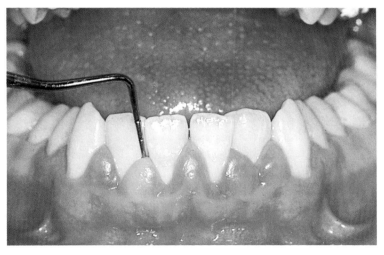

**730  Mandible after initial therapy**
Elimination of inflammation reduced the pseudopocket depths to 3–5 mm. The gingivae remain fibrotically enlarged and home care is still difficult.

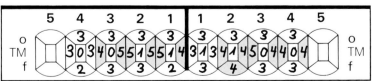

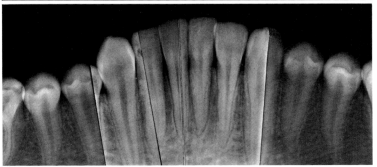

**731  Probing depths and tooth mobility (TM)**
The remaining pseudopockets are the result solely of redundant tissue; there is no true attachment loss or osseous defect. Tooth mobility (TM) values are normal.

**Radiographic findings**
No bone loss is detectable in the radiograph.

### 732 Gingival hyperplasia and pseudopockets

A blast of air from the syringe reflects an enlarged papilla away from the tooth surface.

*Right:* Histology of the area indicated by the black line in the clinical view demonstrates that the apical extent of the junctional epithelium is at its normal position at the CEJ.

A mild inflammatory infiltrate is still apparent even after initial therapy (H & E, x10).

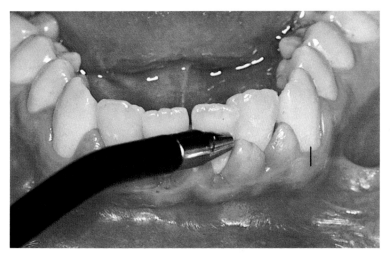 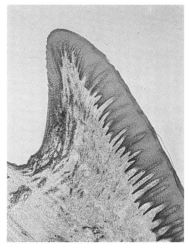

### 733 Anesthesia

Profound anesthesia is accomplished by injections in the mucobuccal fold. To reduce hemorrhage during the procedure, each interdental papilla destined for resection is injected directly.

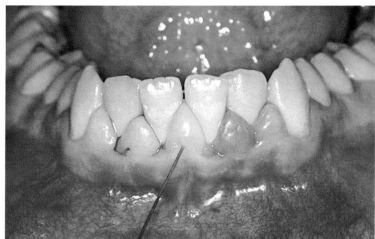

### 734 Marking the base of pockets

The pocket marking forceps is used on papilla and on the midfacial marginal gingivae to indicate the course of the sulcus base between teeth 43 and 33.

*Right:* The schematic depicts the bleeding point at the level of the pocket bottom (black arrow). The periodontal probe depicts the incision (red arrow) and the incision line.

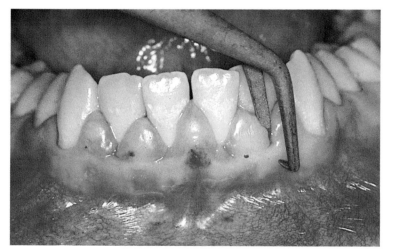 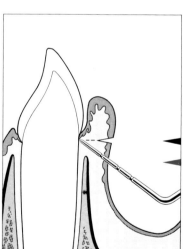

### 735 Planned gingivectomy/ gingivoplasty

The hatched lines indicate the hyperplastic tissue that will be removed by an oblique incision with subsequent recontouring.

The *lingual* aspect of the mandible in this case exhibited no pseudopockets and the gingival contour was normal. Therefore in this case the gingivectomy was limited to the facial aspect.

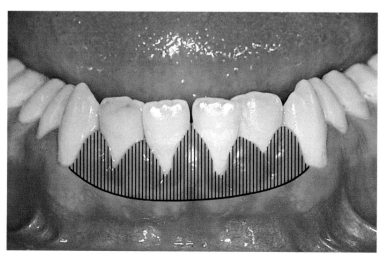

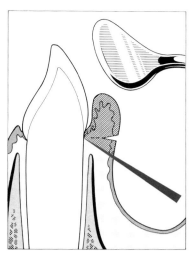

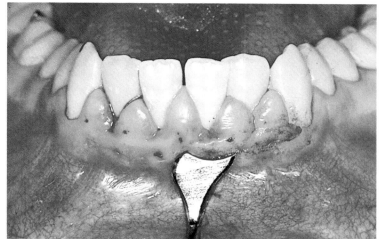

**736 Uninterrupted bevelled incision with the Kirkland knife**
The incision line is totally within the attached gingiva. The mucogingival line is nowhere approached.

*Left:* The schematic depicts the marked pocket fundus and the incision line (red) on the facial aspect.

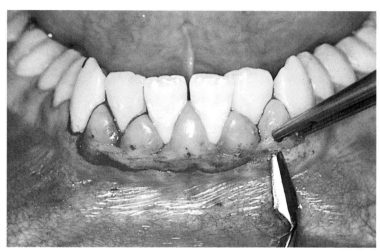

**737 Use of the Orban papilla knife**
The pointed papilla knife is used at the same 45° angle as the GV knife to release the excised tissue by cutting through the papilla to the col region. The tissue should not be *torn* away!

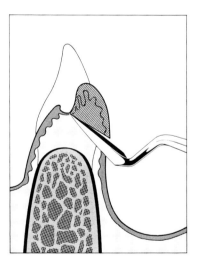

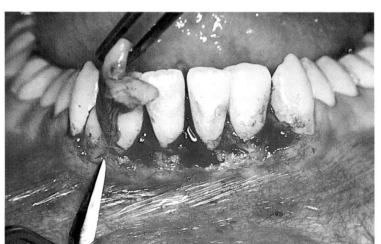

**738 Removal of the tissue**
Using gentle pressure on the surgical forceps, the incised tissue is teased free.

The papilla knife is used to sever any remaining tissue.

*Left:* Definitive release of the excised tissue (red, hatched) using the papilla knife in the interdental area.

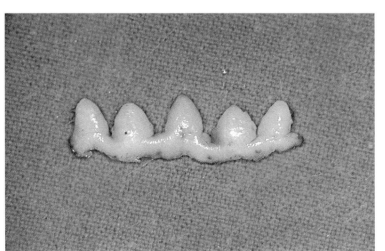

**739 Excised tissue**
In this case it was possible to remove the redundant tissue as a single piece.

If the etiology of the lesion is known, histopathologic evaluation is seldom indicated.

### 740 Scaling and root planing with direct vision

Even when scaling during initial therapy has been performed with great care, residual plaque and calculus may be revealed after tissue removal.

Therefore the most important step in treatment during gingivectomy is cleaning and smoothing of any exposed root surfaces. In this way, a biologically compatible surface is created for the new junctional epithelium that must form.

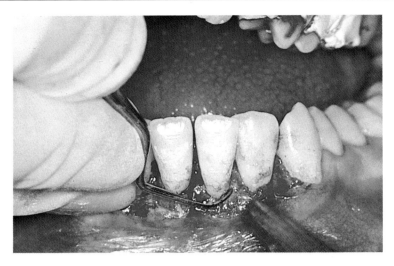

### 741 Gingivectomy wound after scaling

The teeth are clean.

The incision line/wound margin remains relatively sharp, despite the 45° angulation of the initial incision. This edge must be rounded in order to provide ideal gingival contour after healing.

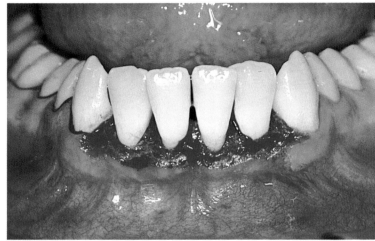

### 742 Smoothing the "sharp edge"

The number 12 electrosurgical loop is indicated for this fine contouring step. Light, smooth and rapid movement of the electrosurgical tip will prevent overheating the tooth and preclude any osseous contact. The electrosurgical instrument should not be adjusted too high. Tissue must not be burned and no "smoke" should develop.

*Right:* Rounding of the incision margin using the electrosurgical loop.

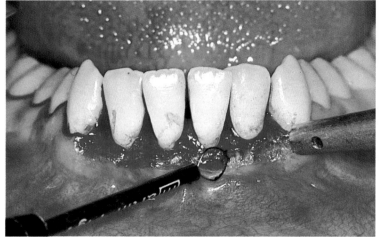

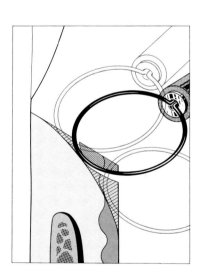

### 743 Cleansing the wound

The Kirkland knife is used to scrape away residual tissue tags or debris. In this case, recontouring extended bilaterally to the first premolars.

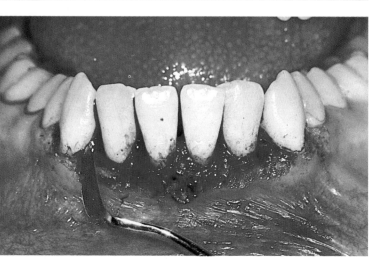

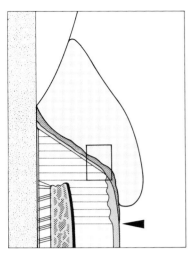

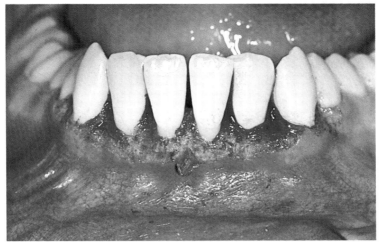

### GV – Wound healing

**744  Clinical view immediately following GV/GP**
The surgical procedure creates a relatively expansive wound surface that must be covered and protected by a periodontal dressing.

*Left:* The GV wound is in the region of the attached gingiva. The black arrow indicates the mucogingival line.
    A very thin blood coagulum separates the dressing from the wound (cf. enlargement, Fig. 745 L).

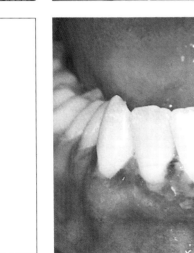

**745  Dressing in place**
Peripac is a rigid dressing that must not encroach upon the mobile mucosa, to prevent pressure and ulceration. The dressing should be left in situ for 7–10 days.

*Left:* Healing two days after GV:

1  Granulation tissue (fibroblasts, new vessels and some PMNs) emigrate from the wound surface into the coagulum
2  Epithelium proliferates from the basal cell layer of the oral epithelium
3  Coagulum

**746  Dressing removal and dental prophylaxis after 7 days**
Careful tooth cleaning by means of rubber cups and very fine abrasive paste (e.g., dentifrice). The wound surface is cleansed using $H_2O_2$ (3%) and a mild spray. The patient is informed that oral hygiene can be reinstituted, carefully at first.

*Left:* The granulation tissue matures into normal connective tissue; it is covered with a thin epithelial layer. A new epithelial attachment begins to form upon the tooth (root) surface.

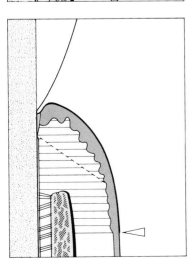

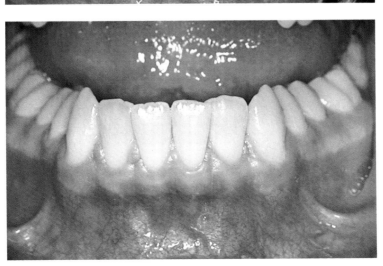

**747  Six months after GV/GP**
The gingivae are inflammation-free and exhibit a generally physiologic morphology. A very slight recurrence of gingival hyperplasia can be detected between 43, 42 and 41 (papillae).

*Left:* The tissue is completely regenerated. Normal oral epithelium with rete ridges and a shallow sulcus. A new, short junctional epithelium has differentiated upon the tooth surface.

# Gingivectomy/Gingivoplasty

## Summary

This 18-year-old patient presented with a very pronounced hyperplastic gingivitis. Oral hygiene, especially in the maxillary interdental areas, ranged from hopeless to nonexistent. The anterior crowding contributed to the poor situation. During initial therapy, it became clear that the young man was very difficult to motivate. Both the patient and his parents initially refused orthodontic treatment, and for this reason selective occlusal grinding was employed to improve the malocclusion as much as possible. Despite these unfavorable circumstances, initial therapy and a subsequent surgical procedure (GV/GP) led to an acceptable result in terms of gingival contour and freedom from gingival pockets. A short recall interval was mandatory to maintain the results of treatment.

Two years later, and motivated by the success of the gingival treatment, the patient sought orthodontic therapy to correct the malocclusion.

**748   Initial clinical view**
Extreme hyperplastic gingivitis, plaque, calculus, absence of home care. The symptoms of disease are limited primarily to the labial surfaces of maxillary and mandibular anterior segments.

Factors contributing to the gingival condition included malocclusion, crowding in the maxilla, and mouth breathing.

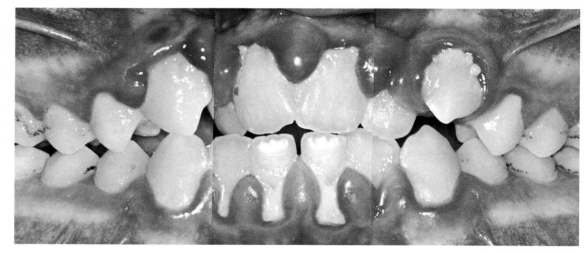

**749   Probing depths and tooth mobility (TM) in the mandible before treatment**
Pseudopockets, but no attachment loss.

Before

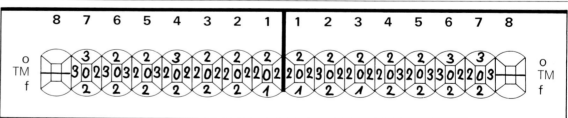

After

**Probing depths and tooth mobility (TM) 7 years later**
Normal probing depths after periodontal therapy and orthodontic treatment.

**750   Clinical findings 7 years postoperatively**
Despite irregular recall there was no recurrence of the hyperplastic gingivitis even though home care by the patient was only moderate. The patient has been able to maintain the area with only minor inflammation. The orthodontic result, while less than optimum, is satisfactory.

*The maxillary arch was also treated by means of GV/GP (see next page).*

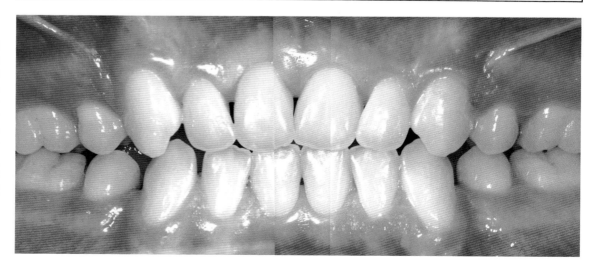

# GV/GP in the Maxilla – Buccal and Palatal

This documented 18-year-old patient (pp. 277–282) also underwent a gingivectomy procedure for treatment of the extreme hyperplastic gingivitis on the labial as well as palatal aspects in the maxillary arch. The surgery was extended to the distal aspect of the second premolars on both sides. In the figures below, only the procedure on the palatal aspect is depicted. The occlusal photographs (Figs. 751–753) depict the severe anterior crowding.

A GV/GP operation can be performed routinely if the palatal vault is high; however, if the palate is flat a GV results in an expansive wound surface that heals slowly (epithelialization occurs at ca. 0.5 mm per day).

Hemorrhage from the incisive foramen can be readily controlled by means of electrocoagulation or injection of a vasoconstrictor-containing anesthetic solution under pressure directly into the canal.

For the maintenance of treatment results in the palatal as well as lingual areas, proper and consistent oral hygiene is especially important (OHI and monitoring). In this regard, observe the difficulties in the final evaluation (Fig. 753).

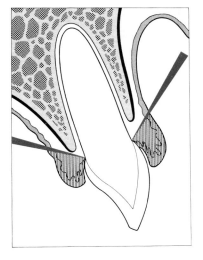

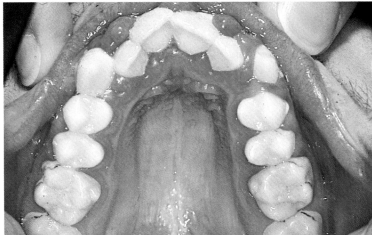

**751   Before initial therapy**
The hyperplastic gingivitis is enhanced on the palatal aspect by the anterior crowding, which also renders oral hygiene very difficult and leads to plaque accumulation and retention.

*Left:* The schematic depicts the anticipated GV incisions labially and palatally. This surgical procedure is performed only *after* initial therapy (not depicted here).

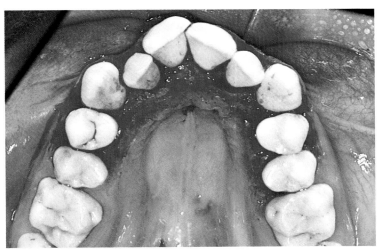

**752   After gingivectomy**
The ideal 45° angle incision is also applied in the palatal area if the anatomic situation permits. This can result in expansive open wound surfaces, which are painful and take longer to heal completely. In such cases, it is often necessary to place a second periodontal dressing one week after the surgical procedure.

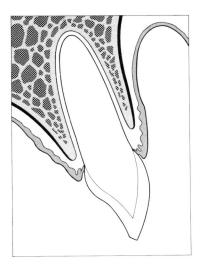

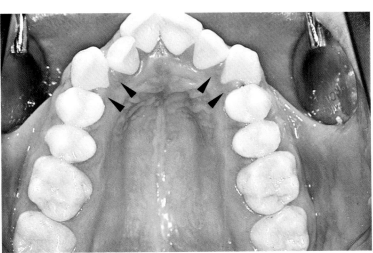

**753   Three months after GV**
The patient's home care has been inadequate, particularly in difficult-to-reach areas occasioned by tooth position anomalies. In these areas hyperplastic gingivitis has begun to recur (arrows).

The clinical situation is remarkably improved in comparison to the initial condition (Fig. 750). These conditions can be maintained with frequent recall. The success of this therapy motivated the patient to seek orthodontic treatment.

*Left:* Healthy postoperative situation.

# GV/GP – Phenytoin-Induced Gingival Overgrowth

Diphenylhydantoin preparations are frequently employed in the treatment of epilepsy. About half of all individuals who ingest hydantoins (generic: phenytoin) on a chronic regimen develop gingival enlargement (pharmacogenetic factor, Hassell 1981). The development of such gingival lesions is enhanced by microbial plaque. Following initial therapy, gingivectomy is the treatment of choice for phenytoin-induced gingival overgrowth. Plaque control is often difficult, especially in mentally or physically handicapped individuals. In such cases, chemical plaque control (chlorhexidine, e.g., Peridex; Low et al. 1989) is indicated as an adjunct to home care.

female who had taken phenytoin for many years and who was incapable of adequate home care.

---

*Initial findings:*

HYG: 0%          PD: to 8 mm, only pseudopockets
PBI:  3.8
Radiographic survey: Incipient bone loss

**754  Phenytoin-induced gingival overgrowth with severe secondary inflammation**
The fibrous gingival overgrowth may have been an etiologic factor in tooth migration. The treatment plan included gingivectomy after initial therapy, with gingivoplasty to improve gingival contour.

*Right:* The radiographs reveal incipient bone resorption, especially in the maxillary anterior area. This is *not* due to phenytoin!

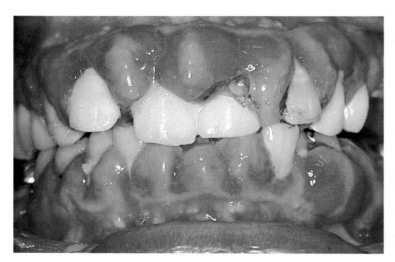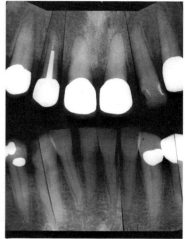

**755  Customized acrylic tray used as a carrier for chlorhexidine gel**
To prevent plaque accumulation and postsurgical recurrence of the gingival enlargement, customized transparent acrylic trays were fabricated for use as medicament carriers in both maxilla and mandible.

The patient, who lacks the dexterity to adequately perform oral hygiene, fills each tray with chlorhexidine gel (1% chlorhexidine digluconate) and wears the trays for 30 minutes each evening.

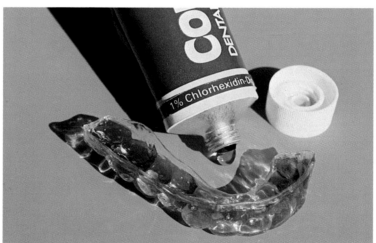

**756  One year after GV/GP – Trays in situ**
The maxillary incisors have spontaneously regained their proper alignment in the dental arch. Recurrence of the gingival overgrowth was completely inhibited by chemical plaque control (CHX gel, once daily).

The acrylic trays extend to the attached gingiva and are well adapted, thus preventing seepage of the gel into the oral cavity.

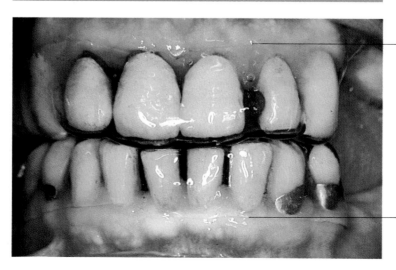

**Borders of medicament carriers**

# GV/ GP – Corrective Operations, Minor Procedures
# Exposing the Margins of Restorations and Cavity Preparations

The point was made earlier in this *Atlas* that GV/GP as definitive therapy (pocket elimination) for periodontitis is virtually never performed today. On the other hand, these procedures maintain their value as corrective measures.

The margins of restorations and crowns should be located supragingivally to avoid irritation of the periodontal tissues. Exceptions to this rule may be considered in anterior regions, for reasons of esthetics.

Tooth preparation and impression taking are technically difficult procedures if the preparation margins are located subgingivally. Also it is considerably easier to place a rubber dam if margins are supragingival.

In the case presented here, carious lesions that extend into the subgingival area are exposed by a labial and palatal gingivectomy procedure. If properly performed, there should be no subsequent esthetic problem.

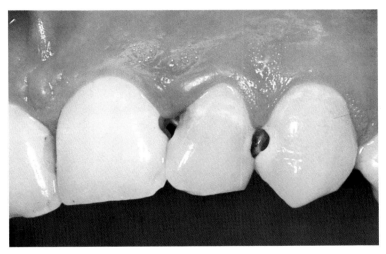

**757  Subgingival caries on teeth 21, 22 and 23**
Without a gingivectomy, it would be impossible to create a proper cavity preparation or apply the rubber dam, which is necessary for elimination of moisture when placing a composite resin restoration.

When treatment is complete the margins of the restoration should be supragingival.

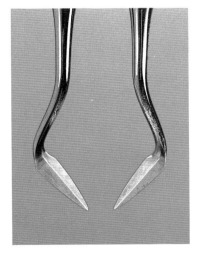
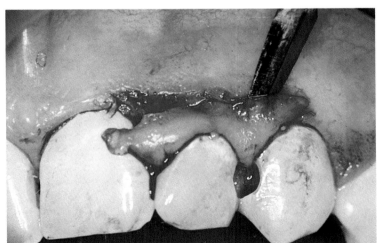

**758  GV/GP using the Orban papilla knife**
The gingiva is excised using a gingivectomy knife (e.g., Kirkland) or, as in this case using a papilla knife (Orban). Electrosurgery may also be used to advantage for such minor procedures. Minimal hemorrhage results, and restorations can be placed at the same appointment.

*Left:* Paired, angled Orban papilla knife (ZI 14 L & R; Deppeler).

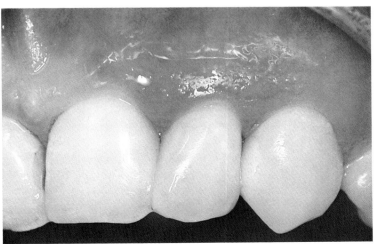

**759  After restorative treatment and healing**
The apical margins of the four scarcely visible composite restorations lie supragingivally and are therefore accessible for oral hygiene by means of toothbrush and dental floss.

This promotes prevention of recurrent caries as well as gingivitis.

Courtesy of *A. Bachmann*

# Gingivectomy – Lengthening the Clinical Crown and Exposure of Preparation Margins

Crown lengthening by means of flap reflection and ostectomy has already been described (pp. 236–237). If pseudopockets exist because of gingival hyperplasia or if suprabony pockets accompany early periodontitis, the gingivectomy procedure can be used to advantage to expose carious lesions, perforation areas or preparation margins for fillings and crowns.

In a 37-year-old female with mild periodontitis (AP) reconstruction is necessary in the mandibular left segment. Tooth 36 exhibits buccal furcation involvement (F1), an open crown margin and cervical caries. Tooth 37 also exhibits secondary caries and cervical lesions. Tooth 38 must be extracted. 36 and 37 are prepared for full coverage restorations. The gingivectomy procedure is employed to expose the restoration margins, thereby lengthening the clinical crowns.

*Initial findings:*

| | |
|---|---|
| HYG: 25% | PBI: 3.6 |
| PD: to 6 mm pockets | TM: to grade 2 |

**760 Initial situation, before and after removal of the old reconstruction**

Caries is detectable beneath the crown on 36, at the cervical area of 37 and around all old restorations on the third molar (which is destined for extraction).

The gingivae are hyperplastic and bleed at the slightest touch.

*Right:* Crown and old cast gold restorations have been removed; the preparation margins were at least 2 mm subgingival. The swollen lingual and buccal papillae are clearly visible.

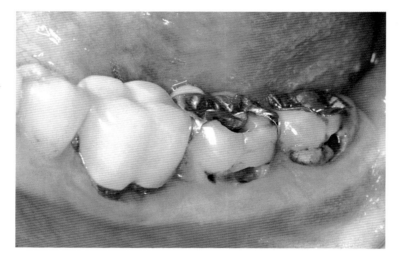

**761 Initial preparation – Gingivectomy**

The carious lesions can be eliminated by initial tooth preparation. Using a 45° oblique incision the hyperplastic gingiva is resected buccally and lingually.

*Right:* Excised tissue.

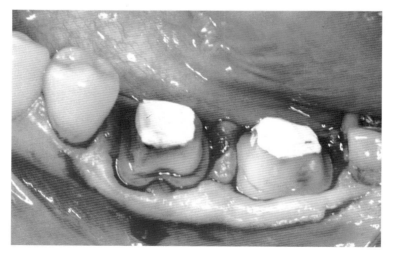
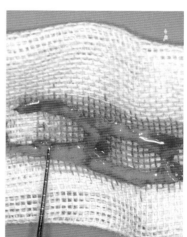

**762 Temporary crowns – Supragingival margins**

After healing of the gingivectomy wound the preparation margin of tooth 37 is close to the marginal gingiva, that of tooth 36 is far removed from it. The furcation entrance is revealed, and must be conscientiously cleaned by the patient (caries!). Special dentifrices and/or fluoride preparations may be required for tooth neck hypersensitivity.

*Right:* Bone loss in the furcation is evident radiographically, but it is not through-and-through clinically.

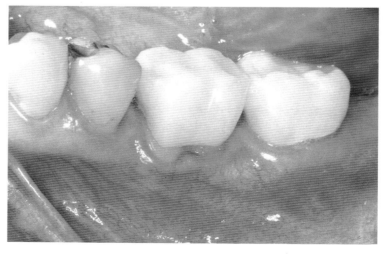
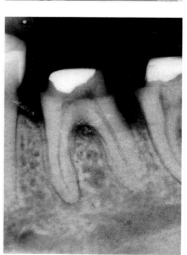

# GV/GP for Prosthetic, Endodontic and Esthetic Reasons

Minor gingivectomy procedures are often indicated for exposure of preparation margins in endodontically treated, severely broken down teeth that must be restored by means of a core or full crown. The GV is indicated more often in these situations than for routine restorations. As with a gingivectomy performed for periodontal reasons, the bone must not be touched. The use of an electrosurgical device is recommended for this type of minor procedure to reduce hemorrhage.

In the case presented here (30-year-old male), a gingivectomy on the labial aspect was necessary to expose a perforation that had occurred subsequent to an endodontic procedure. The GV not only revealed the margins of the post-and-core and the new metal/ceramic crown, but also effectively adjusted the length of tooth 11 to correspond to 21. Furthermore the procedure improved gingival contour in the area.

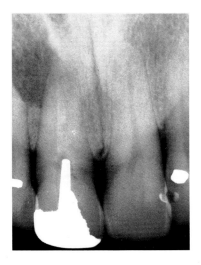
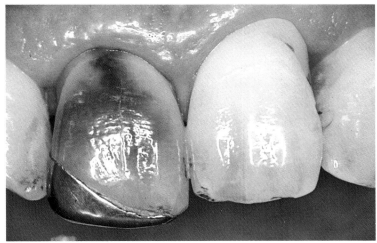

**763 Perforation, corrosion**
The old post-inlay covering the incisal edge must be replaced. The clinical crown had discolored excessively due to metal corrosion. A perforation was detected about 2 mm subgingivally. The adjacent tooth, 21, exhibits recession of ca. 2 mm.

*Left:* The radiograph reveals the short, corroding post, but no bone loss. There is but scant evidence of root canal filling.

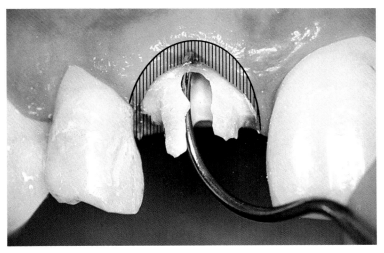

**764 Exposure of the perforation via GV**
The procedure of choice is a half moon-shaped gingivectomy (indicated by lines) using electrosurgery to expose the perforation site, demonstrated by the explorer tip.
The GV procedure can equalize the clinical crown lengths of 11 and 21.

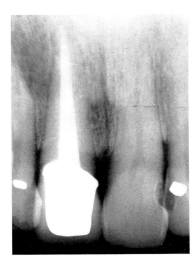
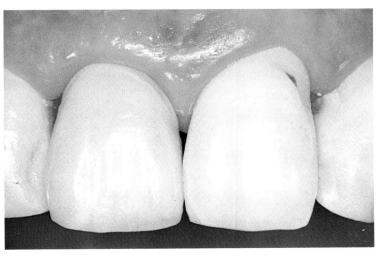

**765 Definitive restoration with a metal/ceramic crown**
The labial porcelain crown margin covers the perforation site and lies slightly subgingivally (for esthetic reasons).
Both central incisors are now approximately the same length.

*Left:* The radiograph reveals the revised root canal filling, the post, and the new crown.

# Gingivoplasty

The gingivoplasty procedure can be used purely to correct tissue morphology, for example to recontour bulbous papillae. This can reduce plaque retention and render oral hygiene easier. The goal of this procedure is the creation of a physiologic gingival contour that fills the interdental area.

The 28-year-old female described below complained of gingival bleeding. In terms of home care, she had never received any professional instruction, motivation or treatment. Her gingivitis was of long duration.

*Initial findings:*

HYG: 40%
PBI: 3.7
TM: 0–1
PD: 5 mm in interproximal areas; pseudopockets

Initial therapy and proper home care essentially eliminated her gingival inflammation; however, some interdental papillae were bulbously enlarged and appeared morphologically unfavorable. This residual situation was corrected by means of electrosurgery.

### 766 Gingivitis
Before initial therapy, the inflammatory hyperplastic enlargement of the interdental papillae was especially pronounced in the mandibular segment. Pseudopockets were shallow. The malocclusion was obvious, with a partial anterior open bite.

Poor home care was demonstrated by application of a plaque-disclosing agent.

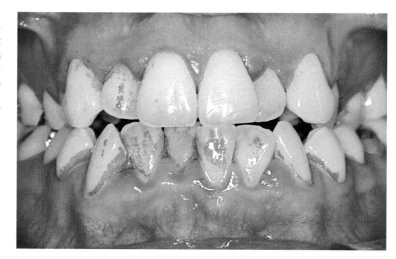

### 767 Gingivoplasty
Following initial therapy and repeated OHI, hyperplastic gingival papillae remained. These were removed using the rhomboid-shaped tip of the electrotome. This modeling procedure should be performed definitively, since partial recurrence is to be expected (healing via granulation tissue). Bone must not be touched.

*Right:* Section at the level of the cervix. The recontouring procedure should eliminate plaque retention, enhance self-cleansing and simplify oral hygiene.

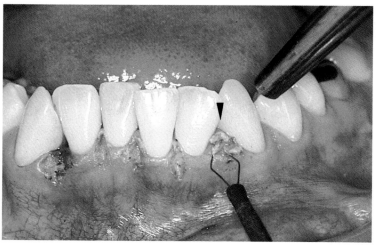
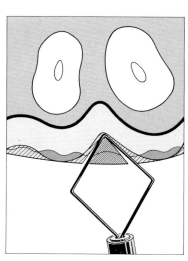

### 768 10 weeks after gingivoplasty
Bulbous gingival papillae are gone. The recreation of physiologic morphology simplifies oral hygiene, as evidenced by the 10-week postoperative clinical data:

| | |
|---|---|
| HYG | 90% |
| PBI | 0.8 |
| TM | 0–1 |
| PD | max. 2 mm |

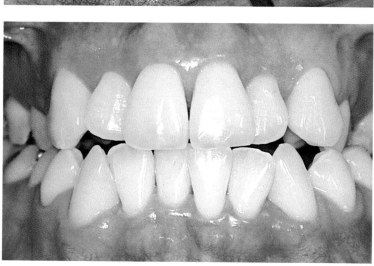

# Mucogingival Surgery

## Stopping Recession – Covering Recession

The indications for mucogingival surgery as a treatment modality for recession have been sharply reduced in scope in recent years. Numerous studies have demonstrated that periodontal health (freedom from inflammation) can be maintained regardless of the finite width of attached gingiva (Wennström 1983, 1985; Wennström & Lindhe 1983 a, b).

The indications for mucogingival surgical procedures today are limited to progressive recession (rarely), frena that insert directly at the gingival margin and elicit recession, and localized severe recession rendering effective oral hygiene impossible. A free gingival graft (FGG) may be indicated prior to orthodontic procedures in the mandibular anterior area (seldom), or around abutment teeth lacking attached gingiva.

Mucogingival surgery consists of the following procedures:

| |
|---|
| **Frenotomy – Frenectomy** |
| **Gingival extension with free gingival graft (FGG)** |
| **Extension operation / Vestibuloplasty** (Edlan-Mejchar, modif. 1963) |
| **Covering a denuded root surface by means of:**<br>  – **Direct free gingival graft (one-step procedure)**<br>  – **Coronal flap repositioning after FGG (two-step procedure)**<br>  – **Sliding flap** (Grupe & Warren 1956, Grupe 1966) |

### General consideration concerning indications

The progress of gingival recession generally ceases spontaneously with institution of careful, non-traumatic plaque control measures and, if necessary, changing the patient's brushing technique, *without* any surgical procedures. In order to avoid unnecessary surgery (overtreatment!) in patients exhibiting gingival recession, the following preventive procedures are recommended:

1. Thorough tooth cleaning and polishing, and elimination of gross functional disturbances.
2. Monitored change of home care techniques. The vertical rotatory method (modified Stillman, cf. p. 153), which involves brushing from the gingiva toward the teeth, has been shown to be effective in patients with recession. The toothbrush should have soft or medium bristles.
3. Preparation of intraoral photographs and/or study models. This makes it possible at subsequent recall appointments to compare the actual situation, and to answer questions about stability or progression of gingival recession.
4. Initially, short-interval recall *without* repeated scaling at areas of recession.

Mucogingival surgery may be indicated if areas of recession persist and progress over months or years despite institution of the preventive measures noted above (Rateitschak et al. 1979).

# Frenotomy – Frenectomy

Frena may exert excessive pull upon the gingival margin and the interdental papillae, resulting in localized recession. For this reason, labial and buccal frena that splay far toward the gingival margin should be eliminated. This can be accomplished by simple separation *(frenotomy)* or by removal of the entire frenum *(frenectomy)*. These represent the least complicated mucogingival surgical procedures.

The triangular or rhomboid wound that exists after frenotomy / frenectomy may be covered using a "mini" free gingival graft if necessary. If no free gingival graft is employed, 20–50% recurrence may be expected.

The frenectomy procedure in the maxilla is demonstrated below in the case of a 17-year-old patient with healthy periodontal conditions.

*Findings:*
HYG: 95%      TM: 0
PBI:   0.4
The figures depict the clinical situation.

**769   Labial frenum**
The pull exerted by the extremely high frenum attachment in this young patient has caused rather severe retraction of the papilla tip between the central incisors (black arrows). This area is routinely injured during toothbrushing.

*Right:* The extent of this frenum becomes visible when the upper lip is reflected. The black arrow demonstrates the position of the receded papilla. The thin red arrow depicts the incision, which can be made using scalpel and/or scissors.

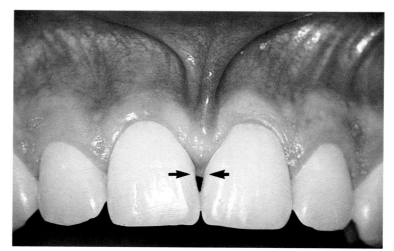
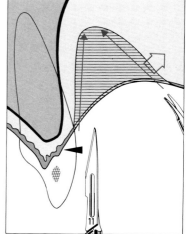

**770   Immediate postsurgical view**
Excision of the frenum creates a rhomboid-shaped wound. A thin elevator or scissors is used to sever muscle and connective tissue fibers from the periosteum of the alveolar process, and the mucosal edges are approximated with sutures.

It was not possible to close the wound completely at its coronal extent due to the immobility of the attached gingiva. A small free gingival graft would be helpful in such a situation.

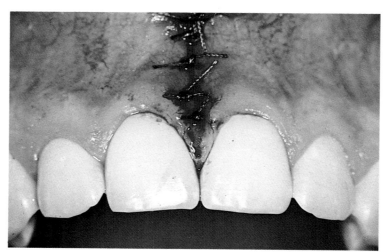

**771   Two years postoperative**
Elimination of the frenum pull led to complete regeneration of the interdental papilla (arrows). The interdental space between the central incisors again became completely filled by gingival tissue.

*Right:* The facial papilla regenerated (open red arrow) and the vestibulum was slightly deepened.

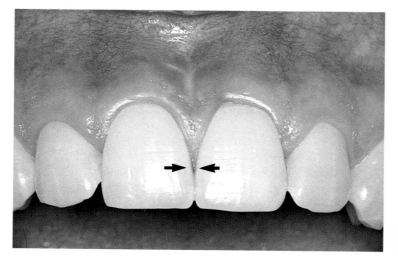
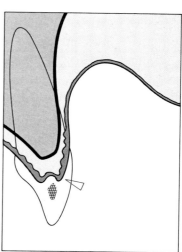

# Gingival Extension with a Free Gingival Graft (FGG)

Extension of the vestibulum by means of a free gingival graft (FGG) remains the most common mucogingival surgical procedure, within the rather limited indications. The technique was first reported by Björn (1963) and was later systematized by Sullivan and Atkins (1968 a, b). The procedure leads to replacement of mobile, non-keratinized oral mucosa by "true" keratinized gingiva or palatal mucosa.

## Indications

There exists consensus today that under the rubric of "indications for mucogingival surgery," gingival recession should not be routinely treated surgically. The generally accepted procedure is to modify and then repeatedly monitor oral hygiene procedures. Generally this is sufficient to bring the progression of recession to a halt. However, if recession continues to progress, a free gingival graft is indicated.

If *localized* recession extends to the mucogingival line or beyond, home care is rendered very difficult, leading in some cases to extremely persistent inflammation. Such situations are common with high frenum attachment or a shallow vestibulum, where the mobile oral mucosa closely approaches the gingival margin. Injury to the gingival margin during toothbrushing is common with such unfavorable morphology. Stopping the recession by means of a free gingival graft is the only available recourse.

Treatment of *generalized* recession by means of free gingival grafting is possible, but is seldom indicated. Because the quantity of palatal donor tissue is limited, repeated operations are often necessary; however, use of a mesh graft (p. 304) can sometimes be employed for successful treatment of larger areas.

Free gingival grafting has been recently suggested as a pre-orthodontic measure. In the chapter "Types of Periodontal Diseases" (p.109), the etiologic role of morphologic-anatomic characteristics in gingival recession was noted, particularly the fact that the bone over the facial root surface may be extremely thin and often fenestrated, or may be altogether absent. If teeth are moved orthodontically in such cases (especially in the mandibular anterior and canine regions), gingival recession may result (Wennström et al. 1987a). The free gingival graft may be indicated as a preventive measure.

## Contraindications

The FGG procedure is not indicated in areas of *stationary* recession that are accessible for oral hygiene, or do not exhibit signs of persistent inflammation, or present no esthetic problems.

A FGG generally is taken from the palate. The whitish color of this highly keratinized mucosa is retained even after transplantation of the tissue. In the often visible maxillary anterior and canine regions, this may create an esthetic concern that must be considered.

## Surgical principles

The surgical procedure is performed with block anesthesia. The anesthetic solution should contain a vasoconstrictor that will inhibit excessive hemorrhage.

The *first phase* of the procedure involves preparation of the recipient bed apical to the recession area. A horizontal incision is made along the mucogingival line. If attached gingiva is completely absent, the incision is made 1–2 mm apical to the gingival margin. The incision is made through the mucosa and submucosal tissues, but does not encroach upon the periosteum. This horizontal incision assumes an arcuate shape as its ends turn towards the vestibular fold. Mucosa, submucosal connective tissue and muscle fibers are carefully separated from the underlying periosteum. In this way, a *recipient bed covered with periosteum* is prepared to receive the free gingival graft (James & McFall 1978).

James et al. (1978) and Caffesse et al. (1979a, b) were able to demonstrate that a FGG can also be successful if it is placed upon an osseous surface that is not covered by periosteum.

The *second phase* of surgery is the removal of a 1 mm thick graft, usually from the palate. Small FGGs may also be excised from an edentulous ridge area. The graft should be taken from the same side of the mouth as the recipient site. This provides the patient with chewing function on the other side during healing.

The *third phase* of the procedure involves fixation of the graft at the recipient site, usually with sutures. Some authors recommend heavy and prolonged pressure upon the transplanted graft, as well as fixation using tissue adhesive (e.g., histoacryl). If a tissue adhesive is employed, care must be taken that it does not flow between the FGG and the periosteal surface; if it does, *loss of the FGG is virtually certain*.

# Instruments for Harvesting a Graft ...

The mucosa for a free gingival graft is usually taken from the palate. Several special and easy-to-use surgical instruments are available for this procedure.

The *hand mucotome* may be used to harvest graft tissue of varying width and thickness.

The *motor-driven mucotome,* on the other hand, always provides a strip of graft tissue of identical width and thickness. The connective tissue undersurface of such a strip is so smooth that it may be confused with the epithelial surface. For this reason, the epithelial surface should be marked before the operation, using a nontoxic, waterproof, felt-tipped pen. A graft transplanted with the wrong side up will not succeed.

For harvesting graft tissue with individual shapes, *scalpels* or *gingivectomy knives* may be used.

**772  Hand mucotomes**
These instruments consist of a handle and a cutting head onto which disposable blades are affixed. The Deppeler mucotomes are available straight (as shown here) or with an angled handle.

- **PR 1**  7 mm wide
- **PR 4**  9 mm wide
- **PR 2**  11 mm wide
- **PR M**  16 mm wide

*Right:* Disposable blades fabricated from razor blade steel.

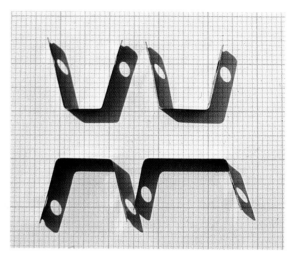

**773  Motor-driven mucotome described by Mörmann**
This instrument (Aesculap Co.) permits removal of uniform grafts.

- **6.5 mm**  width
- **0.75 mm**  thickness

The apparatus resembles a contraangle handpiece, and is driven by the micromotor. The instrument head can be positioned as desired.

*Right:* The blades are removed laterally from the cutting head using a special plunger, and can be resharpened.

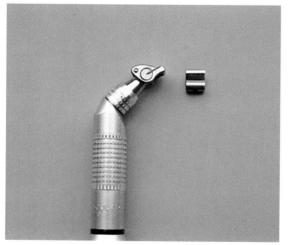
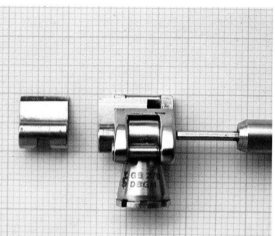

**774  Scalpel, gingivectomy knife, surgical forceps, minihook**
An individualized free graft can be obtained using fine scalpels (no.15 or 15C) or the gingivectomy knife.
For lifting the graft out of the palate, the mini-hook (Gillis) can be less traumatic to the tissue than a forceps, which can crush tissue. A suture can also be used to lift the graft.

*Right:* Magnification of the instruments' working tips.

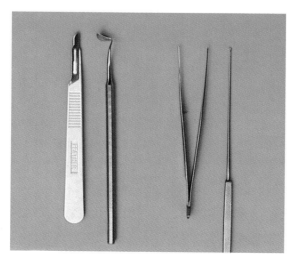
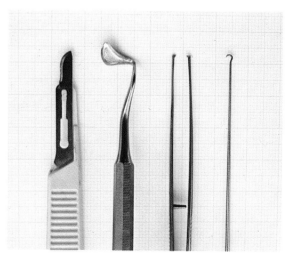

# ... and Their Use

The hand- or motor-driven mucotomes provide rectangular strips of graft tissue that must be trimmed to fit the prepared recipient bed.

If the surgeon desires a perfectly fitting graft of special shape, it must be obtained using the scalpel or GV knife plus a pattern or template made of aluminum foil or wax. The method for harvesting an individual graft is indicated especially when the recession to be treated is severe and must be covered with arcuate grafts. This is also true when a graft is to be placed around a lone-stand-ing tooth or a tooth at the distal end of the arch. In these instances the graft itself must be adapted around the tooth, toward the alveolar ridge (p. 303).

Removal of palatal tissue is accomplished with profound local anesthesia. If the anesthetic solution is injected with elevated pressure, the palatal mucosa will be lifted somewhat and may prove easier to remove after the incisions are completed. The depth of incision during palatal tissue removal must be carefully monitored in order to avoid injury to the major palatal arteries.

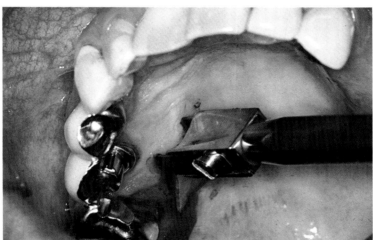

**775   Removing a graft from the palate using a hand muco-tome PR 1 (7 mm)**
The cutting head is moved slightly back and forth as the incision is made. To provide a precise cut, the index finger of the left hand is used for guidance and application of pressure. The ideal graft is uniform and less than 1 mm thick.

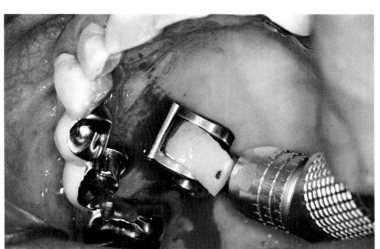

**776   Graft harvest using the motor-driven mucotome**
The head of the instrument must be pressed lightly against the palatal mucosa so that the blade engages tissue fully and a uniformly thick graft is achieved. Marking the epithelial surface precludes suturing the graft incorrectly into the recipient bed.

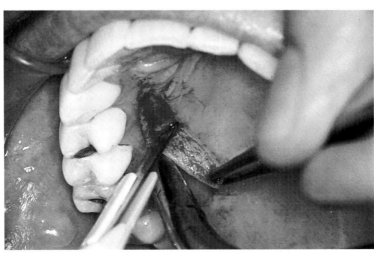

**777   Harvesting an individual graft**
Using a template prepared at the recipient site, palatal tissue is harvested using a scalpel. The first incision is made around the periphery of the graft, to a depth of 1 mm. The GV knife can then be used (without the template) to undermine the graft margins, before teasing out the graft with forceps and scalpel.

# Free Gingival Graft Thickness and Shape

The structure of the epithelium (keratinization pattern, cell layers) is determined by its subjacent connective tissue. It is for this reason that a free graft must contain subepithelial connective tissue; this is ensured if the graft is 1 mm thick (Fig. 778).

As a free gingival graft heals, the original graft epithelium is almost completely desquamated, while the subjacent connective tissue is "accepted" (see Revascularization, p. 301). New epithelialization occurs from the surrounding mucosa (Bernimoulin & Lange 1972). Even epithelium that grows in over the free graft from the non-keratinized oral mucosa will differentiate into *keratinized* mucosa upon the transplanted connective tissue. Palatal rugae must not be transplanted, because they would be visible in the attached gingiva even after complete healing.

Taking a graft using a hand mucotome or scalpel carries with it the danger of penetrating too deeply and severing branches of the palatine artery. Profuse hemorrhage may ensue.

**778 Histology of the palate**
The soft tissue overlying the palatal bone is about 3–5 mm thick. The ideal graft should be no more than 1 mm thick, so that it contains both epithelium and subepithelial connective tissue.

The cross-hatched area at the bottom of the histologic section represents a graft that is 6 mm wide and 0.8 mm thick.

**A** Thin graft
**B** Medium graft
**C** Thick graft

Courtesy *H. E. Schroeder*

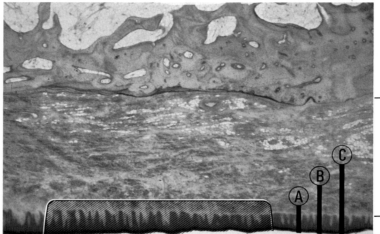

**779 Thinning an excessively thick graft**
Excessively thick grafts contain fatty tissue and glandular tissue. Following removal, such thick grafts must be thinned using the mucotome, a scalpel or scissors on a sterile glass slab under saline irrigation.

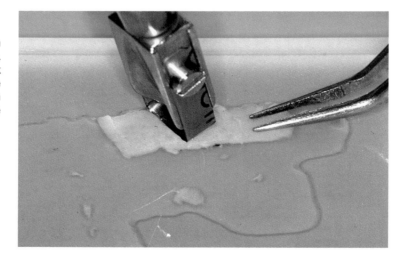

**780 Trimming the graft**
Grafts harvested with mucotomes are rectangular and often must be appropriately trimmed to fit the recipient bed. Such trimming is obviated if the graft is taken from the palate using a scalpel and a template of aluminum foil or wax.

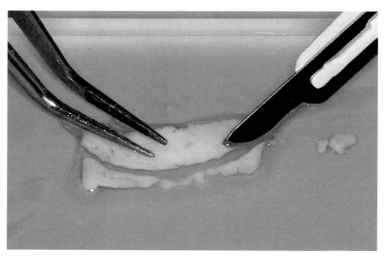

# Gingival Extension with Free Gingival Graft (FGG)

## Operative procedure

In this 43-year-old female with excellent oral hygiene, *generalized buccal recession* had been diagnosed 3 years previously. Mild interdental recession, perhaps related to the patient's use of interdental stimulators, was also noted. The patient's brushing method had been horizontal scrubbing, but was changed to modified Stillman 3 years ago. With this, the progression of recession in the maxilla came to a halt.

However, in the mandible the recession became more severe, especially in the canine and premolar area, until attached gingiva was completely absent. In the following series of photos, the indicated surgical procedure for gingival extension with FGG is portrayed.

*Presurgical findings:*
   HYG: 93%      PBI: 0.8      TM: 0–1
   The clinical picture, radiographic findings, recession and width of attached gingiva are presented below.

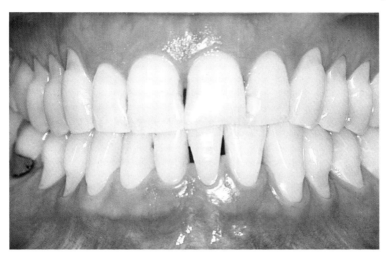

**781   Initial clinical view**
Areas of recession are visible in maxillary and mandibular canine and posterior areas. Teeth with recession exhibit wedge-shaped defects at the CEJ, probably as a result of improper traumatic toothbrushing.

The areas of recession in the mandible, especially in canine and premolar regions are *progressing*. No McCall's festoons are seen.

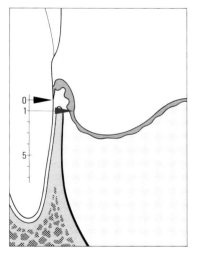

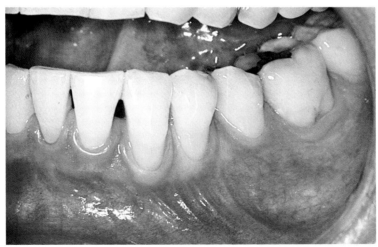

**782   Surgical site in lower left segment**
There is no attached gingiva present on the buccal aspect of teeth 33, 34 and 35. Tension applied to the vestibular mucosa causes blanching of the gingival margin. A FGG in this area is indicated because the recession is progressively worsening.

*Left:* The schematic depicts that practically no attached, keratinized gingiva remains (area between red and black arrows).

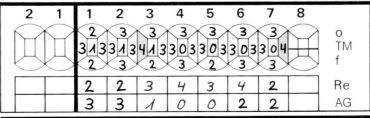

| 2 | 1 | 1 | 2 | 3 | 4 | 5 | 6 | 7 | 8 | | |
|---|---|---|---|---|---|---|---|---|---|---|---|
| | | 2 | 3 | 3 | 3 | 3 | 3 | 3 | | | o |
| 3 1 3 | 3 1 3 | 4 1 3 | 3 0 3 | 3 0 3 | 3 0 3 | 3 0 4 | | | | | TM |
| | | 2 | 3 | 2 | 3 | 2 | 3 | 3 | | | f |
| | | 2 | 2 | 3 | 4 | 3 | 4 | 2 | | | Re |
| | | 3 | 3 | 1 | 0 | 0 | 2 | 2 | | | AG |

**783   Probing depths, tooth mobility (TM), recession (Re), width of attached gingiva (AG)**
From a periodontal standpoint the main problem was the buccal recession. Probing depths were normal and tooth mobility was not increasing.

**Radiographic findings**
The facial recession areas are not apparent in the radiograph. Nevertheless, slight horizontal bone loss is apparent in the interdental regions.

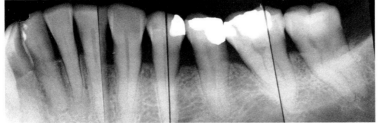

**784 Planning the incision**
A horizontal incision will be performed along the mucogingival border. If no attached gingiva is present the incision is made 1–2 mm apical to the gingival margin. The incision curves apically at its mesial and distal extents, toward the vestibulum into areas where sufficient attached gingiva is present.

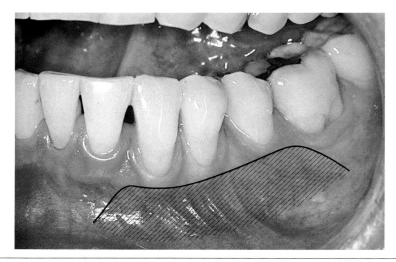

**First surgical phase: Extension**

**785 Horizontal incision**
The chairside assistant pulls on the lip to create tension in the vestibular mucosa. Then the no. 15 scalpel is used to make the horizontal incision about 1 mm deep along the mucogingival line, without encroaching upon the periosteum.

*Right:* Schematic depiction of the incision at the approximate position of the mucogingival line.

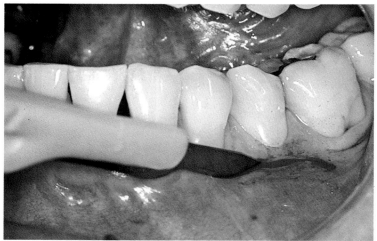
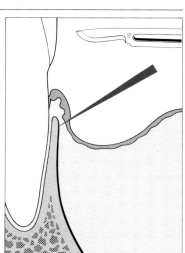

**786 Horizontal incision complete**
The extent to the incision corresponds to the plan. Hemorrhage is slight as a result of local anesthetic containing a vasoconstrictor.

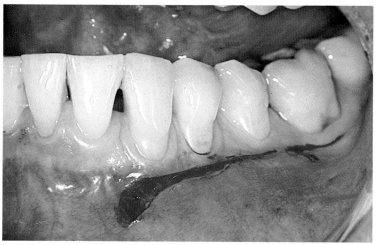

**787 Preparation of the recipient site (extension)**
Connective tissue and muscle fibers are sharply dissected. The scalpel is maintained at an oblique angle to the periosteum.
     The recipient bed should consist of periosteum freed of all submucosal tissues so that the graft will firmly attach.

*Caution:* Mental nerve.

*Right:* Lip and cheek are reflected (arrow), opening the wound to permit clean preparation.

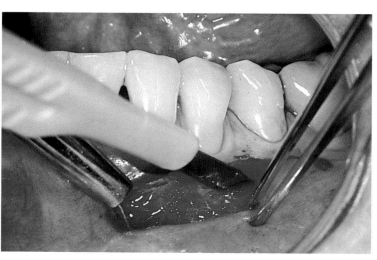
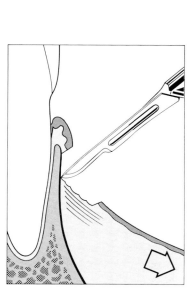

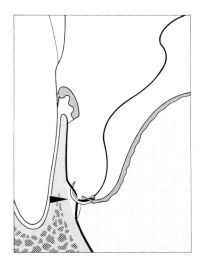

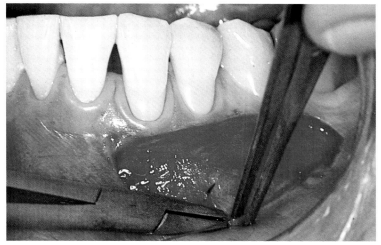

### 788  Suturing the mucosa apically to the periosteum (optional)

The recipient bed should be wider at its apical extent than the planned graft. The free margin of the vestibular mucosa can be affixed to the periosteum using resorbable catgut or vicryl sutures; however, this is *not mandatory*.

*Left:* A small, curved, atraumatic needle traverses the mucosa and the periosteum (arrow). This suture must not be pulled excessively, to avoid tearing the periosteum.

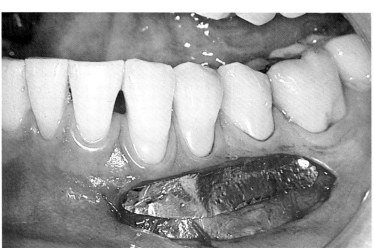

### 789  Pattern for the free graft

Sterilized aluminum foil is used to create a pattern that precisely fits into the recipient bed. The apical edge of the pattern should be about of 2 mm short of the border of the bed.

If the graft is to be relatively straight and symmetrical (quadratic) a pattern may not be necessary and the free gingival graft can be taken using a mucotome.

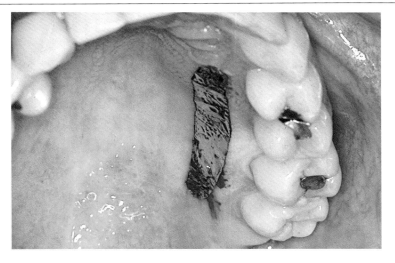

### Second surgical phase: Harvesting an individual palatal free graft

### 790  Aluminum foil pattern on the palate

The foil is placed onto the palate, about 2–3 mm removed from the gingival margin. A scalpel is used to incise around the pattern to a depth of 1 mm.

For patient comfort, the donor site should be on the same side of the mouth as the recipient site.

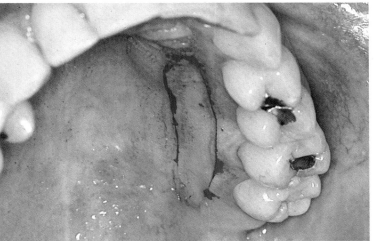

### 791  Palatal graft outlined by 1 mm incision

The graft must not contain rugae from the anterior palatal area as these would be transplanted with the graft.

Posteriorly, the graft must not encroach on the soft palate.

**792  Mobilization of the graft margin**
A gingivectomy knife is used to undermine and reflect the margins of the graft. A surgical forceps or the mini-hook (e. g., Gillis) can then be used to lift the tissue.

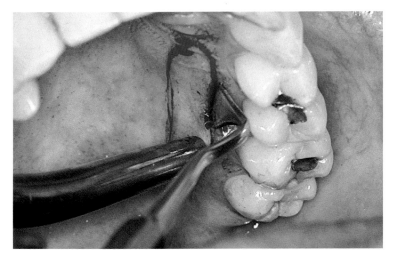

**793  Removing the graft**
The no. 15 scalpel is used to completely free the graft from the underlying tissue. Visible in the clinical view is yellow fatty tissue on the undersurface of the graft, indicating that it is somewhat too thick.

*Right:* After removal, the graft is placed on a sterile glass or wooden slab next to the foil pattern. The graft is thinned appropriately and trimmed to correspond exactly to the pattern.

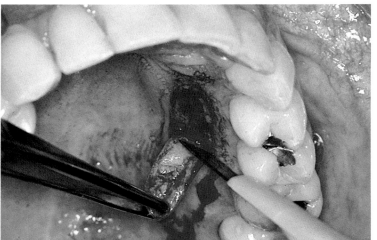
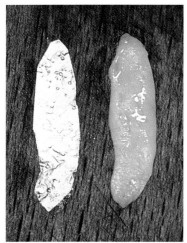

**794  Palatal donor site after graft removal**
Hemorrhage is generally slight, but if it is persistent, pressure applied over a gauze square, or repeated forceful injection of anesthetic with vasoconstrictor will stop it. In the extremely rare instance of excessive hemorrhage, the severed vessel may need to be ligated with resorbable suture.

A tissue adhesive such as cyanoacrylate may be applied directly to cover the donor site.

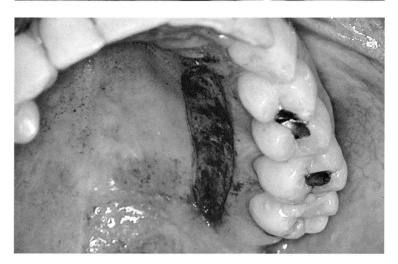

**795  Acrylic stent**
Covering the palatal wound with a "miniplast" stent requires more effort but is better insurance than coverage using a tissue adhesive. If severe bleeding occurs – which is relatively rare – the stent can be used with anticoagulant gauze as a pressure dressing. It inhibits painful mechanical contact with tongue and saliva, and protects the wound during eating.
The expanse of a miniplast stent can be seen on this model. Anterior teeth and palatal rugae remain uncovered.

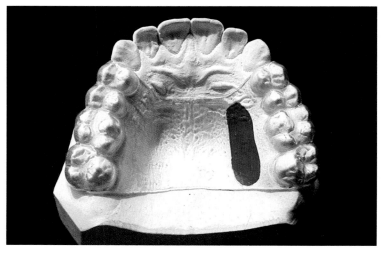

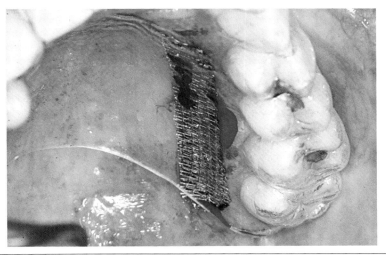

**796 Covering the donor site with coagulant-impregnated gauze and an acrylic stent**
Most patients wear the stent continuously for only the first few postoperative days, and thereafter only while eating or sleeping.

Re-epithelialization of the palatal wound begins at the wound margins. The rate of regrowth is about 0.5 mm per day. Thus, depending upon the expanse of the donor site, complete re-epithelialization can be expected in 10–14 days.

**Third operative phase: Graft placement**

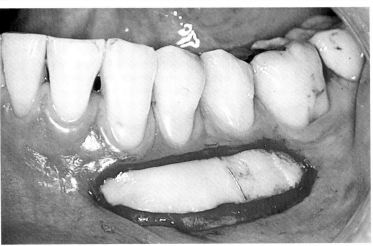

**797 FGG "in bed"**
The border of the FGG approximates the incision line. Apically, the extension wound is ca. 2 mm wider than the FGG.

*Caution:* The graft must be placed with its connective tissue side toward the periosteum.

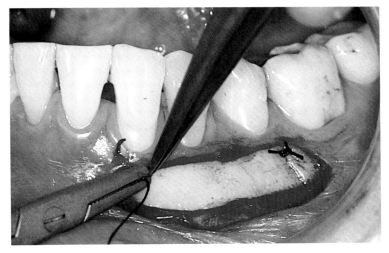

**798 Suturing the graft to place**
In this case sutures are first placed at the mesial and distal ends of the graft, then one additional suture is placed at each interdental area on the coronal graft margin. Thin, sharply curved, atraumatic needle/suture combinations are indicated (e.g., 4–0 or 5–0 silk).

*Alternative:* The FGG is held in place with finger pressure, then sealed at its coronal border using tissue adhesive, without sutures.

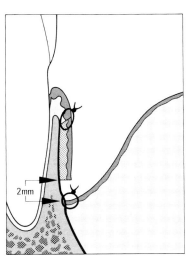

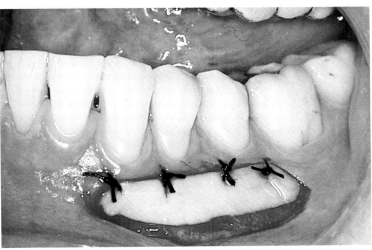

**799 End of surgical phase**
The finished graft should be held to place on the periosteum for 2–3 minutes using a moist gauze square under finger pressure. This prevents formation of a thick blood clot beneath the graft, which would tend to lift the graft from the bed. Periodontal dressing is generally not used. The patient is instructed not to brush in the area for 8 days.

*Left:* The FGG is about 2 mm smaller in coronoapical dimension than the extension wound.

# FGG – Wound Healing, Clinically …

The healing of a FGG generally proceeds without complications if the graft (ca. 1 mm thick) contains portions of the lamina propria in addition to epithelium (ca. 0.5 mm). About 2 days after transplant, portions of the epithelium are exfoliated. At this point the FGG is unsightly and appears necrotic. However, success of a FGG depends not upon the epithelium but upon the subepithelial connective tissue. New epithelialization occurs from the margin of the graft bed. Epithelium that grows in over the FGG from the mucosa differentiates upon the transplanted connective tissue into a kerati-nized "palatal" epithelium.

After one week, the graft has definitively healed into the recipient bed and is covered with a new epithelial layer. Complete keratinization is accomplished after ca. 4 weeks. The palatal wound re-epithelializes ca. 1–2 weeks later, depending upon the width of the graft.

Clinical *failure* is possible if the graft is placed with the epithelial surface apposed to the recipient bed, if a fixed coagulum forms between graft and bed, or if the graft is mechanically dislodged within the first two days after transplant (Sullivan & Atkins 1968a).

### FGG – Wound healing

**800  FGG immediately after surgery**
The graft appears quite pale. It has no circulation. Nutritive transfer occurs early on only via plasma that diffuses throughout the coagulum from the periosteal bed into the FGG. It is important that the FGG not be dislodged within the first few days.

*Right:* A blood coagulum exists between the transplant (**T**) and the surrounding tissues (periosteum, mucosa). The coagulum should be as thin as possible.

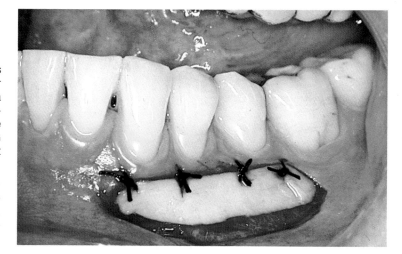
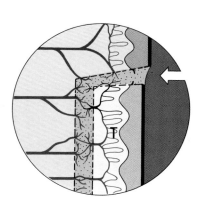

**801  2–3 days after surgery**
The surgical field generally appears "unpleasant" several days after the operation. The necrotic superficial layers (epithelium) of the graft are desquamating as the FGG becomes thinner.

Plaque accumulates because of the lack of home care, causing gingivitis in the surgical area.

*Right:* New vessels begin to penetrate into the transplant via the coagulum. At this point, the FGG has "taken."

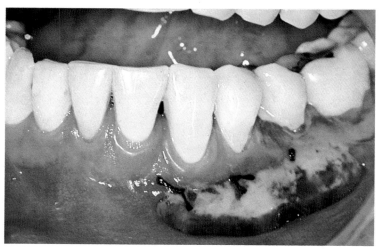

**802  7–8 days postoperative**
Sutures have been removed. The site is cleansed using 3% $H_2O_2$, the teeth using a rubber cup and toothpaste. The graft is firmly adherent to the recipient bed, but the epithelial layer is still very thin. The patient may now be permitted to begin home care in the area; gently at first, using a soft toothbrush.

*Right:* Vascular elements from the recipient bed have made contact with the vascular system of the graft. The circulatory continuity of the graft is again intact.

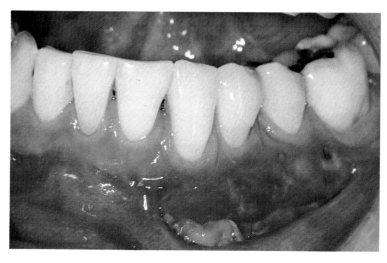
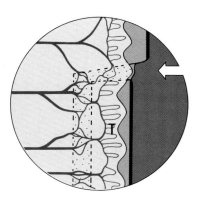

## ... and via Fluorescence Angiography

Fluorescence angiography is a technique that can be used to visualize the re-vascularization and healing in a free gingival graft (Mörmann et al. 1975).

Fifteen seconds after an i.v. injection of sodium fluorescein (20%), the infiltrated capillaries of the periodontal tissues can be photographed under ultraviolet light.

Immediately after surgery, the FGG remains vital thanks only to tissue fluid. The actual "healing in" (vascularization) begins on about the second postoperative day. One week later the healing process is almost complete. Apical to the graft, in the region of overextension, regeneration is not yet complete. A narrow zone is not yet vascularized.

Only after ca. 4 weeks does the graft exhibit the typical pale pink color of palatal mucosa. In some cases, e.g., in visible areas of the maxilla, this pale pink color of the graft may present esthetic problems.

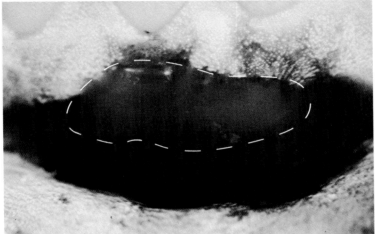

**FGG – Fluorescence angiographic study**

**803  Immediately after surgery**
The entire extension area is devoid of blood circulation (no fluorescence). Nutritive supply to the free graft occurs only by diffusion of tissue fluid from the recipient bed.

The dashed line demonstrates the margin of the FGG, ca. 6 mm in width.

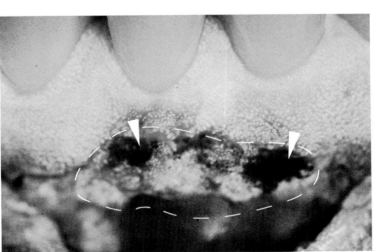

**804  Two days postoperative**
Initial vascularization of the free graft is noted, but several areas of ischemia persist (arrows). Extensive areas of the periosteum in the recipient bed apical to the free graft have not yet vascularized, while the marginal gingiva exhibits normal blood circulation.

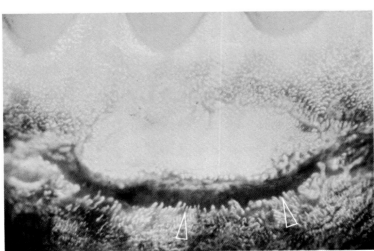

**805  Seven days postoperative operative**
The free graft is completely "accepted" and vascularized.

The apical region of the extension wound (not covered by the graft) appears to be closing slowly, with a narrow band (empty white arrows) still devoid of vasculature.

Courtesy W. Mörmann

# Gingival Extension Using Free Gingival Graft

## Summary

The 43-year-old female had employed a gross but intensive horizontal scrub toothbrushing technique for years. Canine and premolar areas exhibited pronounced, progressing recession with wedge-shaped defects at the CEJ. The dentition was almost plaque-free and there were no signs of inflammation.

Following a change to the modified Stillman technique and a subsequent 3-year period of observation (compared models), recession in the maxilla came to a halt; however, in the mandible the recession had continued to worsen.

Mucogingival surgery involving free gingival grafts was performed bilaterally in the mandible, thereby halting the recession. The newly created 5–6 mm of attached gingiva prevented further recession and made it possible for the patient to practice atraumatic home care.

### 806 Initial findings
Recession in the maxilla remained stable for 3 years after the toothbrushing technique was changed to modified Stillman.

However, recession in the mandible progressed, especially in canine and premolar areas. Eventually almost all of the attached gingiva was lost (to the mucogingival line, red arrow).

*Right:* The remaining attached gingiva between the black and red (MGL) arrows is only 1 mm wide. *No attached gingiva remains on the second premolar.*

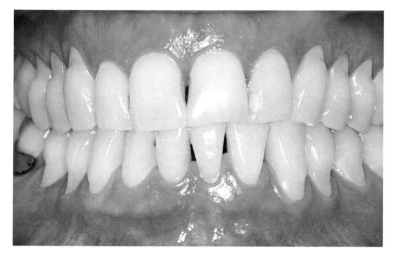
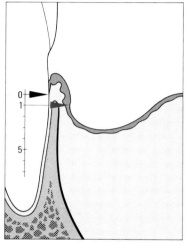

### 807 Facial recession (Re) and width of attached gingiva (AG) in the mandible
Before FGG: In the region of the planned graft, the gingival width is scarcely 1 mm (red), with 3–4 mm of recession.

Before

| | | 8 | 7 | 6 | 5 | 4 | 3 | 2 | 1 | 1 | 2 | 3 | 4 | 5 | 6 | 7 | 8 | | |
|---|---|---|---|---|---|---|---|---|---|---|---|---|---|---|---|---|---|---|---|
| Re Mand. | ✕ | | 2 | 3 | 3 | 4 | 3 | 2 | 2 | 2 | 2 | 3 | 4 | 3 | 4 | 2 | ✕ | Re Mand. |
| AG | ✕ | | 3 | 1 | 0 | 0 | 2 | 3 | 3 | 3 | 3 | 1 | 0 | 0 | 2 | 2 | ✕ | AG |

After

### Re and AG 5 years later
Gingival width in the treated areas is 5–6 mm. The progress of recession has been halted.

| | | 8 | 7 | 6 | 5 | 4 | 3 | 2 | 1 | 1 | 2 | 3 | 4 | 5 | 6 | 7 | 8 | | |
|---|---|---|---|---|---|---|---|---|---|---|---|---|---|---|---|---|---|---|---|
| Re Mand. | ✕ | | 2 | 3 | 3 | 4 | 3 | 2 | 2 | 2 | 2 | 3 | 4 | 3 | 4 | 2 | ✕ | Re Mand. |
| AG | ✕ | | 3 | 5 | 5 | 5 | 2 | 3 | 3 | 3 | 3 | 5 | 6 | 6 | 2 | 2 | ✕ | AG |

### 808 Five years postoperative
The surgical outcome (increased amount of attached gingiva) has halted the recession in the mandible. The rest of the mouth exhibits no further recession, probably as a result of the change in toothbrushing technique. The recall interval for recession cases is variable, usually every 6 months or longer.

Nine years after surgery the clinical picture remains identical.

*Right:* The attached gingiva has been extended and the vestibulum deepened (cf. Fig. 806).

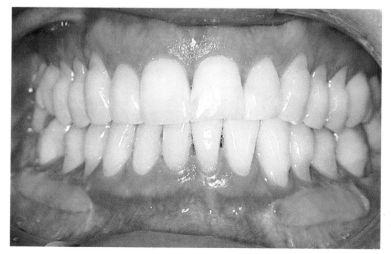
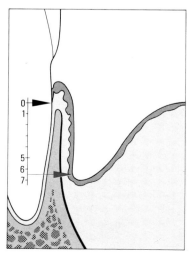

# FGG – Abutment Teeth

Abutment teeth for fixed bridges and removable partial dentures represent areas of particular concern because plaque accumulation is enhanced by crown margins and clasps. Oral hygiene is often difficult. If gingival recession occurs around an abutment tooth or if the width of attached gingiva is minimal, adequate plaque control may become extremely difficult. The free gingival graft offers one opportunity to resolve at least a portion of the problem.

In the case depicted below, a 30-year-old female was to be treated by means of a fixed bridge seated over an intraosseous implant in the edentulous mandibular molar region using the premolar and canine (43–44) as mesial abutments with full cast crowns. No periodontal pockets were present around 43 and 44, but attached gingiva was practically nonexistent, and an FGG procedure was planned.

*Findings:*

| | |
|---|---|
| HYG: 93% | PBI: 0.5 |
| TM: 0 at 43; 1 at 44 | |

The figures below depict the procedure.

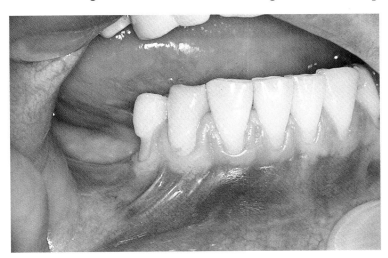

**809 Initial clinical appearance**
Teeth 43 and 44 exhibit severe recession. Attached gingiva is completely absent on 44. This tooth also exhibits a deep wedge-shaped defect. The treatment plan includes 43 and 44 as mesial abutments for a fixed bridge, which will be seated distally on an intraosseous implant.

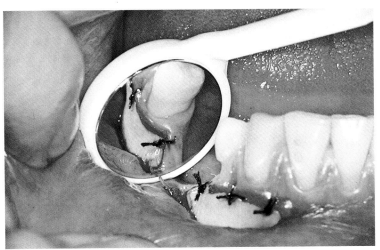

**810 Extension operation with FGG**
The arcuate free graft was taken as a customized explant from the palate. The graft extended from anterior of 43, around the distal surface of 44, and was sutured to place at its coronal margin. No periodontal dressing was placed.

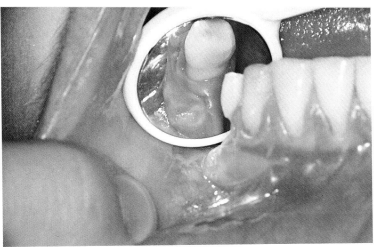

**811 Two months post-operatively**
The newly created 5 mm band of immobile attached gingiva created a favorable periodontal condition around the prospective abutments.
When the reconstruction is complete, patient home care will be simple and atraumatic.

# FGG Over Large Areas – The Mesh Graft

The palate does not provide an unlimited expanse of mucosa for free grafting procedures. The rugae area is not indicated as graft material, and an expansive palatal wound would be extremely uncomfortable for the patient. For these reasons it is advisable to refrain from trying to cover very large defects with a FGG in a single surgical procedure. The mesh graft provides a method whereby a free graft can be "stretched" to cover a larger area. By placing alternating incisions on either edge of the graft, it can be expanded as much as 50%.

In the case depicted, a 35-year-old female presented with progressing areas of recession and Stillman's clefts in the upper left quadrant. The treatment plan included use of a free gingival mesh graft to halt the recession. No periodontal pockets were present after initial therapy.

*Findings:*
HYG: 80%      PBI: 0.7      TM: 0
Clinical appearance is depicted in the figure.

**812  Recession and Stillman's clefts**
The initial clinical view exhibits the progressive recession and Stillman's clefts on teeth 22, 23 and 24. The mucogingival line is clearly visible because the area has been stained with Schiller's iodine solution.

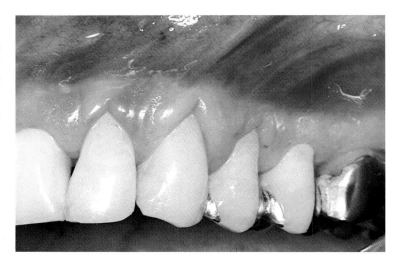

**813  Mesh graft before and after expansion**
In this 17 × 7 mm free graft, a scalpel was used to make alternating incisions on each edge. The tissue can be expanded to cover the recipient bed, which is 1.5 times longer than the graft.

*Right:* The expanded mesh graft is sutured at the mucogingival border. The "gaps" are immediately coronal to the interdental papillae, while grafted tissue is adjacent to the Stillman's clefts.

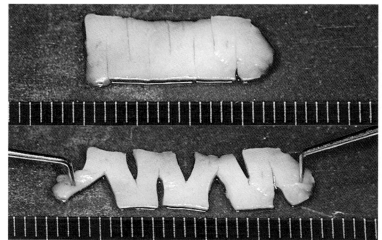

**814  Two years postoperative**
The original shape of the clearly visible free graft is not discernible. Keratinized epithelium has filled in the "gaps" in the original mesh graft.

*Right:* The biopsy is indicated by the black line in the clinical picture. **A** depicts the border between mucosa and graft. **B** shows *keratinized* epithelium from the region of the denuded area. The arrow indicates the mucogingival border.

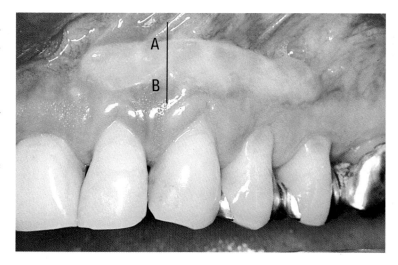

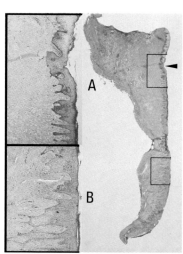

# Covering Areas of Recession?

By means of an extension operation with free gingival graft, the progress of recession can be stopped and the position of the gingival margin can be maintained at a given site. This represents the most important goal of mucogingival surgery.

In contrast, the indications for attempting to *cover* a denuded area are limited indeed. With few exceptions, they usually relate more to the esthetic aspirations of the patient than to biologic necessity.

## Indications

– Extremely advanced areas of recession which, despite treatment via free gingival grafting, are still difficult to clean adequately
– Esthetic concerns, especially in the maxilla. In such cases, however, it is prudent to remember that the often whitish, keratinized graft from the palate may itself represent an esthetic problem.
– Severe and persistent hypersensitivity of root surfaces.

## Contraindications

A denuded area that is not becoming larger or that has been successfully treated via free gingival graft does *not* require coverage. Attempting to cover such an area would have to be viewed as overtreatment or "l'art pour l'art" if one of the rare indications noted above were not present.

## Treatment options

The literature contains many surgical methods and techniques for covering areas of recession. These are discussed briefly below. Coronal repositioning after FGG will be depicted "step by step" in a clinical case (Bernimoulin 1973).

---

– **Laterally repositioned flap (sliding flap)**
– **Direct coverage via free gingival graft (FGG)**
– **Coronal repositioning subsequent to FGG**

---

1. One of the oldest methods for covering an area of recession is the *sliding flap* (Grupe & Warren 1956). It is only indicated for use in areas of localized recession. The principle of the operation is to elevate and reflect the gingiva and mucosa from a tooth exhibiting *no* reces-

sion, and then reposition it laterally as a pedicle graft onto the adjacent tooth to cover the exposed root surface. This method is plagued by a relatively high rate of recurrence. Furthermore, the donor site, which previously exhibited no recession, may develop recession after the sliding flap procedure. Because of this complication, Grupe (1966) modified his method by creating the pedicle flap with "stair step" incisions in the region of the adjacent gingiva. The gingival margin of the adjacent tooth thus remains undamaged. This procedure is not possible, however, if the adjacent tooth exhibits inadequate attached gingiva.

2. *Direct coverage* of a denuded area with a free gingival graft was described by Sullivan and Atkins (1968 a, b). According to the authors this procedure can only be successful in patients with very mild recession and Stillman clefts.

Holbrook and Ochsenbein (1983), on the other hand, showed direct coverage of expansive areas of recession that extended over several teeth. Using a relatively thick graft and a particular suture technique that ensured that the graft would be held firmly onto the underlying tissues, good results were achieved.

3. *Coronal repositioning* subsequent to free grafting, as described by Bernimoulin (1973) is one of the most promising methods for covering root surfaces denuded by recession (see pp. 307–310). An initial surgical procedure is performed to position a free gingival graft just apical to the area of recession. A waiting period of at least 2–3 months follows. In some cases "creeping attachment" occurs without any additional surgery, i.e., the gingiva simply grows coronally (see p. 306). If this does not occur, the denuded root surface can be covered by a second surgical procedure that involves repositioning the grafted tissue coronally.

Follow-up studies have shown that 70% of all denuded roots treated in this manner remain covered without formation of a periodontal pocket (Bernimoulin et al. 1975, Löst 1984 b). No histologic studies have been performed to demonstrate whether the attachment of the gingiva to the root surface occurs via a long junctional epithelium or by means of apposition of new connective tissue. Despite some claims, it is also unclear whether conditioning of the tooth/root surface with citric acid improves the soft tissue attachment to the root surface. It appears unlikely that true new attachment with the formation of new cementum and inserting fibers occurs.

## "Creeping Attachment" After FGG

A 38-year-old female presented with a chief complaint of "worsening denudation" of the cervical area of tooth 34. This tooth had been restored with a full cast crown four years previously during the course of the construction of a fixed bridge. The etiology of recession could not be immediately ascertained, although one could suspect that tension from the mobile mucosa played a part as there was practically no attached gingiva present. In addition, oral hygiene was rendered difficult by the high buccal frenum attachment.

A free gingival graft halted the progress of recession.

At the same time, the patient's home care regimen was modified to the vertical-rotatory method (modified Stillman). The gingival margin spontaneously migrated coronally, a process known as "creeping attachment."

This type of creeping attachment after FGG is not the norm and can only be expected in favorable cases (Matter 1980, Dorfman et al. 1982, Pollack 1984). The mechanism of creeping attachment is wholly unknown. One possible explanation is that the frenum pull on the mobile mucosa is eliminated.

**815 Initial clinical situation**
2 mm of gingival recession are observed on the buccal aspect of the crowned abutment tooth (34). The crown margin is clearly supragingival.

Only a narrow band of attached gingiva remains.

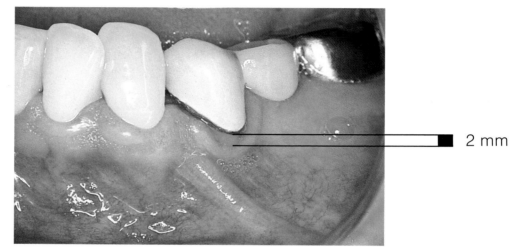

2 mm

**816 One month after free gingival graft**
The clinically visible exposed root surface is now only 1 mm wide.

A spontaneous coronal migration of the stabilized attached gingiva has occurred. The sulcus on the buccal aspect of 34 is not deepened.

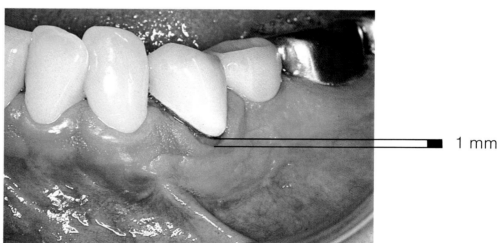

1 mm

**817 Two years after free gingival graft**
The recession on tooth 34 has almost completely disappeared. Less than 0.5 mm of root surface is exposed on the facial surface.

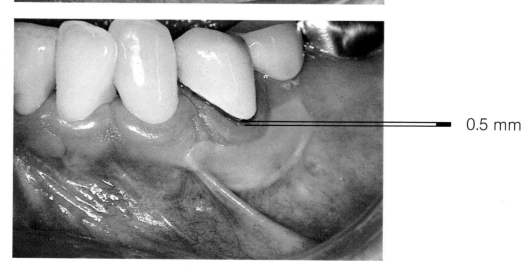

0.5 mm

# Coronal Repositioning After FGG

### Surgical procedure for the two-step operation

This 26-year-old complained of a pronounced, secondarily inflamed and esthetically disturbing area of recession on the facial aspect of tooth 41. The recession extended into the mobile oral mucosa.

Home care was above average, but in the area of 41 oral hygiene was difficult. In the area of exposed root surface there was plaque, calculus and a resultant mild chronic gingivitis. Lip movement caused direct tension on the gingival margin at 41 (pumping effect?).

Although it was possible to *halt* the progress of recession by means of a FGG, the patient also wished to have the existing defect *covered*.

*Findings after FGG:*
HYG: 88%
PBI: 0.8
TM: 0 except tooth 41 (TM = 1)
No periodontal pockets were present. The figures below depict clinical and radiographic findings.

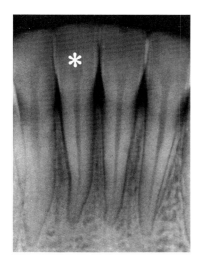
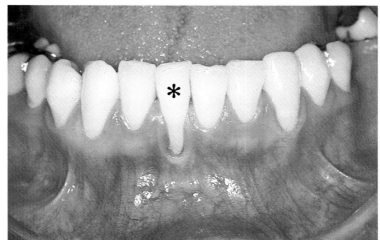

**818 Initial clinical view**
The entire mandible exhibits mild facial recession of 1–3 mm.

Pronounced 6 mm recession is clinically obvious on the facial surface of 41 (∗), extending to the mobile oral mucosa and manifesting marginal inflammation. No periodontal pocketing was detected.

*Left:* The radiograph does not reveal the facial osseous dehiscence on tooth 41.

**First procedure: FGG**

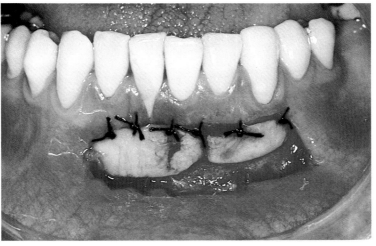

**819 Free gingival graft**
Two small free gingival grafts have been sutured to place in the anterior area between 42 and 33. This would be expected to halt the recession.

The FGG near tooth 41 would have been adequate for treatment of this tooth alone; however, because tooth 33 also exhibited only minimal attached gingiva, the FGG was extended distally.

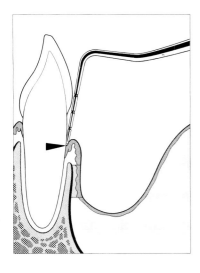
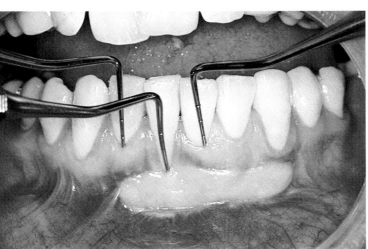

**820 Two months after FGG**
The clinical situation is one of freedom from inflammation and pockets.

It would be reasonable to wait 1–2 years for the possibility of creeping attachment. However, the patient demanded an immediate covering of the defect, which she found esthetically disfiguring. Hypersensitivity of the exposed root surface was also a significant concern.

*Left:* No pockets are present (arrow). The attached gingiva has been widened by the FGG.

## Second surgical procedure: Coronal repositioning

### 821 Surgical plan – Incisions

**1** *Marginal*
An arcuate incision is planned for the facial surface of 41. The "new papillae" are outlined laterally by this initial incision.

**2** *Vertical*
The horizontal incision is carried vertically over teeth 42 and 31.

**3** *Gingivectomy*
Only the epithelium of the papillae coronal to the horizontal incision is excised to prepare a recipient bed.

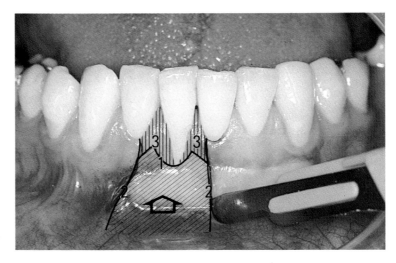

### 822 Incisions 1 + 2

– *Horizontal incision* (**1**): A scalloped incision outlines the shape of the future gingival margin.

– *Vertical incisions* (**2**): These extend from the adjacent teeth (paramedial) into the free mucosa. These incisions outline the tissue flap, which is repositioned coronally (Fig. 821).

*Right:* The schematic depicts the recession, the sulcus (arrow), the free gingival graft and the horizontal internal bevel incision at the cervix of the tooth.

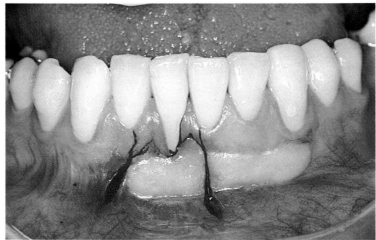
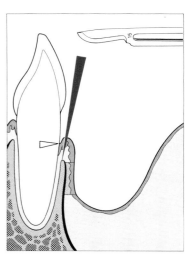

### 823 Creating a flap – Gingivectomy of the "old" papillae

After reflection of a mucoperiosteal flap, only the facial epithelium of the adjacent papilla is excised almost vertically using a gingivectomy knife (see incision 3 in Fig. 821). This provides a connective tissue bed for the flap that will be repositioned coronally.

*Right:* Using a papilla knife, only the facial aspect of the "old" papilla is removed. This creates the recipient bed upon which the coronally repositioned flap will be affixed.

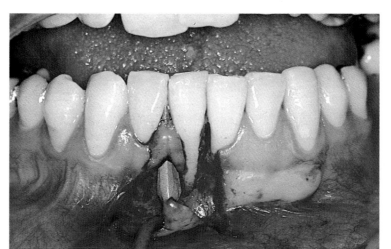
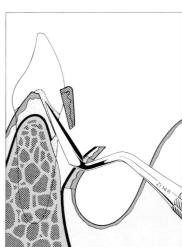

### 824 Root planing

After reflection of the soft tissue flap, it became clear that the osseous facial dehiscence was even more pronounced than the gingival recession.

The root surface exposed by the gingival recession is thoroughly cleaned and planed. Root surfaces exposed by flap reflection should not be treated, however, because the tissue can reattach to pre-existing healthy fibers.

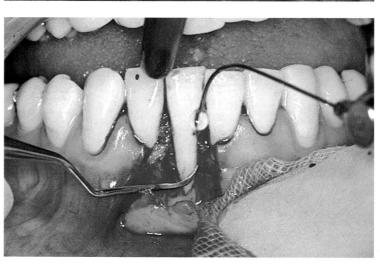

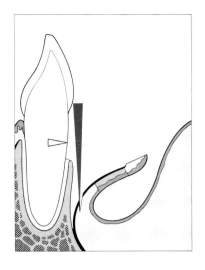

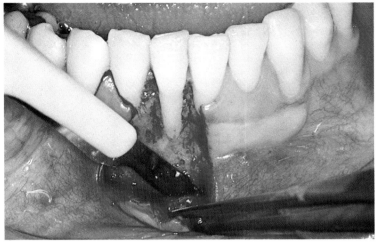

### 825  Severing the periosteum
At the base of the flap, in the area of the mobile oral mucosa, the resilient periosteum is incised completely along the entire extent of the flap, using a no. 15 scalpel. This permits coronal repositioning of the flap without tension.

This incision must be made with care to avoid severing the supraperiosteal blood vessels or the flap itself.

*Left:* Schematic representation of the periosteal incision (red.) The empty black arrow depicts the former position of the gingival margin.

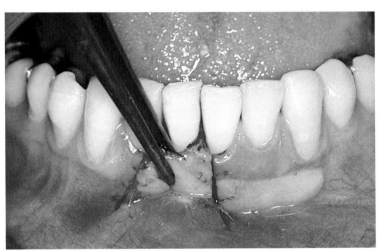

### 826  Coronal repositioning
The flap has been completely mobilized and can be positioned coronally without tension.

If tension exists, e.g., because the periosteal incision was incomplete, the flap may become necrotic and the recession will recur.

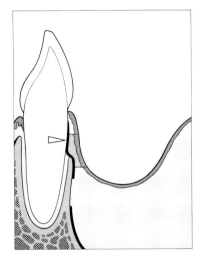

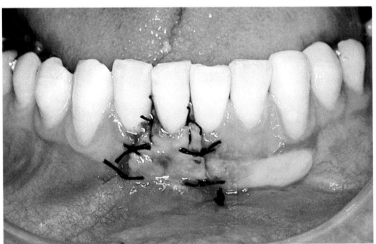

### 827  Immediately after surgery
The incision described above led to the creation of a new gingival margin and new papillae. After coronal repositioning of the flap, the new papillae lie directly upon the highly vascular recipient beds prepared by the gingivectomy. The flap is secured by interrupted sutures interdentally and over the vertical incisions.

*Left:* The effect of evening the periosteum (extending the flap coronally) becomes clear. The empty black arrow depicts the former position of the margin.

### 828  6 months after coronal repositioning
The denuded area on 41 is completely covered, and *no* pocket can be probed on the facial aspect. The step-like indentation in the free graft (line) demonstrates the degree of coronal repositioning of the attached gingiva.

# Coronal Repositioning After FGG

### Summary

A localized area of recession was noted on tooth 41, extending into the oral mucosa. Home care in the area was difficult and the gingival margin was inflamed. A free gingival graft was placed to halt the progression of recession. Nine weeks after graft placement, a second surgical procedure involving coronal repositioning of the grafted tissue was performed at the patient's request (esthetics, hypersensitivity of the exposed root surface) in an attempt to cover the root surface of 41. Eight years later, no recurrence of the recession has occurred.

This degree of success is not always achieved by coronal repositioning. Recurrent recession of about 30% may be expected (Bernimoulin et al. 1975).

The labial plate of bone will not regenerate. Attachment of the gingiva to the root surface is probably via a long junctional epithelium (epithelial attachment with basal lamina and hemidesmosomes).

**829   Initial clinical view**
The mandible exhibits mild generalized recession, while the labial root surface of 41 is exposed by the pronounced 6 mm recession that extends beyond the mucogingival line. No attached gingiva remains in this region nor are there any periodontal pockets.

*Right:* Initial conditions in orofacial section. Gingival recession without periodontal pocketing (black arrow).

Before

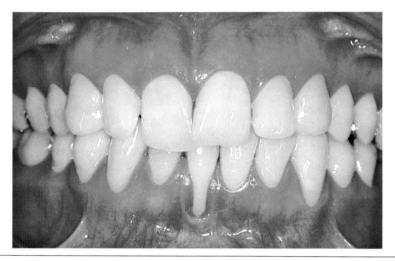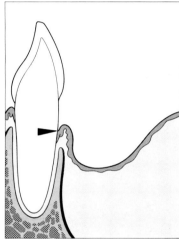

After

**830   8 years after surgery**
The 6 mm defect on tooth 41 that was covered by coronal flap repositioning remains free of recession, and there is no periodontal pocket on the labial surface. The zone of attached gingiva in the area is now 5 mm wide.

*Right:* The coronal repositioning, as indicated by the red and black arrows, remains stable. The connection between tooth and soft tissue is probably by means of a long junctional epithelium.

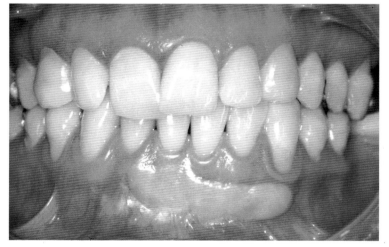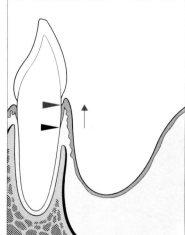

# Periodontics – Endodontics

The relationship of the periodontium to the endodontium (pulp contents) is indeed an intimate one (Ketterl 1984). These two anatomic entities are quite literally connected to each other at the apical foramen and via lateral canals. Thus, pulp pathology may directly effect the periodontal tissues. On the other hand, but less often, advanced periodontitis or severe recession may occasion pulpal inflammation or necrosis by way of the apex, lateral canals or the furcation.

In their comprehensive textbook, Guldener and Langeland (1982) proposed a classification of the possible pathologic relationships between the periodontium and endodontium:

| | |
|---|---|
| Class I | Primarily endodontic problems |
| Class II | Primarily periodontal problems |
| Class III | Combined endodontic and periodontal problems |

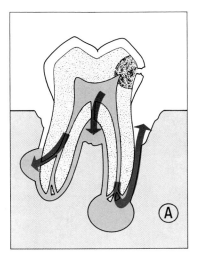 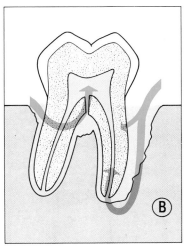 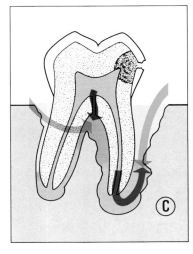

**831  Endo/perio problems – Classification**

**A  Class I, primarily endodontic**
Infection via apex or accessory canals (furcation). Usually a quite narrow and difficult to probe "drainage canal" exists near the gingival margin.

**B  Class II, primarily periodontal**
Infection of the pulp from the pocket via furcation, apex, lateral canals. A "wide" pocket can usually be probed.

**C  Class III, combined endo/perio problem**
Fusion of endodontic and periodontal lesions.

This classification system includes infectious and inflammatory processes of the dental pulp and the periodontium, as well as combined forms of these pathologic processes in both structures. In a broader sense, endodontic/periodontic problems also include iatrogenically caused damage such as perforation and traumatic influences through accidents. Perforation may lead to peri- or intraradicular lesions that may communicate with a periodontal pocket, especially if the perforation is coronally located or if the periodontitis has already progressed far apically. Accidental trauma can injure and contaminate the periodontium, and can also lead to infection, necrosis or trauma within the pulp.

Here we will discuss only the "classic," infectious endo/perio problems. Frequently in such cases the practitioner must decide early on whether a tooth can be saved or whether it might more prudently be extracted.

Clinical data gathering in endo/perio problems is often complex, requiring special medical-dental history, vitality testing, pocket and furcation probing, tooth mobility determination as well as critical examination of radiographs. Findings from all these sources must be synthesized in order to formulate a diagnosis and the appropriate treatment plan.

## Endo/Perio, Class I

The acute inflammatory manifestations in the case shown below are of primarily endodontic origin. There is a simultaneous pronounced loss of attachment. The pulp is necrotic, beneath a large amalgam restoration. The inflammatory process at the apex has expanded coronally, especially on the mesial root but also toward the furcation. The apical lesion communicates with a periodontal pocket.

During clinical data gathering, only the coronal portion of the mesial (periodontal) pocket could be probed, and the tooth was not vital ($CO_2$-test). Diffuse demineralization is clearly visible in the radiograph, which does not portray the usual periodontal pocket.

In terms of therapy, endodontic treatment should always be performed first. Remnants of the attachment apparatus that may have been affected by the endodontic pathology should never be disturbed by deep scaling procedures. A waiting period of at least several months should be observed after endodontic therapy, at which time the periodontal lesions can be treated by closed or open (furcation) scaling.

The prognosis is generally good with regular recall.

**832   Class I**
**Acute endodontic problem in a periodontally involved tooth**
A *Initial findings:* Periodontal attachment loss. Radiolucency on mesial root, extending to apex. Therapy: Initial medicinal root canal filling.
B *Interim finding:* Overfilling with resorbable iodoform paste.
C *Final view:* Three months after definitive root canal filling, the lesion on the mesial root exhibits significant regeneration. Periodontal therapy (scaling) can now be undertaken.

Courtesy *H. M. Meyer*

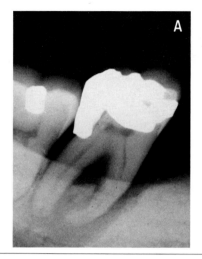
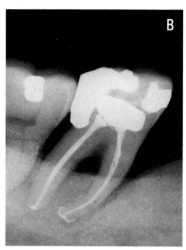
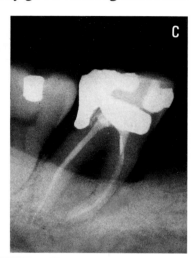

## Endo/Perio, Class II

Lesions of primary periodontal origin are usually encountered on teeth with very deep pockets that approach the apically located lateral pulp canals or even the apex of the tooth itself. This can lead to retrograde pulpitis or pulpal necrosis. Such teeth are often hopeless and should be extracted if they are not of special esthetic or functional significance for the total treatment plan. In the case described below the involved tooth is number 21; the decision was made to attempt to retain this tooth, because extraction would necessitate a costly and complicated bridge construction.

During clinical data gathering a very deep and broad infrabony pocket was detected, from which pus exuded after probing. The tooth was nonvital (the patient had experienced pulpitis several weeks previously). The radiograph revealed the typical shape of a periodontal pocket (see also p. 77, Fig. 176).

*Therapy* was initiated, including initial root canal therapy and subsequent periodontal treatment.

The *prognosis* is questionable with such severe periodontal involvement and a Class II perio-endo lesion.

**833   Class II**
**Primarily periodontal problem**
A *Initial findings:* The localized 11 mm pocket on the mesiopalatal aspect of tooth 21 has occasioned retrograde pulpitis.
B *Interim finding:* Following endodontic treatment, root planing was performed with a flap procedure and the mobile tooth was temporarily splinted by connecting the adjacent restorations.
C *Final view:* Twelve years later, new bone formation is observed. The splint has been in situ for 11 years.

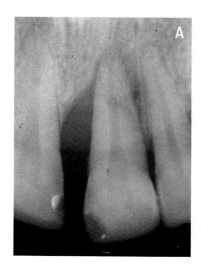
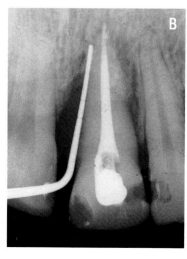
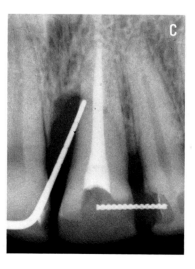

# Endo/Perio, Class III

A true combined lesion results from fusion of endodontic and periodontal lesions that developed independently. Clinical probing usually reveals a more or less broad and continuous defect extending from the gingival margin to the tooth apex. Retention and maintenance of such teeth is questionable and should only be undertaken if loss of the tooth would necessitate extensive reconstruction or if the tooth is an important abutment for bridgework.

In the case depicted here, a 55-year-old female presented with untreated, severe periodontitis (AP). If the questionable tooth 32 were extracted, it is possible that the other mandibular front teeth would also be lost since these would be insufficient as bridge abutments.

Clinical examination revealed generalized periodontitis, heavy plaque accumulation, and a pocket extending to the apex of tooth 32.

The combined periodontal and endodontic therapy must be viewed as a heroic experiment.

The *prognosis* is generally questionable. In the case presented here, however, the long-term success was good.

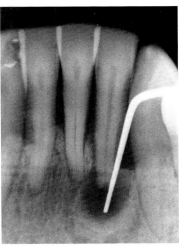
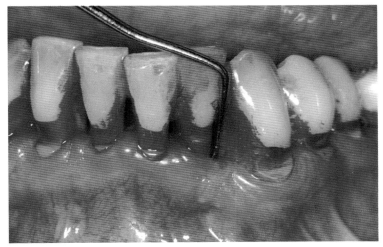
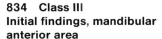

**834 Class III
Initial findings, mandibular anterior area**
Generalized, advanced periodontitis with gingival shrinkage. The patient was not motivated nor had she ever received oral hygiene instructions. Heavy plaque accumulation (disclosing agent). 12 mm pocket on the distobuccal of 32.

*Left:* Pronounced periapical lesion on 32, communicating with the deep distobuccal pocket. Advanced horizontal bone loss.

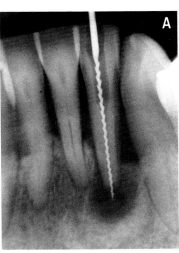
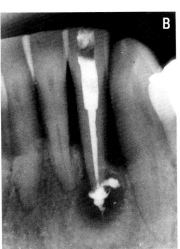
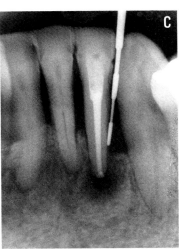

**835 Sequence of the endodontic therapy**
A Broad instrumentation of the canal using Hedstrom files.
B Filling the radiolucency with resorbable iodoform paste (Caution: iodine allergy). Scaling of the coronal aspect of the root surface.
C Definitive root canal filling 8 months after initial therapy. Probing which previously reached the apex (cf. Fig. 834 left), now stops at the alveolar margin.

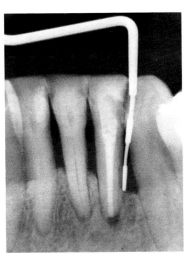
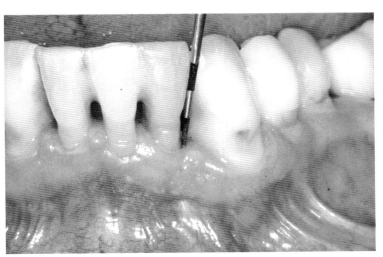

**836 Situation 3 years later**
The pocket has been reduced (CP 12 periodontal probe).

Since initiation of therapy, this patient continued exceptional home care. Teeth 41, 31 and 32 were splinted using composite resin.

*Left:* The apical radiolucency and the draining pocket appear to be almost completely resolved.

# Medicaments

Medicaments are frequently used before, during and after periodontal therapy. The specific mechanisms of action, side effects, indications and contraindications as well as possible interactions of such medicaments must be understood by the dentist. Patients today, especially elderly patients, frequently are already taking various medicines prescribed by physicians for systemic conditions, and these must be taken into consideration before any additional medicines are employed for dental reasons. The spectrum of activity of the medicaments permits their classification into the following four groups:

| |
|---|
| Gingivitis/periodontitis treatment (topical, systemic) |
| Relief of pain and swelling, wound treatment |
| Antibiotic coverage |
| Systemic medications |

## Medicaments for Treatment for Gingivitis and Periodontitis

There exist today no medicaments or vaccines that are effective over the long term for prevention or treatment of gingivitis and periodontitis. As adjuncts to purely mechanical therapy, however, topical as well as some systemic medications may be employed (Helldén et al. 1979, 1981; Müller et al. 1986; Hartmann et al. 1986; Gjermo 1986; Quee et al. 1987; Wolff et al. 1987; Addy 1988).

Most of the agents may be regarded as nonspecific *"causal therapy"* directed generally at the microorganisms of supra- and subgingival plaque.

Medicaments may be used in periodontitis patients:

- For treatment of acute conditions
- For pre-treatment and post-treatment in conjunction with local mechanical therapy
- For support of local therapy in juvenile periodontitis (LJP) and rapidly progressive periodontitis (RPP) as well as "refractory" forms
- For treatment of symptoms that develop after periodontal therapy, e.g., hypersensitive teeth.

### Therapy for acute conditions

Acute infections, especially periodontitis with ANUG, may be treated in the initial stages by means of *topically* applied ointments and mouthwashes containing disinfectant and anti-inflammatory agents. Simultaneously, however, or at the latest during the second appointment, local mechanical therapy including professional tooth cleaning and home care by the patient must also be instituted. Systemic drugs are only extremely rarely employed.

### Medicinal treatments before, during and after local (mechanical) periodontitis therapy

● *Treatment for gingivitis and slowly progressing adult periodontitis (AP)*

In such cases, mechanical therapy is the most important, but *topically* applied rinsing solutions that inhibit plaque (chlorhexidine, hexetidine, $H_2O_2$) may be pre-scribed as adjunctive therapy for short-term use. *Systemic* administration of antibiotics is *not* indicated for treatment of gingivitis or adult periodontitis (AP).

- *Treatment for juvenile (LJP) and rapidly progressive (RPP) periodontitis*

Systemic therapy for these relatively rare periodon-tal diseases is possible today because research has clari-fied the nature of the bacterial infection.

Thus, systemic tetracycline has been recommended as an adjunct to mechanical/surgical therapy for LJP, although Saxen et al. (1986) achieved equally good results with and without use of antibiotics. During mechanical therapy tetracycline may be adminstered over a 10-day course (1 g/day, in 2 doses of 0.5 g). The course of therapy can be repeated using an identical dose several months later, i.e., at the first recall visit or if follow-up therapy becomes necessary.

In RPP patients with repeated destructive episodes, imidazole derivatives such as *metronidazole (Flagyl)* or *ornidazol* (Tiberal) have also been shown effective as ad-juncts to local therapy,when administered over a 10-day course (1 g/day, in 2 doses of 0.5 g). The practitioner must be aware of side effects and contraindications for all systemic medications (see Table, pp. 316–317).

Topical application of these otherwise systemic medicaments is extremely rare today, but experiments with impregnated fibers are providing promising data. Such fibers are inserted into the periodontal pocket and release medicaments slowly (Goodson et al. 1979, 1985; Lindhe et al. 1979; Addy et al. 1982).

### Treatment of problems resulting from periodontal therapy

The most unpleasant consequence of local/mech-anical periodontitis therapy is hypersensitively of ex-posed root surface, which is common.

Despite the availability of several OTC products, hypersensitivity of exposed root surfaces often takes a long time to combat. Most frequently, *topically* applied agents are recommended. Most of these are protein-denaturing astringents, or agents that enhance min-eralization (closure of dentinal tubules). For home care, dentifrices with *formalin* ("Emoform"), *strontium chloride* ("Sensodyne"), or *calcium nitrate* ("Denquel") are available. The same chemical agents are available in more concentrated forms for use in the dental practice as topical agents. Attempts have also been made to use iontophoresis to impel various medicaments (e.g., NaF) intensively into dentin.

## Prevention of Pain and Swelling – Wound Treatment

If surgical intervention is necessary after the com-pletion of initial therapy, the approach favored today is selective and atraumatic (e.g., open curettage, ENAP, modified Widman). Such procedures usually require neither pre-operative nor postoperative systemic medi-cations.

If surgery is more complex or of longer duration, a pain medication may be required, such as *Paracetamol* (Seymour 1983).

For prevention of postoperative edema after exten-sive surgical procedures, medicaments from the *antiph-*

*logistic* and *antirheumatic* categories may be adminis-tered immediately prior to surgery and for several days thereafter. Examples: *Motrin* 400, *Ponstan* 500, *Volta-ren* 50 etc. During the first few days after surgery it is advisable to suggest application of cold compresses over the site.

Two of the most important aspects of periodontal surgery are good flap adaptation and tight suture clo-sure. Various periodontal dressings are also available to protect the surgical site.

## Antibiotic coverage

The hemorrhage that always accompanies scaling, root planing and surgery routinely leads to bacteremia. This is usually of no consequence in a healthy individual, but for patients with certain systemic disorders it can be life threatening. High risk patients include those with heart valve replacement, in whom bacterial endocarditis may occur. Somewhat less critical are patients with con-genital cardiac arrhythmia, mitral valve prolapse with mitral insufficiency, or hypertropic cardiomyopathy.

Antibiotic coverage for such patients may include the following medicaments and dosages:

- *Amoxycillin* 3 g per os 1 h before surgery, then q 6 h 750 mg per os for 36 h.

- *Clindamycin* (600 mg per os) 1 h before surgery, then 300 mg every 6 h (for 36 h) if the patient has a history of allergy to penicillin.

(continued p. 318)

# Periodontitis Therapy – Medicaments for Local Use

| Medicament (Concentration) | Effect Indication (Ind.) | Side effects Contraindication (Contr.) |
|---|---|---|
| **Chlorhexidine (CHX)** | Inhibits plaque formation | Reversible staining of teeth and tongue Influences taste sensation Desquamation of mucosa and disturbance of wound healing with excessive CHX concentration |
| – **CHX digluconate** mouthwash (p. 158), 0.1–0.2% | | |
| Products: – **Peridex** 0.12% *(Procter & Gamble)* – **Corsodyl** 0.2% *(ICI)* – **Chlorhexamed** 0.1% *(Blend-a-Med)* – **Plak-Out** concentrate 10% *(Hawe)* | *Ind.:* Adjunct to mechanical plaque control before and after periodontal surgery | *Contr.:* Exposed bone Long-term use |
| – **CHX digluconate** gel Products: – **Corsodyl** 1% – **Plak-Out** 0.1% | | |
| – **CHX dihydrochloride** powder (p. 159) Product: – **pure substance** 100% *(ICI)* | *Ind.:* Use under periodontal dressing | *Contr.:* Exposed bone |
| **Hexetidine** | Plaque inhibition (less effective than CHX, but research shows it to be extremely effective when used in combination with ZnF$_2$) | Slight, reversible staining Mild influence on taste sensitivity |
| Product: – **Hextril** *(Warner-Chilcott)* 0.1% rinsing solution | *Ind.:* Instead of CHX | *Contr.:* – |
| **Hydrogen peroxide (H$_2$O$_2$)** Products: – 3–10% solution for topical application – 0.3–0.5% rinsing solution | Cleansing and disinfection Some plaque inhibition | Tissue damage with long-term use? "Emphysema" if applied under pressure (syringe) |
| | *Ind.:* Wound clean-up Perio pocket rinsing Initial therapy for ANUG | *Contr.:* – |
| **Sodium perborate in a combined preparation** Products: – **Amosan** *(Cooper),* – **Kavosan** *(Cooper)* sodium perborate, sodium bitartrate, menthol, powder for making rinsing solution | Analgesic | Tissue damage with long-term use? |
| | *Ind.:* For home use by patient Initial therapy for ANUG | *Contr.:* – |
| **Sodium bicarbonate concentrate (NaHCO$_3$)** Product: – paste made from powder, H$_2$O$_2$ and water | Some disinfectant and plaque inhibitory action | None known |
| | *Ind.:* "Keyes technique" (1978a, b) as a dentifrice in gingivitis and periodontitis | *Contr.:* Effectiveness? |
| **Tetracycline** (ointment) | Antibacterial Bacteriostatic | Hypersensitivity reaction |
| Products: – **Achromycin ophthalmic ointment** *(Lederle)* (tetracycline-HCl, 1%) – **Aureomycin ointment** *(Lederle)* (chlortetracycline-HCl, 1% or 3%) | *Ind.:* Acute pocket exacerbation Under periodontal dressing In combination with an adherent salve (e.g., Oratran, Orabase) to cover aphthae or infected ulcerations | *Contr.:* ANUG lesions (necrosis, gram-negative anaerobes!) |
| **Corticosteroids in combination with antibiotics** (ointments) (formula: prednisone) | Anti-inflammatory Analgesic (Antibacterial) | Hypersensitivity reaction Overgrowth of resistant strains |
| Products: – **Terracortril** with tetracycline-HCl *(Pfizer)* – **Locacorten** with neomycin *(Ciba)* – **Dontisolon** with neomycin *(Hoechst); and others* | *Ind.:* Initial therapy for ANUG Acute, painful lesions of gingiva and mucosa | *Contr.:* Acute infections (inflammation) that do not heal within a few days (mycotic, luetic, tuberculous or viral lesions) |

# Periodontitis Therapy – Medicaments for Systemic Adjunctive Treatment

| Medicament<br>(Dosage: Number × tablets × days) | Effect<br>Indication (Ind.) | Side effects<br>Contraindication (Contr.) |
|---|---|---|
| **Tetracycline**<br>(tablets, capsules)<br><br><br><br>Products: – **Hostacyclin 500** (*Hoechst*, 500 mg tetracycline-HCl)<br>2×1×8 to 2×1×14<br>– **Ledermycin** (*Lederle*, 300 mg demethylchlortetracycline)<br>2×1×8 to 2×1×14<br>– **Vibramycin** (*Pfizer*, 100 mg doxycyclin)<br>2×1×8 to 2×1×14 | Variably effective against *gram-positive* and *-negative* organisms, incl. Actinobacillus actinomycetemcomitans (Aa) (broad spectrum antibiotic)<br><br>Bacteriostatic<br>Reduces collagen breakdown<br><br>*Ind.:* Adjunct to local mechanical treatment in *juvenile periodontitis* **(LJP)**<br>Possibly also effective in rapidly progressive periodontitis **(RPP)** | Sensitivity to light<br>Hypersensitivity reactions<br>Often ineffective due to resistant strains<br><br>*Contr.:* Severe liver or kidney disfunction (acidosis)<br>Reduces effect of contraceptives<br>Not in combination with penicillin<br><br>*Relative contr.:* Children to age 8<br>Pregnancy |
| **Imidazoles**<br>– **Metronidazole**<br>(tablets)<br><br><br><br>Product: – **Flagyl** (*Specia*, 250 mg metronidazole)<br>3×1×8 to 4×1×14<br><br>– **Ornidazole**<br>(tablets)<br><br><br><br>Product: – **Tiberal** (*Roche*, 500 mg ornidazole)<br>2×1×8 to 2×1×14 | Especially effective against *gram-negative anaerobes* such as Bacteroides, Fusobacteria, Spirochetes and Protozoa<br><br>Bactericidal<br>*Ind.:* Adjunctive to local mechanical therapy in rapidly progressive periodontitis **(RPP)** and possibly in ulcerative periodontitis **(ANUG)**<br><br>(In combination with *penicillin* for antibiotic coverage [p. 315], and for protection against osteomyelitis etc.) | Digestive disturbance<br>Nausea<br>Reversible leukopenia<br><br><br>*Contr.:* CNS disorders<br>Blood dyscrasias<br>1st trimester of pregnancy<br>Alcohol intolerance<br>(metronidazole)<br><br>*Interaction with hydantoin!* |
| **Spiramycin**<br>(tablets)<br><br><br><br>Product: – **Rovamycin 500** (*Specia*, 500 mg spiramycin)<br>3×1×8 to 4×1×10 | Effective against *gram-positive* (and *-negative*) organisms<br><br>Bactericidal<br><br>*Ind.:* Adjunctive to local mechanical therapy in *rapidly progressive periodontitis* **(RPP)** and possibly during *active, suppurating phases of adult periodontitis* **(AP)** | Gastrointestinal disturbance including nausea, vomiting, diarrhea<br>Allergy (rare)<br><br>*Contr.:* None known |
| **Combined preparations:**<br><br>**Antibiotic & chemotherapeutic**<br>(tablets)<br><br>Product: – **Rodogyl** (*Specia*, 250 mg spiramycin plus 125 mg metronidazole)<br>4×1×8 to 6×1×10 | Effective against *gram-positive* and *-negative aerobes* such as Staphylococci and Streptococci, and against *gram-negative anaerobes* such as Bacteroides, Spirochetes etc.<br><br>Bactericidal<br><br>*Ind.:* Adjunctive to mechanical therapy in *progressive* **(RPP)** and *juvenile* **(LJP)** periodontitis<br>(Also indicated for presurgical antibiotic coverage) | Nausea, vomiting<br>Digestive disturbances<br>Diarrhea<br>Allergic reaction (rare)<br><br><br>*Contr.:* Neurologic disorders<br>Hematopoietic disturbances<br>*(Alcohol intolerance)* |

(continued from p. 315)

These suggestions are taken from recommendations by the American Heart Association, the British Society of Antimicrobial Chemotherapy and the Swiss Working Group for Endocarditis Prevention. *The recommendations are continually modified by these organizations to keep pace with the current state of knowledge.*

Because gram-negative Bacteroides sp. and *Actinobacillus actinomycetemcomitans* may also play a role in endocarditis, more recent recommendations for coverage have included a combination of the above-mentioned antibiotics with metronidazol (Mühlemann 1983, Slots et al. 1983).

## Systemic Medications

Many individuals, especially the elderly, take systemic medications continually or occasionally (Seymour & Heasman 1988). This fact must be considered during the planning of periodontal therapy. Each patient's medical history is of special importance. Some of the most significant considerations include:

● *Patients on anticoagulants*

Surgical procedures should be avoided, but if surgery is imperative the patient's "Quick time" should be slightly increased for a short period in collaboration with the physician.

– Quick time below 10%: Danger of spontaneous hemorrhage
– Quick time above 30%: Danger of thrombosis

Certain medications among those used in dentistry can potentiate the effects of anticoagulants by *lowering* the prothrombin value (Newman & Goodman 1984, AAP 1987b):

Chloramphenicol (Chlormycetin), co-trimoxazol (Bactrim etc.), sulfonamide, mefenamino acids (Ponstan), metronidazole (Flagyl), oxyphenbutazone (Tanderil), phenylbutazone (Butazolidine), salicylate (aspirin).

The effects of anticoagulant medications may be reduced by the following medications, which *increase* the prothrombin time: barbiturates, carbamazepine (Tegretol), also chronic alcoholism.

● *Patients on corticosteroid therapy*

It may be necessary to consult with the physician before periodontal treatment in such patients, whose host response may be reduced or in whom wound healing may be disturbed. Additional dangers in this group include diabetes, hyperglycemia, reduced stress reaction and circulatory collapse.

● *Patients on immunosuppressant drugs,* which are commonly prescribed for autoimmune diseases and following organ transplantation (azathioprine, corticosteroids, cyclosporine). These drugs may lead to reduced host response to infection (bacterial, mycotic, viral, protozoan), increased susceptibility to tumor formation, and gingival overgrowth (cyclosporine; p. 60).

● *Patients on antihypertensive drugs*

If blood pressure is normal, the use of local anesthetics containing small amounts of adrenaline (1:100,000) is permissible. Adrenaline-containing retraction strings or hemostyptics should not be used, nor should noradrenalin-containing local anesthetics. Vasopressin as vasoconstrictor in local anesthetics can be recommended.

● *Diabetes patients taking oral or injectable insulin*

They exhibit reduced host response (Staphylococcus, soor), disturbances of wound healing, spontaneous oral ulcers, and insulin-related hypoglycemia.

Local anesthetic solutions containing adrenaline must not be used (insulin antagonist). Vasopressin is permissible. Patients should be covered antibiotically before any surgical procedures.

Sulfonamides should not be given to patients being treated with sulfonyl urea derivatives, because of the additive effect and possible hypoglycemia.

● *Patients taking phenytoin* (anti-seizure), cyclosporine (immunosuppressive), dihydropyridines (antihypertensive), bleomycin (anticarcinogen, cytostatic) often exhibit gingival enlargement/overgrowth.

● *Many other medications,* which cannot be discussed here in any detail, may cause lesions of the oral mucosa (sulfonamides, barbiturates, analgesics, tetracycline etc.). Medications may also lead to decreased saliva flow or xerostomia (antidepressants, antihistamines, neuroleptics, tranquilizers, antihypertensives, bronchodilators, appetite suppressants, ganglion blockers etc.). Periodontal therapy is rendered more difficult by "dry mouth," and wound healing may be painful or delayed.

Periodontitis therapy for the *patient with a systemic disorder* may have to include some compromises. In some cases, the only course is to provide exclusively palliative treatment. If the patient can be treated normally, the course of periodontal therapy should be performed in coordination with the patient's physician.

# Maintenance Therapy – Recall

The long-term success of periodontal therapy depends less on the manner in which the case was treated than on rigorous follow-up of the wound healing process immediately after therapy and on how well the case is maintained in subsequent recall (Rosling et al. 1976b, Nyman et al. 1977, Knowles et al. 1979, Ramfjord et al. 1982, Westfelt et al. 1985).

Research by Axelsson and Lindhe (1981a, b) showed dramatically the effects of preventive measures during recall (Fig. 837). This study demonstrated that regular and short-interval (2–3 months) prophylaxis by the dental hygienist leads to *freedom from caries and attachment loss.* This 6-year study casts some serious doubts about "classical" reparative dentistry!

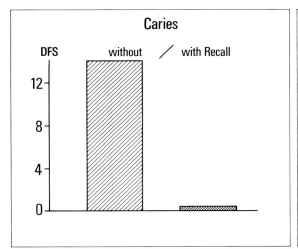

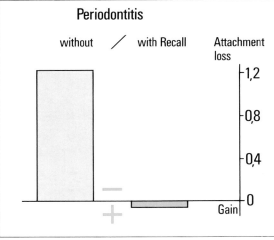

**837 Axelsson study: Caries and attachment loss with and without recall**

Patients who received neither home care motivation nor preventive measures at "one visit to the dentist per year" exhibited 14 new carious lesions and progressive attachment loss over a 6-year period.

Similar patients who received intensive professional prophylaxis every 2–3 months developed essentially no new carious lesions and actually exhibited some attachment gain.

---

*The primary goals of maintenance therapy* are:

- Maintenance of oral health
- Maintenance of optimum chewing function
- Prevention of new infection (gingivitis, periodontitis)
- Prevention of re-infection of inactive residual pockets (periodontitis)
- Prevention of dental caries

*These goals can be achieved through:*

- Re-examination and re-evaluation
- Re-motivation and new information for the patient
- Re-instruction in home care procedures
- Supragingival plaque and calculus removal
- Professional root cleaning and root planing in areas exhibiting renewed disease activity
- Topical fluoride application

# Recall in the Practice – Recall Effect

The introduction of a recall system into the dental practice demands particular organization that can only be accomplished using auxiliary personnel (p. 322).

Viewed realistically, however, even the presence of appropriate personnel and infrastructure within the dental practice cannot ensure that recall will be consistent and effective for *all* patients. Some patients will not accept the recommended recall schedule, preferring to make their own appointments at an interval of their own choosing. One factor that may play a role in such choice is proximity of the patient to the dental office. A factor of concern to the dentist is that with a growing number of recall patients there will be less and less time for accepting new patients and performing initial therapy.

With initiation of a comprehensive recall system, the practice gradually makes a transition from *reparative dentistry* to *preventive dental medicine*. Such a transition is a laudable goal, but it is achieved even today by too few preventive-minded practitioners.

Both private and governmental medical/dental insurance programs must come to accept that preventive measures are more meaningful and, in the long run, more cost effective than reparative dentistry.

It is eminently wiser for a third party payor to cover the cost of prevention than to repeatedly pay out large sums for treatment of disease that could have been prevented. It may be prudent for preventive services to eventually take precedence over restorative measures.

A recall interval may vary between 2–12 months depending on severity of the case, degree of motivation and manual dexterity of the patient, as well as the capacity of the dental practice team.

The time necessary for a recall appointment is routinely *underestimated*. It is certainly more than a short "scraping" of calculus (which is not a primary pathogen). The many tasks to be performed during a recall appointment may require an entire hour.

The challenge presented by a regular recall system and a preventive approach to dentistry is not yet accepted in all western countries. Even some university dental schools include preventive dentistry only peripherally in the curriculum, and periodontology is not yet a separate department in some European schools. The capacity for training dental auxiliary personnel is lacking or inadequate in many universities.

Certain clinical data must be gathered at every recall appointment, before professional prophylaxis is performed and before any necessary follow-up therapy. Other data need to be re-evaluated at longer intervals.

**838 Recall effect**
Initial therapy (blue line) enhanced by surgical intervention (red line) leads to healthy periodontal tissues when plaque control is optimum. If the patient is left on his own, the original suboptimal status will be quickly achieved (dashed black line).

With regular re-motivation and professional prophylaxis at recall appointments (**R1, R2, R3** etc.), the successes achieved by initial therapy and/or surgery can be maintained for years.

Modified from *M. Leu* 1977

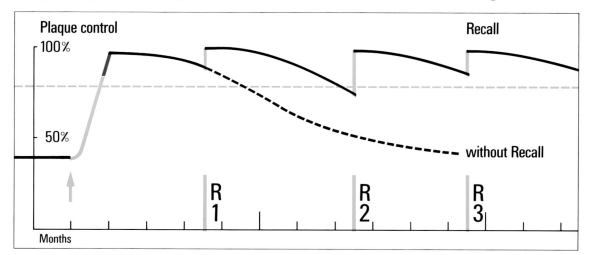

## Recall – Data gathering

- *At each recall appointment* (e.g., every 3–6 months):
  - Gingival condition (PBI; GI-S, bleeding on probing)
  - Plaque accumulation (HYG, HI, disclosing agent)
- *In addition,* every 6–12 months:
  - Probing depths and attachment loss
  - Activity of residual pockets (exudate, pus; possible microbiologic evaluation)
  - Occlusion, reconstructions, caries
- *In addition,* every 3–4 years:
  - Complete radiographic survey, vitality testing

## Recall – Procedures

Depending on the findings at data gathering, the following procedures may be necessary:
- *At every recall appointment:*
  - Re-motivation of the patient
  - Repeated OH instruction and correction of brushing and interdental cleaning techniques
  - Plaque and calculus removal only *where indicated*
- *As necessary:*
  - Treatment of recurrence (root planing, curettage, flap procedures)
  - Restorative work

Patients must be *re-motivated* at every appointment. It is well documented that patient home care wanes with time.

*Oral hygiene procedures* should be monitored and corrected at *each* recall appointment. Errors often creep insidiously into the home care technique, and certain areas of the dentition or certain tooth surfaces may be neglected. Any new restorative work may require alteration of home care practices.

In light of today's knowledge, the dentist and auxiliary personnel must seriously reconsider the question of *professional plaque and calculus removal:* It is not simply a matter of "scraping" all surfaces of all teeth. Rather, teeth that have been neglected and which exhibit plaque and calculus should first be ascertained via a disclosing agent. Pathology in gingival and periodontal tissues must be ascertained by probing. *These* are the areas that must be aggressively pursued by the dental hygienist.

Teeth that exhibit neither plaque nor gingivitis and periodontitis are included only in the *final polishing* procedure and, if indicated, topical fluoridation.

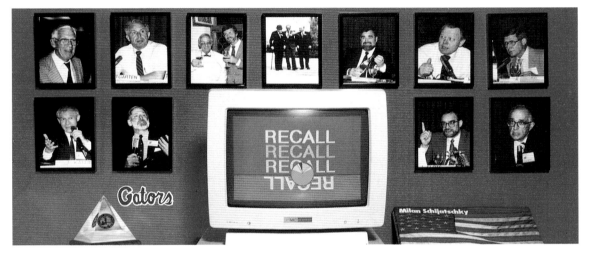

**839   Recall**
– *Remember:* Research findings, important discoveries
– *Remember:* Re-appoint a patient for maintenance.

Today the computer provides the perfect mechanism for scheduling patient recalls at the appropriate interval. Pictured here is the monitor of a computerized patient record system in a periodontal practice.

(In the background is part of a gallery of well-known basic science and clinical researchers in periodontology.)

**840   The "prophy hour"**
The standard length of a recall appointment is one hour. This diagram depicts the work to be accomplished by the dentist (black) and by the dental hygienist (blue) during the hour, and the time required for each task (cf. Fig. 842).

Removal of plaque and calculus requires about 40 minutes. More time is allocated to teeth exhibiting local factors or disease activity. Other teeth may receive only a "polish."

Check by dentist
Fluoride application
Polishing

Examination
Motivation
Reinforcement
Reinstruction

Plaque and calculus removal

Prophy-Hour

60 | 0
– 45 –
– 15 –
30

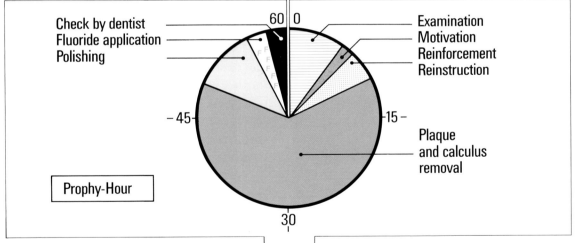

**841   Plaque and/or calculus removal?**
Before starting treatment, data gathering is performed (plaque accumulation, bleeding on probing).

All teeth are cleaned using rubber cups and prophy paste. Curettes or scalers are used on individual tooth/root surfaces only where indicated, e.g., where bleeding on probing or active residual pockets or deposits are present.

Continual scaling on healthy surfaces can lead to further attachment loss and to massive loss of substance from root surfaces!

# Dentist and Auxiliary Personnel

Modern preventive dentistry and a periodontal orientation in dental practice would be impossible today without highly qualified auxiliary personnel such as the dental hygienist (DH). The DH can actually *replace* the dentist at chairside in many procedures such as data gathering, prophylaxis, initial treatment and maintenance therapy.

A fulltime dental hygienist can provide care and maintenance for over 500 periodontitis patients per year, based on an average 4-month recall interval. Such care is, of course, performed under the supervision and control of the dentist. The dental hygienist and other auxiliary personnel can also be of significant assistance to the dentist in the care and maintenance of all other dental patients, e.g, those with extensive prosthodontic work.

**842 Relief of the dentist (gray and black) by the dental hygienist (blue)**
The dental hygienist is responsible for approximately 90% of each recall appointment; the DH can also be of assistance to the dentist in other areas.

For example, during data gathering and initial therapy for most patients, the DH assumes approximately half of the responsibility.

Even during the surgical phase of therapy, the DH plays a significant role in wound management, dressing removal etc.

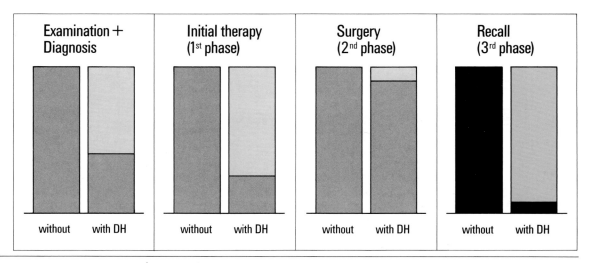

| Examination + Diagnosis | Initial therapy (1st phase) | Surgery (2nd phase) | Recall (3rd phase) |
| without    with DH | without    with DH | without    with DH | without    with DH |

# Auxiliary Personnel and Treatment Needs

The need for periodontal treatment is great. For example, 97% of individuals examined in Hamburg (Fig. 843) required some form of care (Ahrens & Bublitz 1987). The type of treatment indicated, however, varied considerably:

– 3% of individuals with healthy gingiva and 9% of patients exhibiting bleeding on probing required repeated home care instruction. 72% of those exhibiting calculus and patients with pocket depths to 5.5 mm required subgingival scaling. In 16% of those examined, deeper pockets were diagnosed, requiring more complex therapy (surgery). Viewed in this way 84% of the population could be treated prophylactically or therapeutically by auxiliary personnel (12% by trained dental assistants, 72% by dental hygienists).

The dentist can delegate and monitor routine (mild) cases, and actively participate in provision of therapy in more complicated situations.

**843 "Treatment need" (TN) in Hamburg, West Germany (Ahrens & Bublitz 1987)**

**TN I** Hygiene instruction and *supragingival* plaque and calculus removal
**TN II** As above plus *subgingival* scaling, root planing
**TN III** As above plus more complex (surgical) therapy

**A** TN I may also be performed by the dental assistant
**B** TN II can be carried out by the dental hygienist
**C** TN III must be performed by the dentist or specialist

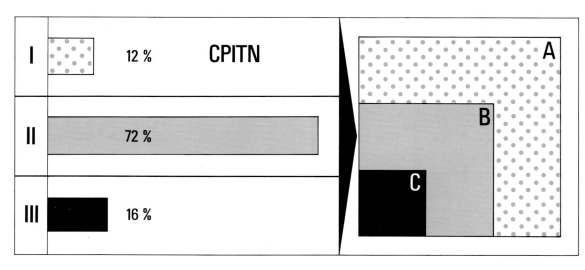

| I | 12 % | CPITN | A |
| II | 72 % | | B |
| III | 16 % | | C |

# Failures – No Maintenance Therapy

## Success in periodontal therapy

– Inflammation (gingival bleeding) eliminated
– Pocket activity eliminated
– Probing depths reduced
– Attachment loss halted
– Tooth mobility stabilized or reduced

## Failure of periodontal therapy

– Persistent bleeding
– Persistent pocket activity
– Increasing probing depths
– Advancing attachment loss, tooth loss
– Increasing tooth mobility

Most failures in the treatment of periodontitis can be explained. The most common causes of failure include: Incorrect local and systemic medical history, incorrect diagnosis and prognosis, incorrect treatment plan, inadequately performed therapy, *insufficient patient cooperation*, and *lack of maintenance* (Rateitschak 1985).

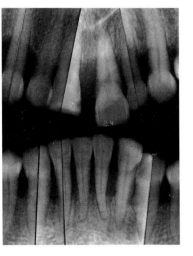
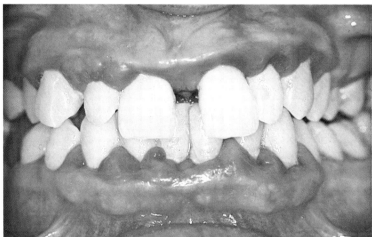

**844 Advanced, rather rapidly progressive periodontitis**
When this 38-year-old woman presented, she had never been instructed in oral hygiene methods. She just wanted a check-up; she had no complaints!

*Clinical findings:*

| | |
|---|---|
| HYG | 0% |
| PBI | 3.8% |
| PD | Active pockets to 8 mm |
| TM | High, with tooth migration |

*Left:* Radiographic finding

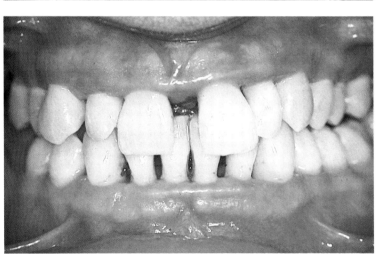

**845 After initial therapy**
The clinical picture is significantly improved after thorough scaling and root planing. The patient's cooperation and home care was inadequate from the beginning. Because of this, no surgical procedures were performed.

Shortly after initial therapy, plaque and calculus accumulations occurred in the mandibular anterior area.

The patient refused to go on regular maintenance recall or to undergo any orthodontic therapy.

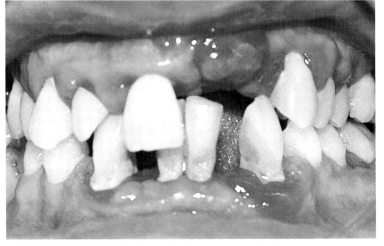

**846 Five years later, without recall**
The patient presented again after teeth 22, 23; 32 and 42 had exfoliated spontaneously.

The dentist elected not to repeat extensive periodontal therapy.

*New treatment plan:*

| | |
|---|---|
| Maxilla: | Complete denture |
| Mandible: | Retain 4 premolars; partial denture |

*Left:* Radiographic finding 5 years later.

# Negative Results of Therapy

Periodontal therapeutic measures such as closed subgingival scaling and, above all, surgical procedures, lead to tissue shrinkage and therefore to "lengthening" of teeth. The consequences include:

- Hypersensitivity of exposed root surfaces
- Poor esthetics (maxillary anterior area)
- Phonetic difficulties

*The patient must be warned of these possible consequences before initiation of periodontal therapy.*

*Sensitive teeth* may be treated by means of desensitizing solutions and dentifrices. In refractory cases, the dentist may attempt electrosurgical fulguration, or may place cervical restorations, or (in extreme situations) the teeth can be devitalized (pulp extirpation). Problems of *esthetics* and *phonetics* may be successfully treated by fabrication of a customized gingival mask ("party gums"; Iselin & Lufi 1983 a, b). Full cast crowns may alleviate the situation in some cases; however, the latter procedure may only exacerbate the poor esthetics, as crown margins may be exposed supragingivally.

**Successful (?) periodontal therapy**

**847 Exposure of the CEJ and coronal root surface ("long teeth")**
This 32-year-old female exhibited gingival recession prior to the surgical procedure, and esthetics became worse still after periodontal surgery. After treatment, the chief complaints were poor esthetics and phonetic difficulties.

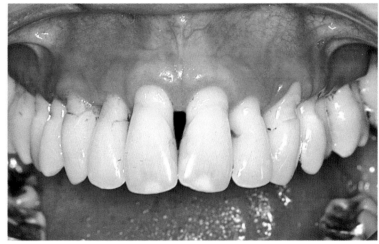

**848 Gingival mask**
A customized impression tray was used to obtain a precise model of the labial part of the anterior maxillary segment, including the attached gingiva to the mucogingival line. The gingival mask was fabricated on the model, finished to a knife edge just short of the mucogingival line. Retention was achieved by extension of the acrylic into interdental areas.

*Right: Denture base acrylic* in various shades and textures can be used to blend the gingival mask perfectly with the patient's own tissues.

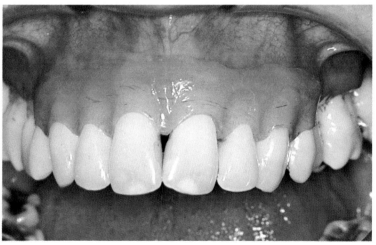
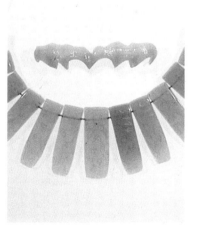

**849 Improved esthetics**
The gingival mask may provide a significant esthetic improvement, especially for patients with a high smile line.

Excellent oral hygiene is a prerequisite for this type of gingival mask; anything less leads quickly to cervical caries!

In addition to the rigid gingival mask made from acrylic, soft gingival prostheses ("Gingivamoll") have also been recommended (Iselin & Lufi 1983 a, b). These generally provide more comfort, which outweighs the fact that they stain easily.

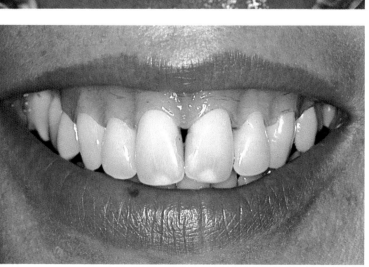

# Function – Occlusal Therapy

The masticatory system is composed of the jaws, the temporomandibular joints, the muscles of mastication, the nervous system, the teeth with their occlusal complex, and the periodontal tissues. These parts are physiologically and morphologically synchronized when function is normal.

Within certain limits of tolerance, the masticatory system can adapt to deviations from the norm. However, if any disturbance, alteration or disease in any one of the component parts of the masticatory system occurs, the other components may also be affected.

Psychic stress situations can accentuate functional disturbances, especially parafunctions. In exceptional cases stress may represent the sole etiology (Graber 1982, 1985; Jäger et al. 1987).

Functional disturbances *do not* elicit periodontitis. Nevertheless, such disturbances must be recognized and treated by the dentist because they elicit alterations in masticatory musculature and temporomandibular joint function, as well as the *progression* of an existing active periodontitis.

This chapter will present:

| |
|---|
| Normal function and physiologic tooth mobility |
| Boundaries of mandibular movement |
| Disturbed function (functional analysis) and occlusal periodontal trauma |
| Therapy for functional disturbances; bite guards, selective grinding |

## Normal Function

The complexity of the stomatognathic system makes it difficult to define the term "normal function." It is only possible to describe physiologic data and norms for the individual components:

### Force
- *The "normal" chewing force* is dependent on the type of food taken. It varies between 100 g during the intake of soup, pudding etc., increases to ca. 15 kg when chewing tough meat, and may reach 20 kg when very hard foodstuffs are taken (Ammann 1980).

### Duration
- *The "normal" temporal loading of the periodontium* is short. The occlusal forces that are imposed upon the periodontium during chewing and swallowing are *intermittent* in character. The duration of a chewing maneuver is only 0.1–0.4 seconds. During swallowing, the periodontium is loaded for only ca. 1 second. If these maneuvers are summed over a 24-hour period, it is revealed that only 15–20 minutes of loading occurs per day (Graf 1969).

### Direction
- *The "normal" direction of forces* that are imposed upon the periodontium during chewing is extremely variable. The "ideal" direction of loading would be vertical/axial, because this would ensure that all periodontal fibers and the alveolar process would be loaded evenly. Such equal loading does not occur even in centric occlusion! During chewing, on the other hand, alternating and combined forces are exerted primarily from the horizontal/orofacial and vertical directions (Graf et al. 1974, Graf & Geering 1977).

# Physiologic Tooth Mobility

The manner in which a tooth is supported within its alveolus, and the elasticity of the entire alveolar process provide for a measurable physiologic tooth mobility in horizontal, vertical and rotational directions (periodontometer, Mühlemann 1967; Periotest, Schulte et al. 1983). Physiologic tooth mobility varies. The teeth are more mobile in the morning than in the evening (Himmel et al. 1957). Variation in tooth mobility also exists among healthy individuals; this is referred to as the normal physiologic range. Nevertheless, each type of tooth will exhibit characteristic mobility depending upon the *surface area* available for insertion of periodontal ligament fibers, and this in turn will depend upon the number of roots, root length and root diameter (Fig. 851).

## Increased tooth mobility

Elevated tooth mobility may result from occlusal trauma or bone loss. However, increased tooth mobility alone is *not* a criterion of periodontal health or pathology.

**850  Physiologic tooth mobility with increasing force (force p = gram)**

**A  Tooth mobility from periodontal ligament deformation**
After orofacial loading with **100 g**, the collagen fibers of the periodontal ligament are stretched: Initial tooth mobility.

**B  Periodontal (alveolar bone) tooth mobility**
Loading with **500 g** force reversibly deforms the entire alveolar process (blue): Secondary tooth mobility.

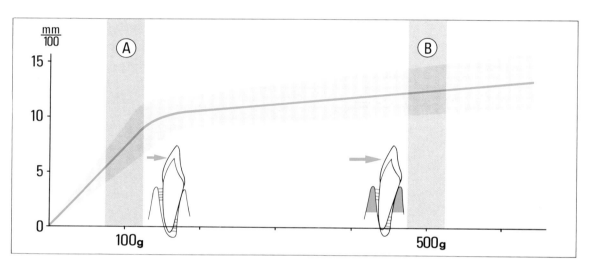

**851  Tooth mobility – Mean values for various tooth types**

|   |   |
|---|---|
| **I** – | Incisors |
| **C** – | Canines |
| **P** – | Premolars |
| **M** – | Molars |

The values depicted here represent *mean mobility figures in health* after application of a constant heavy force (500 g) to elicit secondary tooth mobility.

These values would be scored as zero in clinical charting (see Diagnosis – Prognosis, p. 115; Tooth Mobility, p. 121).

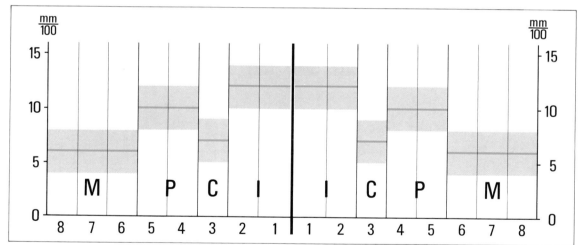

## Initial tooth mobility (A)

This is defined as the first phase of movement of a tooth after loading. It is measured after application of a 100 g force applied in the orofacial direction. The tooth moves relatively easily within the alveolus. Some periodontal ligament fiber bundles are stretched, others relaxed, but significant deformation of the alveolar process does not occur.

Initial tooth mobility is relatively high. It is a function of the width of the periodontal ligament space and the histologic structure of the periodontium. It may range from 5–10 mm x $10^{-2}$, depending on the tooth being measured.

## Secondary tooth mobility (B)

This is measured after application of 500 g of force to a tooth in a orofacial direction. At this magnitude of force, the entire alveolar process is deformed due to the tension on periodontal fibers, and any further movement of the tooth requires much higher forces.

Variations in secondary tooth mobility in a healthy periodontium result from the mass and the quality of the alveolar bone.

Normal periodontal (secondary) tooth mobility ranges from 8–15 mm x $10^{-2}$.

# Idealized Mandibular Border Movement

Man's two temporomandibular joints permit 3-dimensional mandibular movements. The *boundaries* of these movements are generally reproducible values that are of value in prosthetics. They are recorded by an incisal reference point between the two mandibular central incisors. The so-called *Posselt figure* describes the border movements (Posselt 1962). These border movements are usually diagrammed in their ideal form (Figs. 852–854). However, especially in the occlusal contact area, significant individual differences exist (Figs. 859–

861) depending on the morphology of the chewing surfaces. Mandibular border movements may also be altered or limited by dental, skeletal or TMJ anomalies, and functional disturbances (muscle spasm) are also commonly involved.

*Minimum physiologic opening* of the mandible is generally accepted as 40 mm (2 fingers wide), while protrusive and lateral movements are 5 mm. However, many patients exhibit excursive movements that are considerably beyond these means.

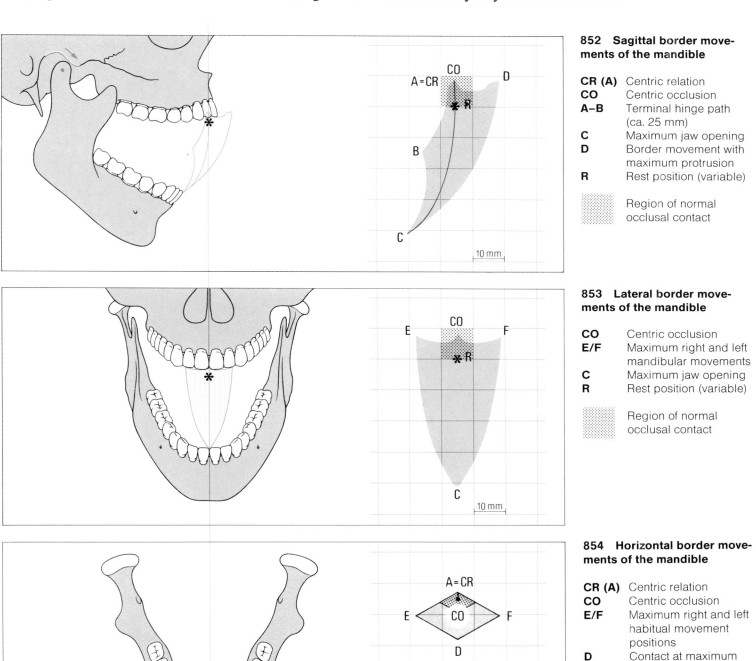

**852  Sagittal border movements of the mandible**

| | |
|---|---|
| **CR (A)** | Centric relation |
| **CO** | Centric occlusion |
| **A–B** | Terminal hinge path (ca. 25 mm) |
| **C** | Maximum jaw opening |
| **D** | Border movement with maximum protrusion |
| **R** | Rest position (variable) |

Region of normal occlusal contact

**853  Lateral border movements of the mandible**

| | |
|---|---|
| **CO** | Centric occlusion |
| **E/F** | Maximum right and left mandibular movements |
| **C** | Maximum jaw opening |
| **R** | Rest position (variable) |

Region of normal occlusal contact

**854  Horizontal border movements of the mandible**

| | |
|---|---|
| **CR (A)** | Centric relation |
| **CO** | Centric occlusion |
| **E/F** | Maximum right and left habitual movement positions |
| **D** | Contact at maximum protrusion |

Region of normal occlusal contact

With increasing jaw opening, the possibility for lateral excursions is progressively limited.

## Effective Mandibular Movements with Tooth Contact

The normal function of the teeth in contact is influenced, often limited or disturbed by interarch relationships of occlusion and articulation.

Joss and Graf (1979) and Graf (1981) registered mandibular movements at contact in normal, healthy, symptom-free subjects using three-dimensional computerized plots. The critical area between centric relation (CR) and maximum intercuspation (CO) was recorded, as well as the border movements of the mandible at initial protrusive and lateral excursion.

Large physiologic variation was detected between *normal bite*, above average *overbite* and abraded dentition, probably as a result of occlusal guidance during mandibular movements.

Significant differences were also detected among test subjects in terms of the distance between CR and CO. A more or less pronounced distance between CR and CO was the rule. This should be kept in mind during selective grinding in the natural dentition when attempting to attain a "long centric" or "freedom in centric." So called "point centric" (CR in CO) is unphysiologic.

**855 Normal bite (model)**
Points of light between the central incisors of maxilla and mandible are the reference marks for the three-dimensional computer plot of mandibular movements at tooth contact. Two Selspot TV cameras (left and right) record the movements of the red (mandibular) point of light. The green light is the stationary reference point (maxilla).

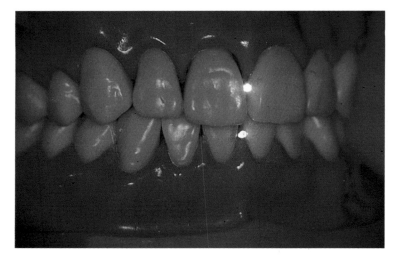

**856 Overbite**
This patient exhibited a true overbite, slight Class II interarch relationship, and pronounced cuspid guidance. The patient was symptom-free.

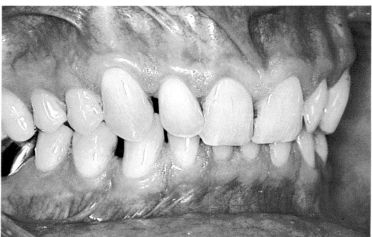

**857 Abraded dentition**
This patient exhibited severe attrition, but was symptom-free despite parafunctions.

No periodontitis could be detected. A protrusive lateral movement is depicted here, demonstrating the patient's bruxing position.

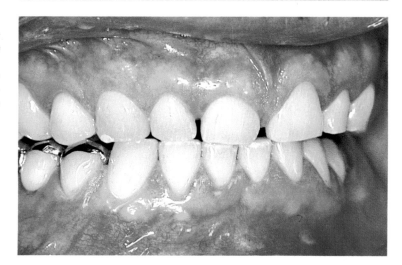

□ Entire field of contact

● CR: Centric relation

○ CO: Centric occlusion

CR: Position at centric relation

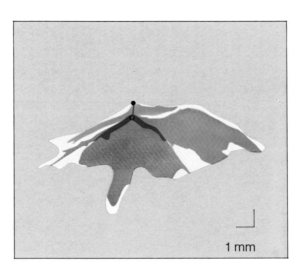

**858 Idealized representation of the horizontal field of movement of the mandible**
Mandibular movements performed with no tooth contact yielded a tracing identical to the *gothic arch* tracing as seen in prosthetics. The only limitation to mandibular movements are the boundaries provided by the anatomic structures of the TMJ.

**Color code for the fields of contact (Figs. 859–861)**
□ Entire field of contact
▨ Incisor contacts
▨ Canine contacts
▨ Premolar contacts

1 mm

1 mm

**859 Normal bite – Computer plot and composite**
The mandibular movement tracing with tooth contact depicts a physiologic distance (0.8 mm, red) between CR and CO. The mandibular movement is guided by incisors and canines in maximum intercuspation, and by premolars in the most retruded position.

*Left:* 3-D Plot
– Elevation 30°
– Angle 75°

Figs. 859–861 courtesy *H. Graf*

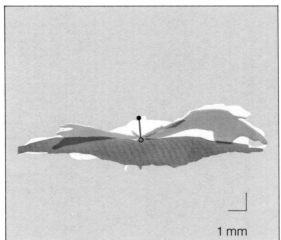

1 mm

1 mm

**860 Overbite – Computer plot and composite**
Only a short guidance path (1 mm, red) exists between CR and CO. The mandible is guided by incisors and canines around the narrow intercuspation region.

*Left:* 3-D Plot
– Elevation 30°
– Angle 75°

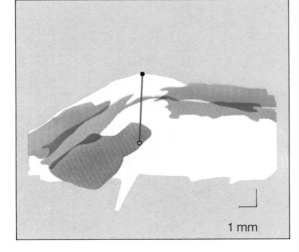

1 mm

1 mm

**861 Abraded dentition – Computer plot and composite**
Excessively expansive *"long centric"* (3 mm, red). Movements to right occur with incisor, canine and premolar guidance; to the left, guidance is primarily on premolars.

*Left:* 3-D Plot
– Elevation 30°
– Angle 75°

**All three variations depicted in Figures 859–861 are within physiologic limits and would require no therapeutic corrections.**

# Functional Disturbances – Causes, Types and Consequences

## General causes of functional disturbances
– *Conditions of psychic stress,* which lead to neuromuscular tension of the jaw musculature can enhance locally elicited functional disturbances. If the patient's level of psychic stress is high, this in itself may be the sole cause of oral parafunctions (frontolateral bruxism; Graber 1985, 1988; Jäger et al. 1987).

## Locally elicited functional disturbances
– *Premature occlusal contacts* in retruded centric, also known as centric relation (CR) and/or in maximum intercuspation, also called habitual closure or centric occlusion (CO).
– *Interferences* in lateral excursions. These occur mostly in the premolar region on the working side, and frequently in the molar areas on the balance side. Functional disturbances caused by balancing interferences during mandibular protrusive movements are rare.
– *Loss of vertical dimension* due to tooth loss or extreme attrition. This can lead to premature contact, interferences or to elevated neuromuscular tone.

## Forms of functional disturbances – Parafunction, bruxism
– *Occlusal parafunctions* elicit periodontal trauma due to unphysiologic loading force and duration. Clenching and bruxing load periodontal structures excessively. Such parafunctions can have varying *consequences* on periodontal health.

## Other forms of functional disturbances
– *Loading in unphysiologic directions,* e.g., tipping forces can lead to migration of teeth.
– *Hypofunction,* e.g., in cases with unilateral chewing, and *afunction* when antagonists are missing. If functional stimulation to the periodontium is lacking, the periodontal ligament space becomes narrower.

Combinations of the various types of functional disturbances are not uncommon.

---

## Functional Analysis

*In the mouth*

The following information should be collected in all cases:
- Wear facets and signs of abrasion (parafunctions)
- Tooth mobility in relation to remaining support (parafunctions, occlusal trauma)
- Premature contacts in centric and in intercuspation
- Articular interference (hyperbalance)
- Neuromuscular symptoms, pressure sensitivity or pain at muscle insertions
- TMJ symptoms

*In the articulator*

An accurate *registration* of bite relationships and an analysis of models mounted in the articulator can enhance the findings collected at chairside. For the planning of major occlusal rehabilitation, such a registration is imperative.

Functional analyses during complete oral rehabilitation has been discussed at length in the literature (Krogh-Poulsen 1968, Bauer & Gutowski 1975, Ramfjord & Ash 1983, Ash & Ramfjord 1988).

---

## Consequences of functional disturbances

Functional disturbances, especially parafunctions (bruxism) may take many forms and may damage one or many aspects of the stomatognathic system:
– *Teeth and occlusal complex:* Excessive attrition of tooth substance; wear facets on restorations or other artificial occlusal surfaces; tooth migration, fracture.
– *Neuromuscular systems:* Neuralgiform complaints, often described as "radiating" pain; muscle spasm and muscle pain, especially at muscle insertion areas; asymmetric or inhibited mandibular movements.

– *TMJ:* Discopathy, abnormal joint mobility, clicking, rubbing, pain, swelling, asymmetric movements as a result of "obstacles" in the joint.
– *Periodontium:* Occlusal trauma, elevated tooth mobility, radiographically visible triangulation in the marginal aspect of the alveolar process, histologic alterations of the periodontium.

The *consequences* of functional disturbances anticipate their *causes.* Of the various consequences of functional disturbances, *occlusal trauma* is the most important for periodontology (p. 331).

# Occlusal Periodontal Trauma

## Definition

Occlusal trauma is defined as *"microscopic altera-tions of periodontal structures in the area of the periodontal ligament, which become manifest clinically in (reversible) elevation of tooth mobility"* (Mühlemann et al. 1956, Müh-lemann & Herzog 1961).

The consequences of occlusal trauma are reflected as histologic alterations in the periodontium: Circula-tory disturbances; thrombosis of periodontal ligament vasculature; edematisation and hyalinisation of collagen fibers; inflammatory cell infiltration; nuclear pyknosis in osteoblasts, cementoblasts and fibroblasts; vascula-ture dilation (Svanberg & Lindhe 1974). The periodontal ligament space adapts to the trauma by becoming wider ("hourglass shape"), and this is manifest clinically by elevated mobility of the traumatized teeth; widening becomes visible radiographically.

The supracrestal (gingival) collagen fibers and the junctional epithelium, however, exhibit *no* histologic alterations.

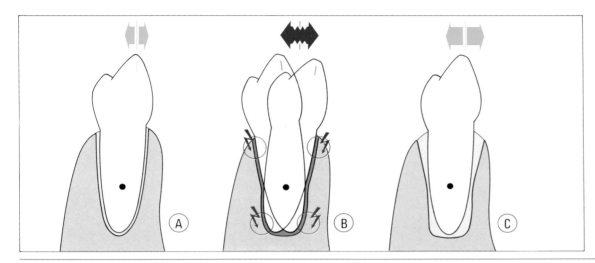

**862  Occlusal trauma – Normal periodontium**

**A** Tooth in healthy periodontium.

**B** If this tooth is unphysiologically loaded (parafunction, jiggling), histologic changes occur in the periodontium (red) and the PDL space becomes wider in areas of pressure (red arrows).

**C** The periodontium can adapt to the improper loading, wherein the hourglass shaped, widened PDL space permits elevated tooth mobility.

Such alterations are reversible if the improper loading is eliminated.

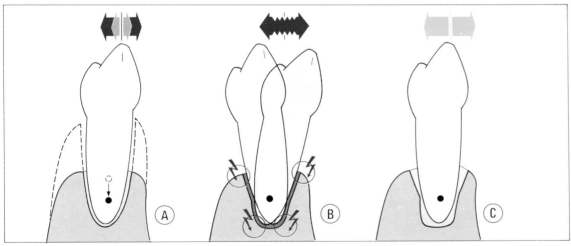

**863  Occlusal trauma – Compromised periodontium**

**A** The periodontium has been compromised by periodontitis (elevated TM).

**B** Additional unphysiologic load-ing leads to further elevation of TM.

**C** If trauma persists, tooth mobility of progressing severity may re-sult. Adaptation in the form of elevated tooth mobility is pos-sible however, even if peri-odontal support has been con-siderably reduced, as long as the remaining tissues are healthy (treated).

Research has proven that abnormal occlusal forces cause neither gingivitis nor periodontitis. However, the *progression* of an already existant periodontitis may be accelerated (Svanberg & Lindhe 1974; Polson et al. 1976 a, b; Lindhe & Ericsson 1982; Pihlstrom 1986; Hanamura et al. 1987).

The histologic alterations in the periodontium and the elevated tooth mobility are *reversible* if the causes of the trauma are eliminated. However, any existing gingivitis or periodontitis will *not* be influenced by elimination of occlusal trauma (Vollmer & Rateitschak 1975).

### Adaptation to unphysiologic forces

Even without treatment the periodontium may adapt to long-standing occlusal trauma. The PDL space remains wide, but regains its normal histologic appear-ance. *Tooth mobility* remains elevated, but does not increase in severity (Nyman & Lindhe 1976).

### Progressive mobility with unphysiologic forces

Heavy, continuous, abnormal occlusal forces may lead to a progressively increasing tooth mobility, and function may be negatively influenced. Trauma may be eliminated via bite plates, selective grinding, splinting or occlusal reconstruction.

# Occlusal Bite Guard – The Michigan Splint

When parafunctional habits (e. g., bruxism) result in occlusal periodontal trauma (increasing tooth mobility), the dentition should undergo selective occlusal grinding and wear facets should be eliminated.

However, selective grinding in CR/CO (p. 335) is often impossible due to masticatory muscle spasms. Reciprocal functional relationships exist among occlusion, periodontium, TMJ, musculature and central nervous system (CNS). The activity of the CNS may also be significantly influenced by psychic components (Fröhlich 1966; Graber 1978, 1985). This central nervous system hyperactivity is relieved through elevated *tone* of the masticatory musculature (clenching or bruxing). In such situations, if occlusal dysharmonies are also present a "vicious circle" is created, which can best be broken through use of an occlusal bite guard, e. g., the Michigan splint (Geering & Lang 1978, Ramfjord & Ash 1983). The result is that the occlusion is taken out of the "circle" and the masticatory musculature relaxes (Graf 1969). In most cases, selective occlusal grinding can then be accomplished after only a few weeks.

**864 Reciprocal influences of the masticatory musculature**

\* Interruption via bite guard

The tone of the masticatory musculature (red) is a product of influences from the central nervous system, the occlusion and the TMJ.

*The feedback mechanisms can be interrupted* through use of a bite guard (blue bar).

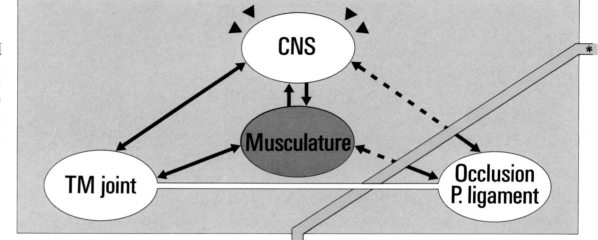

**865 Spasm (left) and normal tone (right)**
Elevated activity of the masticatory musculature (masseter, temporalis) is an etiologic factor for occlusal trauma.

Insertion of an occlusal bite guard (blue) can elicit immediate and dramatic reduction of this hyperactivity. The heavy, destructive forces exerted upon the periodontium by clenching or bruxing are reduced to more physiologic levels. The bite guard also distributes forces evenly over the entire dental arch.

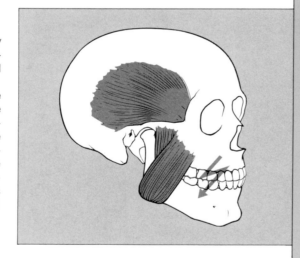
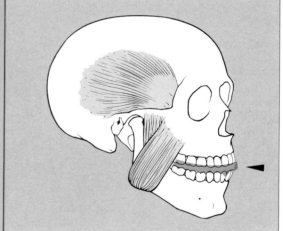

**866 Electromyography before and after insertion of a bite guard**
The electromyograms *before* (red) and *after* (blue) insertion of a bite guard reveal the quieting of the hyperactivity of masticatory muscles.

If the patient's level of psychic stress is very high, however, clenching and bruxism on the bite guard itself may ensue. The possibilities for alleviating this situation include oral physiotherapy or the administration of tranquilizers to calm the CNS component.

Courtesy *H. Graf*

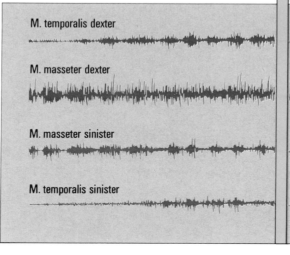

M. temporalis dexter

M. masseter dexter

M. masseter sinister

M. temporalis sinister

1 sec. 300 µV

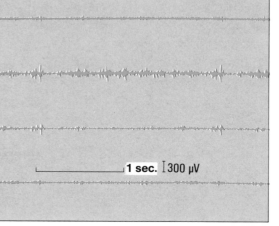

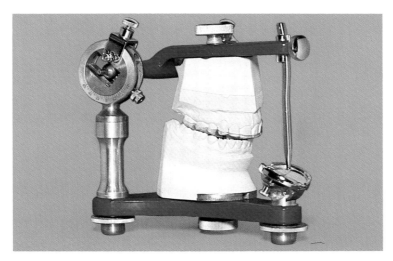

**867  Michigan splint in the articulator**
Fabrication of a bite guard (the Michigan splint is depicted) out of clear acrylic is performed only after registration of the occlusal relationships in an adjustable articulator. This usually means only slight alterations will have to be made on the bite guard at the time of insertion. The thickness of the occlusal surface of the bite guard should be minimized to avoid opening the bite excessively. The Michigan splint is almost always seated in the maxilla.

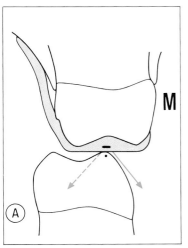

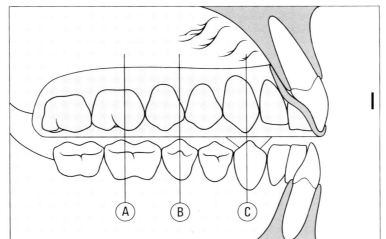

**868  Characteristics of the Michigan splint**
The buccal cusps of mandibular molars and premolars, as well as canines and incisors (**I**), occlude onto the smooth acrylic surface.

*Left:* Transverse section (A). In the *molar* region, where the cusps are relatively flat (**M**) the splint can be flat, without opening the bite excessively (compare plate thickness).
During lateral excursions (working and balance sides, blue arrows) contact is lost immediately due to cuspid guidance.

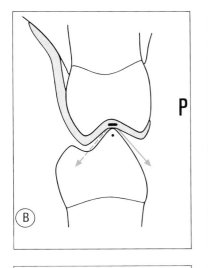

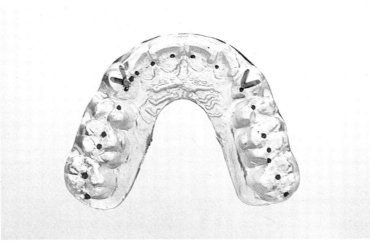

**869  Michigan splint – removable bite guard**
Occlusal contacts of the mandibular buccal cusp tips are marked in red, cuspid guidance pathways for protrusive and lateral excursion in green.

*Left:* Transverse section through the steep cusps of the *premolars* (**P**), the profile of the splint is not flat or horizontal but *indented* in order to avoid excessive opening of the bite. Nevertheless lateral excursion (arrow) is associated with virtual immediate loss of occlusal contact.

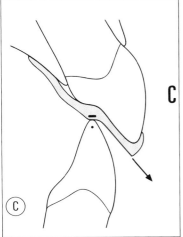

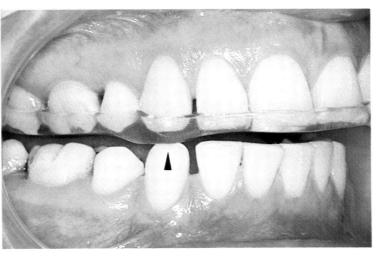

**870  Cuspid rise**
Cuspid rise incorporated into the Michigan splint opens the occlusion during lateral excursions.

*Left:* Transverse section (C). In the canine region (**C**), a *"cuspid rise"* is incorporated: This steep incline in the splint represents the sole guidance of the mandible during lateral and protrusive movement. It forces the mandible to open the occlusion.

---

*The principles of "freedom in centric" (p. 337, Fig. 884) are also observed in the splint occlusion.*

# Goals of Occlusal Adjustment

Occlusal trauma cannot cause periodontitis; however, it may compromise periodontal health and therefore weaken the defense capabilities of periodontal tissue. An already existant periodontitis may be promulgated. For this reason it remains important to eliminate any recognizable causes of the occlusal trauma (as indicated by elevated tooth mobility) during the course of periodontitis therapy (Ramfjord & Ash 1979, 1981, 1983; Ash & Ramfjord 1982).

The therapy of choice involves selective grinding of occlusion and articulation, often after previous relaxation of the musculature by means of a bite guard. Selective occlusal grinding has additional effects in addition to elimination of occlusal trauma:

- Prevention or elimination of parafunctions
- Creation of symmetrical left/right chewing function
- Stabilization of the occlusal plane
- Adjustment of occlusion *after* orthodontic treatment
- Adjustment of occlusion *before* prosthetic replacement.

No effort should be made to achieve any sort of "ideal" occlusion!

**871 Contact of antagonists in intercuspation (CO)**
With maximum closure there exist point-type contacts of the buccal cusps of mandibular teeth in the fossae of the maxillary teeth, or of the maxillary palatal cusps in the mandibular fossae. In the ideal, non-abraded dentition, these contacts may be two- or three-point in nature, i.e., the cusps of maxillary teeth may occlude at more than one point (e.g., on second molar).

*Right:* Sagittal border movement of the mandible (Posselt figure). Movement of the mandible into CO.

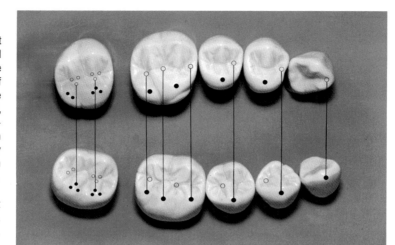
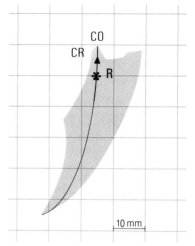

**872 "Tapping test" for determination of tooth-tooth contacts in centric relation (CR)**
The patient's mandible is moved by the dentist along the joint-guided hinge axis without pressure, until first contact between maxillary and mandibular teeth occurs.
*Caution:* Application of pressure can force the condyle dorsally and inferiorly, into an unphysiologic, unstable position.

*Right:* Using this technique the head of the condyle achieves its zenith in the fossa (radiograph).

Courtesy *H. Graf*

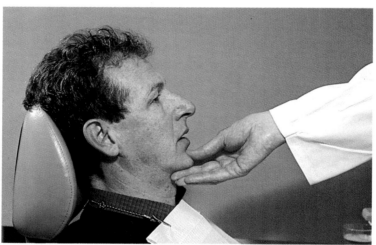
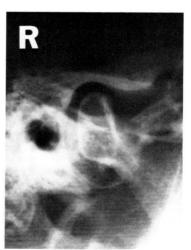

**873 Slide from premature contact in CR into intercuspation (CO)**
When the mandible is manipulated by the dentist along its hinge axis, the movement may be inhibited by one or more premature contacts. If the patient then bites into full intercuspation, the mandible shifts (usually in an anterior direction, and many times anterior-lateral).

*Right:* Posselt figure. Deviation of the mandible from a premature contact in CR into CO.

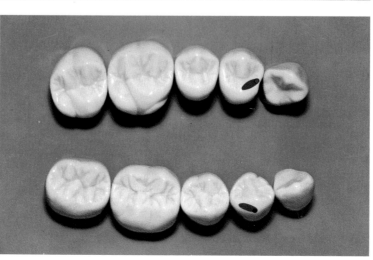
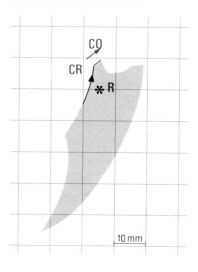

# Practical Occlusal Adjustment – Premature Contacts

*Premature contacts* in centric relation are detected using the "tapping test." A rule of thumb is that if the test reveals that at least three pair of opposing teeth on each side of the arch make contact at the same instant, and if a *sagittal,* interference-free slide in centric of no more than 1 mm occurs, *no* corrective occlusal adjustment is indicated.

If only one or two pair make contact initially, and/or if subsequent *lateral slide* occurs, selective grinding is indicated.

An experienced dentist can perform selective grind-ing immediately. Only in difficult cases or with complex and expansive rehabilitation is it necessary to first mount the case in an articulator to study the precise interarch relationships.

The goal of selective grinding is the creation of *"free-dom in centric"* (Ramfjord & Ash 1983), i.e., free horizontal guidance of the cusps between CR and CO (see complete description in Ramfjord & Ash 1983, Ash & Ramfjord 1988). "Point centric" in retruded contact position is unphysiologic, especially in elderly periodon-titis patients.

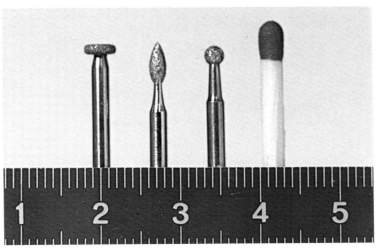

**874   Instrumentarium for selective grinding**
Selective grinding is performed using fine wheel, flame and ball-shaped diamonds. The occlusal surfaces of the teeth are dried thoroughly, then the premature contacts are marked with ribbons of various colors.

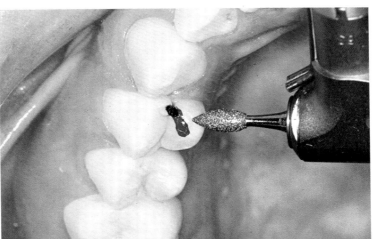

**875   Premature contact in CR, with slide (red) into CO (black)**
The red marking is shaped into a gentle depression using a flame-shaped diamond, without en-croaching upon the palatal cusp tip of 14 or the contact point in CO (black dot).

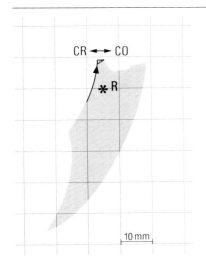
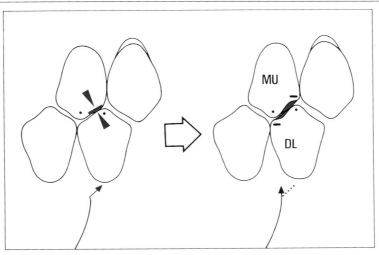

**876   Premature contact on mesiodistal cusp inclines**
This results in a forward/sagittal mandibular shift. The mesial cusp incline is recontoured on the maxil-lary tooth (**MU**) and the distal cusp incline in the mandible (**DL**; **M**esial **U**pper and **D**istal **L**ower).

It is necessary to repeatedly check the selective grinding by re-marking with color ribbon (elimina-tion of secondary contacts).

*Left:* A "long centric" is created be-tween CO and CR, i.e., a horizontal-ly located sagittal guide path not more than 1 mm in extent.

## 877 Premature contact on orofacial cusp inclines

Teeth 15 and 45 exhibit premature contact (red) in centric on the buccal cusp inclines. This causes a lateral shift of the mandible, and must be eliminated because at maximum intercuspation the TMJ position is asymmetric (see Situation 1, Fig. 878).

*Right:* Mandibular shift (red arrow) in the frontal segment of the Posselt figure.

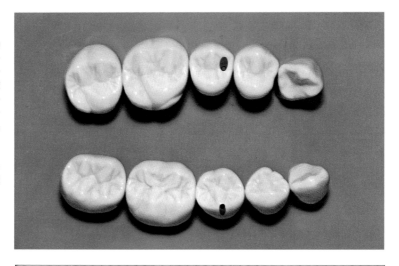

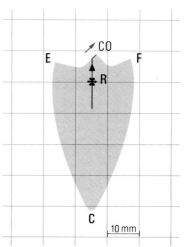

## 878 Buccal-lingual inclines – Possible premature contacts (right):

**1** Inner aspect of maxillary facial and outer aspect of mandibular facial cusp
**2** Inner aspect of maxillary palatal and inner aspect of mandibular facial cusp
**3** Outer aspect of palatal and inner aspect of mandibular lingual cusp

### Correction of situation 1 (left):
Widening the maxillary fossa facially. It also may be necessary to reduce the mandibular tooth.

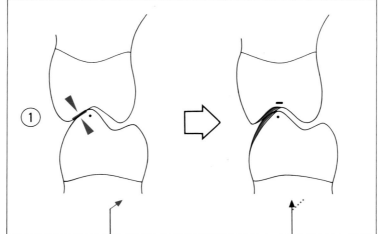

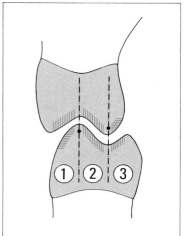

## 879 Correction of situation 2:
The premature contact is eliminated through minimal widening and lateral shifting of the fossae of both teeth. Neither *cusp tip* is altered in any way.

It is wise to keep in mind that the contacting surfaces often represent balancing side interferences (p. 339).

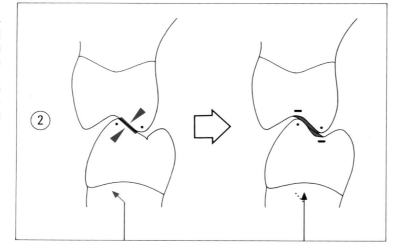

## 880 Correction of situation 3:
The fossa of the mandibular tooth is widened somewhat to accommodate the cusp of the maxillary tooth. The outer aspect of the palatal cusp may also be slightly reduced at the point where it contacts the fossa of its antagonist.

*Right:* By eliminating the prematurities (Situations 1–3), a *wide centric* is created (see Posselt figure).

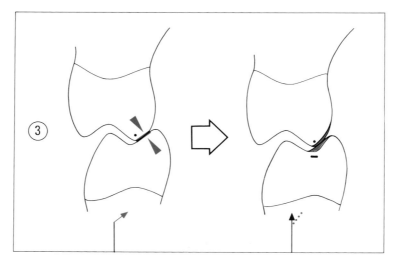

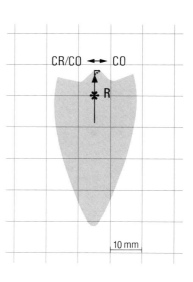

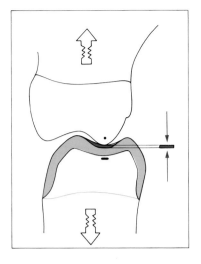

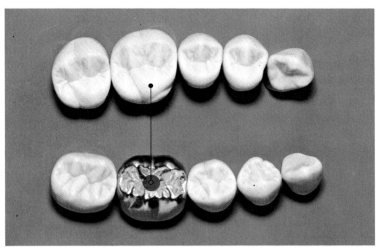

### 881 Premature contact between cusp and fossa

This type of prematurity is often detected after seating a filling, a crown or a bridge, and may occur in CR or CO.

*Left:* The two involved teeth are depressed into their sockets each time the jaws are closed, often resulting in increased axial tooth mobility.

The procedure for eliminating this situation involves *deepening the fossa* by occlusal grinding. The corresponding cusp may be reduced if it also represents a balancing side interference.

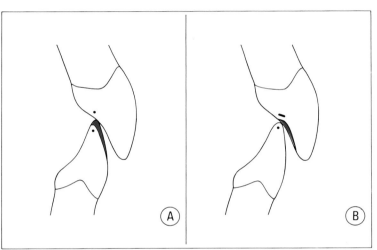

### 882 Anterior prematurity

Naturally occurring prematurities in the anterior segment are rare, but may be detected after a crown or bridge is seated.

The contacts during mandibular protrusive movement should be checked before any selective grinding is performed. If the effected teeth are found to exert an interference during protrusive, then selective grinding is performed on the mandibular tooth (**A**).

If interference does not occur during protrusive movement, the palatal surface of the maxillary tooth (**B**) is reduced.

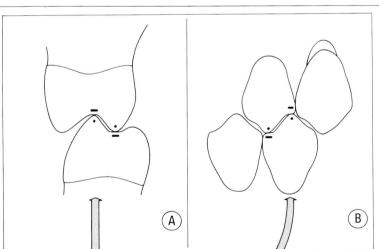

### 883 Selective grinding of "centric" completed

The patient can now assume a multipoint occlusion in both CR and CO without any interference or slide. A mesiodistal *long centric* has been created (**B**) that permits a degree of mandibular movement against the maxillary teeth.

Similarly (**A**), a *wide centric* has been created that permits ca. 0.5 mm of free mandibular movement buccolingually.

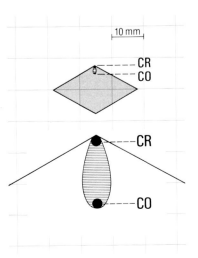

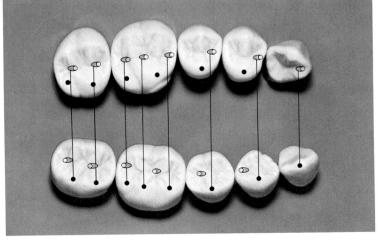

### 884 "Freedom in centric"

There exists between CR and CO a tear-shaped field measuring about 1 x 0.5 mm within which free movement of mandible, i.e., of the cusps within their respective fossae is possible *(freedom in centric)*. These areas are depicted on the occlusal surfaces of opposing teeth in this figure, with lines connecting the cusp tips to their CR position in the fossae.

*Left:* This horizontal section through the Posselt figure depicts the relatively short distance of the "long centric," which is magnified below.

# Working Side

The goals of selective grinding in the posterior segments of the dental arch are the creation of interference-free harmonic movements in intercuspation and the elimination of broad guidance surfaces that are the sites of parafunctions (clenching, bruxism).

Physiologic, non-traumatic posterior segment guidance on the working side is left unchanged; this situation may be characterized by anterior guidance or group function.

Interferences are usually removed by selective reduction and flattening of the interfering, excessively steep cusp inclines ("BULL" rule, Fig. 886). The goal is to achieve *cuspid guidance* during lateral mandibular movements if possible.

The posterior segment guidance pathways that are created by selective occlusal grinding should be contact *lines*, not broad contact surfaces, for example the line contact of the buccal cusp inclines of the mandibular teeth against their maxillary antagonists. Expansive contact areas between antagonists may provide the stimulus for renewed parafunction.

**885  Interference – Dysharmonious lateral movement**
The most commonly encountered interferences on the working side (see green pathway, right) are found on premolars. The involved surfaces are usually the buccal cusp in the mandible and the inner aspect of the buccal cusp in the maxilla (e.g., between 14 and 44 as depicted here).

*Right:* Unharmonic lateral movement guidance in the premolar region.

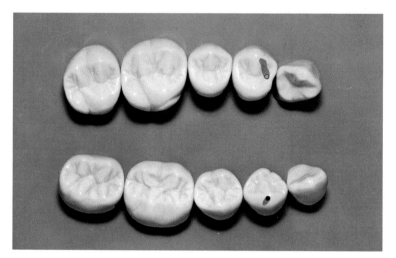
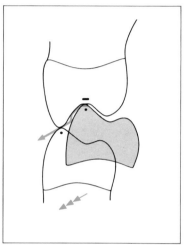

**886  Selective grinding of interference on the working side – "BULL" rule**
The contacts in centric must *not* be eliminated ("long centric") during the selective grinding procedure. Above all the cusp tips (black dot) must not be touched.

This can be accomplished by performing selective grinding in the maxilla (**BU**) to eliminate an interference on the buccal aspect, and by grinding in the mandible (**LL**) to eliminate an interference on the lingual aspect (the BULL rule: **B**uccal **U**pper, **L**ingual **L**ower).

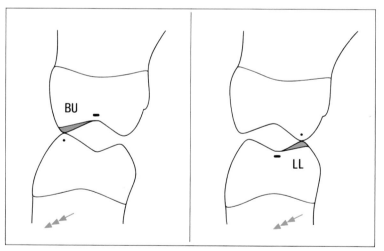

Contact on working side

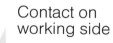

**887  Harmony in the posterior segment after selective grinding**
The goal in elimination of an interference on the working side is to integrate *cuspid guidance* into posterior segment guidance. *Group function*, e.g., guidance involving incisors, canines and premolars is acceptable in the fully dentulous situation, but is not a goal to be sought aggressively.

*Right:* Harmonic, straight line cuspid guidance (green arrow).

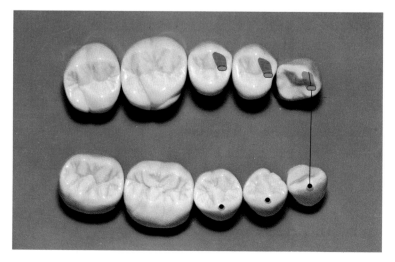
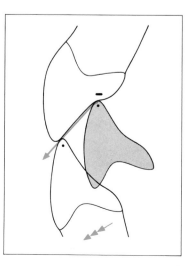

# Balancing Side

In the natural dentition balancing side contacts are neither necessary nor desirable. *Balancing side interferences* are, in fact, injurious. They elicit parafunctions, particularly clenching. Balance antagonists are usually the second molars and, if present, the third molars, which become abraded or mobile (i.e., periodontally damaged) because they must bear the clenching forces. All balancing side interferences should be *eliminated* by means of selective grinding of the balance pathway. However, centric contacts and guidance contacts on the working side must be maintained. The centric contacts will determine whether the balance pathway to be eliminated by grinding is on the inner aspect of the palatal cusp or on the inner aspect of the mandibular buccal cusp. If both upper and lower cusps are involved simultaneously in the balancing side interference, it will be necessary to relieve the situation with maintenance of at least one cusp-fossa contact in centric.

Heavy balancing side interference on a third molar may be an indication for extraction.

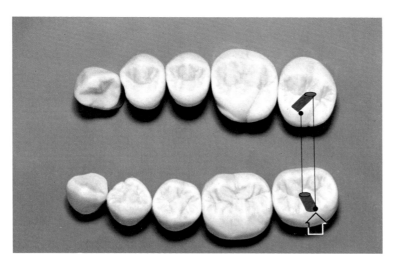

**888 Balancing side interference in posterior segment**
A balancing side interference (red marking) exists during lateral mandibular movement to the right, between the inner aspect of the buccal cusp of the lower second molar and the inner aspect of the palatal cusp of the upper second molar.

Centric contacts exist on the palatal cusp in the maxilla and on the buccal cusp in the mandible; the latter should preferentially be maintained (arrow).

No contact on working side

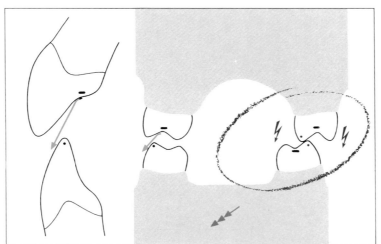

**889 Balancing side interference in the left molar area during mandibular excursion to the right**
The excessively steep cusp inclines on the balance side (circled red) prevent any tooth contact on the working side (green).

Even the canine region (left) is devoid of guiding contact (see long green arrow).

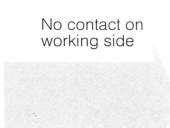
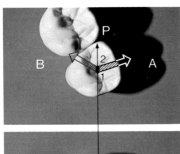
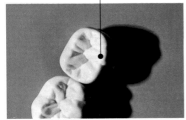

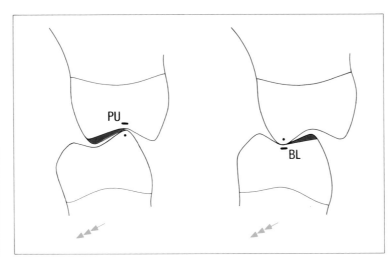

**890 Elimination of balancing interference – "PUBL" rule**
If centric contact is between the mandibular buccal cusp and the maxillary fossa, the upper palatal balance pathway (**PU**) should be eliminated.

If centric contact consists of the upper palatal cusp in the lower fossa, the balancing side interference is removed by grinding the inner aspect of the lower buccal cusp (**BL**).

*Left:* Grinding the palatal cusp while retaining the centric contact between the mandibular buccal cusp and the maxillary fossa.

## Protrusive Movement – Interferences

If interferences occur on anterior teeth during protrusive movements, they must be eliminated. Any interferences in the posterior segments should also be eliminated via selective occlusal grinding, analogous to mesiodistal elimination of balancing side interferences as described above.

In patients with anterior open bite, no attempt should be made to achieve anterior contacts by grinding in the posterior segment.

## Reduction of Wear Facets

Broad surface contacts between antagonists, which occur due to bruxism, represent trigger zones that can elicit parafunctions ("vicious circle"). Such wear facets should therefore be removed according to the principles of Jankelson (1960) during selective grinding (see also Removal of Premature Contacts, p. 336, Fig. 878, Situation 1 and Fig. 880, Situation 3).

Whenever possible such selective grinding should be performed only in enamel. Surfaces should be polished subsequently and fluoridated topically.

**891   Selective grinding in protrusive movement**
Centric contacts on the anterior teeth should occur only in CO (not in CR). Occasionally the teeth make contact only when a slight mandibular protrusive movement is made from CO. These contacts (black dots) must be maintained when selective grinding is performed during protrusive movement:

**A** In the maxilla
**B** In maxilla and mandible, maintaining a centric contact in the middle
**C** In the mandible

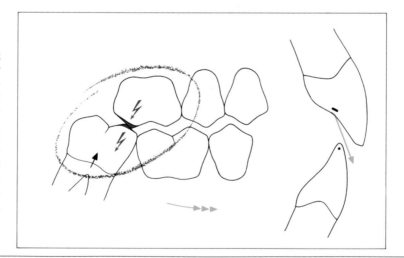

**892   Elimination of balancing contact during protrusive movement**
Molars that are tipped or that lack antagonists (circled in red) may make it impossible to achieve contact in the anterior segment during mandibular protrusion (green arrows).

Extraction of such molars will eliminate the interference, but selective grinding can achieve the same goal. The procedure is similar to eliminating a balancing side interference in the posterior area, but in a mesiodistal plane.

**893   Re-shaping wear facets**
Parafunctional habits can result in expansive attrition in the area of the maxillary buccal cusps and mandibular oral cusps (wear facets). (**A**: blue bar = *widening* of occlusal field).

By selective occlusal grinding of the external surfaces of the cusps (Jankelson), the wide facets can be reduced to point contacts with the newly created cusp tips (arrows); the field of occlusion is thereby reduced (**B**: *narrowing*, coronoplasty).

*Right:* Reduction of wear facets by coronoplasty.

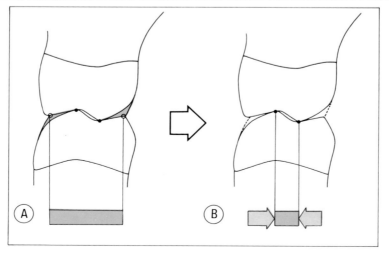

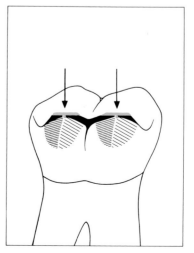

# Orthodontics

Anomalies of tooth position in a periodontally compromised dentition may be characterized as:

| Anomalies that have existed since tooth eruption |
| --- |
| Anomalies that have resulted from periodontitis (or functional disturbances) |

A causal relationship between existing dental malocclusion and periodontitis is difficult to document (Ainamo 1972; Geiger et al. 1973, 1974; Stahl 1975; Ingerval et al. 1977; Buckley 1972, 1981; Hug 1983). However, dental crowding may make plaque removal difficult, and this favors the progression of inflammatory disease in the periodontal supporting tissues.

Drifting that occurs as a consequence of periodontitis may include tipping, rotation, extrusion and protrusion. Realignment of teeth in a dentition manifesting periodontitis can usually be accomplished by means of simple orthodontic movement.

### Diagnosis – Etiology

The factors involved in the development of dental malocclusion following loss of periodontal support are not always obvious. Possible causes include oral parafunctions such as tongue thrust or lip biting, occupation-related peculiarities such as holding nails or pins between the teeth, and tipping of adjacent teeth into an extraction site resulting in occlusal imbalances. It has also been speculated that the granulation tissue present in deep periodontal pockets may exert a force that causes drifting, or that the intact fiber structure on the side of a tooth opposite a deep pocket may exert a *pull* that results in tipping or drifting of a tooth.

### Treatment planning

Orthodontic treatment of a periodontally compromised dentition should never be started until the initial therapy phase is completed and the infection has been brought under control. The rationale for various treatment options should be considered: Is the proposed tooth movement for functional or esthetic reasons? Could the patient's problem be solved by other means, for example by recontouring teeth (odontoplasty) to correct functional, morphologic or esthetic problems? Is a prosthetic solution feasible?

### Apparatus

If the final decision is to proceed with orthodontic treatment, an array of possible methods including simple wire ligatures, removable plates and fixed appliances is available. The choice will depend in large measure on the diagnosis, the goals of therapy and the difficulty of the tooth movement desired.

Another factor in selection of treatment modality is the concerns of the patient, especially the adult patient, who is often neither prepared nor willing to submit to long-term orthodontic therapy with fixed appliances.

### Risks

Compromises often have to be made. In a dentition that has been ravaged by periodontal disease, orthodontic treatment represents a particular trauma for the remaining supporting structures. It has been amply demonstrated that orthodontic treatment results in temporarily increased tooth mobility, which is similar to the increased TM caused by occlusal trauma. For this reason, if the destruction in the periodontium is severe, major orthodontic treatment may be contraindicated.

Following orthodontic therapy, long-term retention is virtually always required in a periodontally compromised dentition; this may take the form of semipermanent splinting (p. 349) or a night guard (p. 342).

# Space Closure in the Maxillary Anterior Segment

Following therapy for moderate periodontitis (AP), the 40-year-old female depicted below requested that the space between 21 and 22 be closed orthodontically for esthetic reasons. The diastema had developed over the previous several years. Gingival shrinkage following the periodontal treatment further enlarged the interdental area, making the esthetic problem greater.

Space closure was accomplished in two months by means of a *removable appliance* with a *labial bow* and finger spring on 21. The entire anterior segment was retracted and tooth 21 was moved distally.

After such treatment, retention is required. This can be accomplished using a *cast metal splint* (Wolf & Rateitschak 1965), a composite resin splint, or a lingual bonded retainer.

Tipping movements of single teeth can be performed by the general practitioner or by the periodontist. An orthodontist is not necessary for this simple tooth movement. Severe anomalies, especially those that have been present since tooth eruption, should be treated in collaboration with an orthodontist.

**894 Before orthodontics – After completion of periodontal therapy**
Protrusion of the anterior segment. Clinical appearance 3 months after periodontal treatment.

*Right:* An unesthetic diastema has developed between 21 and 22. The brown staining is due to chlorhexidine rinse, which was prescribed for plaque control postsurgically.

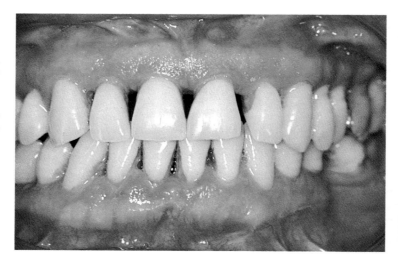
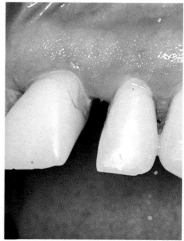

**895 Removable appliance**
Acrylic palatal plate with a labial bow for correction of the anterior protrusion and a finger spring for distal movement of 21.

*Right:* In order to avoid elongation (supereruption) of the anterior teeth or apical movement of the arch wire, small "bumps" of acid-etched composite resin (yellow) can be placed on the facial surfaces of some teeth above the arch wire.
One force vector of the appliance is thereby directed in an apical direction (small red arrow).

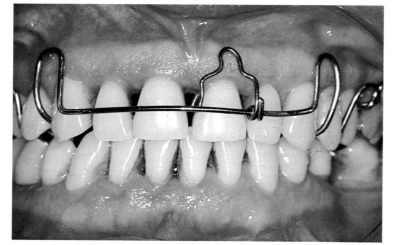
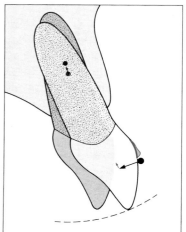

**896 Retention after completion of orthodontic treatment – Two possibilities**
*Cast metal splint:* A chrome-cobalt splint can be worn at night. It is anchored on the premolars by means of flexible clasps that grasp the tooth crown.

*Right:* An alternative to a removable retainer is the use of acid-etched resin for semipermanent splinting of groups of teeth (here 21, 22, 23). This also enhances esthetics by decreasing the size of the interdental spaces.

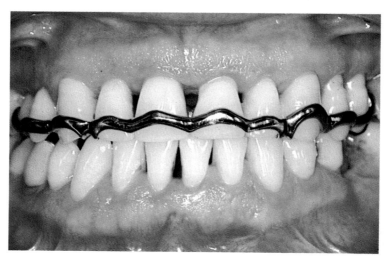
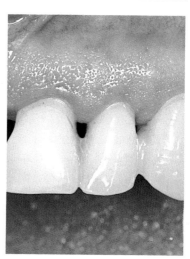

# Treatment for Protrusion

This 41-year-old female suffered from generalized periodontitis of moderate severity. Some drifting of the anterior teeth had occurred, and maxillary anterior protrusion had become noticeably more severe in the last several years. The patient requested periodontal therapy, but also desired esthetic improvement.

Orthodontic treatment would be indicated in a patient of this age solely on the basis of her functional problems, which included overbite, overjet and anterior protrusion in both maxilla and mandible. The goals of the orthodontic treatment, following completion of initial periodontal therapy were 1) bite opening and 2) retraction of the anterior segments. The treatment was accomplished using fixed appliances in both arches, a transpalatal arch to expand the maxilla, and posterior *high pull headgear* with bite-opening torque. Following orthodontic treatment, restorative procedures are to be performed to stabilize the occlusion. Also, the initial therapy phase of periodontal treatment is *repeated,* to eliminate inflammation resulting from compromised oral hygiene during the 8-month orthodontic phase.

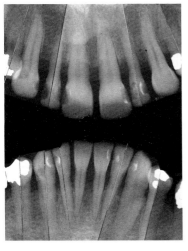

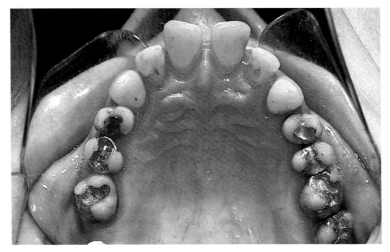

**897 Initial clinical view**
The patient presented with moderate periodontitis, as well as protrusion and rotation of the anterior teeth. The situation was probably enhanced by the patient's lip biting habit. Erythema of the palate was caused by a removable orthodontic "plate" worn by the patient for some time, but without success.

*Left:* The radiograph reveals horizontal bone loss and diastemata in both anterior segments, which may have been caused by a tongue thrust habit.

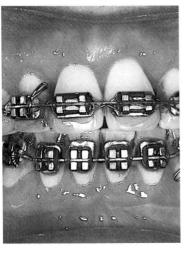

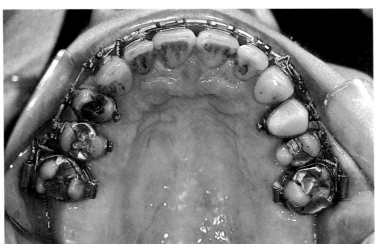

**898 Fixed orthodontic appliance**
Brackets were affixed by means of acid-etched resin; the treatment involved edgewise technique and headgear. All maxillary and mandibular teeth were included in the orthodontic therapy.

These clinical views were taken immediately before removal of the appliances at the termination of active treatment.

*Left:* Maxillary and mandibular anterior teeth following orthodontic treatment.

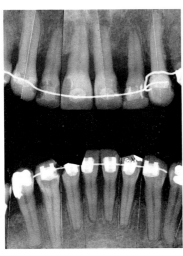

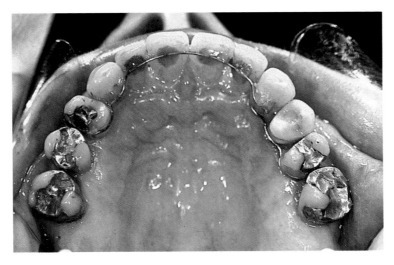

**899 Retention**
Acid-etched resin was used with a palatal arch wire for retention in the maxillary anterior segment; its esthetic value is obvious.

The necessary restorative work and follow-up treatment for periodontitis may now begin. The patient should be placed on a short-interval recall initially due to enhanced plaque accumulation caused by the appliances.

*Left:* In the mandible, retention was achieved by means of a wire in the already present facial brackets.

Courtesy P. Stöckli

# Uprighting the Mandibular Second Molar

It is not necessary to prosthetically close every space in the dental arch. If the occlusion is stable and there is adequate periodontal support, no drifting of teeth should occur.

Tipping of a second molar into a first molar extraction sight is a common occurrence, and is accelerated in a dentition manifesting periodontal destruction. The mesial surface of the tipped molar becomes an excellent area for plaque accumulation, which promotes the development of a still deeper periodontal pocket on this surface (Ericsson 1986). This was the situation presented by a 48-year-old female with adult periodontitis (AP), whose case is depicted below.

Tooth 38 was extracted during initial therapy, for endodontic reasons. Both lower second molars were uprighted during a 7-month period before seating fixed 3-unit bridges bilaterally.

The tooth movement was accomplished with an appliance incorporating a bite plane extending distally to the bicuspid area, a labial bow, and uprighting springs mesial to both second molars.

**900 Initial panoramic radio-graph – Mesially tipped second mandibular molars**
Following extraction of the first molars years ago, the second molars had tipped severely into the spaces. Periodontal pockets had formed on the mesial surfaces of the second molars (plaque retention, difficult home care). The development of mesial pockets may have been accelerated by the change in occlusion that occurred with the initial tipping of the molars, resulting in nonphysiologic forces on the molars and further tipping.

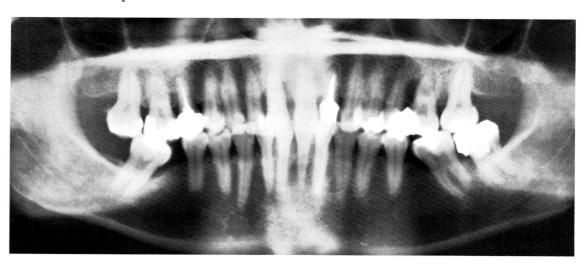

**901 Removable appliance – Lateral views**
Mandibular appliance was fabricated from clear acrylic and incorporated an anterior bite plane, labial bow with adjustment loops and uprighting springs for the molars.

Opening the bite was necessary to eliminate occlusal interferences on the molars during uprighting.

Although clumsier and less precise than a fixed appliance, the removable appliance is often preferred by adult patients.

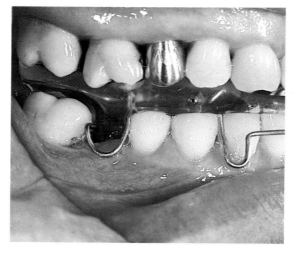
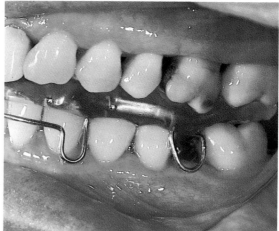

**902 Panoramic radiograph after completion of orthodontic and prosthetic treatment**
Tooth 38 was extracted and the two lower second molars were uprighted.

The 3-unit bridges were prepared and seated soon after completion of orthodontic therapy, serving as retainers for the uprighted molars. The pontics of the bridges permit adequate access for oral hygiene on the mesial surfaces of the second molars.

Courtesy P. Stöckli

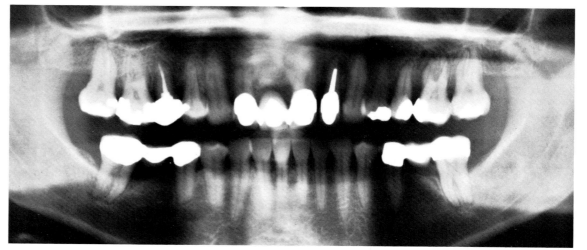

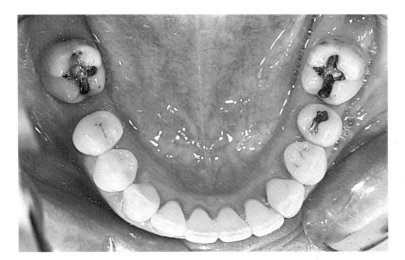

**903 Initial occlusal view**
The second molars (47; 37) are severely tipped mesially.

The tipping has narrowed the extraction site, making adequate oral hygiene difficult and promoting plaque retention (gingivitis, periodontitis). Pockets exist mesial to both second molars.

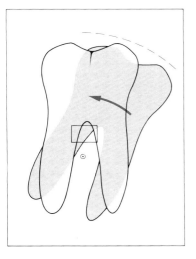

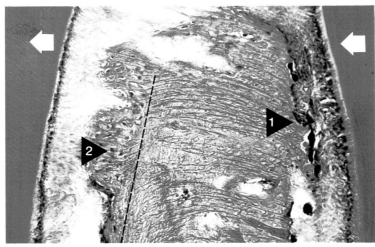

**904 Bone resorption and deposition during orthodontic treatment – Histology**
The white arrows indicate direction of uprighting a mandibular molar (furcation area). In the pressure zone (black arrow **1**), one notes osteoclastic bone resorption, while in the tension zone (black arrow **2**) bone apposition is observed (van Gieson, x 25).

Courtesy *N. P. Lang*

*Left:* The diagram depicts the center of rotation during uprighting of a 2-rooted molar, located between the roots, near the bifurcation.

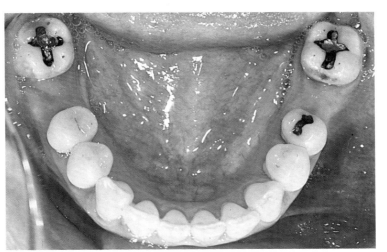

**905 Molar uprighting complete**
Definitive prosthetic work should begin immediately, to maintain the space created.

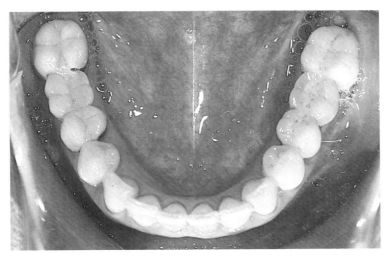

**906 Space closure – Retention**
Fixed bridgework maintains the uprighted molars and affords replacement of the missing teeth.

The interdental spaces and the area beneath the pontics are contoured to permit and facilitate home care by the patient, who can use interdental brushes in these areas.

Courtesy *P. Stöckli*

## Treatment of the Malpositioned Canine

A 14-year-old female was referred because of extremely severe gingivitis and malpositioning of the maxillary right canine, which caused a plaque retentive area. However, oral hygiene was not substandard only in *this* region! The patient proved extremely difficult to motivate. The erythematous, edematous, swollen gingiva bled at the slightest touch. Following initial therapy, a removable orthodontic appliance was selected over a fixed appliance because of the unreliable patient cooperation in home care. Fixed appliances require a high level of patient cooperation and motivation for plaque control around brackets and wires. A removable appliance can be easily cleaned at the sink, and the oral cavity is easier to keep clean as well.

Financial considerations may also be a factor in the selection of fixed or removable orthodontic appliances. In this case, during the course of orthodontic treatment the patient's oral hygiene improved considerably, after repeated OHI.

**907 Initial view – Malpositioned canine**
The maxillary right canine was severely malpositioned. The use of a plaque disclosing agent revealed the very poor oral hygiene. The canine and the palatally displaced left lateral incisor created especially difficult plaque-retentive areas. The result was extremely severe gingivitis with pseudopockets.

*Right:* Detail of the area around 13, 12. When the gingiva is reflected with an instrument the massive subgingival plaque accumulations are visible.

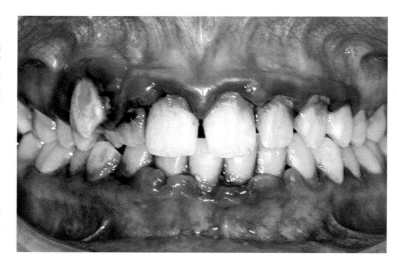
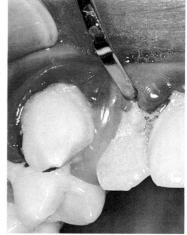

**908 Removable orthodontic appliance**
Subsequent to periodontal initial therapy, a palatal plate with a labial arch wire was fabricated. The appliance incorporated a finger spring on 11 and a modified adjustment loop for vertical and lingual forces on the canine (13).

Extraction of the first premolar (14) was necessary to create space for the malpositioned canine. The orthodontic treatment lasted about one year.

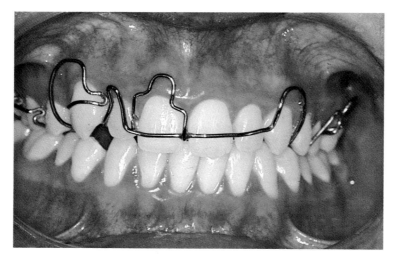

**909 Final result 3 years after initiation of therapy**
The orthodontic result is acceptable. The patient (now 17 years old) performs home care effectively using the Bass technique and dental floss. Use of a disclosing agent reveals plaque in only a few locations.

*Right:* Bringing the maxillary right canine into line makes maintaining oral hygiene in the area easier (use of dental floss is depicted).

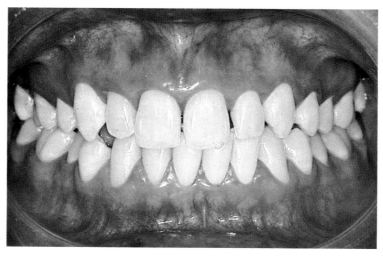
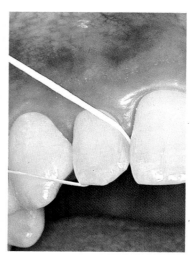

# Splinting – Stabilization

The significance and the value of immobilizing mobile teeth by splinting as a periodontal therapeutic technique remain controversial. In order to clarify whether there exist any true indications for splinting, one must first consider the causes of tooth mobility:

*Quantitative* loss of supporting structure due to periodontitis

*Qualitative* alterations of supporting structures due to trauma from occlusion

Short-term trauma to the periodontium due to treatment of periodontitis

Combinations of the above

Mobile teeth whose degree of mobility is not increasing *do not* generally require splinting. Teeth with increased mobility traced to occlusal trauma should be treated by occlusal adjustment, not by splinting (Vollmer & Rateitschak 1975). While it is true that mobile teeth can be immobilized by splinting, and that this may provide some comfort for the patient, it does not lead to any long-term biologic stabilization of teeth (Galler et al. 1979, Rateitschak 1980).

Depicted below is a classification of splinting possibilities:

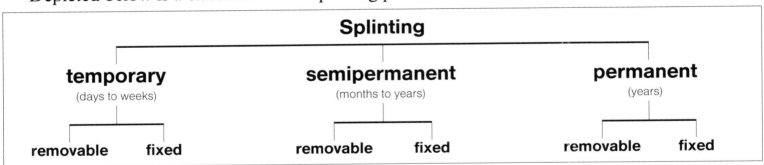

**Indications for the various types of splinting**

*Temporary or semipermanent* splinting is indicated for severely mobile teeth before or during periodontal therapy. Such splinting can reduce treatment trauma.

*Semipermanent or permanent* splinting may be used to stabilize highly mobile teeth that impair the patient's chewing. Splinting may be employed during an observation period before determination of the long-term prognosis. Orthodontic retention may also be viewed as a type of semipermanent splinting.

*Permanent* splinting is employed during complex oral rehabilitation where abutments are highly mobile or where a few abutments must support the entire prosthesis, particularly when such abutment teeth have minimal periodontal support but have been successfully treated periodontally. Splinting may also be necessary in cases of intractable parafunctions. If such teeth are not splinted, the danger of progressively increasing tooth mobility exists (Nyman & Lindhe 1979).

# Temporary Splinting

The simple wire ligature (Fig. 910) may serve as a *fixed* splint for a few days to several weeks. Wire ligatures are seldom used today, primarily because of the esthetic considerations. A more commonly used fixed temporary splint is the acid-etch composite resin splint without tooth preparation (Fig. 911). Such a splint can be applied quickly and easily with the rubber dam in place; however, it is a temporary measure because adhesion of the resin to tooth structure is not very strong without the additional mechanical retension provided by a cavity preparation, grooves etc. Fracture of the splint is common if more than 3–4 teeth are included in a single splinted unit.

A *removable* temporary splint may be fabricated of clear acrylic pulled under vacuum over a study model (Fig. 912). Such splints are often indicated for temporary stabilization of individual teeth for short periods of time. This type of splint was formerly used as a "bite guard" in the treatment of oral parafunction, but with very little success.

**910 Wire splint**
Soft steel wire (0.4 mm dia) is wrapped around the facial and oral surfaces of the teeth to be splinted, and the ligature is tightened by twisting the ends.

Stabilization of individual teeth is accomplished by application of interdental ligatures. Acid-etch resin "stops" may be applied to the labial surface of each tooth (cf. Fig. 895) to prevent the wire from slipping apically.

A wire splint affords no protection against occlusal forces, but it can reinforce periodontal dressings and acrylic splints.

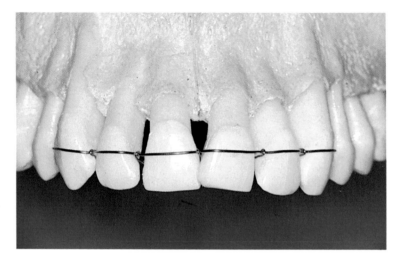

**911 Composite resin splint, no tooth preparation**
After thoroughly cleaning the teeth, the interproximal surfaces are acid-etched and resin is applied. The apical area of the interdental space must be left open for oral hygiene.

*Right:* Above, incisal view of resin splint in place; below, scanning EM view of an acid-etched enamel surface (red = etched enamel; yellow = composite resin).

SEM Courtesy *F. Lutz*

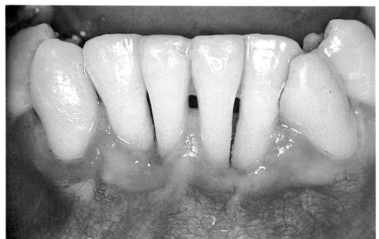
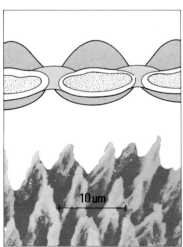
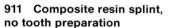

10 μm

**912 Vacuum formed removable acrylic splint**
This splint can be used for short-term retention or stabilization of teeth.

*Right:* The margin of the splint should extend just beyond the height of contour of each tooth (black arrows) on both labial and lingual surfaces, to provide secure retention.

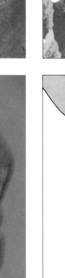
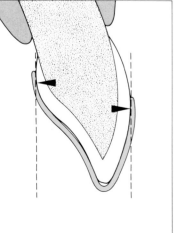

# Semipermanent Splinting – Anterior Area

The most commonly employed *fixed* semipermanent splint in the anterior area is the acid-etch composite resin splint applied after tooth preparation. It may serve for several months or even years. Often it is possible to remove old anterior restorations and utilize the cavity preparations in the splint. The technique of application is identical to placement of composite resin restorations using the acid-etch pretreatment.

The procedure is generally performed using the rubber dam, because even the slightest moisture con-tamination after etching the enamel and application of the composite material could compromise the result of the procedure. Light-polymerized resin is used for this type of splint because of its long working time.

*Removable* semipermanent splints may be fabricated as cast chrome-cobalt alloy frameworks incorporating finger clasps for retention. This type of splint generally is indicated only for wear at night, as a retention applicance after orthodontic treatment (see Fig. 896).

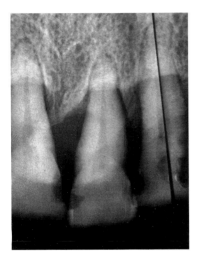

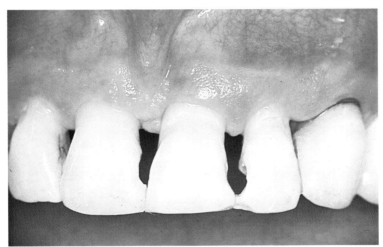

**913 Composite resin splint with tooth preparation**
This 38-year-old female was adamant in her wish that the almost hopelessly involved maxillary anterior teeth be maintained.

Following initial therapy, the highly mobile teeth 11, 21 and 22 were stabilized by removing the old Class III resins and using the cavity preparations for retention.

*Left:* Radiographic view. Pronounced attachment loss. The root of tooth 21 exhibits approximately 75% attachment loss.

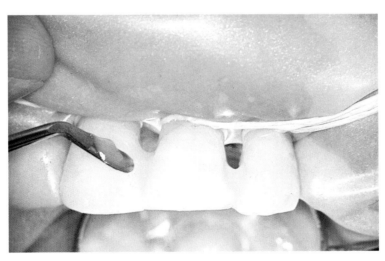

**914 Splint application with rubber dam**
After etching the cavity margins with phosphoric acid, the cavity preparations and the coronal portion of the interdental spaces are filled with light-cured composite resin, which is permitted to set and is then definitively polished.

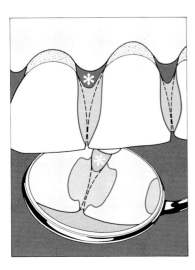

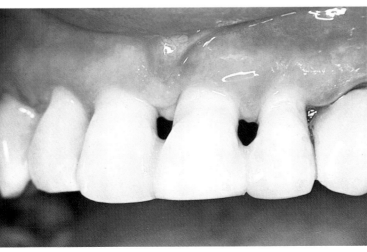

**915 Three years later**
The interdental spaces were left open beneath the contact areas; this permitted good interdental hygiene using toothpicks and interdental brushes.

*Left:* Schematic depiction of the splint. Red = acid-etched areas, yellow = composite resin.

The resin is retained by both the acid-etching and by the undercuts of the cavity preparations. The asterisk (*) denotes the open interdental space (hygiene).

# Semipermanent Splinting – Posterior Area

The question of whether a tooth with pronounced attachment loss should be retained or extracted can often not be answered at the initial examination. Even following initial therapy or after surgical intervention, the estimation of long-term prognosis may be difficult. The decision concerning whether to retain or to remove a tooth becomes even more problematic if the extraction would reconcile the patient to an extensive prosthetic solution, or to a free-end partial denture situation. It is in such situations that semipermanent splinting may be indicated. Such splints may remain for months or even years in the posterior segments. Two such cases are presented here.

**Case 1:** In this 50-year-old patient attachment loss and trauma have led to severe mobility of tooth 14. Following initial therapy and before planning the rehabilitation for the entire dentition, the decision was made to employ semipermanent splinting for several months and to observe whether stabilization and/or osseous regeneration would occur, especially mesial to 14.

**Case 1**

**916   After initial therapy**
Despite initial therapy and selective grinding, tooth 14 remains highly mobile. The old amalgam restoration presents an opportunity for semipermanent splinting.

*Right:* The radiograph depicts the rather severe attachment loss, especially on the mesial aspect of tooth 14.

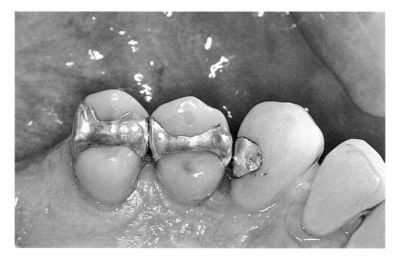
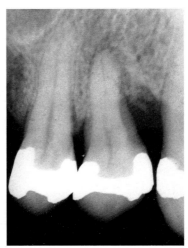

**917   Occlusal groove and wire placement**
A groove is cut into the occlusal amalgams in teeth 13, 14 and 15 with retentive undercuts. A stiff stainless steel wire (ca. 1 mm dia.) is adapted into the groove for reinforcement.

The groove is subsequently filled with composite resin.

*Right:* The schematic depicts how the strong metal reinforcement (black) is completely surrounded by the composite material (yellow). The old amalgam restoration (black) is also visible.

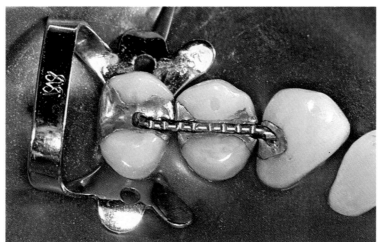
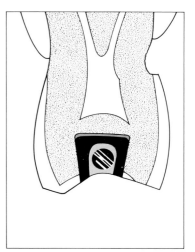

**918   Semipermanent splint**
It is imperative that the interdental space beneath the splint be left open for cleaning. Here, for example, interdental brushes can be conveniently used.

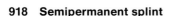
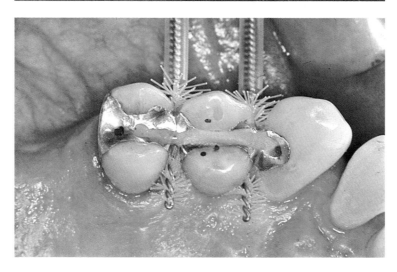

**Case 2:** In this 35-year-old patient, tooth 17 was lost and 16 appeared hopeless, with severe attachment loss, especially distally and palatally. An abscess (fistula) had formed from the palatal root. This apical process was confluent with the deep palatal pocket.

In order to spare the patient an expansive fixed bridge or a partial denture, the decision was made to attempt to maintain tooth 16. Tooth 17 was extracted, root canal therapy was performed on 16, whose palatal root was also resected. The splinting was performed antecedent to these operations. Relatively deep cavities were prepared on teeth 16, 15 and 14; the vital teeth were treated with a thin cement base. The rubber dam was applied, and the enamel etched occlusally. After placing a small amount of composite resin onto the floor of each cavity preparation, a twisted, stainless steel wire was placed. The cavities were then filled, layer by layer using light-sensitive material. Occlusal "stops" should be on sound tooth structure; if this is not universally possible, small amalgam "stops" may have to be placed in the acrylic to oppose the occluding cusps.

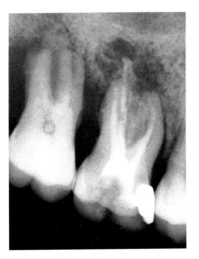
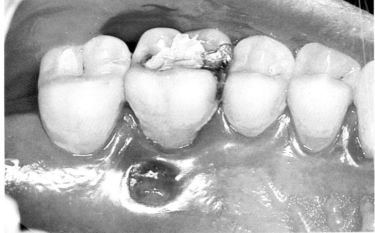

**Case 2**

**919  Emergency: Apical abscess with palatal fistula**
Virtually hopeless situation for teeth 16 and 17.

Tooth 17 will be extracted, and an attempt will be made to retain 16 by endodontics and resection of the palatal root.

*Left:* Radiograph before extraction of 17. Tooth 16 has already been treated endodontically.

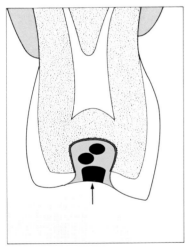
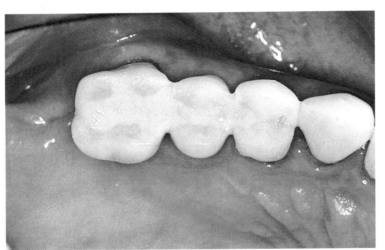

**920  Splint complete**
The occlusion must be checked and adjusted appropriately.

*Left:* If centric contacts from opposing teeth fall onto the resin splint, and the splint is destined for long-term use, the dentist may elect to put amalgam "stops" in the occlusal surface at the contact areas (black arrow). Such "stops" will be more resistant to abrasion.

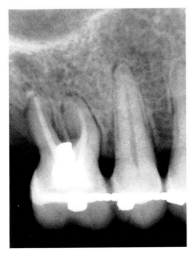
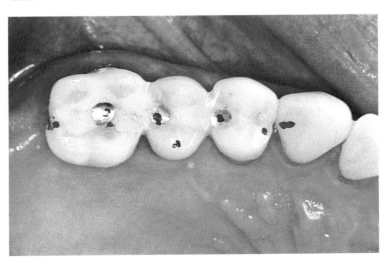

**921  Amalgam stops**
All of the major occlusal contact (red marks) of mandibular cusp tips with the splinted unit are either on enamel or on the amalgam stops.

*Left:* Visible in the radiograph are the remaining buccal roots and the amalgam used in the pulp chamber before resection of the palatal root, one year after treatment.

The definitive treatment plan includes restorations on 14 and 15, a crown on 16, with reduction of the orofacial width of the tooth from the palatal (*no* palatal root).

# Permanent Splinting – Adhesive Technique

Soon after introduction of the acid-etch technique for anterior restorations, the so-called adhesive bridges and adhesive splints were propagated (Rochette 1973). In recent years, this technique has been refined. Methods for preparation of enamel have been developed that ensure adequate retention of such constructions after conservative tooth preparation (Holste & Renk 1985; Besimo & Jäger 1986a, b; Livaditis 1986; Marinello et al. 1987, 1988). When splinting in the anterior region, the proximal surfaces of the teeth are rendered parallel and fine grooves are prepared. Shallow depressions at the margin provide occlusal support. The incisal edges are not included, for esthetics reasons.

In contrast to the semipermanent splints that simply bond adjacent teeth with acid-etch resin, bridges and splints prepared with the acid-etch technique can serve as definitive immobilization for mobile teeth.

The acid-etch splinting technique is demonstrated below in the mandible of a 46-year-old patient.

**922 Mandibular anterior area following initial periodontal therapy**
All four front teeth are mobile. The high degree of mobility of 31 and 41 is particularly disturbing to the patient (insecurity, fear of tooth loss). In order to minimize the trauma of the subsequent therapy and to improve patient comfort, a cast splint is planned.

*Right:* Radiographic findings. Particularly pronounced attachment loss between 31 and 32, and between 41 and 42.

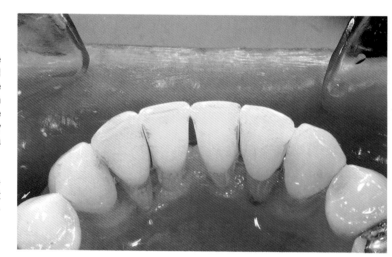
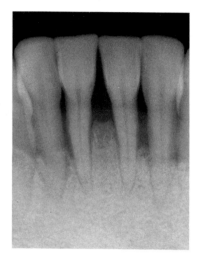

**923 Before seating the splint**
A rubber dam must be placed in the area of operation before acid-etch and subsequent seating of the splint. The elegant preparations (only in enamel!) are scarcely visible in the clinical picture.

*Right:* Preparation and splint form. The occlusal and lateral aspects depict the careful and minimal tooth preparation. Enamel must be maintained at all prepared surfaces, otherwise adhesion after acid-etching is not guaranteed.

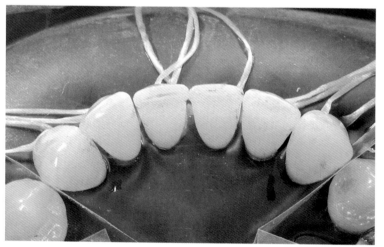
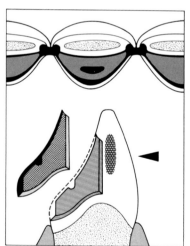

**924 After seating the splint with composite resin**
The periodontitis therapy (subgingival scaling, surgical intervention if necessary) can be continued without compromise; the healing process can be observed over months or even years (long-term prognosis).

*Right:* Clinical picture 3 months after subgingival scaling.

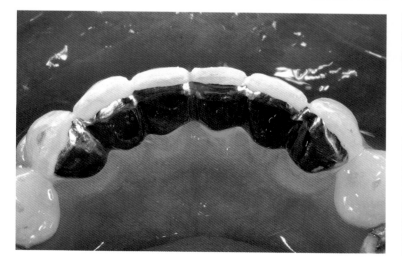
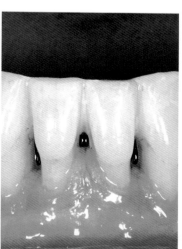

Courtesy *W. Iselin*

# Reconstruction – Prosthetics

Dental caries morbidity continues in a slow but steady decline in all western countries. On the other hand, periodontitis has not yet shown such a tendency to decline. These facts create a situation wherein, especially in the elderly, teeth are extracted more often for periodontal reasons. Furthermore, prosthetic replacement of such lost teeth must almost always be accomplished using as abutments remaining teeth that have lost tooth-supporting structure.

The primary goal of *all* dental procedures must be maintenance of the natural dentition, accomplished through regular *preventive measures* and, whenever necessary, early *periodontal treatment*. Extensive and costly prosthetic partial replacements that more often than not damage the remaining dentition and periodontium more than helping them, can be avoided (Strub & Belser 1978)!

## Problems in Periodontal Prosthetics

### Replacement: yes or no?

If periodontal therapy is instituted too late, or if individual teeth are lost despite periodontal therapeutic efforts, the question becomes: Should such teeth be replaced at all? Dentistry has progressed beyond the "feeling" that a healthy, functional dentition must contain 28 teeth (sans wisdom teeth). The fact is that in many cases molars are lost due to furcation involvement and the dental arch is reduced in many cases (especially in elderly patients) to solely *premolar occlusion,* which may be completely tolerable (Helkimo et al. 1978; Käyser 1981; Lang 1982; DeBoever 1978, 1984).

The most important feature is not the "tooth replacement," but the reinstatement of chewing function, esthetics and speech; in short, the *oral health oft the patient.*

### Temporal sequence

*Definitive prosthetic treatment* in a periodontally compromised dentition may only begin several months after conclusion of the treatment for periodontitis. It is only at this time that the periodontal tissue relationships have consolidated. The patient's level of home care cooperation is known. The prognosis for the individual abutment teeth can be established with some certainty after re-evaluation. In the interim between conclusion of periodontal therapy and definitive prosthetic treatment, a dentally-born temporary replacement of the highest possible quality should be provided.

The path that leads to successful and long-term prosthetic replacement is predicated in many instances upon:

- Periodontal therapy
- Seating a temporary prosthesis

The length of time that a temporary replacement will be used will vary from case to case depending upon the remaining dentition, the remaining support around abutment teeth, the long-term prognosis etc.; it may range from a few months to several years.
The decision must also be made concerning whether the temporary should be *removable* or *fixed.* Such a decision is based upon the strategic locations of remaining teeth as well as the planned lifespan of the temporary. Removable temporaries (plates with clasps) are generally less "friendly" to the periodontium than *fixed* temporaries.

- Re-evaluation and definitive prosthetic planning
- Definitive reconstruction that promotes hygiene accessibility and therefore periodontal health
- Regular recall

# Fixed Provisional Restoration

Temporary replacements for lost teeth must be "friendly" to the periodontium. This is especially true when the temporary is to be inserted immediately after extraction of hopeless teeth and periodontal surgery on the remaining teeth. Any temporary replacement must not negatively influence the healing process. Fixed temporary replacement is preferable whenever this is possible. Generally speaking, spaces created by tooth extraction should be closed immediately; lone-standing molars may be an exception to this rule.

Prepared teeth should be provided immediately with temporaries that provide satisfactory chewing function.

Immediate temporaries must often be replaced after a few weeks by more precise long-term temporaries. Such temporaries should correspond in position, contour, interdental space relationships and occlusal surfaces to the definitive replacements that will follow.

Depicted is a 42-year-old with adult periodontitis who was treated with a fixed temporary after extractions and periodontal therapy.

**925   After initial therapy**
The corrective treatment phase begins with the extraction of 12; 21 and 22. During the same surgical procedure, the abutment teeth 13, 11 and 23 are treated periodontally for pocket elimination, and a fixed temporary is incorporated.

During the appointment before the surgical procedure, the *abutment teeth* are grossly prepared and an impression is made of the prepared teeth; in the laboratory the "extracted" teeth are eliminated and an acrylic bridge is prepared.

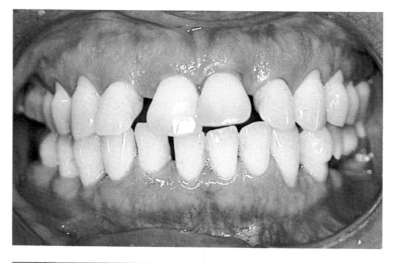

**926   Immediately after surgery**
The extractions and the periodontal procedures on the prepared abutment teeth are performed simultaneously. A frenotomy is also performed.

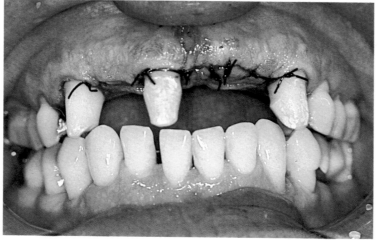

**927   Long-term temporary bridge**
The acrylic bridge that had been fabricated in the laboratory is adjusted and seated. All crown margins are clearly supragingival.

Definitive tooth preparation and construction and seating of the final bridgework can only begin after complete healing of the periodontal surgical areas and the extraction wounds; this is generally a matter of months.

*Right:* The schematic clearly shows that the crown margins (e.g., tooth 23) remain supragingival.

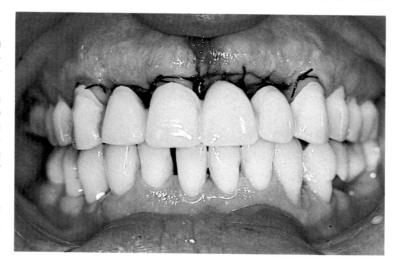
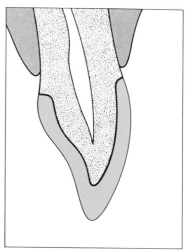

# Removable Provisional Appliance

A removable temporary is indicated when the definitive prosthetic treatment is to be a cast framework partial denture or one incorporating telescope crowns, or if only a few abutment teeth remain for anchorage.

The requirements of a definitive removable partial denture should also be fulfilled by the temporary denture: Clasps must hold the abutment teeth bodily, occlusal rests (dental/periodontal support) must prevent apical depression of saddles, the marginal gingiva must not be traumatized by clasps or the denture base.

A temporary denture fabricated before the surgery often requires adjustment upon insertion, because the postoperative conditions are seldom exactly like those "estimated" in the lab. It is often necessary to reline the denture immediately for good tissue adaptation.

Even a precisely constructed removable temporary may irritate the periodontal structures of the remaining teeth (especially a palatal plate).

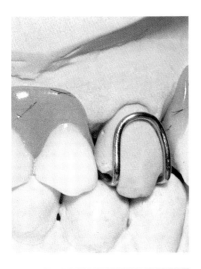
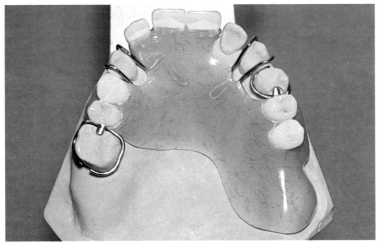

**928   Removable maxillary temporary denture on model**
The retentive elements grasp the abutment teeth bodily. The canine incisal edges were reduced mesially and distally to provide space for the cast arms. This was permissible because the treatment plan calls for canines to receive full cast telescope crowns. The ledges created on the canines provide dental support for the temporary denture.
Neither the denture base nor the clasps must be permitted to impinge on the marginal gingiva.

*Left:* Detail of the clasp on tooth 13.

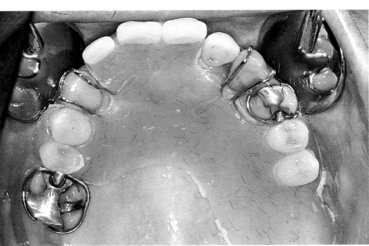

**929   Temporary denture after relining**
Immediately following the periodontal surgery, which included extractions and flap procedures, the temporary denture is adapted in the mouth and relined using a soft material.
The soft reliner also serves as a wound dressing.

*Left:* The wire clasp on tooth 13 prevents apical displacement of the temporary denture.

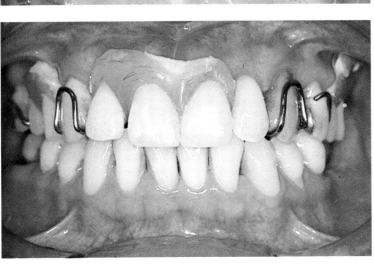

**930   Frontal view of relined upper temporary denture**
The canine clasps are optimum in terms of function, but minimal in terms of esthetics.

# Long-Term Temporaries – Adhesive Bridges

Under the rubrik "Permanent Splinting – Adhesive Technique," the development and the clinical aspects of this procedure were described (p. 352).

In the anterior area, especially in the maxilla, adhesive bridges are indicated relatively frequently as long-term temporaries or even as definitive replacement for individual teeth. Mandibular anterior teeth often exhibit severe but irregular attachment loss. If, for example, an individual mandibular incisor cannot be retained, and its neighbor is equally periodontally compromised but still treatable, the treatment of choice over the long term is often extraction of all four front teeth. An appropriate prosthetic solution would then be the seating of an 8-unit bridge from 44, 43 to 33, 34. This kind of excessively costly treatment may be avoided by use of adhesive bridges. The esthetics is exceptionally good and the costs are relatively moderate. The abutment teeth adjacent to the space need only be lightly prepared.

An adhesive bridge to replace tooth 21 is depicted below in a 41-year-old patient.

**931   Extraction of 31**
Tooth 31 exhibits pronounced attachment loss and is highly mobile. The tooth-supporting structures of the adjacent teeth are endangered. The treatment plan includes periodontitis therapy for the entire dentition. Tooth 31 will be extracted.

*Right:* The radiograph depicts a Williams probe within the 10 mm pocket.

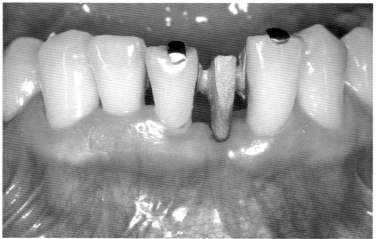
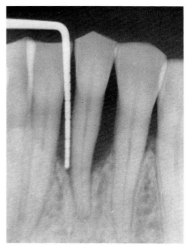

**932   Try-in of the bridge framework**
The bridge framework spans all four anterior teeth. The "hooks" over teeth 41 and 32 guarantee precise positioning during the try-in. The hooks are removed before definitive seating.

*Right:* Adhesive bridge immediately before seating, with etched adhesive surfaces. The relief of the minimal tooth preparation can hardly be observed.

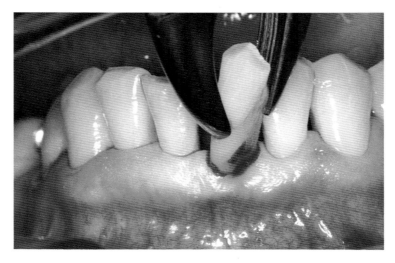
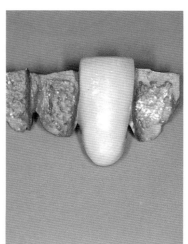

**933   Seated adhesive bridge**
Before cementation, e.g., during framework try-in, the color and shape of the pontic is checked. Here it is too wide and a bit too long apically (red mark).

Following etching of the lingual surfaces of the three remaining anterior teeth under the rubber dam, the bridge is seated using chemical and light-polymerized composite resin.

*Right:* Radiograph 2 months after extraction of 31; one month after seating the bridge.

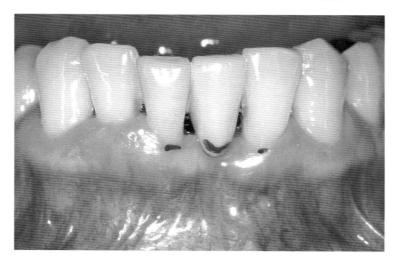
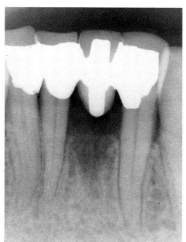

# Definitive Reconstruction – Fixed or Removable

## Prerequisites

The absolute prerequisite for any definitive reconstruction is a healthy periodontium.

The term *healthy* in this context does not only refer to connective tissue attachment at the physiologic level of youth (cf. pp. 1–10), but also a successfully *treated* periodontium whose marginal niveau may, in fact, be located considerably apically.

Periodontal therapy today is considered successful if shallow, non-active "pockets" remain; however, complete pocket elimination is desirable before construction of definitive reconstructions.

After periodontal therapy the following criteria must be met for any prosthetic reconstruction:

- Compulsory
  - Patient cooperation in home care
  - Clinical freedom from inflammation in the periodontium
  - Presence of only shallow, inactive sulci/pockets
- Optional
  - Freedom from periodontal pockets
  - Normal gingival and osseous contours
  - Adequate (1–2 mm) attached gingiva

## Fixed replacement – Possibilities and limitations

When fixed bridgework is planned today, even in a periodontally compromised dentition, one must deviate from ancient dogma! The "classic" Ante's law (Ante 1926, 1936, 1938) demanded that whenever a fixed bridge is seated, the abutment's root surfaces anchored in periodontal supporting tissues must be at least as expansive as that of the teeth to be replaced. This theory dominated the thinking of teachers, clinicians and practitioners for decades. The unnecessary inclusion of additional abutment teeth in bridge constructions is often associated more with damage than with advantage: Healthy teeth are ground down (with loss of vitality), subgingival crown margins elicit periodontal damage, increased plaque retention, unnecessary splinting.

The clinical studies from the Gothenburg school (Nyman & Lindhe 1976, Nyman & Ericsson 1982) have clearly shown that even long-span bridges and total reconstructions can serve adequately for many years even when seated upon few abutments that exhibit compromised, but healthy (treated) periodontal conditions.

The limitations of fixed replacements can certainly be reached when only very few (3–5) abutments are available in a dental arch.

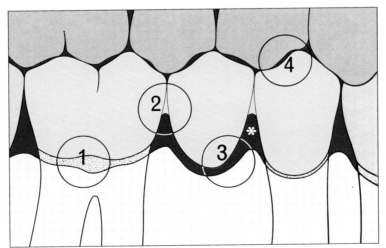

**934  Periodontal problem zones with fixed replacements**

**1** Supragingival crown margins, precise marginal adaptation

**2** Open interdental spaces, crown contour

**3** Point- or line-shape contact of pontic with tissue

**4** Occlusion, articulation

Points 1–3 permit ideal plaque control by dentist and patient.

## Removable replacement – Possibilities and limitations

In a dentition that is seriously compromised periodontally, the few teeth that can be successfully retained after periodontal therapy should serve as abutments for a removable ("hybrid") prosthesis. In such cases, the so-called telescope (coping) reconstructions have been shown to be compatible with periodontal health (Körber 1974). Hybrid prosthetic reconstructions often serve the function of transition to total prosthetic replacement (Geering & Kundert 1986, Graber 1986). The accessibility of individual abutments makes plaque control relatively easy.

The removable cast framework partial denture may serve well in patients who are to be treated palliatively and in those for whom financial considerations play a significant role in the treatment plan (Bergmann et al. 1982; see also Treatment Planning, p. 138).

The dentist should never attempt to exceed the wishes of the patient; don't "over treat." There is no reason to refuse a complete denture to a patient with advanced periodontitis, if that patient is prepared to accept that form of treatment or even desires it! This may be particularly true for elederly patients, who often require an extended adaptation period for any prosthetic replacement.

# Fixed Reconstructions

In this context "fixed" reconstruction denotes primarily crowns and bridges. In a broader view, however, the term also includes combinations of fixed and removable reconstructions, e.g., an anterior bridge that extends to the canines or premolars, and on which precision attachments or clasps of a removable free-end prosthesis are attached. Fixed replacements may also incorporate cantilevered extensions, e.g., extending a bridge into the second premolar or molar region without any distal abutment. This solution spares the patient from a removable free-end prosthesis (Figs. 937, 940;

Nyman & Lindhe 1979; Nyman & Ericsson 1982).

The requirements shown in Figure 934 are supported and discussed below. It quickly becomes clear that (with the exception of occlusion) the most important criteria are plaque control and the possibility for maintaining cleanliness in the marginal periodontal area.

– *Crown margins:* Whenever possible the apical extent of any crown should lie supragingivally and be accessible for hygiene. Partial crowns fulfill this requirement very well. With full crowns, step preparations

**935  Minimal reconstruction 13 (12) – Minimal demands of the patient!**
The 55-year-old patient demanded replacement for the missing tooth 12 after periodontal therapy. A porcelain-fused-to-metal crown with a cantilever off of 12 was prepared.

Additional indicated treatment was refused (extraction of the retained 35, space closure in the mandible, replacement of inadequate crowns on 37 and 38).

*The primary concern (red circle):* The cantilever bridge, which has now been in place for 7 years.

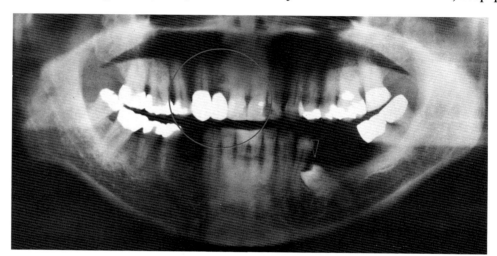

**936  Total reconstruction – High patient demands**
The 54-year-old refused a removable prosthesis in the maxilla. His problems included:
– Free-end situation (left)
– Furcation involvement (F2) on 16
– Moderate home care

*Planning:* Total rehabilitation in three phases. Total splint in the anterior area with two symmetrical lateral segments, connected to the anterior segment via milled and screw-retained attachments.

*The primary concern (red circle):* The 3-unit cantilever.

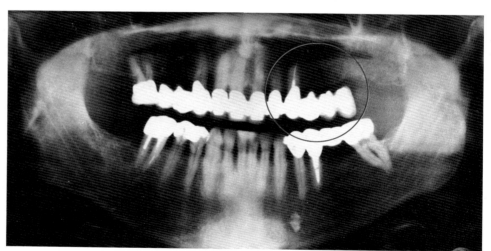

**937  Premolar occlusion with cantilever bridges in maxilla and mandible**
In a 66-year-old patient several hopeless premolars and molars were lost. She refused removable replacement, exhibited excellent home care and demanded maximum esthetics.

Problems: Relatively short clinical crowns (retention, space for interdental hygiene).

*The primary concern (red cirle):* The cantilevers in both maxilla and mandible.

Bridgework in situ for 4 years.

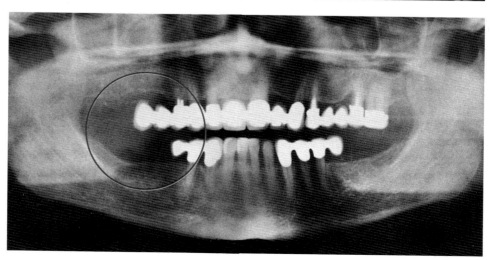

with tapered margins are preferred.

– *Interdental space, crown contour:* It is critical that adequate interdental hygiene be possible beneath soldered and nonsoldered contact points between crowns, between crowns and pontics, and between crowns and cantilevers. *Crown contour* must not be accentuated.

– *Pontics:* Pontics and cantilevered elements should generally be reduced in orofacial dimension (Finger et al. 1981). Pontics should contact the gingiva at a point or along a fine line, to ensure adequate cleansibility (e.g., Super-Floss). Exception to these general rules may have to be made for esthetic reasons in the anterior area (Fig. 938).

– *Occlusion:* If the expanse of a fixed bridge is short, its occlusal form should correspond to that of the remaining dentition, assuming that the patient exhibits no general stomatognathic symptoms or difficulties. If this is not the case, preliminary treatment may be required. In the case of long-span reconstructions, mounting of the case in a regulatable articulator is required, with occlusion adjusted according to the principles of "freedom in centric" (Ramfjord & Ash 1983, Ash & Ramfjord 1988).

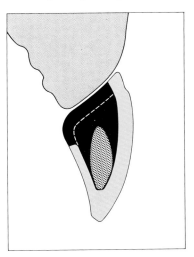

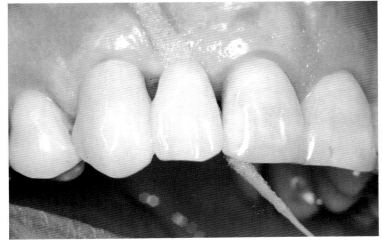

**Plaque control by:**

**938 Super-Floss –
Crown on 13, cantilevered 12**
Tooth 13: Porcelain-fused-to-metal crown, whose margins are at the gingival margin.
Tooth 12: Cantilevered pontic which contacts the ridge lightly (natural tooth length). The interdental spaces are accessible.

*Left:* As a compromise for esthetic and phonetic reasons, the pontic contacts the alveolar ridge over a rather broad surface; cleansibility with Super-Floss is maintained.

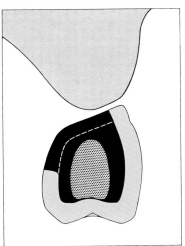

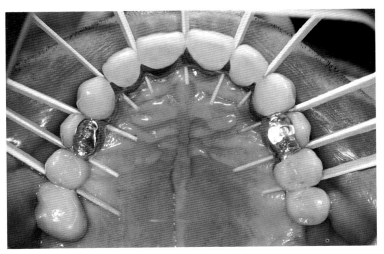

**939 Toothpicks –
Complete maxillary rehabilitation in 3 segments**
Precision attachments on teeth 14 and 24 (pontics) with massive connections to the anterior bridge. Nevertheless the possibility exists for using toothpicks in all interdental spaces for hygiene.

*Left:* The pontics and cantilevered units contact the alveolar ridge along a narrow line. The compromise of the anterior region (Fig. 938) is not indicated in premolar and molar regions.

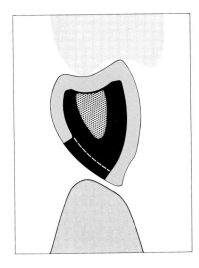

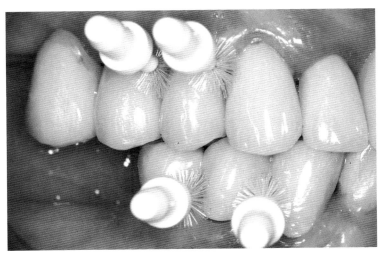

**940 Spiral brushes – Cantilever bridge in maxillary right segment and in the mandible**
The cantilevered units in the mandible do not contact the alveolar ridge and are thus accessible for cleaning with Super-Floss. The interdental spaces are open for cleaning with spiral brushes. The cantilevered pontics (15 & 16, no occlusion) sever only an esthetic function. This construction has been in place for 4 years.

*Left:* In the mandibular posterior region, pontics and cantilevers should not contact the alveolar mucosa, to enhance cleansibility.

# Removable Prosthetics – Cast Framework Partial Denture

The partial denture with a cast framework represents the minimal solution in terms of prosthetic replacement in a treated, periodontally compromised dentition. It is never as precise as a telescope construction or a combination of fixed and removable replacements. Nevertheless, *socioeconomic circumstances* frequently demand its use.

Bergmann et al. (1983) demonstrated that the useful life of a cast framework partial denture can approach 10 years in a patient with treated periodontitis who performs adequate home care.

Prerequisites for a long and complication-free partial denture lifespan include maintaining the proper occlusal relationships (selective grinding), precise construction, taking perfect impressions using customized trays, maintaining the interdental areas of remaining teeth (for hygiene), and keeping the patient on a regular recall schedule. In addition, the partial denture should be rigid, should have clasps that hold abutment teeth bodily, and should be tooth-borne (e.g., through use of occlusal rests). The major connector (palatal strap or lingual bar) should be strong yet not obtrusive (Graber 1986).

**941 Initial view**
Generalized, mild to moderate periodontitis (AP), with severe involvement of the maxillary anterior segment. These teeth are hopelessly involved. All other teeth can be treated periodontally and maintained.

The entire dentition exhibits extremely heavy deposits of plaque and calculus both supra- and subgingivally.

*Right:* The radiograph depicts the significant involvement of the anterior teeth. Extremely heavy calculus accumulation is obvious.

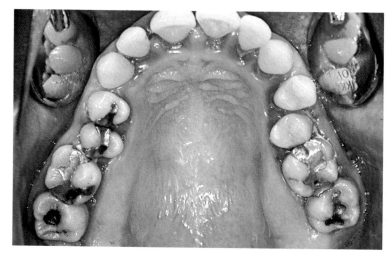
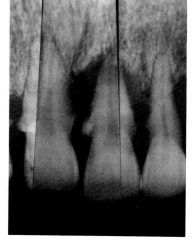

**942 After periodontal therapy**
The patient was completely informed of the alternatives available for replacement of the anterior teeth, including the prognosis for remaining teeth and expected costs. He elected the cast framework partial denture rather than a fixed anterior bridge.

Before taking the final impression, all old restorations were smoothed and polished. The teeth were recontoured according to the requirements of a removable framework partial denture (occlusal rests, parallelism, space for minor connectors, retention).

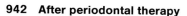
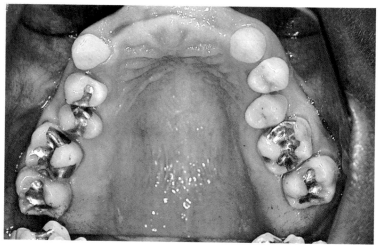

**943 Cast framework partial denture**
The gingival margins of all remaining teeth are not encroached upon by the major connector or the clasps. The unit does not add new plaque retentive areas. All clasps and retainers are kept away from the gingival margin insofar as this was possible.

*Right:* Clasps do not approach the gingival margin; the interdental spaces are open for cleaning.

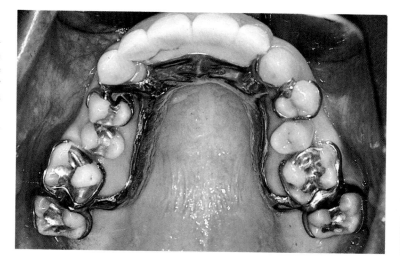
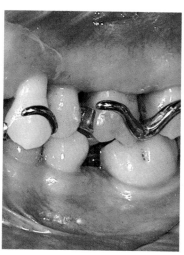

# Removable Prosthetics – Construction of Telescopes

The telescope ("coping") replacement is costly in terms of time and effort, but is especially "friendly" to the periodontal tissues. It permits perfect hygiene for the individual un-splinted primary abutment teeth.

A telescope construction can be made to resemble a *removable bridge* or a *partial denture*. The decision to use one or the other form will depend on the number and distribution of remaining teeth. If only very few abutments remain, a prosthesis incorporating a palatal strap is indicated to ensure transverse strength. Esthetic considerations may also influence the decision between telescope bridges or removable partial dentures. Problems often arise in anterior and canine areas, where abutment teeth must be severely reduced during tooth preparation in order to preclude overcontouring the final restoration.

The margin of the telescope crown should be located *supragingivally*. The denture base and any connectors (e.g., palatal strap) must not encroach upon gingival margin tissues. The occlusion must be functional, noninterfering and consistent with the patient's mandibular movements.

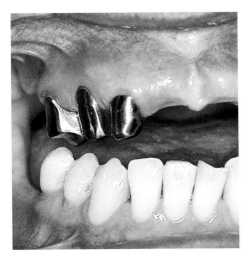
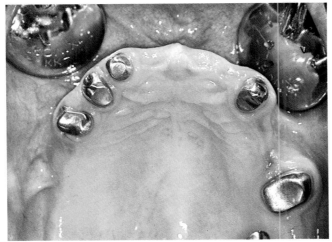

**944  Primary anchors for a telescoping construction**
Maxillary teeth 14, 13, 12; 23 and 26 received telescope caps 6 months after completion of periodontal therapy (pp. 253–257). All crown margins are located just supragingivally.

The prosthesis that seats onto the primary anchors may be either a removable bridge (**A**) or a removable partial denture (**B**).

In the 45-year-old patient depicted here, *both* types were fabricated and evaluated.

*Left:* Detail of the telescope crowns.

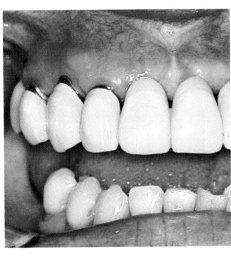
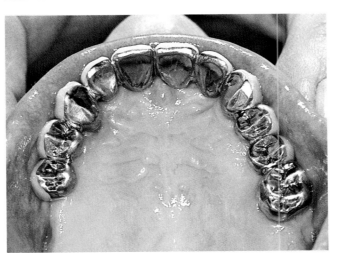

**945  A – Telescoping bridge (removable)**
The gingiva must not receive any irritation from the bridgework. The patient found the central incisors esthetically objectionable (too long).

*Left:* Detail of bridge construction.

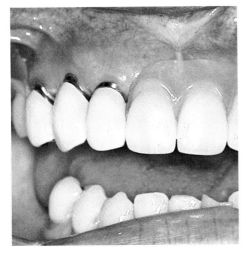
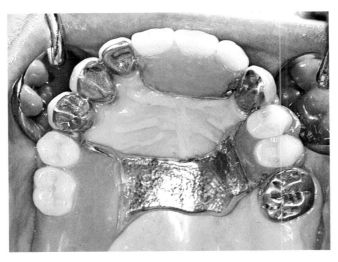

**946  B – Telescoping partial denture**
It was possible to improve the esthetics in the anterior region. Neither the saddle nor the palatal strap encroach on the gingival margin.

When the partial denture is removed, perfect oral hygiene is easy on the 5 lone-standing abutments.

The *opinion of the patient* (not the dentist!) was that the partial denture variation was superior to the removable bridgework because of stability and esthetics.

*Left:* Detail of the prosthesis.

# Geriatric Periodontology? – The Periodontium in the Elderly

## Different circumstances

In the chapter on therapy it was stated that a scientific basis exists for the treatment of gingivitis, periodontitis and recession. The importance of patient cooperation in home care as a prerequisite to successful therapy was emphasized.

Such statements may have to be altered because of changing demographics: Decline in birth rate, longer life expectancy. Elderly individuals may suffer somatic as well as psychic changes, which may force physicians and dentists to deviate from conventional plans for treatment. This may not be taken to mean, however, that elderly individuals should be treated in any way "poorer" than younger persons, but that the treatment may simply be different.

It is also worthy of note that aging is not always associated with reductions in all bodily and psychic function and coordination (Geering 1986).

The following, as a general rule, are *decreased in the elderly:*

– Immune status, host resistance
– Muscular strength and coordination of movement

– Long-term resistance
– Perceptual speed
– Auditory, visual (color) and taste perception
– Adaptability to new situations (prostheses!)
– Short-term memory, complex learning

The following generally are *unaffected by age or may even be enhanced:*

– Long-term memory and ability to learn
– Experience, discrimination
– Healthy attitude towards one's fellow man
– Speaking ability, vocabulary, fluency
– Trainability of psychic and somatic functions
– Reliability, stability

It has been repeatedly emphasized that the following prerequisites must be fulfilled by patients before any extensive periodontal therapy:

1) Time, understanding and ability to withstand stress, 2) continual and proper cooperation in terms of home care and 3) good general health (immune status).

It is precisely these prerequisites that may be partially or totally absent in elderly individuals. Such patients may be less receptive ("It's not worth it any more"!).

**947 Age pyramids in 1920 and in the year 2000 – Switzerland**
*Left:* The age pyramid in 1920 was well balanced and even. The length of the bars depict the number of individuals in five age categories.

*Right:* By the year 2000 the "pyramid" is unequal and actually resembles a thick pear. This is due to slowing of the birth rate on the one hand as well as aging of the population. The length of the bars represents the percentage of citizens in five age categories. The darker color represents the working population; men (blue), women (red).

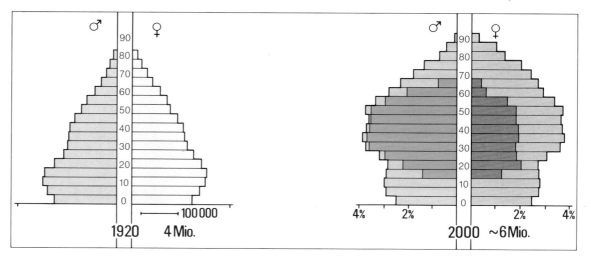

This attitude often leads to compromises during therapy. Despite understanding and good intentions, frequently the manual dexterity is lacking to achieve optimum plaque control. Plaque accumulation and gingival inflammation develop more rapidly, and periodontal bone loss appears to occur more quickly in old persons (Imfeld 1985).

## Changes in treatment planning

These facts may lead to more radical planning. Teeth with questionable prognoses (advanced attachment loss) are more likely candidates for extraction. Some would take the extreme position that only those teeth that can be expected to last to the end of life should be treated periodontally at all. It is better to provide an elderly patient with a prosthesis, perhaps even a complete denture (to which he can adapt) instead of maintaining such a patient for years or decades during periodontal therapeutic heroism, and then finally reconcile the patient to a complete denture that the patient does not accept or cannot any longer accept.

In the elderly patient it is not the type of therapy or even the saving of teeth at any price that is of prime importance, rather it is the maintenance of the patient's oral well being (health, function, esthetics, phonetics).

# Periodontology: Quo Vadis?

## Summary and Predictions

In the discipline of periodontolgy the evolution of new knowledge has progressed extremely rapidly in recent years. However, careful evaluation of the progress made reveals that many problems remain unsolved, many questions remain unanswered. These relate to etiology and pathogenesis and therefore also to diagnosis and therapy. Despite these reservations, treatment concepts exist today that are practice-proven and scientifically supported. Knowledge of and adherence to these concepts of gingivitis and most forms of periodontitis can predict successful prevention and treatment.

The utopian long-term goals of "causal" periodontal prevention and therapy remain vaccination against the disease and *Restitutio ad integrum* after treatment. Unfortunately, these goals are still a long way off! Where we stand today and which of our problems can likely be solved in the near future will be presented and discussed in this section.

### Etiology and pathogenesis

Fact: *Gingivitis can be defined clinically only by means of rather gross parameters* such as bleeding upon probing, visible inflammation (reddening) and edematous swelling. The causal relationship between microorganisms and the initiation of gingivitis was proven in 1965 (Löe et al.). Even today, however, the border between gingivitis and healthy gingiva is often difficult to discern. This may be explained by the fact that bacteria can *always* be found in the oral cavity, and even with good oral hygiene a very thin layer of plaque accumulates on the tooth surface in only a few hours. The exquisite host response mechanisms are responsible for the histologic picture, which exhibits some polymorphonuclear leukocytes within the junctional epithelium, as well as a discrete infiltrate containing a few lymphocytes, plasma cells and macrophages in the subepithelial conncective tissues. This is the case even in gingiva that appears "clinically healthy."

Fact: *Clinically manifest gingivitis does not always progress into periodontitis.* When such conversion does occur, it is likely due to the *combined* effects of a gram-negative, anaerobic, pathogenic flora (e. g., Bacteroides species, *A. actinomycetemcomitans*) and the response of the host (immune status) to such infectious attack. Host response is primarily a defense reaction; it can vary in intensity, it may be compromised in various ways, or it may become excessive (immunopathology).

The enormous importance of the immune system in defense against infection becomes dramatically clear when one considers how it can be weakened by the HIV virus (AIDS). This virus destroys but a single link (T-helper cells) in the extremely complex chain of host defense (p. 27), yet the consequences are so critical that the patient sooner or later *dies,* usually as the result of opportunistic infection or tumor.

Genco (1987) characterized the host response to periodontal infection in two forms: The "antibody-complement-PMN axis" and the "lymphocyte-macrophage-lymphokine axis." To date only the significance of the PMN has been well researched. Current dogma holds that PMNs play a key role in the progression of periodontitis. It has been demonstrated, for example, that in cases of extremely aggressive forms of disease the PMNs are injured by the leukotoxins produced by bacteria (e.g., Aa) and in this way lose their protective function. This may also be the mechanism by which bacteria actually penetrate into tissue. Congenital (hereditary) and acquired PMN defects in severe systemic syndromes (e.g., Chediak-Higashi) and systemic diseases (e.g., myeloid leukemia and juvenile diabetes) are always associated with rapidly progressive periodontitis.

In such conditions the PMNs do not respond to the bacterial chemotaxins, or their adherence and mobility are disturbed, or they are incapable of ingesting and phagocytosing bacteria. The capacity of PMNs to phagocytize may also be reduced by insufficient opsonization of bacteria by antibodies and/or complement.

Elevations of the antibody titer to specific bacteria have been reported, especially in LJP and RPP. However, no protective function has yet been attributed to these antibodies, which seem to be only polyclonal and non-specific.

In terms of the bacterially elicited inflammatory process, specific mediators (e.g., IL-1, TNF, $PGE_2$; p. 30) are known to exist in the "lymphocyte-macrophage-lymphokine axis." Some of these have been shown to be responsible for the destruction of periodontal tissues (e.g., collagen loss and bone resorption).

Research in bacterial and viral immunology is constantly leading to new knowledge that broadens our understanding of the pathogenesis of periodontal disease. It must, however, be acknowledged that all of these highly interesting results that have appeared in hundreds of basic science publications have as yet had essentially no significant therapeutic consequences in the practice of periodontics. We are learning more and more about the immune system, but we remain impotent in our effort to influence it for any periodontal therapeutic purposes. Periodontitis therapy via vaccination is not even a topic for discussion today, nor is the development of any drug capable of "favorably" influencing the immune response.

In the pathogenesis of periodontitis, "environmental" factors (microorganisms) have been studied in considerable depth, but very little is currently known about *genetic susceptibility* to periodontitis. The classical *human twin model* provides a straightforward method of considerable power for incorporating questions of genetic susceptibility or resistance to disease. In addition to detection and estimation of genetic contributions to individual differences, the effects of specific environmental factors may be evaluated.

Identical (monozygous) and fraternal (dizygous) twins represent a unique resource for studies of the origin and natural history of disease, because the genetic similarities are well-defined and easily understood. The twin paradigm has been successfully utilized in studies of dental caries (Goodman et al. 1959) and craniofacial disorders (Nakata 1985), and very recently attempts have been made to apply it in periodontology (Cockey et al. 1987, Michalowicz et al. 1988). Targeted approach to studies of genetics in periodontology is to be found also

in the recent research on juvenile periodontitis, whose hereditary basis has been well documented (Boughman et al. 1986, Long et al. 1987). Through comparisons of similar or clonal genotypes with documentation of naturally occurring environmental differences, it should be possible in the near future to elucidate specific factors that might indicate predisposition to destructive disease, so that preventive measures might be focused on individuals with these factors.

## Types of disease

*Gingivitis* is no longer viewed today as a serious disease. Furthermore it is widely acknowledged that even a clinically manifest gingivitis need not progress into periodontitis, if the host immune response is normal and adequate to the microbiologic challenge. Evidence is accumulating, in fact, that gingivitis is a predecessor only of *adult periodontitis (AP)* and not of the rapidly progressive forms such as RPP and LJP.

Such new knowledge does not mean, however, that the gingivae (and oral mucosa) should now be discounted or disregarded clinically. Both gingiva and oral mucosa often manifest clinical alterations in cases of hormonal imbalance or disturbance, systemic diseases and general infections (AIDS and others). This fact demands more and more the full attention of the dentist.

*Periodontitis* as a disease entity has become better understood in recent years, due primarily to advances in microbiology, immunology, epidemiology and connective tissue biochemistry. Various quite well delineated and clinically characterized types of disease have been differentiated:

● Prepubetal periodontitis (PP), which is extremely rare

● Localized juvenile periodontitis (LJP)

● Rapidly progressive periodontitis of young adults (RPP)

● Slowly progressive adult periodontitis (AP)

Most recently a therapy-resistant periodontitis (Refractory Periodontitis, RP) has been differentiated from the other types (AAP 1986 a, b). Future research should reveal whether "RP" is truly an independent disease entity or whether it is identical to RPP.

Clinical differentiation among the various types of periodontitis remains indistinct. This is particularly true between LJP and RPP. One may thus speak of *post-juvenile* periodontitis if the special localization of the affected teeth in LJP (incisors and molars) spreads to other teeth and becomes generalized in young adults. But the problem is even more complex, and raises additional questions: Why doesn't periodontitis *spread* to healthy sites by inoculation from diseased sites? Why do only some surfaces of some teeth undergo attachment loss? Do site-to-site differences in "resistance" exist?

The basis for the varying course of disease is understood today to be a reflection of the varying pathogenicity of microorganisms and the differences or even defects in the immune status of individual patients. It is certainly conceivable that additional knowledge of the etiology and pathogenesis of periodontitis will lead to a modification of the clinical classification of the various types of disease.

*Recession* is no longer characterized as a periodontal "disease" today. Anatomic peculiarities such as absent or very thin facial bone, although within the anatomic norm, are responsible for the receding gingival margin. Local trauma including vigorous horizontal toothbrushing will, in such cases, initiate or intensify gingival recession. Other morphologic variations including high labial frena also enhance recession. If recession extends to the mobile oral mucosa, localized secondary inflammation will complicate the clinical picture.

## Diagnosis and prognosis

Using conventional diagnostic measurements (probing depths, gingival indices, radiographs etc.), one can measure only the "historical" *results* of periodontitis. Such static observations permit only the experienced practitioner to estimate the course of disease, its dynamics and the prognosis.

Fact: *The practitioner has no reliable method to determine either the presence of attachment loss or its likelihood in the future.* Evaluation of gingival bleeding tendency (e.g., bleeding upon probing, bleeding indices) as well as fluid flow from the pocket have been widely used as indicators of disease *activity,* at least at the time of the examination. Unfortunately, these parameters are not strongly correlated with attachment loss activity.

Research continues to seek new avenues that will permit reliable prediction of the dynamics of the disease process. In the early 1980s, microbiologic dark-field diagnosis was in vogue. It was recommended for routine daily practice. This method, however, can only reveal bacterial morphotypes, and the microorganisms detected correlate only imprecisely with the clinical condition. In short, they do not reveal any useful, *predictable* information about the *activity* of a periodontal pocket.

The removal of anaerobic bacteria from the pocket and their culture and metabolic differentiation are possible. These have become standard methods for research; however, for a practice situation this remains too costly. Already available – perhaps prematurely recommended for routine practice use – are diagnostic tests, e.g., the $DMD_x$-test, which utilize genetic technology to demonstrate particular periodontopathic bacteria in periodontal pockets. Whether such tests will become routine and whether they truly represent progress in diagnosis has yet to be proved.

In truth, the practitioner today still has only *clinical observation* to estimate of periodontal disease activity. He can record clinical signs of crevicular inflammation, but must also monitor attachment levels longitudinally. Connective tissue attachment loss is the final clinical expression of periodontitis!

Clinical experience and individual diagnostic/prognostic accumen continue to be important, in the absence of more objective, scientifically-based criteria.

## Therapy

Fact: *Tissue regeneration is not yet a part of routine periodontal therapy.* Since the turn of the century, the periodontal therapeutic pendulum has swung – depending upon the author and the spirit of the time – between conservative and surgical treatment methods. The recommendation for surgical therapy often predominated, because the primary symptom, the *pocket,* could be eliminated by means of gingivectomy, flap operations, ostectomy and apical repositioning. Such resective methods were "successful" because the primary harbor for pathogenic pocket flora was eliminated. The disadvantages of such radical surgical procedures included often *massive* loss of periodontal tissue, lack of any possibility for tissue regeneration, lengthening of the clinical crown and exposure of cervical areas, with consequences such as hypersensitivity, root caries as well as esthetic and phonetic problems.

Today, on the other hand, we try to eliminate the "cause" of the disease. Our primary goal is complete removal of subgingival plaque. This is accomplished, as always, mechanically, and may be supported in severe cases of LJP or RPP by topically and/or systemically administered antibiotics.

The removal of endotoxins from the root surface may involve removal of cementum or even dentin. This enhances healing and partial spontaneous regeneration of the periodontal tissues. Such cleaning of the root surface may be performed closed (scaling, curettage) or open with direct vision (open curettage, modified Widman operation, flap procedures). The selection of a procedure depends less on the primary diagnosis than upon the morphologic/anatomic characteristics, including localization and access to pockets, tooth morphology, technical difficulties, dexterity of the operator etc.

## Healing:
## Classic therapy or guided tissue regeneration

In most cases periodontal therapy results in healing of the pocket by means of a *long junctional epithelium with epithelial attachment*.

More desirable would be a healing process whereby new connective tissue attachment occurred, with new collagen fibers inserting into newly formed cementum. Early investigations attempted to enhance this type of connective tissue regeneration by means of "conditioning" the root surfaces (e.g., with citric acid, pH 1). The results were neither dramatic nor reproducible and therefore cannot be recommended for routine use in clinical practice today.

In recent years attempts have been made to inhibit the apical proliferation of junctional epithelium by placing *membranes* (e.g., Gore-Tex) immediately after flap surgery. The membranes cover all planed root surfaces that were infected. The goal is to provide time for the *periodontal connective tissue* to proliferate and regenerate. This type of "guided tissue regeneration" (GTR) has received wide praise recently (Nyman et al. 1982 a, b; Gottlow 1986; Gottlow et al. 1986; Becker et al. 1987; Pontoriero et al. 1987). The principle of the surgical GTR procedure is depicted in Fig. 949. This method can, at

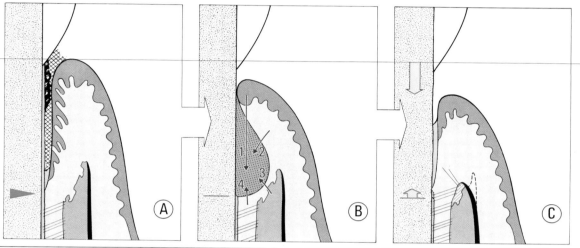

**948   Healing following classical therapy (cf pp. 136–137)**
**A**   Initial finding – Periodontitis with infrabony pockets

Original gingival margin

**B**   Situation immediately after conservative or surgical treatment (scaling and root planing). Regeneration of the tissues (arrows **1–4**) proceeds at various speeds.
**C**   Healing by means of long junctional epithelium. Minimal connective tissue regeneration, severe shrinkage of the gingiva.

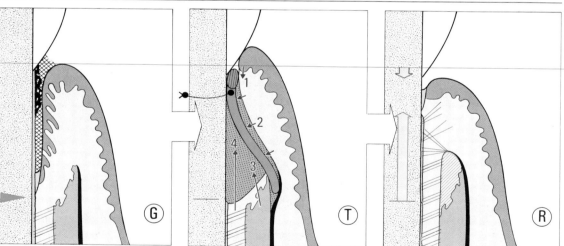

**949   Guided Tissue Regeneration (GTR)**
**G**   Initial findings as in **A**, above.

Original gingival margin

**T**   After flap procedure and membrane placement. It separates oral epithelium (**1**) and gingival connective tissue (**2**) from tooth and bone (**3**). PDL (**4**) and bone regenerate.
**R**   New PDL near new bone. New cementum with dentogingival fibers (blue arrow). Minimal gingival shrinkage.

this time, only be recommended to periodontal specialists for "saving" strategically important abutment teeth. The operative site must be opened a second time for removal of the membrane, and the price for such membranes remains excessively high. This surgical GTR technique cannot yet be recommended for routine practice application in periodontitis therapy.

*Resorbable* membranes will probably simplify the procedure (Magnusson et al. 1988).

It is possible that in some cases transplants or alloplastic implants can enhance *osseous regeneration* in periodontal pockets. The results of such procedures, however, are neither predictable nor overwhelmingly successful. Following periodontal therapy, regeneration or remineralization of bone often occurs spontaneously.

One might therefore quite reasonably conclude that research into guided tissue regeneration appears to offer more promise than do alloplastic implants.

## Maintenance therapy and recall

Fact: *Patient compliance controls the outcome of periodontal therapy.* A treated periodontitis patient *"should never leave"* the dentist and his auxiliaries. The maintenance of treatment success is only possible through constant vigilance and recall. The patient's oral hygiene must be monitored and professional tooth cleaning must be performed. In contrast to earlier times, the recall intervall is not static, e.g., "every 3 months." In most cases the recall interval is dependent upon the original diagnosis (AP, RPP etc.), the initial severity of the disease, the results of treatment, as well as the cooperation of the patient in home care. The latter may decrease over the years, and necessitate a change in the recall interval, which may range from two to 12 months depending upon the circumstances.

The treatment performed during a routine recall appointment is viewed today somewhat differently than in earlier times: Each and every surface of a tooth is *not* necessarily subjected to scaling and root planing procedures. More frequently, after use of a plaque-disclosing agent, cleaning is performed only in those areas where plaque is present and scaling is performed only where calculus is present. More intensive treatment of residual pockets is performed only when symptoms of activity are observed or when the pockets have deepened in comparison to the previous appointment.

The mechanical tooth and root cleaning procedures on indicated sites that must be performed at each recall appointment will be unavoidable until a substance is found that can completely inhibit new plaque formation and therewith calculus accumulation. Whether this will ever occur is more than questionable. To date *all* effective plaque inhibitors (e.g., chlorhexidine etc.) are associated with adverse side effects that prohibit long-term continuous use.

## "Occlusal therapy"

There is still no consensus even today concerning the value of "functional" therapy in periodontitis. Dysfunctional improper loading, parafunctions and bruxism cause neither gingivitis nor periodontitis. They do, however, often lead to dramatic changes in the periodontium (widening of the periodontal ligament space, mild inflammatory infiltrate, circulatory disturbances, edema and hyalinization of collagenous structures, activation of cementoclasts and osteoclasts). Whether these types of changes can intensify an already existent periodontitis remains a subject of controversy, but it is well documented scientifically that it leads to increased tooth mobility. Ramfjord and Ash (1979) declared:

*"Periodontal trauma from occlusion constitutes an aberration in periodontal health; therefore, the treatment of traumatic lesions in the periodontium always should be included in the periodontal therapy."*

Occlusal trauma and its consequences can be eliminated for the most part by selective grinding or by splinting. Therefore, "functional therapy" signifies treatment of the traumatized periodontal ligament, but not treatment of periodontitis *per se.*

## Reconstruction, splinting

Consideration of periodontal relationships must become part of every prosthetic treatment plan. Most recent research results have led to the abandonment of old dogma (e. g., Ante's law etc.). In a periodontally treated dentition today, it is possible to consider the use of rather more complicated (also fixed) reconstructions than was previously the case, given good cooperation by the patient in home care and regular recall.

*Principles of reconstruction and concepts of occlusion* have become somewhat simpler today ("long centric," cuspid as well as anterior tooth guidance). Of course, every reconstruction must take into consideration the entire stomatognathic system (muscles of mastication, TMJ etc.) with the choice of a concept of occlusion.

*Splinting* should be avoided whenever possible in a complete dentition or when planning reconstruction. Splinting does *not* lead to tightening of mobile teeth in any biologic sense. It is for this reason that splinting should only be considered for stabilization of extremely mobile teeth to enhance patient comfort or to ensure stability of critical abutments in reconstructions.

## "The road away from reparative, towards preventive ..."

"Curative" dentistry is developing more and more toward "preventive" dentistry. While preventive measures are associated with certain costs, these are relatively small in comparison to the significant costs associated with major periodontitis therapy and are tiny in comparison to the grotesque costs associated with periodontal and prosthetic treatment of a dentition that has been neglected for too long. The dentist and his/her team would save time, and the patient would be spared a long course of suffering and economic hardship, if periodontitis could be prevented. These facts must become known to patients, public health officials, insurance companies and the media.

# Acknowledgements for Figures

Approximately ten percent of all the *photographs* in this *Atlas* were graciously provided by our colleagues around the world, whose names appear below. Because many Figures contain more than one photograph, each acknowledgement contains an exact description of the donor's contribution (e.g.: L, M or R for left, middle or right; A, B, C etc.).

The remaining 90 percent of the illustrative material derived either from the authors or from their departments or practices.

*Photographs of objects* were made exclusively by co-author Dr. Herbert F. Wolf.

## Universities

### University of Basle

**Dr. B. Maeglin,** Department of Oral Surgery and Pathology
135 L, 136 R, 139, 140 L, 140 R, 141 L, 141 R, 142 L, 142 R, 149 R, 150 L, 150 R, 151, 153 L, 153 R, 154, 155 L, 155 R, 163, 164 R, 165, 168 R

and his coworkers
**Dr. C. Bassetti**
385, 386

**Dr. B. Daicker,** Clinic for Ophthalmology, Eye Hospital
253 L, 253 R, 254 L, 254 R

**Dr. R. Guggenheim,** Scanning Electron Microscope Laboratory, Geology Institute
132 R

**Dr. B. Speck,** Hematology Department, Medical School
143 L, 143 R, 144 L, 144 R, 145 L, 145 R

**Dr. H.-J. Müller,** Pediatric Clinic, Children's Hospital
258

**Dr. B. Widmer,** Department of Orthodontics and Pedodontics
239

### University of Berne

**Dr. H. Graf,** Department of Periodontology
859 L, 859 R, 860 L, 860 R, 861 L, 861 R, 866, 872 R

**Dr. N. P. Lang,** Department of Crown and Bridge Prosthodontics
13 R, 15, 17 L, 156, 292, 509 L, 904 R

and his coworkers
**Dr. M. Grassi**
168 L, 168 M

### University of California, San Francisco

**Dr. G. C. Armitage,** Department of Periodontology
292

**Dr. J. R. Winkler,** Department of Stomatology
161, 164 L, 166

### University of Geneva

**Dr. G. Cimasoni,** Department of Periodontology
32 R, 287, 692 L, 693 L, 694 L

**Dr. J.-M. Meyer,** Department of Dental Materials
358 L

### Loma Linda University / University of Malmö

**Dr. J. Egelberg,** Department of Periodontology
24 R, 98 R, 101 L

### University of Pennsylvania, Philadelphia

**Dr. M. A. Listgarten,** Department of Periodontics
30 R, 31 L, 31 R, 39 L

All *histologic preparations* (except as noted) were generously provided by Dr. Alice Kallenberger (emeritus), Histology Department, University of Basle Dental Institute, and Dr. Arthur Hefti, Department of Cariology and Periodontology Dental Institute, University of Basle.

All *diagrams and illustrations* were prepared by Mr. Bernhard Struchen and Partners in the Atelier for Scientific Illustrations, Zurich, Switzerland, from drafts created by Dr. Herbert Wolf.

## University of Zurich

**Dr. B. Guggenheim,** Department of Oral Microbiology and General Immunology
41L, 41R, 42R, 43L, 43R, 44, 49, 50, 51, 52

**Dr. F. Lutz,** Department of Cariology, Periodontology and Preventive Dental Medicine
36L, 911R (SEM)

and his coworkers
**Dr. W. Mörmann**
25, 356L, 357L, 803, 804, 805

**Dr. Th. Götsch**
167

**Dr. W. Iselin**
922L, 922R, 923L, 924L, 924R

**Dr. H. R. Mühlemann (Professor emeritus)**
4R, 147R
and his former coworkers
**Dr. A. Bachmann**
757, 758R, 759

**Dr. C. Schweizer-Hirt**
356R, 357R, 359L, 360L

**Dr. H. E. Schroeder,** Department of Oral Structural Biology
10L, 10R, 11R, 15L, 18R, 19L, 33R, 62, 328, 778

**Dr. P. Stöckli,** Department of Orthodontics
897L, 897R, 898L, 898R, 899L, 899R, 900, 901L, 901R, 902, 903, 905, 906

## Dental Hygiene School, Zurich

**Dr. E. T. Egloff,** St. Gallen
5L, 5R

## Private Practitioners

**Dr. M. Ebneter,** Zurich
278R

**Dr. E. T. Egloff,** St. Gall
5L, 5R

**Dr. U. Hersberger,** Frenkendorf/BL
226, 227L

**Dr. M. Leu,** Zurich
519, 520

**Dr. H.-M. Meyer,** Zurich
832A, 832B, 832C

**Dr. F. Wolgensinger,** Kilchberg/ZH
3L

# References

The massive clinical and scientific literature in periodontology and its related fields continues its relentless growth. For the practitioner and even for the academic periodontologist, it is fast becoming scarcely possible to embrace.

In this *Atlas* the authors have cited from the literature only those articles with immediate pertinence to the problem being discussed; these articles are listed below *without asterisk*.

References listed *with* an *asterisk* (*) are not cited in the text, but represent further valuable reading on selected topics.

For these reasons, this Reference section makes no pretense of being complete. Indeed, many significant and valuable articles, as well as classic historical publications and some recent works are not included.

At the beginning of the Reference section is a separate listing of valuable *textbooks* and the most important *periodicals* that are recommended for more intensive study of periodontology. Within the Reference section, textbooks, conference proceedings etc. are also indicated (°).

## Books – Textbooks

**Ash, M. M., Ramfjord, S. P.:** An Introduction to Functional Occlusion. Saunders, Philadelphia 1982

**Baer, P. N., Morris, M. L.:** Textbook of Periodontics. Lippincott, Philadelphia 1977

**Bhaskar, S. N.:** Synopsis of Oral Pathology. 7th ed. Mosby, St. Louis 1986

**Carranza, F. A., Jr.:** Glickman's Clinical Periodontology. 6th ed. Saunders, Philadelphia 1984

**Fedi, P. F., Jr.:** The Periodontic Syllabus. Lea & Febiger, Philadelphia 1985

**Frandsen, A.:** Public Health Aspects of Periodontal Disease. Quintessence, Chicago 1984

**Genco, R.:** Contemporary Periodontics. Mosby, St. Louis 1989

**Goldman, H. M., Cohen, D. W.:** Periodontal Therapy. 6th ed. Mosby, St. Louis 1980

**Grant, D. A., Stern, I. B., Listgarten, M. A.:** Periodontics. 6th ed. Mosby, St. Louis 1988

**Greenspan, D., Greenspan, J. S., Pindborg, J. J. Schiött, M.:** AIDS and the Dental Team. Year Book Medical Publishers, 1986

**Hassell, T. M.:** Epilepsy and the Oral Manifestations of Phenytoin Therapy. Karger, Basel 1981

**Holm-Pedersen, P., Löe, H.:** Geriatric Dentistry. Munksgaard, Copenhagen 1986

**Lindhe, J.:** Textbook of Clinical Periodontology. 2nd ed. Munksgaard, Copenhagen 1989

**Manson, J. D.:** An Outline of Periodontics. PGS, Littleton/MA 1983

**Newman, M. G., Goodman, A. D.:** Guide to Antibiotic Use in Dental Practice. Quintessence, Chicago 1984

**Page, R. C., Schroeder, H. E.:** Periodontitis in Man and Other Animals. A Comparative Review. Karger, Basle 1982

**Pattison, G. L., Pattison, A. M.:** Periodontal Instrumentation. A Clinical Manual. Reston, Reston/VA 1979

**Pindborg, J. J., Hjörting-Hansen, E.:** Atlas of the Diseases of the Jaws. Munksgaard, Copenhagen 1974

**Pindborg, J. J.:** Atlas of Diseases of the Oral Mucosa. Munksgaard, Copenhagen 1985

**Posselt, U.:** Physiology of Occlusion and Rehabilitation. Davis, Philadelphia 1962

**Prichard, J. F.:** The Diagnosis and Treatment of Periodontal Disease. Saunders, Philadelphia 1979

**Ramfjord, S. P., Ash, M. M.:** Periodontology and Periodontics. Saunders, Philadelphia 1979

**Ramfjord, S. P., Ash, M. M.:** Occlusion. 3rd ed. Saunders, Philadelphia 1983

**Robertson, P., Greenspan, J. S.:** Perspectives on Oral Manifestations of AIDS. PGS, Littleton/MA 1988

**Roitt, I. M.:** Essential Immunology. 6th ed. Blackwell, Oxford, Boston, Melbourne 1988

**Schijatschky, M. M.:** Life-Threatening Emergencies in Dental Practice. Quintessence, Chicago 1979

**Schluger, S., Yuodelis, R., Page, R. C., Johnson, R.:** Periodontal Disease, 2nd ed. Lea & Febiger, Philadelphia 1989

**Schroeder, H. E., Listgarten, M. A.:** Fine Structure of the Developing Epithelial Attachment of Human Teeth. 2nd ed. Karger, Basle 1977

**Schroeder, H. E.:** The Periodontium. Springer, Berlin 1986

**Stahl, S. S.:** Periodontal Surgery. Thomas, Springfield 1976

**Ten Cate, A. R.:** Oral Histology, Development, Structure and Function. Mosby, St. Louis 1980

**Ward, H. L., Simring, M.:** Manual of Clinical Periodontics. 2nd ed. Mosby, St. Louis 1978

## Periodicals

**Journal of Clinical Periodontology** (Munksgaard, Copenhagen)

**Journal of Periodontology** (American Academy of Periodontology, Chicago)

**Journal of Periodontal Research** (Munksgaard, Copenhagen)

**The Journal of the Western Society of Periodontology – Periodontal Abstracts** (Western Society of Periodontology)

## Information – Atlases

**Ebneter, M., Wolf, H. F., Wolgensinger, A.:** Dental Atlas. Quintessence Publishing Co., Inc. Chicago, London, Tokyo, Berlin 1984

## References

## A

\* **AAP, American Academy of Periodontology:** New Approaches to the Diagnosis and Chemotherapeutic Management of the Periodontal Diseases. Spec. issue 1985

**AAP, American Academy of Periodontology:** Glossary of Periodontic Terms. J. Periodontol., Suppl. November 1986a

**AAP, American Academy of Periodontology:** Current Procedural Terminology for Periodontics and Insurance Reporting Manual, 5th ed. 1986b

**AAP, American Academy of Periodontology:** Periodontal Diseases of Children and Adolescents. Approved by the Executive Council, 1987a

° **AAP, American Academy of Periodontology:** Perspectives on Oral Antimicrobial Therapeutics. PSG Publishing, Littleton, Massachusetts 1987b

\* **AAP, American Academy of Periodontology:** Periodontal Therapy: A Summary Status Report 1987–1988

**Addy, M., Rawle, L., Handley, R., Newman, H. N., Coventry, R.:** The development and in vitro evaluation of acrylic strips and dialysis tubing for local drug delivery. J. Periodontol. 53: 693–699, 1982

\* **Addy, M., Dowell, P.:** Dentine hypersensitivity – A review. II. Clinical and in vitro evaluation of treatment agents. J. clin. Periodontol. 10: 351–363, 1983

\* **Addy, M.:** Chlorhexidine compared with other locally delivered antimicrobials. A short review. J. clin. Periodontol. 13: 957–964, 1986

° **Addy, M.:** Rational for chemotherapy in the treatment of periodontal disease. Periodontology Today. Int. Congr., Zürich. Karger, Basel 1988 (pp. 281–289)

**Adriaens, P. A., De Boever, J. A., Loesche, W. J.:** Bacterial invasion in root cementum and radicular dentin of periodontally diseased teeth in humans – A reservoir of periodontopathic bacteria. J. Periodontol. 59: 222–230, 1988

\* **AHA, American Heart Association:** Prevention of bacterial endocarditis. Circulation 56: 139–A, 1977

**Ahrens, G., Bublitz, K. A.:** Parodontalerkrankungen und Behandlungsbedarf der Hamburger Bevölkerung. Eine epidemiologische Studie an 11'305 Probanden. Dtsch. zahnärztl. Z. 42: 433–437, 1987

**Ainamo, A., Ainamo, J., Poikkeus, R.:** Continuous widening of the band of attached gingiva from 23 to 65 years of age. J. periodont. Res. 16: 595–599, 1981

**Ainamo, J.:** Relationships between malalignment of the teeth and periodontal disease. Scand. J. dent. Res. 80: 104–110, 1972

**Ainamo, J., Bay, I.:** Problems and proposals for recording gingivitis and plaque. Int. dent. J. 25: 229–235, 1975

\* **Ainamo, J., Talari, A.:** The increase with age of the width of attached gingiva. J. periodont. Res. 11: 182–188, 1976

**Ainamo, J., Barmes, D., Beagrie, G., Cutress, T., Martin, J., Sardo-Infirri, J.:** Development of the World Health Organization (WHO) Community Periodontal Index of Treatment Needs (CPITN). Int. dent. J. 32: 281–291, 1982

**Ainamo, J.:** New perspectives in epidemiology and prevention of periodontal disease – Implications for practical application. Dtsch. zahnärztl. Z. 43: 623–630, 1988

°\* **Ainamo, J.:** What are the problems in defining periodontal diseases? Periodontology Today. Int. Congr., Zürich. Karger, Basel 1988 (pp. 50–58)

\* **Allen, E. P., Gainza, C. S., Farthing, G. C., Newbold, D. A.:** Improved technique for localized ridge augmentation: A report of 21 cases, J. Periodontol. 56: 195–199, 1985

\* **Allenspach-Petrzilka, G. E., Guggenheim, B.:** Bacteroides melaninogenicus ss intermedius invades rat gingival tissue. J. periodont. Res. 17: 456–459, 1982

**Allenspach-Petrzilka, G. E., Guggenheim, B.:** Bacterial invasion of the periodontium; an important factor in the pathogenesis of periodontitis. J. clin. Periodontol. 10: 609–617, 1983

**Amman, H.:** Experimentelle Untersuchungen zur Kybernetik der Okklusion. Med. Diss., Basel 1980

\* **Amsterdam, M., Vanarsdall, R. L.:** Periodontal prosthesis. Twenty-five years in retrospect. Alpha Omegan Dec. 1974 (pp. 9–52)

\* **Amsterdam, M., Purdum, L. C., Purdum, K. L.:** The occlusal graph: A graphic representation of photocclusion data. J. prosth. Dent. 57: 94–98, 1987

**Ante, I. H.:** The fundamental principles of abutments. Thesis. Mich. St. dent. Soc. Bull. 8: 14–23, 1926

**Ante, I. H.:** Abutments. J. Canad. dent. Ass. 2: 249–260, 1936

**Ante, I. H.:** The fundamental principles, design and construction of bridge prosthesis. J. Canad. dent. Ass. 10: 1–9, 1938

\* **Arbeitsgruppe für Prophylaxe der bakteriellen Endokarditis, der Schweizer Kinderkardiologen und der Schweizerischen Zahnärztegesellschaft:** Prophylaxe der bakteriellen Endokarditis. Schweiz. Mschr. Zahnmed. 96: 724–725, 1986

**Armitage, G. C., Svanberg, G. K., Löe, H.:** Microscopic evaluation of clinical measurements of connective tissue attachment levels. J. clin. Periodontol. 4: 173–190, 1977

° **Ash, M. M., Ramfjord, S. P.:** An Introduction to Functional Occlusion. Saunders, Philadelphia 1982

° **Ash, M. M., Ramfjord, S. P.:** Funktionelle Okklusion. Eine Anleitung. Quintessenz, Berlin 1988

\* **Asikainen, S.:** Occurrence of actinobacillus actinomycetemcomitans and spirochetes in relation to age in localized juvenile periodontitis. J. Periodontol. 57: 537–541, 1986

\* **Asikainen, S., Jousimies-Somer, H., Kanervo, A., Summanen, P.:** Certain bacterial species and morphotypes in localized juvenile periodontitis and in matched controls. J. Periodontol. 58: 224–230, 1987

**Atkinson, D. R., Cobb, C. M., Killoy, W. J.:** The effect of an air-powder abrasive system on in vitro root surfaces. J. Periodontol. 55: 13–18, 1984

\* **Attström, R.:** Presence of leukocytes in crevices of healthy and chronically inflamed gingivae. J. periodont. Res. 5: 42–47, 1970

°\* **Attström, R.:** Does supragingival plaque removal prevent further breakdown? Periodontology Today. Int. Congr., Zürich. Karger, Basel 1988 (pp. 251–259)

**Axéll, T.:** A prevalence study of oral mucosal lesions in an adult Swedish population. Thesis. Odontol. Revy 27: Suppl. 36, 1976

**Axéll, T., Holmstrup, P., Kramer, I. R. H., Pindborg, J. J., Shear, M.:** International seminar on oral leukoplakia and associated lesions related to tobacco habits. Community dent. oral Epidemiol. 12: 145–154, 1984

**Axelsson, P., Lindhe, J.:** The effect of a plaque control program on gingivitis and dental caries in school children. J. dent. Res., Spec. issue C. 56: C 142–148, 1977

**Axelsson, P., Lindhe, J.:** Effect of controlled oral hygiene procedures on caries and periodontal disease in adults. Results after 6 years. J. clin. Periodontol. 8: 239–248, 1981 a

**Axelsson, P., Lindhe, J.:** The significance of maintenance care in the treatment of periodontal disease. J. clin. Periodontol. 8: 281–294, 1981 b

**Axelsson, P.:** Periodontal diseases. Can they be provided? Dtsch. zahnärztl. Z. 37: 540–544, 1982

**Aziz-Gandour, I. A., Newmann, H. N.:** The effects of a simplified oral hygiene regime plus supragingival irrigation with chlorhexidine or metronidazole on chronic inflammatory periodontal disease. J. clin. Periodontol. 13: 228–236, 1986

## B

**Badersten, A.:** Nonsurgical Periodontal Therapy. Thesis, Malmö 1984

**Badersten, A., Nilvéus, R., Egelberg, J.:** Effect of nonsurgical periodontal therapy. II. Severely advanced periodontitis. J. clin. Periodontol. 11: 63–76, 1984 a

**Badersten, A., Nilvéus, R., Egelberg, J.:** Effect of nonsurgical periodontal therapy. III. Single versus repeated instrumentation. J. clin. Periodontol. 11: 114–124, 1984 b

* **Baehni, P., Tsai, C. C., McArthur, W. P., Hammond, B. F., Taichman, N. S.:** Interaction of inflammatory cells and oral microorganisms. VIII. Detection of leukotoxic activity of a plaque-derived gram-negative microorganism. Infect. Immun. 24: 233–243, 1979

* **Baehni, P.:** Interactions between plaque microorganisms and human oral epithelial cells. In Lehner, T., Cimasoni, G.: The Borderland Between Caries and Periodontal disease III. Editions Médecine et Hygiène, Genève 1986 (pp. 143–153)

**Baer, P. N., Morris, M. L.:** Textbook of Periodontics. Lippincott, Philadelphia 1977

**Barak, S., Engelberg, I. S., Hiss, J.:** Gingival hyperplasia caused by Nifedipine – Histologic findings. J. Periodontol. 58: 639–642, 1987

° **Barmes, D. E.:** Prevalence of periodontal disease. In Frandsen, A.: Public Health Aspects of Periodontal Disease. Quintessence, Chicago 1984

**Barmes, D. E., Leous, P. A.:** Assessment of periodontal status by CPITN and its applicability to the development of long-term goals on periodontal health of the population. Int. dent. J. 36: 177–181, 1986

**Bass, C. C.:** An effective method of personal oral hygiene, Part II. J. La. med. Soc. 106: 100–112, 1954

**Bassetti, C., Kallenberger, A.:** The influence of chlorhexidine rinsing on the healing of oral mucosa and osseous lesions. A histomorphometric study on experimental animals. J. clin. Periodontol. 7: 443–456, 1980

° **Bauer, A., Gutowski, A.:** Gnathologie. Einführung in Theorie und Praxis. Quintessenz, Berlin 1975

* **Becker, W., Berg, L. E., Becker, B. E.:** Untreated periodontal disease: a longitudinal study. J. Periodontol. 50: 234–244, 1979

* **Becker, W., Becker, B. E., Berg, L. E.:** Periodontal treatment without maintenance – A retrospective study in 44 patients. J. Periodontol. 55: 505–509, 1984

* **Becker, W., Becker, B. E., Prichard, J. F., Caffesse, R., Rosenberg, E., Gian-Grasso, J.:** A surgical and suturing method: Three case reports. J. Periodontol. 58: 819–826, 1987

**Belting, C. M., Hiniker, J. J., Dummett, C. O.:** Influence of diabetes mellitus on the severity of periodontal disease. J. Periodontol. 35: 476–480, 1964

° **Bengel, W.:** Die Photographie in Zahnmedizin und Zahntechnik. Quintessenz, Berlin 1984

° **Bengel, W., Veltman, G.:** Differentialdiagnostik der Mundschleimhauterkrankungen. Quintessenz, Berlin 1986

* **Bergenholtz, G., Nyman, S.:** Endodontic complications following periodontal and prosthetic treatment of patients with advanced periodontal disease. J. Periodontol. 55: 63–68, 1984

**Bergman, B., Hugoson, A., Olsson, C.:** Caries, periodontal and prosthetic findings in patients with removable partial dentures. A ten year longitudinal study. J. prosth. Dent. 48: 506–514, 1982

**Bernick, S., Cohen, D. W., Baker, L., Laster, L.:** Dental disease in children with diabetes mellitus. J. Periodontol. 46: 241–245, 1975

**Bernimoulin, J.-P., Lange, D. E.:** Freie Gingivatransplantate – klinische Aspekte und Zytologie ihrer Einheilung. Dtsch. zahnärztl. Z. 27: 357–364, 1972

**Bernimoulin, J.-P.:** Deckung gingivaler Rezessionen mit koronaler Verschiebungsplastik. Dtsch. zahnärztl. Z. 28: 1222–1226, 1973

**Bernimoulin, J.-P., Lüscher, B., Mühlemann, H. R.:** Coronally repositioned periodontal flap. J. clin. Periodontol. 2: 1–13, 1975

**Bernimoulin, J.-P., Curilović, Z.:** Gingival recession and tooth mobility. J. clin. Periodontol. 4: 107–114, 1977

**Besimo, C., Jäger, K.:** Die Klinik der Adhäsivbrückentechnik. Teil I. Schweiz. Mschr. Zahnmed. 96: 1126–1136, 1986 a

**Besimo, C., Jäger, K.:** Die Klinik der Adhäsivbrückentechnik. Teil II. Schweiz. Mschr. Zahnmed. 96: 1259–1272, 1986 b

° **Bhaskar, S. N.:** Synopsis of Oral Pathology, 7th ed. Mosby, St. Louis 1986

**Björn, A., Björn, H., Grkovic, B.:** Marginal fit of restorations and its relation to periodontal bone level. I. Metal fillings. Odontol. Revy 20: 311–322, 1969

**Björn, A., Björn, H., Grkovic, B.:** Marginal fit of restorations and its relation to periodontal bone level. II. Crowns. Odontol. Revy 21: 337–346, 1970

**Björn, H.:** Free transplantations of gingiva propria. Symposium in Periodontology in Malmö. Odontol. Revy 14: 323, 1963

**Bogle, G., Claffey, N., Egelberg, J.:** Healing of horizontal circumferential periodontal defects following regenerative surgery in beagle dogs. J. clin. Periodontol. 12: 837–849, 1985

**Borel, J. F., Feurer, C., Gubler, H. U., Stähelin, H.:** Biological effects of cyclosporin A: A new antilymphocytic agent. Agents and Actions 6: 468–475, 1976

* **Bössmann, K.:** In-vitro-Experimente zur Plaquebildung. Dtsch. zahnärztl. Z. 34: 437–439, 1979

**Boughman, J., Halloran, S., Roulston, D., Schwartz, S., Suzuki, J., Weitkamp, C., Wenk, R., Wooten, R., Cohen, M.:** An autosomal dominant form of juvenile periodontitis (JP): its localization to chromosome No. 4 and linkage to dentinogenesis imperfecta (DG I–III). J. Craniofac. Genet. Dev. Biol. 6: 341–350, 1986

* **Bowers, G. M., Schallhorn, R. G., Mellonig, J. T.:** Histologic evaluation of new attachment in human intrabony defects. A literature review. J. Periodontol. 53: 509–514, 1982

**Boyd, R. L., Leggott, P., Quinn, R., Buchanan, S., Eakle, W., Chambers, D.:** Effect of self-administered daily irrigation with 0.02% SnF2 on periodontal disease activity. J. clin. Periodontol. 12: 420–431, 1985

**Brägger, U., Lang, N. P.:** Chirurgische Verlängerung der klinischen Krone. Schweiz. Mschr. Zahnmed. 98: 645–651, 1988

°* **Brandtzaeg, P.:** Role of the immune system – Dangers of a nonholistic approach in explaining health and disease. Periodontology Today. Int. Congr., Zürich. Karger, Basel 1988 (pp. 196–208)

* **Brånemark, P. I., Zarb, G., Albrektsson, T.:** Tissue Integrated Prostheses. Osseointegration in Clinical Dentistry. Quintessence, Chicago 1985

* **Brecx, M. C., Holm-Pederson, P., Theilade, J.:** Early plaque formation in young and elderly individuals. Gerodontics 1: 8–13, 1985

* **Brecx, M. C., Lehmann, B., Siegwart, C. M., Gehr, P., Lang, N. P.:** Observations on the initial stages of healing following human experimental gingivitis. A clinical and morphometric study. J. clin. Periodontol. 15: 123–129, 1988

* **Breininger, D. R., O'Leary, T. J., Blumenshine, R. V. H.:** Comparative effectiveness of ultrasonic and hand scaling for the removal of subgingival plaque and calculus. J. Periodontol. 58: 9–18, 1987

**Breitenmoser, J., Mörmann, W., Mühlemann, H. R.:** Zahnfleischverletzung durch Zahnbürstenborsten. Acta parodont., in Schweiz. Mschr. Zahnheilk. 88: 79/1–89/11, 1978

* **Buchanan, S. A., Robertson, P. B.:** Calculus removal by scaling/root planing with and without surgical access. J. Periodontol. 58: 159–163, 1987

**Buckley, L. A.:** The relationship between malocclusion and periodontal disease. J. Periodontol. 43: 415–417, 1972

**Buckley, L. A.:** The relationship between malocclusion, gingival inflammation, plaque and calculus. J. Periodontol. 52: 35–40, 1981

**Buckley, L. A., Crowley, M. J.:** A longitudinal study of untreated periodontal disease. J. clin. Periodontol. 11: 523–530, 1984

* **Budtz-Jörgensen, E.:** Bruxism and trauma from occlusion. An experimental model in Macaca monkeys. J. clin. Periodontol. 7: 149–162, 1980

## C

**Caffesse, R. G., Burgett, F. G., Nasjleti, C. E., Castelli, W. A.:** Healing of free gingival grafts with and without periosteum. Part I. Histologic evaluation. J. Periodontol. 50: 586–594, 1979 a

**Caffesse, R. G., Nasjleti, C. E., Burgett, F. G., Kowalski, C. J., Castelli, W. A.:** Healing of free gingival grafts with and without periosteum. Part II. Radiographic evaluation. J. Periodontol. 50: 595–603, 1979 b

* **Caffesse, R. G., Sweeney, P. L., Smith, B. A.:** Scaling and root planing with and without periodontal flap surgery. J. clin. Periodontol. 13: 205–210, 1986

* **Caffesse, R. G., Smith, B. A., Nasjleti, C. E., Lopatin, D. E.:** Cell proliferation after flap surgery, root conditioning and fibronectin application. J. Periodontol. 58: 661–666, 1987

* **Carnevale, G., Freni Sterrantino, S., Di Febo, G.:** Soft and hard tissue wound healing following tooth preparation to the alveolar crest. Int. J. Periodont. Restor. Dent. 3: 36–53, 1983

**Carranza, F. A., Jr.:** Glickman's Clinical Periodontology. 6th ed. Saunders, Philadelphia 1984

**Carter, H. G., Barnes, G. P.:** The gingival bleeding index. J. Periodontol. 45: 801–805, 1974

**Caton, J., Nyman, S.:** Histometric evaluation of periodontal surgery. I. The modified Widman flap procedure. J. clin. Periodontol. 7: 212–223, 1980

**Caton, J., Nyman, S., Zander, H.:** Histometric evaluation of periodontal surgery. II. Connective tissue attachment levels after four regenerative procedures. J. clin. Periodontol. 7: 224–231, 1980

* **Caton, J., Proye, M., Polson, A.:** Maintenance of healed periodontal pockets after a single episode of root planing. J. Periodontol. 53: 420–424, 1982

**Cercek, J. F., Kiger, R. D., Garrett, S., Egelberg, J.:** Relative effects of plaque control and instrumentation on the clinical parameters of human periodontal disease. J. clin. Periodontol. 10: 46–56, 1983

° **Chaikin, R. W.:** Elements of Surgical Treatment in the Delivery of Periodontal Therapy. Quintessenz, Berlin 1977

* **Cheetham, W. A., Wilson, M., Kieser, J. B.:** Root surface debridement – An in vitro assessment. J. clin. Periodontol. 15: 288–292, 1988

**Cianciola, L. J., Park, B. H., Bruck, E., Mosovich, L., Genco, R. J.:** Prevalence of periodontal disease in insulin-dependent diabetes mellitus. J. Amer. dent. Ass. 104: 653–670, 1982

* **Christersson, L. A., Albini, B., Zambon, J., Slots, J., Genco, R. J.:** Demonstration of actinobacillus actinomycetemcomitans in gingiva of localized juvenile periodontitis lesions. J. dent. Res. 62, Abstract 255: 198, 1983

* **Ciancio, S. G., Genco, R. J.:** The use of antibiotics in periodontal diseases. Int. J. Periodont. Restor. Dent. 3: 54–71, 1983

**Ciancio, S. G.:** Current status of indices of gingivitis. J. clin. Periodontol. 13: 375–378, 1986

* **Ciancio, S. G.:** Chemotherapeutic agents and periodontal therapy: Their impact on clinical practice. J. Periodontol. 57: 108–111, 1986

° **Cimasoni, G.:** Crevicular Fluid Updated. Karger, Basel 1983

°* **Cimasoni, G., Giannopoulu, C.:** Can crevicular fluid component analysis assist in diagnosis and monitoring periodontal breakdown? Periodontology Today. Int. Congr., Zürich. Karger, Basel 1988 (pp. 260–270)

**Claffey, N., Russell, R., Shanley, D.:** Peripheral blood phagocyte function in acute necrotizing ulcerative gingivitis. J. periodont. Res. 21: 288–297, 1986

**Cockey, G., Boughman, J., Hassell, T. M.:** Genetic regulation of drug-induced connective tissue disorder: An in vitro model. In Vitro 23: 23 A, 1987

**Cohen, B.:** Morphological factors in the pathogenesis of periodontal disease. Brit. dent. J. 107: 31–39, 1959

**Cohen, B.:** A study of the periodontal epithelium. Brit. dent. J. 112: 55–65, 1962

**Cohen, D. W., Friedman, L. A., Shapiro, J., Kyle, G. C., Franklin, S.:** Diabetes mellitus and periodontal disease. Part I. J. Periodontol. 41: 709–712, 1970

**Cole, R., Nilvéus, R., Ainamo, J., Bogle, G., Crigger, M., Egelberg, J.:** Pilot clinical studies on the effect of topical citric acid application on healing after replaced periodontal flap surgery. J. periodont. Res. 16: 117–122, 1981

**Curilović, Z., Mazor, Z., Berchtold, H.:** Gingivitis in Zurich school children. A re-examination after 20 years. Helv. odont. Acta, in Schweiz. Mschr. Zahnheilk. 87: 801/41–808/48, 1977

**Cutress, T. W.:** Periodontal health and periodontal disease in young people: global epidemiology. Int. dent. J. 36: 146–151, 1986

## D

**Davenport, R. H., Simpson, D. M., Hassell, T. M.:** Histometric comparison of active and inactive lesions of advanced periodontitis. J. Periodontol. 53: 285–295, 1982

**Davies, G. E., Francis, J., Martin, A. R., Rose, F. L., Swain, G.:** 1:6-di-4-chlorophenyl-diguanidohexane (Hibitane). Laboratory investigation of a new antibacterial agent of high potency. Brit. J. Pharmacol. 9: 192, 1954

**Dayoub, M. B.:** A new filter for osseous coagulum collection. J. Periodontol. 52: 45–46, 1981

**De Boever, J. A.:** Prinzipien der prothetischen Versorgung nach systematischer Parodontalbehandlung. Quintessenz 11: 101–105, 1978

**De Boever, J. A.:** Basis und Grenzen der rationalen Paro-Prothetik. Acta parodont., in Schweiz. Mschr. Zahnmed. 94: 355/59–366/70, 1984

**De Boever, J. A., Vande Velde, F.:** Pulverstrahlgerät zur Belagsentfernung. Eine klinische und rasterelektronenmikroskopische Studie. Dtsch. zahnärztl. Z. 40: 725–729, 1985

* **DGP, Deutsche Gesellschaft für Parodontologie:** Neue PAR-Nomenklatur. DGP-Nachrichten 1: 1–8, 1987

* **Diedrich, P.:** Die Unterstützung der Parodontalbehandlung durch kieferorthopädische Maßnahmen im Erwachsenengebiß. Dtsch. zahnärztl. Z. 39: 570–580, 1984

* **Diedrich, P., Erpenstein, H.:** Die Distalisierung endständiger Prämolaren zur Vermeidung von Freiendsätteln. Dtsch. zahnärztl. Z. 39: 644–649, 1984

* **Di Febo, G., Carnevale, G., Freni Sterantino, S.:** Treatment of a case of advanced periodontitis: Clinical procedures utilizing the "combined preparation technique". Int. J. Periodont. 1: 52–62, 1985

**Dorfman, H. S., Kennedy, J. E., Bird, W. C.:** Longitudinal evaluation of free autogenous gingival grafts. A four-year report. J. Periodontol. 53: 349–352, 1982

**Dzink, J. L., Tanner, A. C. R., Haffajee, A. D., Socransky, S. S.:** Gram negative species associated with active destructive periodontal lesions. J. clin. Periodontol. 12: 648-659, 1985

* **Dzink, J. L., Socransky, S. S., Haffajee, A. D.:** The predominant cultivable microbiota of active and inactive lesions of destructive periodontal diseases. J. clin. Periodontol. 15: 316–323, 1988

## E

**Eaton, K. A., Kieser, J. B., Davies, R. M.:** The removal of root surface deposits. J. clin. Periodontol. 12: 141–152, 1985

**Ebersole, J. L., Frey, D. E., Taubman, M. A., Haffajee, A. D., Socransky, S. S.:** Dynamics of systemic antibody responses in periodontal disease. J. periodont. Res. 22: 184–186, 1987

* **Ebersole, J. L., Taubman, M. A., Smith, D. J., Frey, D. E., Haffajee, A. D., Socransky, S. S.:** Human serum antibody responses to oral microorganisms. IV. Correlation with homologous infection. Oral Microbiol. Immunol. 2: 53–59, 1987

°* **Ebersole, J. L., Holt, S. C.:** Serum antibodies to periodontopathic microorganisms: Specific induction. Periodontology Today. Int. Congr., Zürich. Karger, Basel 1988 (pp. 169–177)

**Edel, A.:** Alveolar bone fenestrations and dehiscences in dry Bedouin jaws. J. clin. Periodontol. 8: 491–499, 1981

* **Edlan, A., Mejchar, B.:** Plastic surgery of the vestibulum in periodontal therapy. Int. dent. J. 13: 593–596, 1963
* **Egelberg, J.:** The blood vessels of the dento-gingival junction. J. periodont. Res. 1: 163–179, 1966
* **Egelberg, J.:** Regeneration and repair of periodontal tissues. J. periodont. Res. 22: 233–242, 1987
○* **Egelberg, J.:** Clinical criteria for evaluation of periodontal therapy. Periodontology Today. Int. Congr., Zürich. Karger, Basel 1988 (pp. 236–243)
**Eichenberger, M.:** Zur Frage der Knochenregeneration nach operativer Entfernung von verlagerten und retinierten Weisheitszähnen. Med. Diss., Basel 1979
* **Ellegaard, B., Karring, T., Löe, H.:** New periodontal attachment procedure based on retardation of epithelial migration. J. clin. Periodontol. 1: 75–88, 1974
* **Ellegaard, B., Borregaard, B., Ellegaard, J.:** Neutrophil chemotaxis and phagocytosis in juvenile periodontitis. J. periodont. Res. 19: 261–268, 1984
**Engelberger, T., Hefti, A., Kallenberger, A., Rateitschak, K. H.:** Correlations among papilla bleeding index, other clinical indices and histologically determined inflammation of gingival papilla. J. clin. Periodontol. 10: 579–589, 1983
* **Ericsson, I., Lindhe, J.:** Recession in sites with inadequate width of keratinized gingiva. An experimental study in the dog. J. clin. Periodontol. 11: 95–103, 1984
**Ericsson, I.:** The combined effects of plaque and physical stress on periodontal tissues. J. clin. Periodontol. 13: 918–922, 1986
* **Erpenstein, H.:** A 3-year study of hemisectioned molars. J. clin. Periodontol. 10: 1–10, 1983
* **Erpenstein, H.:** Was erwartet der „Parodontologe" vom „Prothetiker"? Dtsch. zahnärztl. Z. 39: 563–569, 1984
* **Erpenstein, H.:** Periodontal and prosthetic treatment in patients with oral lichen planus. J. clin. Periodontol. 12: 104–112, 1985
* **Erpenstein, H.:** Wie funktioniert Parodontologie in der Praxis? Schweiz. Mschr. Zahnmed. 97: 67–74, 1987
**Essex, M., Kanki, P. J.:** The origins of the AIDS virus. Scientific American, Vol. 259, No. 4, 44–51, October 1988
**Evian, C. I., Rosenberg, E. S., Listgarten, M. A.:** Bacterial variability within diseased periodontal sites. J. Periodontol. 53: 595–598, 1982

---

# F

**Falkler, W. A., Martin, S. A., Vincent, J. W., Tall, B. D., Nauman, R. K., Suzuki, J. B.:** A clinical, demographic and microbiology study of ANUG patients in an urban dental school. J. clin. Periodontol. 14: 307–314, 1987
○ **Fedi, P. F. Jr.:** The Periodontic Syllabus. Lea & Febiger, Philadelphia 1985
**Feneis, H.:** Gefüge und Funktion des normalen Zahnfleischgewebes. Dtsch. zahnärztl. Z. 7: 467–476, 1952
* **Fesseler, A.:** Die Effektivität der medikamentösen Behandlung bei Parodontalbehandlungen. Dtsch. zahnärztl. Z. 38: 829–835, 1983
**Finger, M., Gusberti, F. A., Lang, N. P.:** Plaque formation on pontics of different design. J. dent. Res. 60, Spec. issue A: 605, 1981
* **Finger, M., Hofstetter, H. W., Gusberti, F. A., Lang, N. P.:** Die Zwischengliedgestaltung bei festsitzenden Rekonstruktionen. In Lange, D. E.: Parodontologie, Implantologie und Prothetik im Brennpunkt von Praxis und Wissenschaft. Quintessenz, Berlin 1985 (S. 235–247)
* **Flores-de-Jacoby, L., Müller, H.-P., Zimmermann, J.:** Der parodontale Zustand bei schmaler keratinisierter Gingiva. Eine klinische und mikrobiologische Studie. Dtsch. zahnärztl. Z. 39: 661–665, 1984
* **Flores-de-Jacoby, L.:** Die Mikrobiologie als Parameter für Diagnose und Verlauf von Parodontalerkrankungen. Dtsch. zahnärztl. Z. 42: 398–404, 1987
* **Flores-de-Jacoby, L.:** Über den Einfluß des gingivalen Bindegewebes auf die Resorption der instrumentell bearbeiteten Wurzeloberfläche. Dtsch. zahnärztl. Z. 42: 505–511, 1987
**Foushee, D. G., Moriarty, J. D., Simpson, D. M.:** Effects of mandibular orthognathic treatment on mucogingival tissues. J. Periodontol. 56: 727–733, 1985
○ **Frandsen, A.:** Public Health Aspects of Periodontal Disease. Quintessence, Chicago 1984
* **Frank, R. M., Voegel, J. C.:** Bacterial bone resorption in advanced cases of human periodontitis. J. periodont. Res. 13: 251–261, 1978

**Frank, R. M.:** Bacterial penetration in the apical pocket wall of advanced human periodontitis. J. periodont. Res. 15: 563–573, 1980
○* **Frank, R. M.:** Is microbial tissue invasion a reality during periodontal breakdown? Periodontology Today. Int. Congr., Zürich. Karger, Basel 1988 (pp. 150–159)
**Freehe, C. L.:** Symposium on dental photography. Dent. Clin. North Am. 27 (no 1): 40–53, 1983
**Frentzen, M., Nolden, R.:** Der CPITN als Hilfsmittel zur Feststellung von Art und Umfang des Behandlungsbedarfs. Eine Studie an mehr als 500 Klinikpatienten. Dtsch. zahnärztl. Z.: 42: 428–432, 1987
* **Frentzen, M., Osborn, J.-F., Nolden, R.:** Anwendung poröser Hydroxylapatitkeramik in der systematischen Parodontaltherapie. Eine klinische Studie über 2 Jahre. Dtsch. zahnärztl. Z. 43: 713–718, 1988
* **Frentzen, M., Osborn, J.-F., Nolden, R.:** Immunchemische und immunhistologische Befunde bei verschiedenen Kalziumphosphatkeramikwerkstoffen im In-vitro-Versuch. Dtsch. zahnärztl. Z. 43: 719–724, 1988
**Fröhlich, F.:** Die okklusionsbedingten Schmerzen im Kiefergesichtsbereich. Schweiz. Mschr. Zahnheilk. 76: 764–776, 1966
* **Froum, S. J., Kushner, L., Stahl, S. S.:** Healing responses of human intraosseous lesions following the use of debridement, grafting and citric acid root treatment. I. Clinical and histologic observations six months postsurgery. J. Periodontol. 54: 67–76, 1983
* **Froum, S. J., Stahl, S. S.:** Human intraosseous healing responses to the placement of tricalcium phosphate ceramic implants. II. 13 to 18 months. J. Periodontol. 58: 103–109, 1987

---

# G

**Gaberthüel, T., Curilović, Z.:** Der Diabetes mellitus – ein Problem für den Zahnarzt? Schweiz. Mschr. Zahnheilk. 87: 579–592, 1977
**Gaberthüel, T.:** So stelle ich die Indikation zur Parodontitisbehandlung. Schweiz. Mschr. Zahnmed. 97: 64–66, 1987
**Galler, C., Selipsky, H., Phillips, C., Ammons, W. F.:** The effect of splinting on tooth mobility. II. After osseous surgery. J. clin. Periodontol. 6: 317–333, 1979
**Gallo, R. C., Montagnier, L.:** The chronology of AIDS research. Nature 326: 435–436, 1987
**Gallo, R. C., Montagnier, L.:** AIDS in 1988. Scientific American, Vol. 259, No. 4, 24–32, October 1988
**Galloway, S. E., Pashley, D. H.:** Rate of removal of root structure by the use of the Prophy-Jet device. J. Periodontol. 58: 464–469, 1987
**Gargiulo, A. W., Wentz, F. M., Orban, B.:** Dimensions and relations of the dentogingival junction in humans. J. Periodontol. 32: 261–267, 1961
○* **Genco, R. J.:** Contemporary Periodontics. Mosby Co., St. Louis 1989
**Geering, A. H., Lang, N. P.:** Die Michigan-Schiene, ein diagnostisches und therapeutisches Hilfsmittel bei Funktionsstörungen im Kausystem. I. Herstellung im Artikulator und Eingliederung am Patienten. Schweiz. Mschr. Zahnheilk. 88: 32–38, 1978
**Geering, A. H.:** Der betagte Mensch als Patient. Schweiz. Mschr. Zahnmed. 96: 1407–1417, 1986
**Geering, A. H., Kundert, M.:** Farbatlanten der Zahnmedizin, Band 2: Total- und Hybridprothetik. Thieme, Stuttgart 1986
**Geiger, A. M., Wassermann, B. H., Turgeon, L. R.:** Relationship of occlusion and periodontal disease. Part VI. Relation of anterior overjet and overbite to periodontal destruction and gingival inflammation. J. Periodontol. 44: 150–157, 1973
**Geiger, A. M., Wassermann, B. H., Turgeon, L. R.:** Relationship of occlusion and periodontal disease. Part VII. Relationship of crowding and spacing to periodontal destruction and gingival inflammation. J. Periodontol. 45: 43–49, 1974
**Gellin, R. G., Miller, C., Javed, T., Engler, W. O., Mishkin, D. J.:** The effectiveness of the Titan-S sonic scaler versus curettes in the removal of subgingival calculus. A human surgical evaluation. J. Periodontol. 57: 672–680, 1986
**Genco, R. J., Slots, J.:** Host responses in periodontal diseases. J. dent. Res. 63: 441–451, 1984
**Genco, R. J.:** Highlights of the conference and perspectives for the future. International Conference on Periodontal Research, Ittingen. J. periodont. Res. 22: 164–171, 1987

°* **Genco, R. J.:** Contemporary Periodontics. Mosby, St. Louis 1989

**Germann, M.:** Eine einfache Methode zur Quasi-Standardisierung der Parodontalfotografie. Parodontologie 25: 16–18, 1971

* **Gessert, R., Krekeler, G., Pelz, K.:** Vergleichende mikrobiologische Studie der bakteriellen Besiedelung marginaler und apikaler parodontitischer Prozesse. Dtsch. zahnärztl. Z. 42: 471–473, 1987

**Gillett, R., Johnson, N. W.:** Bacterial invasion of the periodontium in a case of juvenile periodontitis. J. clin. Periodontol. 9: 93–100, 1982

**Gilmore, N., Sheiham, A.:** Overhanging dental restorations and periodontal disease. J. Periodontol. 42: 8–12, 1971

**Gislén, G., Nilsson, K. O., Matsson, L.:** Gingival inflammation in diabetic children related to degree of metabolic control. Acta odont. scand. 38: 241–246, 1980

**Gjermo, P., Rise, J.:** Chemotherapy in juvenile periodontitis. J. clin. Periodontol. 13: 982–986, 1986

°* **Gjermo, P.:** Validity and reliability of clinical measurements. Periodontology Today. Int. Congr., Zürich. Karger, Basel 1988 (pp. 95–103)

**Glavind, L., Zeuner, E.:** The effectiveness of a rotary electric toothbrush on oral cleanliness in adults. J. clin. Periodontol. 13: 135–138, 1986

* **Gloerfeld, H., Müller, H.-P., Flores-de-Jacoby, L.:** Stabilisierung parodontalgeschädigter Zähne mit dem „Anterior-Splint-Grid"-System. Dtsch. zahnärztl. Z. 40: 811–816, 1985

° **Goldman, H. M., Cohen, D. W.:** Periodontal Therapy. 6th ed. Mosby, St. Louis 1980

* **Goldman, M. J., Ross, I. F., Goteiner, D.:** Effect of periodontal therapy on patients maintained for 15 years or longer – A retrospective study. J. Periodontol. 57: 347–353, 1986

**Goodman, J., Luke, J., Rosen, S., Hackel, E.:** Heritability in dental caries, certain microflora and salivary components. Am. J. Hum. Genet. 11: 263–273, 1959

**Goodson, J. M., Haffajee, A., Socransky, S. S.:** Periodontal therapy by local delivery of tetracycline. J. clin. Periodontol. 6: 83–92, 1979

**Goodson, J. M., Tanner, A. C. R., Haffajee, A. D., Sornberger, G. C., Socransky, S. S.:** Patterns of progression and regression of advanced destructive periodontal disease. J. clin. Periodontol. 9: 472–481, 1982

* **Goodson, J. M., Haffajee, A. D., Socransky, S. S.:** Association between disease activity and therapeutic response. J. dent. Res. 64, Abstract 1661: 359, 1985

**Goodson, J. M., Offenbacher, S., Farr, D. H., Hogan, P. E.:** Periodontal disease treatment by local drug delivery. J. Periodontol. 56: 265–272, 1985

* **Goodson, J. M.:** Clinical measurements of periodontics. J. clin. Periodontol. 13: 446–455, 1986

* **Gordon, J. M., Walker, C. B., Murphy, J. C., Goodson, J. M., Socransky, S. S.:** Concentration of tetracycline in human gingival fluid after single doses. J. clin. Periodontol. 8: 117–121, 1981

**Gorman, W. J.:** Prevalence and etiology of gingival recession. J. Periodontol. 38: 316–322, 1967

* **Götte, H.:** Zahnbeweglichkeit vor und nach Wurzelkanalbehandlungen an Zähnen mit apikalen Veränderungen. Dtsch. zahnärztl. Z. 34: 461–462, 1979

°* **Gottlieb, B., Orban, B.:** Zahnfleisch-Entzündung und Zahnlockerung. Berlinische Verlagsanstalt, Berlin 1933

**Gottlow, J.:** New attachment formation by guided tissue regeneration. Thesis, Göteborg 1986

**Gottlow, J., Nyman, S., Lindhe, J., Karring, T., Wennström, J.:** New attachment formation in the human periodontium by guided tissue regeneration. J. clin. Periodontol. 13: 604–616, 1986

° **Graber, G.:** Psychosomatik und Okklusion. In Singer, F., Schön, F.: Europäische Prothetik heute. Quintessenz, Berlin 1978 (S. 169–176)

**Graber, G.:** Was leistet die funktionelle Therapie und wo findet sie ihre Grenzen? Dtsch. zahnärztl. Z. 40: 165–169, 1985

° **Graber, G.:** Color Atlas of Dental Medicine 2: Removable Partial Dentures. Thieme, Stuttgart, New York 1988

° **Graber, G.:** Der Einfluß von Psyche und Streß bei dysfunktionsbedingten Erkrankungen des stomatognathen Systems. In Hupfauf, L.: Praxis der Zahnheilkunde, Band 8: Myoarthropathien. Urban & Schwarzenberg, München 1989 (im Druck)

**Graf, H.:** Bruxism. Dent. clin. N. Amer. 13: 659–665, 1969

**Graf, H., Grassl, H., Aeberhard, H. J.:** A method for measurement of occlusal forces in three directions. Helv. odont. Acta 18: 7–11, 1974

**Graf, H., Geering, A. H.:** Rationale of clinical application of different occlusal philosophies. Oral Sci. Rev. 10: 1–10, 1977

* **Graf, H.:** Physiologie der Zahnbeweglichkeit. Dtsch. zahnärztl. Z.: 35: 678–679, 1980

° **Graf, H.:** Analysis of human jaw movement patterns by graphic computer display. In Kawamura, Y., Dubner, R.: Oral-facial Sensory and Motor Function. Quintessenz, Berlin 1981

°* **Grant, D. A., Stern, I. B., Listgarten, M. A.:** Periodontics. 6th ed. Mosby, St. Louis 1988

**Grassi, M., Winkler, J. R., Murray, P. A., Greenspan, D., Greenspan, J. S.:** Orale Manifestationen der HIV-Infektionen: Gegenwart und Perspektiven. Schweiz. Mschr. Zahnmed. 97: 1537–1544, 1987 a

**Grassi, M., Tellenbach, R., Lang, N. P.:** Periodontal conditions of teeth adjacent to extraction sites. J. clin. Periodontol. 14: 334–339, 1987 b

* **Greene, J. C., Vermillon, J. R.:** Oral hygiene index: A method for classifying oral hygiene status. J. Amer. dent. Ass. 61: 172–179, 1960

**Greenspan, D., Greenspan, J. S., Pindborg, J. J., Schiøt, M.:** AIDS and the Dental Team. Munksgaard, Copenhagen 1986

* **Greenspan, J. S.:** The problem – Etiology, pathogenesis and epidemiology of HIV-infection. J. Calif. dent. Ass. 15: 15–18, 1987

* **Greenspan, J. S., Greenspan, D.:** Oral aspects of the acquired immunodeficiency syndrome. J. oral Pathol. (in press)

**Greenstein, G.:** Effects of subgingival irrigation on periodontal status. J. Periodontol. 58: 827–836, 1987

* **Griffiths, G. S., Addy, M.:** Effects of malalignment of teeth in the anterior segments on plaque accumulation. J. clin. Periodontol. 8: 481–490, 1981

°* **Grün, L.:** Zur Entwicklung von Seuchen und infektiösen Krankheiten. In Knolle, G.: HTLV-III-Infektion. Quintessenz, Berlin 1986 (S. 11–16)

**Grupe, H. E., Warren, R. F.:** Repair of gingival defects by a sliding flap operation. J. Periodontol. 27: 92–95, 1956

**Grupe, H. E.:** Modified technique for the sliding flap operation. J. Periodontol. 37: 491–494, 1966

* **Guggenheim, B.:** Können neue Erkenntnisse der Immunologie und der Mikrobiologie die praktische Parodontalbehandlung verändern? Dtsch. zahnärztl. Z. 43: 631–634, 1988

° **Guldener, P. H. A.:** Beziehung zwischen Pulpa- und Parodontalerkrankungen. In Guldener, P. H. A., Langeland, K.: Endodontologie. Thieme, Stuttgart 1982 (S. 368–378)

**Gülzow, H.-J.:** Vergleichende klinische Untersuchungen zum Reinigungseffekt einer herkömmlichen und einer gelförmigen Zahnpasta. Dtsch. zahnärztl. Z. 42: 725–727, 1987

* **Günay, H.:** Juvenile Parodontitis: Heilung nach Transplantation von allogener kältekonservierter Knochenspongiosa. Dtsch. zahnärztl. Z. 42: 450–457, 1987

* **Gusberti, F. A., Brecx, M. C., Lang, N. P.:** Microscopic evaluation of bacterial colonization of interdental subgingival sites prior to and during experimental gingivitis in man. Schweiz. Mschr. Zahnmed. 98: 619–623, 1988

* **Gusberti, F. A., Sampathkumar, P., Siegrist, B. E., Lang, N. P.:** Microbiological and clinical effects of chlorhexidine digluconate and hydrogenperoxide mouthrinses on developing plaque and gingivitis. J. clin. Periodontol. 15: 60–67, 1988

# H

* **Haffajee, A. D., Socransky, S. S.:** Frequency distributions of periodontal attachment loss. Clinical and microbiological features. J. clin. Periodontol. 13: 625–637, 1986

* **Haffajee, A. D., Socransky, S. S., Dzink, J. L., Taubman, M. A., Ebersole, J. L., Smith, D. J.:** Clinical, microbiological and immunological features of subjects with destructive periodontal diseases. J. clin. Periodontol. 15: 240–246, 1988

**Hammer, B., Hotz, P.:** Nachkontrolle von 1- bis 5jährigen Amalgam-, Komposit- und Goldgußfüllungen. Schweiz. Mschr. Zahnheilk. 89: 301–314, 1979

**Hammond, B. F.:** The microbiology of periodontal diseases with emphasis on localized juvenile periodontitis. Alpha Omegan 76: 27–31, 1983

**Hamp, S. E., Nyman, S., Lindhe, J.:** Periodontal treatment of multirooted teeth. Results after 5 years. J. clin. Periodontol. 2: 126–135, 1975

**Hanamura, H., Houston, F., Rylander, H., Carlsson, G. E., Haraldson, T., Nyman, S.:** Periodontal status and bruxism – A comparative study of patients with periodontal disease and occlusal parafunctions. J. Periodontol. 58: 173–176, 1987

**Haneke, E.:** The Papillon-Lefèvre syndrome: Keratosis palmoplantaris with periodontopathy. Hum. Genet. 51: 1–35, 1979

**Hansen, G. C.:** An epidemiologic investigation of the effect of biologic aging on the breakdown of periodontal tissue. J. Periodontol. 44: 269–277, 1973

* **Harndt, R.:** Beziehungen zwischen Endodont und Parodont. Dtsch. zahnärztl. Z. 34: 453–455, 1979

* **Hartmann, J., Müller, H.-P., Flores-de-Jacoby, L.:** Systemische Metronidazoltherapie und/oder subgingivale Zahnreinigung mit Wurzelglättung. Teil II. Entwicklung klinischer Parameter in Relation zu Veränderungen in der Zusammensetzung der assoziierten subgingivalen Mikroflora. Dtsch. zahnärztl. Z. 41: 579–584, 1986

* **Hartmann, J., Müller, H.-P., Flores-de-Jacoby, L.:** Einige klinische und mikrobiologische Parameter zur Vorhersage klinischer Attachmentveränderungen nach nichtchirurgischer Parodontalbehandlung. Dtsch. zahnärztl. Z. 42: 663–666, 1987

° **Hassell, T. M.:** Epilepsy and the Oral Manifestations of Phenytoin Therapy. Karger, Basle 1981

**Hassell, T. M., Jacoway, J. R.:** Über die klinischen Verlaufsformen und neueren Forschungsergebnisse von Gingivavergrößerungen (I). Quintessenz 4: 721–730, 1981 a

**Hassell, T. M., Jacoway, J. R.:** Über die klinischen Verlaufsformen und neueren Forschungsergebnisse von Gingivavergrößerungen (II). Quintessenz 5: 903–911, 1981 b

* **Hefti, A., Widmer, B.:** Reduktion des Keimpegels in der Mundhöhle vor zahnärztlichen Behandlungen durch Mundwässer und Mundantiseptika. Acta parodont., in Schweiz. Mschr. Zahnheilk. 90: 73/1–78/6, 1980

**Hefti, A., Engelberger, T., Büttner, M.:** Gingivitis in Basel schoolchildren. Helv. odont. Acta, in Schweiz. Mschr. Zahnheilk. 91: 1087/25–1092/30, 1981

**Helkimo, E., Carlsson, G. E., Helkimo, M.:** Chewing efficiency and state of dentition. Acta odont. scand. 36: 33–41, 1978

**Helldén, L. B., Listgarten, M. A., Lindhe, J.:** The effect of tetracycline and/or scaling on human periodontal disease. J. clin. Periodontol. 6: 222–230, 1979

**Helldén, L. B., Camosci, D., Hock, J., Tinanoff, N.:** Clinical study to compare the effect of stannous fluoride and chlorhexidine mouthrinses on plaque formation. J. clin. Periodontol. 8: 12–16, 1981

° **Hellwege, K.-D.:** Die Wurzelglättung. Instrumentelle und medikamentöse Therapie infizierter Wurzeloberflächen. Quintessenz, Berlin 1987

**Henne, H.-A., Flores-de-Jacoby, L., Zafiropoulos, G. G.:** Epidemiologische Untersuchungen des Parodontalzustandes bei Bundeswehrsoldaten nach Anwendung des CPITN. Dtsch. zahnärztl. Z. 43: 696–700, 1988

* **Herforth, A.:** Der laterale Verschiebelappen – modifizierte Operationstechnik. Dtsch. zahnärztl. Z. 35: 750–753, 1980

**Herrmann, D.:** Gingivostomatitis herpetica (Stomatitis aphthosa) bei Erwachsenen. Dtsch. zahnärztl. Z. 27: 870–875, 1972

**Heyward, W. L., Curran, J. W.:** The epidemiology of AIDS in the U.S.: Scientific American, Vol. 259, No. 4, 52–59, October 1988

**Himmel, G. K., Marthaler, T. M., Rateitschak, K. H., Mühlemann, H. R.:** Experimental changes of diurnal periodicity in the physical properties of periodontal structures. Helv. odont. Acta 1: 16–18, 1957

* **Hirschfeld, L., Wassermann, B.:** A long term survey of tooth loss in 600 treated patients. J. Periodontol. 49: 225–237, 1978

**Holbrook, T., Ochsenbein, C.:** Complete coverage of denuded root surface with a one-stage gingival graft. Int. J. Periodont Restor. Dent. 3: 8–27, 1983

° **Holm-Pedersen, P., Löe, H.:** Geriatric Dentistry. Munksgaard, Copenhagen 1986

° **Holste, T., Renk, A.:** Klebebrücken in der Zahnheilkunde, Hanser, München 1985

**Holton, W. L., Hancock, E. B., Pelleu, G. B., Jr.:** Prevalence and distribution of attached cementicles on human root surfaces. J. Periodontol. 57: 321–324, 1986

**Hormand, J., Frandsen, A.:** Juvenile periodontitis. Localization of bone loss in relation to age, sex, and teeth. J. clin. Periodontol. 6: 407–416, 1979

**Hug, H. U.:** Periodontal status and its relationship to variations in tooth position. An analysis of the findings reported in the literature. Helv. odont. Acta, in Schweiz. Mschr. Zahnheilk. 92: 1073/11–1086/24, 1982

**Hugoson, A.:** Effect of the Water Pik device on plaque accumulation and development of gingivitis. J. clin. Periodontol. 5: 95–104, 1978

* **Hüttmann, J., Plagmann, H.-C.:** Vergleichende In-vitro-Untersuchungen verschiedener druckluft-betriebener Zahnsteinentfernungsgeräte. Dtsch. zahnärztl. Z. 40: 749–754, 1985

* **Hüttemann, R. W.:** Ultraschallaktivierte Instrumente zur Belagsentfernung. Dtsch. zahnärztl. Z. 40: 721–724, 1985

* **Hüttemann, R. W., Dönges, H.:** Untersuchungen zur Therapie überempfindlicher Zahnhälse mit Hydroxylapatit. Dtsch. zahnärztl. Z. 42: 486–488, 1987

# I

**Imfeld, T.:** Oligosialie und Xerostomie. I. Grundlagen, Ätiologie, Pathologie. Acta parodont., in Schweiz. Mschr. Zahnmed. 94: 741/81–754/94, 1984

**Imfeld, T.:** Alterszahnmedizin – Herausforderung der Zukunft. Swiss Dent 6, Nr. 7/8: 21–33, 1985

* **Imperiali, D., Grunder, U., Lang, N. P.:** Mundhygienegewohnheiten, zahnärztliche Versorgung und subjektive Kaufähigkeit bei sozioökonomisch unterschiedlichen Bevölkerungsschichten in der Schweiz. Schweiz. Mschr. Zahnmed. 94: 612–624, 1984

**Ingber, J. S., Rose, L. F., Coslet, J. G.:** The biologic width – a concept in periodontics and restorative dentistry. Alpha Omega 10: 62–65, 1977

**Ingerwall, B., Jacobsson, U., Nyman, S.:** A clinical study of the relationship between crowding of teeth, plaque and gingival condition. J. clin. Periodontol. 4: 214–222, 1977

* **International Conference on Research in the Biology of Periodontal Disease.** B. Klavan (ed.). Chicago Ill. 1977 (pp. 226–288)

**Iselin, W., Lufi, A.:** Die flexible Zahnfleischepithese I. Quintessenz 2: 275–280. 1983 a

**Iselin, W., Lufi, A.:** Die flexible Zahnfleischepithese II. Quintessenz 3: 483–494, 1983 b

**Iselin, W., Lutz, F., Mörmann, W.:** Iatrogene Reize: Vorkommen, Wirkung und Eliminationstechnik. Dtsch. zahnärztl. Z. 40: 730–738, 1985

**Iselin, W., Dvoracek, J., Lutz, F.:** Qualitative und quantitative Untersuchungen von Zahn- und Füllungsoberflächen nach der Anwendung eines Pulver-Wasserstrahlgerätes. Schweiz. Mschr. Zahnmed. 99: 1989 (in Vorbereitung)

* **Isidor, F., Attström, R., Karring, T.:** Regeneration of alveolar bone following surgical and non-surgical periodontal treatment. J. clin. Periodontol. 12: 687–696, 1985

**Isidor, F., Karring, T., Nyman, S., Lindhe, J.:** New attachment – reattachment following reconstructive periodontal surgery. J. clin. Periodontol. 12: 728–735, 1985

# J

* **Jackson, H.-K., Lin, C. T., Kwan, H.-W.:** Treatment of a patient with Papillon-Lefèvre-Syndrome – A case report. J. Periodontol. 58: 789–793, 1987

**Jäger, K., Borner, A., Graber, G.:** Epidemiologische Untersuchungen über die Ätiologiefaktoren dysfunktioneller Erkrankungen im stomatognathen System. Schweiz. Mschr. Zahnmed. 97: 1351–1356, 1987

**James, W. C., McFall, W. T., Jr.:** Placement of free gingival grafts on denuded alveolar bone. Part I. Clinical evaluations. J. Periodontol. 49: 283–290, 1978

**James, W. C., McFall, W. T., Jr., Burkes, E. J.:** Placement of free gingival grafts on denuded alveolar bone. Part II. Microscopic observations. J. Periodontol. 49: 291–300, 1978

**Jankelson, B.:** Technique for obtaining optimum functional relationship for the natural dentition. Dent. N. Clin. Amer. 4: 131–141, 1960

**Johnson, B. D., Engel, D.:** Acute necrotizing ulcerative gingivitis – A review of diagnosis, etiology and treatment. J. Periodontol. 57: 141–150, 1986

**Joss, A., Graf, H.:** A method for analysis of human mandibular occlusal movement. Helv. odont. Acta, in Schweiz. Mschr. Zahnheilk. 89: 1211/41–1220/50, 1979

# K

* **Kalkwarf, K. L.:** Mucogingival considerations prior to replacement of removable partial prostheses. Compend. continu. Educ. Dent. 5: 69–75, 1984

* **Karring, T., Isidor, F., Nyman, S., Lindhe, J.:** New attachment formation on teeth with a reduced but healthy periodontal ligament. J. clin. Periodontol. 12: 51–60, 1985

° **Karring, T.:** Repair or regeneration, does it matter? Periodontology Today. Int. Congr., Zürich. Karger, Basel 1988 (pp. 271–280)

**Käyser, A. F.:** Shortened dental arches and oral function. J. oral Rehabil. 8: 457–462, 1981

**Ketterl, W.:** Wechselbeziehungen der Endodontie und Parodontologie. Dtsch. zahnärztl. Z. 39: 585–588, 1984

**Keyes, P. H., Wright, W. E., Howard, S. A.:** The use of phase-contrast microscopy and chemotherapy in the diagnosis and treatment of periodontal lesions – An initial report. I. Quintessence int. 1: 51–56, 1978a

**Keyes, P. H., Wright, W. E., Howard, S. A.:** The use of phase-contrast microscopy and chemotherapy in the diagnosis and treatment of periodontal lesions – An initial report. II. Quintessence int. 2: 69–76, 1978b

* **Khatiblou, F. A., Ghodssi, A.:** Root surface smoothness or roughness in periodontal treatment. J. Periodontol. 54: 365-367, 1983

**Knight, G. M., Wade, A. B.:** The effects of hormonal contraceptives on the human periodontium. J. periodont. Res. 9: 18–22, 1974

°* **Knolle, G.:** HTLV-III-Infektion. Problem für die zahnärztliche Praxis? Quintessenz, Berlin 1986

**Knowles, J. W., Burgett, F. G., Nissle, R. R., Shick, R. A., Morrison, E. C., Ramfjord, S. P.:** Results of periodontal treatment related to pocket depth and attachment level. Eight years. J. Periodontol. 50: 225–233, 1979

**Knowles, J. W., Burgett, F. G., Morrison, E. C., Nissle, R. R., Ramfjord, S. P.:** Comparison of results following three modalities of periodontal therapy related to tooth type and initial pocket depth. J. clin. Periodontol. 7: 32–47, 1980

° **Koch, M. G.:** AIDS. Vom Molekül zur Pandemie. Spektrum der Wissenschaft, Heidelberg 1987

* **Kocher, T., Topoll, H.:** Experimentelle Untersuchungen über die Auswirkungen eines supra- und subgingivalen Scalings mit Handinstrumenten oder Ultraschall-Geräten auf die Entzündungsreaktion der marginalen Gingiva bei unterschiedlicher Mundhygiene. Dtsch. zahnärztl. Z. 40: 771–774, 1985

**Kocher, T., Plagmann, H. C.:** Der radektomierte Molar als Pfeilerzahn. Dtsch. zahnärztl. Z. 43: 725–728, 1988

**Koivuniemi, J., Savoff, K., Rateitschak, K. H.:** Gingivitis- und Plaquebefall bei Schulkindern in städtischen und ländlichen Gemeinden. Acta parodont., in Schweiz. Mschr. Zahnheilk. 90: 682/74–694/86, 1980

° **Körber, K. H.:** Konuskronen – Teleskope. Einführung in Klinik und Technik. Hüthig, Heidelberg 1974

* **Kornman, K. S., Karl, E. H.:** The effect of long-term low-dose tetracycline therapy on the subgingival microflora in refractory adult periodontitis. J. Periodontol. 53: 604–610, 1982

* **Kornman, K. S.:** Nature of periodontal diseases: Assessment and diagnosis. J. periodont. Res. 22: 192–204, 1987

* **Kraal, J. H., Kenney, E. B.:** The response of polymorphnuclear leukocytes to chemotactic stimulation for smokers and non-smokers. J. periodont. Res. 14: 383–389, 1979

* **Krekeler, G.:** Ist die Verbindung parodontal-chirurgischer Maßnahmen mit zahnärztlich-chirurgischen Maßnahmen sinnvoll? Dtsch. zahnärztl. Z. 39: 581–584, 1984

* **Krekeler, G., Pelz, K., Chuba, P. J., Göbel, U. B.:** Evaluation molekularbiologischer Sonden zum Direktnachweis anspruchsvoller Bakterien bei entzündlichen Parodontalerkrankungen. Dtsch. zahnärztl. Z. 43: 665–667, 1988

* **Kremers, L., Daliemunthe, S. H., Lampert, F.:** Zahnsteinreduktion mit HEDP? Eine klinische Langzeitstudie. Dtsch. zahnärztl. Z. 35: 729–731, 1980

* **Krill, D. B., Fry, H. R.:** Treatment of localized juvenile periodontitis (periodontosis) – A review. J. Periodontol. 58: 1–8, 1987

° **Krogh-Poulsen, W. G.:** Management of the occlusion of the teeth. Part II. Examination, diagnosis, treatment. In Schwartz, L., Chayes, C. M.: Facial Pain and Mandibular Dysfunction. Saunders, Philadelphia 1968 (pp. 249–280)

**Kronauer, E., Borsa, G., Lang, N. P.:** Prevalence of incipient juvenile periodontitis at age 16 years in Switzerland. J. clin. Periodontol. 13: 103–108, 1986

° **Krüger, E.:** Operationslehre für Zahnärzte. Quintessenz, Berlin 1977

* **Krüger, W.:** Sind für den Erfolg einer Parodontalbehandlung funktionsanalytische und funktionstherapeutische Maßnahmen notwendig? Dtsch. zahnärztl. Z. 39: 599–605, 1984

* **Krüger, W., Donath, K., Mayer, H.:** Knochenersatzmittel mit Zusatz eines Wachstumsfaktors: Ein neuer Weg für die Regeneration von parodontalen Knochendefekten? I. Induzierte Knochenregeneration im Tierexperiment. Dtsch. zahnärztl. Z. 43: 709–712, 1988

* **Kundert, E., Palla, S.:** Mundhygiene beim älteren Patienten. Schweiz. Mschr. Zahnmed. 98: 654–660, 1988

# L

**Lamezan, R. L., Rateitschak, K. H.:** Häufigkeit von parodontalem Knochenschwund bei erwachsenen Patienten – Eine röntgenologische Studie. Schweiz. Mschr. Zahnmed. 98: 231–238, 1988

* **Lampert, F., Berger, K.:** Die zytologische Prüfung des Parodontaltherapeutikums „Spezial Parodontosesalbe". Dtsch. zahnärztl. Z. 41: 585–588, 1986

**Lang, N. P., Löe, H.:** The relationship between the width of keratinized gingiva and gingival health. J. Periodontol. 43: 623–627, 1972

**Lang, N. P., Cumming, B. R., Löe, H.:** Toothbrushing frequency as it relates to plaque development and gingival health. J. Periodontol. 44: 396–405, 1973

**Lang, N. P., Ramseier-Grossmann, K.:** Optimal dosage of chlorhexidine digluconate in chemical plaque control when applied by the oral irrigator. J. clin. Periodontol. 8: 189–202, 1981

**Lang, N. P.:** Was heißt funktionelle Rekonstruktion im parodontal reduzierten Gebiß? Acta parodont., in Schweiz. Mschr. Zahnheilk. 92: 365/41–377/53, 1982

**Lang, N. P., Kiel, R. A., Anderhalden, K.:** Clinical and microbiological effects of subgingival restorations with overhanging or clinically perfect margins. J. clin. Periodontol. 10: 563–578, 1983

° **Lang, N. P.:** Checkliste Zahnärztliche Behandlungsplanung. 2. Aufl. Thieme, Stuttgart 1988

°* **Lang, N. P., Hofstetter, H., Gerber, C.:** Extensionsbrücken – eine Alternative zur Freiendprothese? In Lange, D. E.: Parodontologie, Implantologie und Prothetik im Brennpunkt von Praxis und Wissenschaft. Quintessenz, Berlin 1985 (S. 249–262)

* **Lang, N. P., Joss, A., Orsanic, T., Gusberti, F. A., Siegrist, B. E.:** Bleeding on probing. A predictor for the progression of periodontal disease? J. clin. Periodontol. 13: 590–596, 1986

* **Lang, N. P., Siegrist, B. E., Brägger, U.:** Strategisch wichtige Pfeiler. Schweiz. Mschr. Zahnmed. 98: 633–641, 1988

* **Langdon-Down, J.:** Observations on an ethic classification of idiots. Clinical Lectures and Reports, London Hospital 3: 259–262, 1966

**Lange, D. E., Schroeder, H. E.:** Cytochemistry and ultrastructure of gingival sulcus cells. Helv. odont. Acta 15: 65–86, 1971

* **Lange, D. E.** Klinische und instrumentelle Probleme bei der Sondierung des Sulcus gingivae und der parodontalen Taschen. Dtsch. zahnärztl. Z. 40: 693–700, 1985

° **Lange, D. E.:** Parodontologie in der täglichen Praxis, 3. Aufl. Quintessenz, Berlin 1986

* **Larato, D. C.:** Furcation involvements: Incidence and distribution. J. Periodontol. 41: 499–501, 1970

* **Leib, A. M., Berdon, J. K., Sabes, W. R.:** Furcation involvements correlated with enamel projections from the cementoenamel junction. J. Periodontol. 38: 330–334, 1967

**Leon, A. R.:** The periodontium and restorative procedures. J. oral Rehabil. 4: 105–117, 1977

**Leu, M.:** Nachsorge parodontalbehandelter Patienten. Dtsch. zahnärztl. Z. 32: 38–43, 1977

**Lie, T., Leknes, K. N.:** Evaluation of the effect on root surfaces of air turbine scalers and ultrasonic instrumentation. J. Periodontol. 56: 522–531, 1985

**Lie, T., Hoff, I., Gjerdet, R.:** Computerized evaluation of the effectiveness of subgingival scaling in jaw models. J. clin. Periodontol. 14: 149–155, 1987

* **Lieser, H., Raetzke, P.:** Der Effekt regelmäßig durchgeführter Prophylaxe-Maßnahmen auf die Gingivitis- und Kariesmorbidität von Kindern in Kindergärten. Dtsch. zahnärztl. Z. 39: 666–668, 1984

**Lindhe, J., Björn, A. L.:** Influence of hormonal contraceptives on the gingiva of woman. J. periodont. Res. 2: 1–6, 1967

**Lindhe, J., Lundgren, D., Nyman, S.:** Considerations on prevention of periodontal disease. Literature review. J. West. Soc. Periodontol. 18: 50–57, 1970

**Lindhe, J., Heijl, L., Goodson, J. M., Socransky, S. S.:** Local tetracycline delivery using hollow fiber devices in periodontal therapy. J. clin. Periodontol. 6: 141-149, 1979

**Lindhe, J., Ericsson, J.:** The effect of elimination of jiggling forces on periodontally exposed teeth in the dog. J. Periodontol. 35: 562–567, 1982

° **Lindhe, J.:** Textbook of Clinical Periodontology. Munksgaard, Copenhagen 1983

* **Lindhe, J., Haffajee, A. D., Socransky, S. S.:** Progression of periodontal disease in adult subjects in the absence of periodontal therapy. J. clin. Periodontol. 10: 433–442, 1983

* **Lindhe, J., Westfelt, E., Nyman, S., Socransky, S. S., Haffajee, A. D.:** Long-term effect surgical/non-surgical treatment of periodontal disease. J. clin. Periodontol. 11: 448–458, 1984

**Listgarten, M. A.:** Electron microscopic observations on the bacterial flora of acute necrotizing ulcerative gingivitis. J. Periodontol. 36: 328–339, 1965

**Listgarten, M. A., Lewis, D. W.:** The distribution of spirochetes in the lesion of acute necrotizing ulcerative gingivitis: An electron microscopic and statistical survey. J. Periodontol. 38: 379–386, 1967

**Listgarten, M. A.:** Normal development, structure, physiology and repair of gingival epithelium. Oral Sci. Rev. 1: 3–63, 1972

**Listgarten, M. A., Mayo, H. E., Tremblay, R.:** Development of dental plaque on epoxy resin crowns in man. A light and electron microscopic study. J. Periodontol. 46: 10–26, 1975

**Listgarten, M. A.:** Structure of the microbial flora associated with periodontal health and disease in man. A light and electron microscopic study. J. Periodontol. 47: 1–18, 1976

**Listgarten, M. A., Helldén, L.:** Relative distribution of bacteria at clinically healthy and periodontally diseased sites in humans. J. clin. Periodontol. 5: 115–132, 1978

**Listgarten, M. A., Rosenberg, M. M.:** Histological study of repair following new attachment procedures in human periodontal lesions. J. Periodontol. 50: 333–344, 1979

**Listgarten, M. A.:** Periodontal probing: What does it mean? J. Periodontol. 7: 165–176, 1980

**Listgarten, M. A., Shifter, C. C., Laster, L.:** 3-year longitudinal study of the periodontal status of an adult population with gingivitis. J. clin. Periodontol. 12: 225–238, 1985

* **Listgarten, M. A.:** A perspective on periodontal diagnosis. J. clin. Periodontol. 13: 175–181, 1986

**Listgarten, M. A.:** Pathogenesis of periodontitis. J. clin. Periodontol. 13: 418–425, 1986

**Listgarten, M. A.:** Nature of periodontal diseases: Pathogenic mechanism. J. periodont. Res. 22: 172–178, 1987

° **Listgarten, M. A.:** Why do epidemiologic data have no diagnostic value? Periodontology Today. Int. Congr., Zürich. Karger, Basel 1988 (pp. 59–67)

**Livaditis, G. J.:** Etched-metal resin-bonded intracoronal cast restorations. Part II. Design criteria for cavity preparation. J. prosth. Dent. 56: 389–395, 1986

* **Lobene, R. R.:** Current status of indices for measuring gingivitis. Discussion. J. clin. Periodontol. 13: 381–382, 1986

**Löe, H., Silness, J.:** Periodontal disease in pregnancy. Prevalence and severity. Acta odont. scand. 21: 532–551, 1963

**Löe, H., Theilade, E., Jensen, S.:** Experimental gingivitis in man. J. Periodontol. 36: 177–187, 1965

* **Löe, H., Theilade, E., Jensen, S. B., Schiött, C. R.:** Experimental gingivitis in man. III. The influence of antibiotics on gingival plaque development. J. periodont. Res. 2: 282–289, 1967

° **Löe, H., Schiött, C. R.:** The effect of suppression of the oral microflora upon the development of dental plaque and gingivitis. In McHugh, W. D.: Dental Plaque. Livingstone, Edinburgh 1970

**Löe, H., Anerud, A., Boysen, H., Smith, M.:** The natural history of periodontal disease in man. The rate of periodontal destruction before 40 years of age. J. Periodontol. 49: 607–620, 1978

* **Löe, H., Anerud, A., Boysen, H., Morrison, E.:** Natural history of periodontal disease in man. J. clin. Periodontol. 13: 431–440, 1986

* **Loesche, W. J., Syed, S. A., Morrison, E. C., Laughon, B. E., Grossman, N. S.:** Treatment of periodontal infections due to anaerobic bacteria with short-term treatment with metronidazole. J. clin. Periodontol. 8: 29–44, 1981

**Loesche, W. J., Syed, S. A., Laughon, B. E., Stoll, J.:** The bacteriology of acute necrotizing ulcerative gingivitis. J. Periodontol. 53: 223–230, 1982

**Long, J., Nance, W., Waring, P., Burmeister, J., Ranney, R.:** Early onset periodontitis: A comparison and evaluation of two proposed modes of inheritance. Cent. Epidemiol. 4: 13–24, 1987

**Loos, B., Kiger, R., Egelberg, J.:** An evaluation of basic periodontal therapy using sonic and ultrasonic scalers. J. clin. Periodontol. 14: 29–33, 1987

**Löst, C.:** Depth of alveolar bone dehiscences in relation to gingival recessions. J. clin. Periodontol. 11: 583–589, 1984 a

**Löst, C.:** Plastische Deckung gingivaler Rezessionen. Ergebnisse einer 6½jährigen Verlaufskontrolle. Dtsch. zahnärztl. Z. 39: 640–643, 1984 b

° **Löst, C.:** Hemisektion/Wurzelamputation. Hanser, München 1985

* **Löst, C., Haubner, C.:** Histologische Studien und klinische Verlaufskontrolle einschließlich vorläufigem Behandlungsergebnis in einem Fall mit Papillon-Lefèvre-Syndrom. Dtsch. zahnärztl. Z. 40: 778–782, 1985

**Löst, C.:** Was ist unter konservativer, was ist unter chirurgischer Parodontalbehandlung zu verstehen? Dtsch. zahnärztl. Z. 41: 539–544, 1986

* **Löst, C.:** Darstellung parodontaler Strukturen per Ultraschall. Verlauf und Ergebnisse eines Forschungsprojektes. Dtsch. zahnärztl. Z. 43: 729–732, 1988

**Low, D., Burtner, P., Smith, R., Hassell, T. M.:** Positive effects of chlorhexidine spray in the mentally retarded. J. Dent. Res. 68: 412, 1989

**Lucas, R. M., Howell, L. P., Wall, B. A.:** Nifedipine-induced gingival hyperplasia. A histochemical and ultrastructural study. J. Periodontol. 56: 211–215, 1985

# M

* **MacFarlane, T. W., Jenkins, W. M. M., Gilmour, W. H., McCourtie, J., McKenzie, D.:** Longitudinal study of untreated periodontitis. (II). Microbiological findings. J. clin. Periodontol. 15: 331–337, 1988

°* **Mackenzie, I. C.:** Factors influencing the stability of the gingival sulcus. Periodontology Today. Int. Congr., Zürich. Karger, Basel 1988 (pp. 41–49)

**MacPhee, I. T., Muir, K. F.:** Dark ground microscopy in relation to 3 clinical parameters of chronic inflammatory periodontal disease. J. clin. Periodontol. 13: 900–904, 1986

**Maeglin, B.:** Orale Manifestationen bei HIV-Infektionen. Schweiz. Mschr. Zahnmed. 97: 97–101, 1987

**Magnusson, I., Runstad, L., Nyman, S., Lindhe, J.:** A long junctional epithelium – A locus minoris resistentiae in plaque infection? J. clin. Periodontol. 10: 333–340, 1983

**Magnusson, I. Batich, C., Collins, B. R.:** New attachment formation following controlled tissue regeneration using biodegradable membranes. J. Periodontol. 59: 1–6, 1988

* **Magnusson, I., Fuller, W. W., Heins, P. J., Rau, C. F., Gibbs, C. H., Marks, R. G., Clark, W. B.:** Correlation between electronic and visual readings of pocket depths with a newly developed constant force probe. J. clin. Periodontol. 15: 180–184, 1988

* **Magnusson, I., Clark, W. B., Marks, R. G., Gibbs, C. H., Manouchehr-Pour, M., Low, S. B.:** Attachment level measurements with a constant force electronic probe. J. clin. Periodontol. 15: 185–188, 1988

* **Mandel, I. D., Thompson, R. H.:** The chemistry of parotid and submaxillary saliva in heavy calculus formers and non-formers. J. Periodontol. 38: 310–315, 1967

**Mandell, R. L.:** A longitudinal microbiological investigation of actinobacillus actinomycetemcomitans and Eikenella corrodens in juvenile periodontitis. Infect. Immun. 45: 778–780, 1984

* **Mandell, R. L., Tripodi, L. S., Savitt, E., Goodson, J. M., Socransky, S. S.:** The effect of treatment an actinobacillus actinomycetemcomitans in localized juvenile periodontitis. J. Periodontol. 57: 94–99, 1986

**Mann, J. M.; Chin, J.; Piot, P.; Quinn, T.:** The international epidemiology of AIDS. Scientific American 259: 82–89, 1988

**Manouchehr-Pour, M., Spagnuolo, P. J., Rodman, H. M., Bissada, N. F.:** Impaired neutrophil chemotaxis in diabetic patients with severe periodontitis. J. dent. Res. 60: 729–730, 1981 a

**Manouchehr-Pour, M., Spagnuolo, P. J., Rodman, H. M., Bissada, N. F.:** Comparison of neutrophil chemotactic response in diabetic patients with mild and severe periodontal disease. J. Periodontol. 52: 410–415, 1981 b

**Manson, J. D.:** An Outline of Periodontics. PGS, Littleton/MA 1983

\* **Marggraf, E.:** Vaskuläre Immunkomplexe bei der Parodontitis marginalis profunda. Dtsch. zahnärztl. Z. 37: 680–684, 1982

\* **Marggraf, E., Wachtel, H., Bernimoulin, J.-P.:** Langzeitergebnisse nach einzeitiger bilateral gestielter koronaler Verschiebeplastik. Dtsch. zahnärztl. Z. 42: 480–485, 1987

**Marinello, C. P., Kerschbaum, T. H., Heinenberg, B., Hinz, R., Peters, S., Pfeiffer, P., Reppel, P. D., Schwickerath, H.:** Experiences with resin-bonded bridges and splints – A retrospective study. J. oral Rehabil. 14: 251–260, 1987

**Marinello, C. P., Soom, U., Schärer, P.:** Präparation in der Adhäsivprothetik. Schweiz. Mschr. Zahnmed. 98: 139–152, 1988

\* **Marks, S. C., Jr., Mehta, N. R.:** Lack of effect of citric acid treatment of root surfaces on the formation of new connective tissue attachment. J. clin. Periodontol. 13: 109–116, 1986

**Marthaler, T. M., Engelberger, B., Rateitschak, K. H.:** Bone loss in Ramfjord's index: Substitution of selected teeth. Helv. odont. Acta 15: 121–126, 1971

\* **Marxkors, R.:** Der Randschluß der Gußkrone. Dtsch. zahnärztl. Z. 35: 913–915, 1980

**Massler, M., Schour, I., Chopra, B.:** Occurrence of gingivitis in suburban Chicago school children. J. Periodontol. 21: 146–164, 1950

\* **Matter, J., Cimasoni, G.:** Creeping attachment after free gingival grafts. J. Periodontol. 47: 574–579, 1976

**Matter, J.:** Creeping attachment of free gingival grafts. A five-year follow-up study. J. Periodontol. 51: 681–685, 1980

**Mazza, J. E., Newman, M. G., Sims, T. N.:** Clinical and antimicrobical effect of stannous fluoride on periodontitis. J. clin. Periodontol. 8: 203–212, 1981

\* **McAlpine, R., Magnusson, I., Kiger, R., Crigger, M., Garrett, S., Egelberg, J.:** Antimicrobial irrigation of deep pockets to supplement oral hygiene instruction and root debridement. I. Bi-weekly irrigation. J. clin. Periodontol. 12: 568–577, 1985

\* **McDonald, F. L., Saari, J. T., Davis, S. S.:** A comparison of tooth accumulated materials from quadrants treated surgically or nonsurgically. J. Periodontol. 48: 147–150, 1977

\* **McFall, W. T., Jr.:** Tooth loss in 100 treated patients with periodontal disease – A long-term study. J. Periodontol. 53: 539–549, 1982

\* **Meffert, R. M., Thomas, J. R., Hamilton, K. M., Brownstein, C. N.:** Hydroxylapatite as an alloplastic graft in the treatment of human periodontal osseous defects. J. Periodontol. 56: 63–73, 1985

\* **Meffert, R. M.:** Endosseous dental implantology from the periodontist's viewpoint. J. Periodontol. 57: 531–536, 1986

\* **Melcher, A. H., McCulloch, C. A. G., Cheong, T., Nemeth, E., Shiga, A.:** Cells from bone synthesize cementum-like and bone-like tissue. J. periodont. Res. 22: 246–247, 1987

°\* **Melcher, A. H.** Does the developmental origin of cementum, periodontal ligament und bone predetermine their behaviour in adults? Periodontology Today. Int. Congr., Zürich. Karger, Basel 1988 (pp. 6–14)

\* **Mellonig, J. T., Bowers, G. M., Cotton, W. R.:** Comparison of bone graft materials. Part II. New bone formation with autografts and allografts. A histological evaluation. J. Periodontol. 52: 297–302, 1981

\* **Merck Index Online,** 10th ed. July 1986

**Merritt, H. H., Putnam, T. J.:** Sodium diphenyl hydantoinate in the treatment of convulsive disorders. J. Amer. med. Ass. 111: 1068–1073, 1938

**Merritt, H. H., Putman, T. J.:** Sodium diphenylhadantoinate in the treatment of convulsive seizures. Toxic symptoms and their prevention. Arch. Neurol. Psychiat. 42: 1053–1058, 1939

\* **Meyle, J.:** Verlaufsstudien der Chemotaxis neutrophiler Granulozyten bei Patienten mit schwerer marginaler Parodontitis. Dtsch. zahnärztl. Z. 42: 463–466, 1987

**Michalowicz, B., Pihlstrom, B., Aeppli, D., Hinrichs, J.:** Periodontal disease in twins. J. dent. Res. 67: Abstract 1450: 294, 1988

\* **Mierau, H.-D.:** Beziehungen zwischen Plaquebildung, Rauhigkeit der Zahnoberfläche und Selbstreinigung. Dtsch zahnärztl. Z. 39: 691–698, 1984

**Mierau, H.-D., Spindler, T.:** Beitrag zur Ätiologie der Gingivarezessionen. Dtsch. zahnärztl. Z. 39: 634–639, 1984

\* **Mierau, H.-D., Schulze, H.-J.:** Untersuchungen zum Schärfen- und Standzeitvergleich von Handinstrumenten für die Zahnreinigung und Wurzelglättung. Dtsch. zahnärztl. Z. 40: 759–766, 1985

**Mierau, H.-D., Fiebig, A.:** Zur Epidemiologie der Gingivarezessionen und möglicher klinischer Begleiterscheinungen, Untersuchungen an 2410 18- bis 22jährigen (1. Mitteilung). Dtsch. zahnärztl. Z. 41: 640–644, 1986

**Mierau, H.-D., Fiebig, A.:** Zur Epidemiologie der Gingivarezessionen und möglicher klinischer Begleiterscheinungen, Untersuchungen an 2410 18- bis 22jährigen (2. Mitteilung). Dtsch. zahnärztl. Z. 42: 512–520, 1987

° **Miller, A. J., Brunelle, J. A., Carlos, J. P., Brown, L. J., Löe, H.:** Oral Health of United States Adults. National Findings. US Department of Health and Human Services, Public Health Service, National Institute of Health 1987

\* **Miller, P. D., Jr.:** Root coverage using a free soft tissue autograft following citric acid application. Part I. Technique. Int. J. Periodont. Restor. Dent. 2: 65–70, 1982

\* **Montagnier, L., Chermann, J. C., Barré-Sinoussi, F., Chamaret, S., Gruest, J., Nugeyre, M. T., Rey, F., Dauguet, C., Axler-Blin, C., Brun-Vézinet, F., Rouzioux, C., Saimot, G. A., Rozenbaum, W., Gluckmann, J. C., Klatzmann, D., Vilmer, E., Griscelli, C., Foyer-Gazengel, C., Brunet, J. P.:** A new human T-lymphotropic retrovirus: characterization and possible role in lymphadenopathy and acquired immune deficiency syndromes. Report from Cold Spring Harbor Meeting, Sep. 15: 363–376, 1983

**Moore, W. E. C., Holdeman, L. V., Smibert, R. M., Good, I. J., Burmeister, J. A., Palcanis, K. G., Ranney, R. R.:** Bacteriology of experimental gingivitis in young adult humans. Infect. Immun. 38: 651–667, 1982 a

**Moore, W. E. C., Holdeman, L. V., Smibert, R. M., Hash, D. E., Burmeister, J. A., Ranney, R. R.:** Bacteriology of severe periodontitis in young adult humans. Infect. Immun. 38: 1137–1148, 1982 b

\* **Moore, W. E. C.:** Microbiology of periodontal disease. J. periodont. Res. 22: 335–341, 1987

**Mörmann, W., Bernimoulin, J. P., Schmid, M. O.:** Fluorescein angiography of free gingival autografts. J. clin. Periodontol. 2: 177–189, 1975

**Mörmann, W., Lutz, F., Curilović, Z.:** Die Bearbeitung von Gold, Keramik und Amalgam mit Composhape-Diamantschleifern und Proxoshape-Interdentalfeilen. Quintessenz 28: 1575–1583, 1983

\* **Mouton, C., Hammond, P. G., Slots, J., Genco, R. J.:** Serum antibodies to oral bacteroides asaccharolyticus (bacteroides gingivalis): Relationship to age and periodontal disease. Infect. Immun. 31: 182–192, 1981

**Mühlemann, H. R.:** Das weibliche Parodont unter dem Einfluß geschlechtsspezifischer Hormone. Stoma 5: 3–23, 1952

**Mühlemann, H. R., Herzog, H., Vogel, A.:** Occlusal trauma and tooth-mobility. Schweiz. Mschr. Zahnheilk. 66: 527–544, 1956

**Mühlemann, H. R., Mazor, Z. S.:** Gingivitis in Zurich school children. Helv. odont. Acta 2: 3–12, 1958

**Mühlemann, H. R., Herzog, H.:** Tooth mobility and microscopic tissue changes produced by experimental occlusal trauma. Helv. odont. Acta 5: 33–39, 1961

**Mühlemann, H. R.:** Tooth mobility: A review of clinical aspects and research findings. J. Periodontol. 38: 686–708, 1967

**Mühlemann, H. R., Son, S.:** Gingival sulcus bleeding – A leading symptom in initial gingivitis. Helv. odont. Acta 15: 107–113, 1971

° **Mühlemann, H. R.:** Patientenmotivation mit individuellem Intensivprogramm für orale Gesundheit. In Peters, S.: Prophylaxe. Quintessenz, Berlin 1978 (S. 137–149)

**Mühlemann, H. R.:** Klinische Innovationen in der präventiven Parodontologie. Acta parodont., in Schweiz. Mschr. Zahnheilk. 93: 559/87–571/99, 1983

**Müller, H.:** Medizinische Genetik: eine Diasammlung mit Begleittext. ROCOM, Basel 1981

**Müller, H. P., Hartmann, J., Flores-de-Jacoby, L.:** Systemische Metronidazoltherapie und/oder subgingivale Zahnreinigung mit Wurzelglättung. Teil I. Klinische Ergebnisse. Dtsch. zahnärztl. Z. 41: 573–578, 1986

\* **Müller, H. P., Hartmann, J., Flores-de-Jacoby, L.:** Clinical alterations in relation to the morphological composition of the subgingival microflora following scaling and root planing. J. clin. Periodontol. 13: 825–832, 1986

\* **Müller, H. P.:** Potentielle Progressionsmuster von entzündlichen Parodontalerkrankungen. Dtsch. zahnärztl. Z. 42: 405–413, 1987

\* **Müller, R. F., Hessling, T., Lange, D. E.:** Rasterelektronenmikroskopische Untersuchungen an Protozoen des parodontalen Taschenexsudates. Dtsch. zahnärztl. Z. 42: 134–137, 1987

**Müller-Glauser, W., Schroeder, H. E.:** The pocket epithelium: A light-and electron-microscopic study. J. Periodontol. 53: 133–144, 1982

**Mutschelknauss, R., von der Ohe, H.-G.:** Behandlung und Prognose der Parodontitis im Bereich von Bi- und Trifurkationen. Dtsch. zahnärztl. Z. 37: 805–810, 1982

* **Mutschelknauss, R.:** Verschiedene Methoden der Taschentherapie im klinischen Vergleich. Dtsch. zahnärztl. Z. 38: 816–828, 1983

´ **Mutschelknauss, R., von der Ohe, H.-G.:** Nachuntersuchungen behandelter Bi- und Trifurkationen bei Parodontitis profunda. Dtsch. zahnärztl. Z. 38: 891–898, 1983

---

## N

* **Nabers, C. L., Stalker, W. H., Esparza, D., Naylor, B., Canales, S.:** Tooth loss in 1535 treated periodontal patients. J. Periodontol. 59: 297–300, 1988

**Nakata, M.:** Twin studies in craniofacial genetics – A review. Acta Genet. Med. Gamello 34: 1–14, 1985

* **Neumann, R.:** Die Alveolar-Pyrrhoe und ihre Behandlung. Meusser, Berlin 1915

* **Neumann, R.:** Die Behandlung der sogenannten Alveolarpyorrhoe und der anderen Paredantosen. Meusser, Berlin 1924

* **Newesely, H.:** Bewertung der Abrasivität von Zahnpflegemitteln und ihrer Auswirkung auf die beteiligten Gewebe. Dtsch. zahnärztl. Z. 40: 767–770, 1985

* **Newman, H. N.:** Update on plaque and periodontal disease. J. clin. Periodontol. 7: 251–258, 1980

* **Newman, H. N.:** Modes of application of anti-plaque chemicals. J. clin. Periodontol. 13: 965–974, 1986

**Newman, M. G., Socransky, S. S.:** Predominant cultivable microbiota in periodontosis. J. periodont. Res. 12: 120–128, 1977

**Newman, M. G.:** The role of bacteroides melaninogenicus and other anaerobes in periodontal infections. Rev. infect. Dis. 1: 313–324, 1979

**Newman, M. G., Goodman, A. D.:** Guide to Antibiotic Use in Dental Practice. Quintessence, Chicago 1984

* **Newman, M. G.:** Current concepts of the pathogenesis of periodontal disease – Microbiology emphasis. J. Periodontol. 56: 734–739, 1985

* **Niedermeier, W., Pröschel, P.:** Die Desmodontometrie – Ein neues Verfahren zur Bestimmung und Analyse der Zahnbeweglichkeit. I. Meßprinzip und Meßanordnung. Dtsch. zahnärztl. Z. 42: 807–812, 1987

* **Niedermeier, W.:** Die Desmodontometrie – Ein neues Verfahren zur Bestimmung und Analyse der Zahnbeweglichkeit. II. Reproduzierbarkeit der Methode und physiologische Einflüsse auf das Meßergebnis. Dtsch. zahnärztl. Z. 42: 1021–1027, 1987

**Niemi, M.-L., Ainamo, J., Etemadzadeh, H.:** Gingival abrasion and plaque removal with manual versus electric toothbrushing. J. clin. Periodontol. 13: 709–713, 1986

* **Nisengard, R. J., Alpert, A. M., Krestow, V.:** Desquamative gingivitis: Immunologic findings. J. Periodontol. 49: 27–32, 1978

**Nisengard, R. J., Bascones, A.:** Bacterial invasion in periodontal disease: A workshop. J. Periodontol. 58: 331–339, 1987

**Nordland, P., Garrett, S., Kiger, R., Vanooteghem, R., Hutchens, L. H., Egelberg, J.:** The effect of plaque control and root debridement in molar teeth. J. clin. Periodontol. 14: 231–236, 1987

**Nyman, S., Lindhe, J.:** Prosthetic rehabilitation of patients with advanced periodontal disease. J. clin. Periodontol. 3: 135–147, 1976

**Nyman, S., Lindhe, J., Rosling, B.:** Periodontal surgery in plaque-infected dentitions. J. clin. Periodontol. 4: 240–249, 1977

**Nyman, S., Lindhe, J.:** A longitudinal study of combined periodontal and prosthetic treatment of patients with advanced periodontal disease. J. Periodontol. 50: 163–169, 1979

**Nyman, S., Ericsson, I.:** The capacity of reduced periodontal tissue to support fixed bridgework. J. clin. Periodontol. 9: 409–414, 1982

**Nyman, S., Gottlow, J., Karring, T., Lindhe, J.:** The regenerative potential of the periodontal ligament. An experimental study in the monkey. J. clin. Periodontol. 9: 257–265, 1982a

**Nyman, S., Lindhe, J., Karring, T., Rylander, H.:** New attachment following surgical treatment of human periodontal disease. J. clin. Periodontol. 9: 290–296, 1982b

* **Nyman, S., Sarhed, G., Ericsson, I., Gottlow, J., Karring, T.:** Role of "diseased" root cementum in healing following treatment of periodontal disease. J. periodont. Res. 21: 496–503, 1986

**Nyman, S., Gottlow, J., Lindhe, J., Karring, T., Wennström, J.:** New attachment formation by guided tissue regeneration. J. periodont. Res. 22: 252–254, 1987

---

## O

* **Ochsenbein, C.:** A primer of osseous surgery. Int. J. Periodont. Restor. Dent. 1: 8, 1986

* **Okada, H., Ito, H., Harada, Y.:** T-cell requirement for establishment of the IgG-dominant B-cell lesion in periodontitis. J. periodont. Res. 22: 187–189, 1987

**O'Leary, T. J., Drake, R. B., Naylor, J. E.:** The plaque control record. J. Periodontol. 43: 38, 1972

* **O'Leary, T. J.:** The inflammation reduction phase of periodontal therapy: Oral hygiene and root planing procedures. Alpha Omegan 76: 32–39, 1983

**O'Leary, T. J.:** The impact of research on scaling and root planing. J. Periodontol. 57: 69–75, 1986

* **O'Leary, T. J., Barrington, E. P., Gottsegen, R.:** Periodontal therapy – A summary status report 1987–1988. J. Periodontol. 59: 306–310, 1988

* **Osborn, J. F., Frentzen, M.:** Grundlagen der Anwendung von Hydroxylapatitkeramik-Implantaten. Dtsch. zahnärztl. Z. 43: 646–655, 1988

**Osborne, W. H., Snyder, A. J., Tempel, T. R.:** Attachment levels and crevicular depths at the distal of mandibular second molars following removal of adjacent third molars. J. Periodontol. 53: 93–95, 1982

* **Ott, P. W., Pröschl, P.:** Zur Ätiologie des keilförmigen Defektes. Dtsch. zahnärztl. Z. 40: 1223–1227, 1985

---

## P

**Page, R. C., Schroeder, H. E.:** Pathogenesis of inflammatory periodontal disease. A summary of current work. Lab. Invest. 33: 235–249, 1976

° **Page, R. C., Schroeder, H. E.:** Periodontitis in Man and Other Animals. A Comparative Review. Karger, Basel 1982

**Page, R. C., Altman, L. C., Ebersole, J. L., Vandesteen, G. E., Dahlberg, W. H., Williams, B. L., Osterberg, S. K.:** Rapidly progressive periodontitis. A distinct clinical condition. J. Periodontol. 54: 197–209, 1983a

**Page, R. C., Bowen, T., Altman, L. C., Vandesteen, G. E., Ochs, H., Makkenzie, P., Osteberg, S. K., Engel, D., Williams, B. L.:** Prepubertal periodontitis. I. Definition of a clinical disease entity. J. Periodontol. 54: 257–271, 1983b

**Page, R. C.:** Gingivitis. J. clin. Periodontol. 13: 345–355, 1986

* **Page, R. C., Beatty, P., Waldrop, T. C.:** Molecular basis for the functional abnormality in neutrophils from patients with generalized prepubertal periodontitis. J. periodont. Res. 22: 182–183, 1987

°* **Page, R. C.:** Are there convincing animal models for periodontal diseases? Periodontology Today. Int. Congr., Zürich. Karger, Basel 1988 (pp. 112–122)

**Pankhurst, C. L., Waite, I. M., Hicks, K. A., Allen, Y., Harkness, R. D.:** The influence of oral contraceptiva therapy on the periodontium – Duration of drug therapy. J. Periodontol. 52: 617–620, 1981

° **Pasler, F. A.:** Zahnärztliche Radiologie. Thieme, 2.Aufl. Stuttgart 1989

**Pasler, F. A.:** Die radiologische Darstellung des Alveolarkammes. Dtsch. zahnärztl. Z. 40: 707–714, 1985

° **Pattison, G. L., Pattison, A. M.:** Periodontal Instrumentation. A Clinical manual. Reston Publishing, Reston/VA 1979

* **Peng, T. K., Nisengard, R. J., Levine, M. J.:** The alteration in gingival basement membrane antigens in chronic periodontitis. J. Periodontol. 57: 20–24, 1986

* **Pertuiset, J. H., Saglie, F. R., Lofthus, J., Rezende, M., Sanz, M.:** Recurrent periodontal disease and bacterial presence in the gingiva. J. Periodontol. 58: 553–558, 1987

°* **Picton, D. C. A.:** Distribution of collagen fibres in the periodontal ligament and their role in tooth support. Periodontology Today. Int. Congr., Zürich. Karger, Basel 1988 (pp. 24–31)

* **Pihlstrom, B. L., McHugh, R. B., Oliphant, T. H., Ortiz-Campos, C.:** Comparison of surgical and nonsurgical treatment of periodontal disease. A review of current studies and additional results after 6½ years. J. clin. Periodontol. 10: 524–541, 1983

**Pihlstrom, B. L., Anderson, K. A., Aeppli, D., Schaffer, E. M.:** Association between signs of trauma from occlusion and periodontitis. J. Periodontol. 57: 1–6, 1986

\* **Pilot, T.:** Economic perspectives on diagnosis and treatment planning in periodontology. J. clin. Periodontol. 13: 889–893, 1986

° **Pindborg, J. J.:** Manifestations of systemic disorders. In Lindhe, J.: Textbook of Clinical Periodontology. Munksgaard, Copenhagen 1983 (pp. 255–284)

° **Pindborg, J. J.:** Atlas of Diseases of the Oral Mucosa. Munksgaard, Copenhagen 1985

° **Pindborg, J. J.:** Atlas der Mundschleimhauterkrankungen. Deutscher Ärzte-Verlag, Köln 1987

\* **Plagmann, H.-C., Jagenow, U.:** Tierexperimentelle Studie zur Reaktion der desmodontalen Gewebe auf intraligamentäre Injektion. Dtsch. zahnärztl. Z. 39: 677–682, 1984

\* **Plagmann, H.-C., Schwardmann, F.:** Untersuchungen zur Hemmwirkung von antiseptischen Mundspüllösungen auf das Bakterienwachstum in der dentalen Plaque und im Speichel. Dtsch. zahnärztl. Z. 40: 806–810, 1985

\* **Plagmann, H.-C., Gleichfeld, A.:** Tierexperimentelle Studie zur Ausbildung und Beeinflussung der befestigten Gingiva hinsichtlich Breite und Keratinisierungsgrad. Dtsch. zahnärztl. Z. 41: 589–596, 1986

\* **Plagmann, H.-C.:** Diagnostische Methoden bei Parodontalerkrankungen. Eine kritische Betrachtung und Forderungen für die Zukunft. Dtsch. zahnärztl. Z. 42: 394–397, 1987

\* **Plagmann, H.-C., Kocher, T., Engelsmann, U.:** Epitheliales Neu-Attachment nach Wurzeloberflächenbearbeitung mit verschiedenen Instrumenten. Dtsch. zahnärztl. Z. 43: 686–692, 1988

**Plüss, E. M., Engelberger, P. R., Rateitschak, K. H.:** Effect of chlorhexidine on dental plaque formation under periodontal pack. J. clin. Peridontol. 2: 136–142, 1975

**Pollack, R. P.:** Bilateral creeping attachment using free mucosal grafts. A case report with 4-year-follow-up. J. Periodontol. 55: 670–672, 1984

**Polson, A. M., Meitner, S. W., Zander, H. A.:** Trauma and progression of marginal periodontitis in squirrel monkeys. III. Adaption of interproximal alveolar bone to repetitive injury. J. periodont. Res. 11: 279–289, 1976a

**Polson, A. M., Meitner, S. W., Zander, H. A.:** Trauma and progression of marginal periodontitis in squirrel monkeys. IV. Reversibility of bone loss due to·trauma alone and trauma superimposed upon periodontitis. J. periodont. Res. 11: 290–298, 1976b

**Polson, A. M., Heijl, L. C.:** Osseous repair in infrabony periodontal defects. J. clin. Periodontol. 5: 13–23, 1978

\* **Polson, A. M., Adams, R. A., Zander, H. A.:** Osseous repair in the presence of active tooth hypermobility. J. clin. Periodontol. 10: 370–379, 1983

**Polson, A. M., Proye, M. P.:** Fibrin linkage: A precursor for new attachment. J. Periodontol. 54: 141–147, 1983

\* **Polson, A. M., Caton, J. G.:** Current status of bleeding in the diagnosis of periodontal diseases. J. Periodontol. 56 (Suppl.): 1–3, 1985

\* **Polson, A. M., Zappa, U. E., Espeland, M. A., Eisenberg, A. D.:** Effect of metronidazole on development of subgingival plaque and experimental periodontitis. J. Periodontol. 57: 218–224, 1986

\* **Polson, A. M., Ladenheim, S., Hanes, P. J.:** Cell and fiber attachment to demineralized dentin from periodontitis-affected root surfaces. J. Periodontol. 57: 235–246, 1986

**Polson, A. M.:** The root surface and regeneration; present therapeutic limitations and future biologic potentials. J. clin. Periodontol. 13: 995–999, 1986

\* **Polson, A. M.:** The relative importance of plaque and occlusion in periodontal disease. J. clin. Periodontol. 13: 923–927, 1986

**Pontoriero, R., Nyman, S., Lindhe, J., Rosenberg, E., Sanavi, F.:** Guided tissue regeneration in the treatment of furcation defects in man. J. clin. Periodontol. 14: 618–620, 1987

\* **Pontoriero, R., Nyman, S., Lindhe, J.:** The angular bony defect in the maintenance of the periodontal patient. J. clin. Periodontol. 15: 200–204, 1988

**Pontoriero, R., Lindhe, J., Nyman, S., Karring, T., Rosenberg, E., Sanavi, F.:** Guided tissue regeneration in degree II furcation-involved mandibular molars. A clinical study. J. clin. Periodontol. 15: 247–254, 1988

**Posselt, U.:** Physiology of Occlusion and Rehabilitation. Davis, Philadelphia 1962

\* **Preus, H. R., Olsen, I., Gjermo, P.:** Bacteriophage infection – A possible mechanism for increased virulence of bacteria associated with rapidly destructive periodontitis. Acta odont. scand. 45: 49–54, 1987

**Preus, H. R., Gjermo, P.:** Clinical management of prepubertal periodontitis in 2 siblings with Papillon-Lefèvre syndrome. J. clin. Periodontol. 14: 156–160, 1987

°\* **Preus, H. R.:** The pathogenicity of haemophilus (actinobacillus) actinomycetemcomitans. A new concept. Periodontology Today. Int. Congr., Zürich. Karger, Basel 1988 (pp. 160–168)

°\* **Prichard, J. F.:** The Diagnosis and Treatment of Periodontal Disease. Saunders, Philadelphia 1979

\* **Prichard, J. F.:** The diagnosis and management of vertical bony defects. J. Periodontol. 54: 29–35, 1983

\* **Purucker, P., Bräuer, G., Bernimoulin, J.-P.:** Auswirkung von Parodontalinstrumenten auf die Wurzeloberfläche und deren bakterielle Besiedelung. Dtsch. zahnärztl. Z. 43: 681–685, 1988

## Q

**Quee, T. C., Gosselin, D., Millar, E. P., Stamm, J. W.:** Surgical removal of the fully impacted mandibular third molar. The influence of flap design and alveolar bone height on the periodontal status of the second molar. J. Periodontol. 56: 625–630, 1985

**Quee, T. C., Chan, E. C. S., Clark, C., Lautar-Lemay, C., Bergeron, M.-J., Bourgouin, J., Stamm, J.:** The role of adjunctive Rodogyl therapy in the treatment of advanced periodontal disease – A longitudinal clinical and microbiologic study. J. Periodontol. 58: 594–601, 1987

## R

\* **Raetzke, P.:** Reaktion der marginalen Gingiva auf den Kontakt mit Kronen und Verblendmaterialien bei Probanden mit exzellenter Mundhygiene. Dtsch. zahnärztl. Z. 40: 1206–1208, 1985

\* **Ralls, S. A., Cohen, M. E.:** Problems in identifying "bursts" of periodontal attachment loss. J. Periodontol. 57: 746–752, 1986

**Ramfjord, S. P.:** Indices for prevalence and incidence of periodontal disease. J. Periodontol. 30: 51–59, 1959

**Ramfjord, S. P., Nissle, R. R.:** The modified Widman flap. J. Periodontol. 45: 601–607, 1974

**Ramfjord, S. P., Knowles, J. W., Nissle, R. R., Burgett, F. G., Shick, R. A.:** Results following three modalities of periodontal therapy. J. Periodontol. 46: 522–526, 1975

**Ramfjord, S. P.:** Present status of the modified Widman flap procedure. J. Periodontol. 48: 558–565, 1977

° **Ramfjord, S. P., Ash, M.:** Periodontology and Periodontics. Saunders, Philadelphia 1979

**Ramfjord, S. P., Ash, M. M., Jr.:** Significance of occlusion in the etiology and treatment of early, moderate and advanced periodontitis. J. Periodontol. 52: 511–517, 1981

**Ramfjord, S. P., Morrison, E. C., Burgett, F. G., Nissle, R. R., Schick, R. A., Zann, G. J., Knowles, J. W.:** Oral hygiene and maintenance of periodontal support. J. Periodontol. 53: 26–30, 1982

° **Ramfjord, S. P., Ash, M. M.:** Occlusion, 3rd ed. Saunders, Philadelphia 1983

\* **Ranney, R. R., Yanni, N. R., Burmeister, J. A., Tew, J. G.:** Relationship between attachment loss and precipitating serum antibody to actinobacillus actinomycetemcomitans in adolescents and young adults having severe periodontal destruction J. Periodontol. 53: 1–7, 1982

\* **Ranney, R. R., Best, A. M., Breen, T. J., Moore, W. E. C., Moore, L. V. H.:** Bacterial flora of progressing periodontitis lesions. J. periodont. Res. 22: 205–206, 1987

**Rateitschak, K. H., Egli, U., Fringeli, G.:** Recession: A 4-year longitudinal study after free gingival grafts. J. clin. Periodontol. 6: 158–164, 1979

**Rateitschak, K. H.:** Indikation, Wert und Unwert der Schienung. Dtsch. zahnärztl. Z. 35: 699–703, 1980

**Rateitschak, K. H.:** Mißerfolge in der Parodontologie. Acta parodont., in Schweiz. Mschr. Zahnmed. 95: 609/81–620/92, 1985

**Rateitschak, K. H.:** Grenzen zwischen konservativer und chirurgischer Parodontalbehandlung aus klinischer Sicht. Dtsch. zahnärztl. Z. 41: 545–551, 1986

**Rateitschak, K. H., Rateitschak-Plüss, E. M., Wolf, H. F.:** Langdon Down-Syndrom: Mongolismus – Trisomie 21. Schweiz. Mschr. Zahnmed. 97: 1145–1148, 1987

* **Rateitschak-Plüss, E. M., Guggenheim, B.:** Effects of a carbohydrate-free diet and sugar-substitutes on dental plaque accumulation. J. clin. Periodontol. 9: 239–251, 1982

**Rateitschak-Plüss, E. M., Hefti, A., Rateitschak, K. H.:** Gingivahyperplasie bei Cyclosporin-A-Medikation. Acta parodont., in Schweiz. Mschr. Zahnheilk. 93: 57/1–65/9, 1983 a

**Rateitschak-Plüss, E. M., Hefti, A., Lörtscher, R., Thiel, G.:** Initial observation that Cyclosporin-A induces gingival enlargement in man. J. clin. Periodontol. 10: 237–246, 1983 b

* **Rateitschak-Plüss, E. M., Schroeder, H. E.:** History of periodontitis in a child with Papillon-Lefèvre syndrome. A case report. J. Periodontol. 55: 35–46, 1984

**Rateitschak-Plüss, E. M.:** Probleme beim instrumentellen subgingivalen Scaling und Root planing. Dtsch. zahnärztl. Z. 40: 715–720, 1985

* **Rateitschak-Plüss, E. M., Rateitschak, K. H., Hefti, A., Lori, A., Gratwohl, A., Speck, B.:** Zahnärztliche Betreuung von Patienten mit Knochenmarktransplantation. Schweiz. Mschr. Zahnmed. 98: 472–477, 1988

* **Rechmann, P., Herforth, A., Chatzigiannis, S.:** Nachuntersuchungsergebnisse nach konservativen und chirurgischen Parodontalbehandlungen bei einem nicht überwachten Patientenkollektiv. Dtsch. zahnärztl. Z. 40: 795–799, 1985

**Redfield, R. R., Wright, D. C., Tramont, E. C.:** The Walter Reed staging classification for HTLV-III/LAV infection. The New England J. Medicine, Vol. 314, No. 2, 131–132, January 1986

**Redfield, R. R., Burke, D. S.:** HIV-infection: The clinical picture. Scientific American, Vol. 259, No. 4, 70–78, October 1988

* **Reich, E., Schmalz, G., Reith, A.:** Vergleich des CPITN mit gebräuchlichen Parodontalindizes. Dtsch. zahnärztl. Z. 41: 610–612, 1986

**Reichart, P., Pohle, H.-D., Gelderblom, H., Strunz, V.:** AIDS – Orale Manifestationen. Dtsch. zahnärztl. Z. 41: 374–376, 1986

**Renggli, H. H., Regolati, B.:** Gingival inflammation and plaque accumulation by well-adapted supragingival and subgingival proximal restorations. Helv. odont. Acta 16: 99–101, 1972

**Renggli, H. H.:** Auswirkungen subgingivaler approximaler Füllungsränder auf den Entzündungsgrad der benachbarten Gingiva. Habilitationsschrift (Thesis), Zürich 1974

° **Rett, A.:** Mongolismus. Biologische, erzieherische und soziale Aspekte, 2. Aufl. Huber, Bern 1983

**Reuland-Bosma, W., Van Dijk, J.:** Periodontal disease in Down's syndrome: A review. J. clin. Periodontol. 13: 64–73, 1986

°* **Reynolds, J.:** Mediators of osteoclast activation in vitro and their relevance to resorption in periodontal diseases. Periodontology Today. Int. Congr., Zürich. Karger, Basel 1988 (pp. 218–226)

* **Rezende, M., Pertuiset, J., Saglie, R.:** The progression of periodontal destruction: The concept of disease activity. J. West. Soc. Periodontol. 34: 89–94, 1986

* **Riemensperger, H.-D., Raetzke, P.:** Breite der befestigten Gingiva und gingivale Gesundheit bei 8- bis 14jährigen Schulkindern. Dtsch. zahnärztl. Z. 42: 131–133, 1987

° **Riethe, P.:** Die Quintessenz der Mundhygiene. Quintessenz, Berlin 1974

**Riethe, P.:** Welche Füllungsmaterialien sind im gingivalen Bereich vertretbar? Dtsch. zahnärztl. Z. 39: 589–598, 1984

° **Riethe, P.:** Farbatlanten der Zahnmedizin, Band 6: Kariesprophylaxe und konservierende Therapie. Thieme, Stuttgart 1988

**Ringelberg, M. L., Dixon, D. O., Francis, A. O. I., Plummer, R. W.:** Comparison of gingival health and gingival crevicular fluid flow in children with and without diabetes. J. dent. Res. 56: 108–111, 1977

**Ririe, C. M., Crigger, M., Selvig, K. A.:** Healing of periodontal connective tissues following surgical wounding and application of citric acid in dogs. J. periodont. Res. 15: 314–327, 1980

**Rivera-Hidalgo, F.:** Smoking and periodontal disease – A review of the literature. J. Periodontol. 57: 617–624, 1986

**Robertson, P., Greenspan, J. S.:** Perspectives on Oral Manifestations of AIDS. PGS, Littleton/MA 1988

**Robinson, R. W.:** Osseous coagulum for bone induction. J. Periodontol. 40: 503–510, 1969

**Rochette, A. L.:** Attachment of a splint to enamel to lower anterior teeth. J. prosth. Dent. 30: 418–423, 1973

° **Roitt, I., Brostoff, J., Male, D.:** Immunology. Gower, London 1985

**Roitt, I. M.:** Essential Immunology. 6th ed. Blackwell, Oxford, Boston, Melbourne 1988

**Rosling, B., Nyman, S., Lindhe, J.:** The effect of systemic plaque control on bone regeneration in infrabony pockets. J. clin. Periodontol. 3: 38–53, 1976 a

**Rosling, B., Nyman, S., Lindhe, J., Jern, B.:** The healing potential of the periodontal tissues following different techniques of periodontal surgery in plaque-free dentitions. A 2-year clinical study. J. clin. Periodontol. 3: 233–250, 1976 b

* **Rosling, B. G., Slots, J., Christersson, L. A., Gröndahl, H. G., Genco, R. J.:** Topical antimicrobial therapy and diagnosis of subgingival bacteria in the management of inflammatory periodontal disease. J. clin. Periodontol. 13: 975–981, 1986

* **Ross, I. F., Thompson, R. H.:** A long-term study of root retention in the treatment of maxillary molars with furcation involvement. J. Periodontol. 49: 238–244, 1978

* **Ross, I. F., Thompson, R. H.:** Furcation involvement in maxillary and mandibular molars. J. Periodontol. 51: 450–454, 1980

* **Roulet, J. F., Roulet-Mehrens, T. K.:** The surface roughness of restorative materials and dental tissues after polishing with prophylaxis and polishing pastes. J. Periodontol. 53: 257–266, 1982

* **Rozanis, J., Johnson, R. H., Haq, M. S., Schofield, I. D.:** Spiramycin as a selective dental plaque control agent. J. periodont. Res. 14: 55–64, 1979

**Rylander, H., Ramberg, P., Blohmé, G., Lindhe, J.:** Prevalence of periodontal disease in young diabetics. J. clin. Periodontol. 14: 38–43, 1987

## S

**Saadoun, A. P.:** Diabetes and periodontal disease. A review and update. J. West. Soc. Periodontol. 28: 116–139, 1980

**Saadoun, A. P.:** Management of furcation involvement. J. West. Soc. Periodontol. 33: 91–125, 1985

**Sabiston, C. B., Jr.:** A review and proposal for the etiology of acute necrotizing gingivitis. J. clin. Periodontol. 13: 727–734, 1986

**Saglie, F. R., Newman, M. G., Carranza, F. A., Jr., Pattison, G. L.:** Bacterial invasion of gingiva in advanced periodontitis in humans. J. Periodontol. 53: 217–222, 1982

* **Saglie, F. R., Carranza, F. A., Jr., Newman, M. G., Cheng, L., Lewin, K. J.:** Identification of tissue-invading bacteria in human periodontal disease. J. periodont. Res. 17: 452–455, 1982

* **Saglie, F. R., Pertuiset, J. H., Rezende, M. T., Sabet, M. S., Raoufi, D., Carranza, F. A., Jr.:** Bacterial invasion in experimental gingivitis in man. J. Periodontol. 58: 837–846, 1987

* **Saglie, F. R., Pertuiset, J. H., Smith, C. T., Nestor, M. G., Carranza, F. A., Jr., Newman, M. G., Rezende, M. T., Nisengard, R.:** The presence of bacteria in the oral epithelium in periodontal disease. III. Correlation with Langerhans cells. J. Periodontol. 58: 417–422, 1987

**Saglie, F. R., Marfany, A., Camargo, P.:** Intragingival occurrence of actinobacillus actinomycetemcomitans and bacteroides gingivalis in active destructive periodontal lesions. J. Periodontol. 59: 259–265, 1988

* **Saladin, R.:** Der parodontal kranke Mensch. Dtsch. zahnärztl. Z. 42: 424–427, 1987

**Salkin, L. M., Freedman, A. L., Stein, M. D., Bassiouny, M. A.:** A longitudinal study of untreated mucogingival defects. J. Periodontol. 58: 164–166, 1987

° **Sauerwein, E.:** Alterszahnheilkunde, 2. Aufl. Thieme, Stuttgart 1983

**Saxby, M. S.:** Prevalence of juvenile periodontitis in a British school population. Community Dent. oral Epidemiol. 12: 185–187, 1984

**Saxby, M. S.:** Juvenile periodontitis: An epidemiological study in the west Midlands of the United Kingdom. J. clin. Periodontol. 14: 594–598, 1987

**Saxén, L.:** Juvenile periodontitis. J. clin. Periodontol. 7: 1–19, 1980

**Saxén, L., Asikainen, S., Sandholm, L., Kari, K.:** Treatment of juvenile periodontitis without antibiotics. A follow-up study. J. clin. Periodontol. 13: 714–719, 1986

**Saxer, U. P., Mühlemann, H. R.:** Motivation und Aufklärung. Schweiz. Mschr. Zahnheilk. 85: 905–919, 1975

* **Saxer, U. P., Turconi, B., Elsässer, C.:** Patient motivation with the papillary bleeding index. J. prev. Dent. 4: 20–22, 1977

**Schallhorn, R. G., Hiatt, W. H., Boyce, W.:** Iliac transplants in periodontal therapy. J. Periodontol. 41: 566–580, 1970

**Schallhorn, R. G.:** Postoperative problems associated with iliac transplants. J. Periodontol. 43: 3–9, 1972

\* **Schallhorn, R. G.:** Present status of osseous grafting procedures. J. Periodontol. 28: 570–576, 1977

\* **Schei, O., Waerhaug, J., Lovdal, A., Arno, A.:** Alveolar bone loss as related to oral hygiene and age. J. Periodontol. 30: 7–16, 1959

° **Schettler, G.:** Innere Medizin, 7. Aufl. Thieme, Stuttgart 1987

**Schijatschky, M. M.:** Life-Threatening Emergencies in Dental Practice. Quintessence, Chicago 1979

**Schluger, S., Yuodelis, R., Page, R. C., Johnson, R.:** Periodontal Disease, 2nd ed. Lea & Febiger, Philadelphia 1989

\* **Schmid, M. O.:** The subperiostal vestibule extension. Literature review, rationale and technique. J. West. Soc. Periodontol. 24: 3, 1976

**Schmid, W.:** Die Prävention des Down-Syndroms (Mongolismus). Neue Zürcher Zeitung, Nr. 15, 20. 1. 1988, S. 77

**Schnetz, H., Franzen, H.:** Zahnärztliche Eingriffe bei Diabetes mellitus und Nebennierenrindeninsuffizienz. Zahnärztl. Rdsch. 77: 35–38, 1968

\* **Schonfeld, S. E., Checchi, L.:** Review of immunology for the periodontist. J. West. Soc. Periodontol. 33: 53–64, 1985

° **Schroeder, H. E., Listgarten, M. A.:** Fine Structure of the Developing Epithelial Attachment of Human Teeth, 2nd ed. Karger, Basel 1977

° **Schroeder, H. E., Attström, R.:** Pocket formation: An hypothesis. In Lehner, T., Cimasoni, G.: The Borderland Between Caries and Periodontal Disease II. Academic Press, London 1980 (pp. 99–123)

° **Schroeder, H. E.:** Pathobiologie oraler Strukturen: Zähne, Pulpa, Parodont. Karger, Basel 1983

\* **Schroeder, H. E., Seger, R. A., Keller, H. U., Rateitschak-Plüss, E. M.:** Behavior of neutrophilic granulocytes in a case of Papillon-Lefèvre syndrome. J. clin. Periodontol. 10: 618–635, 1983

**Schroeder, H. E., Rateitschak-Plüss, E. M.:** Focal root resorption lacunae causing retention of subgingival plaque in periodontal pockets. Acta parodont., in Schweiz. Mschr. Zahnheilk. 93: 1033/179–1041/187, 1983

° **Schroeder, H. E.:** The Periodontium. Springer, Berlin 1986

° **Schroeder, H. E.:** Orale Strukturbiologie. Entwicklungsgeschichte, Struktur und Funktion normaler Hart- und Weichgewebe der Mundhöhle und des Kiefergelenks, 3. Aufl. Thieme, Stuttgart 1987 a

**Schroeder, H. E.:** Klinik und Pathologie verschiedener Formen von Parodontitis. Dtsch. zahnärztl. Z. 42: 417–421, 1987 b

**Schroeder, H. E., Scherle, W. F.:** Warum die Furkation menschlicher Zähne so unvorhersehbar bizarr gestaltet ist. Schweiz. Mschr. Zahnmed. 97: 1495–1508, 1987

°\* **Schroeder, H. E.:** Origin, structure and distribution of cementum and its possible role in local periodontal treatment. Periodontology Today. Int. Congr. Zürich. Karger, Basel 1988 (pp. 32–40)

**Schulte, W., d'Hoedt, B., Lukas, D., Mühlbradt, L., Scholz, F., Bretschi, J., Frey, D., Gudat, H., König, M., Markl, M., Quante, F., Schief, A., Topkaya, A.:** Periotest – neues Meßverfahren der Funktion des Parodontiums. Zahnärztl. Mitt. 11: 1229–1240, 1983

**Schulte, W.:** Was leistet das Periotestverfahren heute? Dtsch. zahnärztl. Z. 40: 705–706, 1985

**Schwarz, J. P., Hefti, A., Rateitschak, K. H.:** Vergleich der Oberflächenrauhigkeiten des Wurzeldentins nach Bearbeitung mit Diamantschleifkörpern und Handinstrumenten. Acta parodont., in Schweiz. Mschr. Zahnheilk. 94: 343/47–354/58, 1984

**Schweizer, B., Rateitschak, K. H.:** Zur Topographie des Knochenschwundes und der Zahnfleischtaschen bei Parodontitis. Acta parodont., in Schweiz. Mschr. Zahnheilk. 82: 1075/101–1089/115, 1972

**Schweizer-Hirt, C., Schait, A., Schmid, R., Imfeld, T., Lutz, F., Mühlemann, H. R.:** Erosion und Abrasion des Schmelzes. Eine experimentelle Studie. Schweiz. Mschr. Zahnheilk. 88: 497–529, 1978

\* **Schweizerische Arbeitsgruppe für Endokarditisprophylaxe:** Prophylaxe der bakteriellen Endokarditis. Schweiz. med. Wschr. 114: 1246–1252, 1984

**Scott-Metsger, D., Driskell, T. D., Paulrud, J. R.:** Tricalciumphosphate ceramic – a resorbable bone implant: Review and current status. J. Amer. dent. Ass. 105: 1035–1038, 1982

\* **Seymour, G. J.:** Possible mechanisms involved in the immunoregulation of chronic inflammatory periodontal disease. J. dent. Res. 66: 2–9, 1987

**Seymour, R. A.:** Efficacy of paracetamol in reducing post-operative pain after periodontal surgery. J. clin. Periodontol. 10: 311–316, 1983

**Seymour, R. A., Heasman, P. A.:** Drugs and the periodontium. Review paper. J. clin. Periodontol. 15: 1–16, 1988

\* **SGP, Schweizerische Gesellschaft für Parodontologie:** Zum Thema Parodontitis, 1986

**Sheiham, A.:** Prevention and control of periodontal disease. In: International Conference on Research in the Biology of Periodontal Disease. June, 12–25, 1977, p. 308

°\* **Shenker, B. J.:** Immunsuppression: An etiopathogenic mechanism. Periodontology Today. Int. Congr., Zürich. Karger, Basel 1988 (pp. 178–186)

\* **Siegrist, B. E., Gusberti, F. A., Brecx, M. C., Weber, H. P., Lang, N. P.:** Efficacy of supervised rinsing with chlorhexidine digluconate in comparison to phenolic and plant alkaloid compounds. J. periodont. Res. 21 (Suppl.): 60–73, 1986

**Silness, J., Löe, H.:** Periodontal disease in pregnancy. II. Correlation between oral hygiene and periodontal condition. Acta odont. scand. 22: 121–135, 1964

**Singletary, M. M., Crawford, J. J., Simpson, D. M.:** Dark-field microscopic monitoring of subgingival bacteria during periodontal therapy. J. Periodontol. 53: 671–681, 1982

**Škach, M., Zábrodský, S., Mrklas, L.:** A study of the effect of age and season on the incidence of ulcerative gingivitis. J. periodont. Res. 5: 187–190, 1970

**Skougaard, M. R.:** Turnover of the gingival epithelium in marmosets. Acta odont. scand. 23: 623–643, 1965

° **Skougaard, M. R.:** Cell renewal, with special reference to the gingival epithelium. In Staple, P. H.: Advances in Oral Biology, Vol. 4. Academic Press, New York 1970 (pp. 261–288)

**Slots, J.:** Comparison of five growth media and two anaerobic techniques for isolating bacteria from dental plaques. Scand J. dent. Res. 83: 274–278, 1975

**Slots, J.:** The predominant cultivable organisms in juvenile periodontitis. Scand. J. dent. Res. 84: 1–10, 1976

**Slots, J.:** The predominant cultivable microflora of advanced periodontitis. Scand. J. dent. Res. 85: 114–121, 1977

**Slots, J.:** Subgingival microflora and periodontal disease. J. clin. Periodontol. 6: 351–382, 1979

**Slots, J., Reynolds, H. S., Genco, R. J.:** Actinobacillus actinomycetemcomitans in human periodontal disease: A cross-sectional microbiological investigation. Infect. Immun. 29: 1013–1020, 1980

**Slots, J., Rosling, B. G., Genco, R. J.:** Suppression of penicillin-resistant oral actinobacillus actinomycetemcomitans with tetracycline. Considerations in endocarditis prophylaxis. J. Periodontol. 54: 193–196, 1983

**Slots, J., Genco, R. J.:** Microbial pathogenicity. Black pigmented bacteroides species, capnocytophaga species, and actinobacillus actinomycetemcomitans in human periodontal disease: Virulence factors in colonization, survival, and tissue destruction. J. dent. Res. 63: 412–421, 1984

**Slots, J., Bragd, L., Wikström, M., Dahlén, G.:** The occurrence of actinobacillus actinomycetemcomitans, bacteroides gingivalis and bacteroides intermedius in destructive periodontal disease in adults. J. clin. Periodontol. 13: 570–577, 1986

**Slots, J.:** Bacterial specificity in adult periodontitis. A summary of recent work. J. clin. Periodontol. 13: 912–917, 1986

\* **Slots, J., Listgarten, M. A.:** Bacteroides gingivalis, bacteroides intermedius and actinobacillus actinomycetemcomitans in human periodontal diseases. J. clin. Periodontol. 15: 85–93, 1988

°\* **Slots, J., Taichman, N. S., Oler, J., Listgarten, M. A.:** Does the analysis of the subgingival flora have value in predicting periodontal breakdown? Periodontology Today. Int. Congr., Zürich, Karger, Basel 1988 b (pp. 132–140)

\* **Smith, B. A., Echeverri, M., Caffesse, R. G.:** Mucoperiosteal flaps with and without removal of the pocket epithelium. J. Periodontol. 58: 78–85, 1987

**Smukler, H., Landsberg, J.:** The toothbrush and gingival traumatic injury. J. Periodontol. 55: 713–719, 1984

**Socransky, S. S.:** Microbiology of periodontal disease – present and future considerations. J. Periodontol. 48: 497–504, 1977

**Socransky, S. S., Haffajee, A. D., Goodson, J. M., Lindhe, J.:** New concepts of destructive periodontal disease. J. clin. Periodontol. 11: 21–32, 1984

**Soh, L. L., Newman, H. N., Strahan, J. D.:** Effects of subgingival chlorhexidine irrigation on periodontal inflammation. J. clin. Periodontol. 9: 66–74, 1982

* **Spranger, H.:** Die Versorgung approximaler Kavitäten aus parodontologischer Sicht. Dtsch. zahnärztl. Z. 36: 251–253, 1981

**Stahl, S. S.:** The need for orthodontic treatment: A periodontist's point of view. Int. dent. J. 25: 242–247, 1975

**Stahl, S. S.:** Periodontal Surgery. Thomas, Springfield 1976

**Stahl, S. S., Froum, S. J., Kushner, L.:** Periodontal healing following open debridement flap procedures. II. Histologic observations. J. Periodontol. 53: 15–21, 1982

**Stahl, S. S., Froum, S. J., Kushner, L.:** Healing responses of human intraosseous lesions following the use of debridement, grafting and citric acid root treatment. J. Periodontol. 54: 325–338, 1983

* **Stahl, S. S.:** Periodontal attachment in health and disease. J. West. Soc. Periodontol. 33: 147–157, 1985

* **Stahl, S. S., Froum, S. J.:** Histological evaluation of human intraosseous healing responses to the placement of tricalcium phosphate ceramic implants. I. Three to eight months. J. Periodontol. 57: 211–217, 1986

**Stamm, J. W.:** Epidemiology of gingivitis. J. clin. Periodontol. 13: 360–366, 1986

**Strub, J. R., Belser, U. C.:** Parodontalzustand bei Patienten mit kronen- und brückenprothetischem Ersatz. Acta parodont., in Schweiz. Mschr. Zahnheilk. 88: 569/35–581/47, 1978

**Strub, J. R., Gaberthüel, T. W., Firestone, A. R.:** Comparison of tricalcium phosphate and frozen allogenic bone implants in man. J. Periodontol. 50: 624–629, 1979

**Sullivan, H. C., Atkins, J. H.:** Free autogenous gingival grafts. I. Principle of successful grafting. Periodontics 6: 121–129, 1968 a

**Sullivan, H. C., Atkins, J. H.:** Free autogenous gingival grafts. III. Utilization of grafts in the treatment of gingival recession. Periodontics 6: 152–160, 1968 b

**Suomi, J. D., Smith, L. W., McClendon, B. J.:** Marginal gingivitis during a sixteen-week period. J. Periodontol. 42: 268–270, 1971

**Svanberg, G. K., Lindhe, J.:** Vascular reactions in the periodontal ligament incident to trauma from occlusion. J. clin. Periodontol. 1: 58–69, 1974

**Svanberg, G. K.:** Hydroxyproline titers in gingival crevicular fluid. J. periodont. Res. 22: 212–214, 1987

## T

* **Takei, H. H., Han, T. J., Carranza, F. A., Jr., Kenney, E. B., Lekovic, V.:** Flap technique for periodontal bone implants – Papilla preservation technique. J. Periodontol. 56: 204–210, 1985

**Tal, H.:** Relationship between the interproximal distance of roots and the prevalence of intrabony pockets. J. Periodontol. 55: 604–607, 1984

* **Tanner, A. C. R., Socransky, S. S., Goodson, J. M.:** Microbiota of periodontal pockets losing crestal alveolar bone. J. periodont. Res. 19: 279–291, 1984

* **Tanner, A. C. R., Dzink, J. L., Socransky, S. S., Des Roches, C. L.:** Diagnosis of periodontal disease using rapid identification of "activity-related" gram-negative species. J. periodont. Res. 22: 207–208, 1987

o* **Tanner, A. C. R.:** Is the specific plaque hypothesis still tenable? Periodontology Today. Int. Congr., Zürich. Karger, Basel 1988 (pp. 123–131)

**Tarnow, D., Fletcher, P.:** Classification of the vertical component of furcation involvement. J. Periodontol. 55: 283–284, 1984

o* **Ten Cate, A. R.:** Oral Histology, Development, Structure and Function. Mosby, St. Louis 1980

* **Tenenbaum, H.:** A clinical study comparing the width of attached gingiva and the prevalence of gingival recessions. J. clin. Periodontol. 9: 86–92, 1982

* **Terranova, V. P., Franzetti, L. C., Hic, S., DiFlorio, R. M., Lyall, R. M., Wikesjö, U. M. E., Baker, P. J., Christersson, L. A., Genco, R. J.:** A biochemical approach to periodontal regeneration: tetracycline treatment of dentin promotes fibroblast adhesion and growth. J. periodont. Res. 21: 330–337, 1986

* **Terranova, V. P., Hic, S., Franzetti, L. C., Lyall, R. M., Wikesjö, U. M. E.:** A biochemical approach to periodontal regeneration – AFSCM: Assays for specific cell migration. J. Periodontol. 58: 247–257, 1987

**Theilade, E.:** The non-specific theory in microbial etiology of inflammatory periodontal diseases. J. clin. Periodontol. 13: 905–911, 1986

* **The Medical Letter on Drugs and Therapeutics:** Prevention of bacterial endocarditis. 26: 3, 1984

* **Thie, B., Steegman, B.:** Die Deckung gingivaler Rezessionen mittels freien Schleimhauttransplantates – zwei ergänzende Verfahren. Dtsch. zahnärztl. Z. 42: 216–219, 1987

**Thornton, S., Garnick, J.:** Comparison of ultrasonic to hand instruments in the removal of subgingival plaque. J. Periodontol. 53: 35–37, 1982

**Tinanoff, N., Tanzer, J. M., Kornmann, K. S., Maderazo, E. G.:** Treatment of the periodontal component of Papillon-Lefèvre syndrome: A case report. J. clin. Periodontol. 13: 6–10, 1986

* **Topoll, H. H.:** Die Bildung eines bindegewebigen Attachments nach Anwendung von Zitronensäure und Fibrinkleber. Dtsch. zahnärztl. Z. 41: 613–618, 1986

* **Topoll, H. H., Zwadlo, G., Lange, D. E., Sorg, C.:** Analyse des entzündlichen Infiltrates verschiedener Entzündungsstadien der marginalen Gingiva mittels monoklonaler Antikörper. Dtsch. zahnärztl. Z. 42: 467–470, 1987

* **Topoll, H. H., Lange, D. E.:** Die Tunnelierung mehrwurzliger Zähne. Ergebnisse 8 Jahre post operationem. Dtsch. zahnärztl. Z. 42: 445–449, 1987

* **Topoll, H. H., Streletz, E., Hucke, H. P., Lange, D. E.:** Furkationsdiagnostik. Ein Vergleich der Aussagekraft von OPG, Röntgenstatus und intraoperativem Befund. Dtsch. zahnärztl. Z. 43: 705–708, 1988

**Totti, N., McCusker, K. T., Campbell, E. J., Griffin, G. L., Senior, R. M.:** Nicotine is chemotactic for neutrophils and enhances neutrophil responsiveness to chemotactic peptides. Science 233: 169, 1984

## V

**Van der Velden, U., de Vries, J. H.:** The influence of probing force on the reproducibility of pocket depth measurements. J. clin. Periodontol. 7: 414–420, 1980

* **Van der Velden, U.:** Location of probe tip in bleeding and non-bleeding pockets with minimal gingival inflammation. J. clin. Periodontol. 9: 421–427, 1982

**Van der Velden, U., Abbas, F., Winkel, E. G.:** Probing considerations in relation to susceptibility to periodontal breakdown. J. clin. Periodontol. 13: 894–899, 1986

* **Van der Velden, U.:** Response to treatment, our chief diagnostic method. Periodontology Today. Int. Congr., Zürich. Karger, Basel 1988 (pp. 244–250)

* **Van Dyke, T. E., Duncan, R. L., Cutler, C. W., Kalmar, J. R., Arnold, R. R.:** Mechanisms and consequences of neutrophil interaction with the subgingival microbiota. Periodontology Today. Int. Congr., Zürich. Karger, Basel 1988 (pp. 209–217)

**Van Palenstein-Helderman, W. H.:** Microbial etiology of periodontal disease. J. clin. Periodontol. 8: 261–280, 1981

* **Van Palenstein-Helderman, W. H.:** Is antibiotic therapy justified in the treatment of human chronic inflammatory periodontal disease? J. clin. Periodontol. 13: 932–938, 1986

* **Van Winkelhoff, A. J., van Steenbergen, T. J. M., de Graaff, J.:** The role of black-pigmented bacteroides in human oral infections. J. clin. Periodontol. 15: 145–155, 1988

* **Villela, B., Cogen, R. B., Bartolucci, A. A., Birkedal-Hansen, H.:** Crevicular fluid collagenase activity in healthy, gingivitis, chronic adult periodontitis and localized juvenile periodontitis patients. J. periodont. Res. 22: 209–211, 1987

* **Visser, H., Krüger, W.:** Gibt es abgesicherte Wirkungen der Soft-Laser bei der Parodontalbehandlung? Dtsch. zahnärztl. Z. 42: 442–444, 1987

**Völk, W., Mireau, H.-D., Biehl, P., Dornheim, G., Reithmayer, Ch.:** Beitrag zur Ätiologie der keilförmigen Defekte. Dtsch. zahnärztl. Z. 42: 499–504, 1987

**Vollmer, W. H., Rateitschak, K. H.:** Influence of occlusal adjustment by grinding on gingivitis and mobility of traumatized teeth. J. clin. Periodontol. 2: 113–125, 1975

**Vouros, I., Frentzen, M., Nolden, R.:** Modifizierte Widman-Plastik und subgingivale Kürettage. Eine klinische Vergleichsstudie. Dtsch. zahnärztl. Z. 41: 605–609, 1986

# W

* **Wachtel, H., Vogeley, E., Purucker, P., Bernimoulin, J.-P.:** Einfluß der Gingivaextension mit freiem Schleimhauttransplantat auf Gingivarezessionen mit klinischen Entzündungszeichen. Dtsch. zahnärztl. Z. 41: 597–604, 1986

**Waerhaug, J.:** Healing of the dento-epithelial junction following subgingival plaque control. II. As observed on extracted teeth. J. Periodontol. 49: 119–134, 1978

* **Waerhaug, J.:** The angular bone defect and its relationship to trauma from occlusion and downgrowth of subgingival plaque. J. clin. Periodontol. 6: 61–82, 1979

* **Waerhaug, J.:** The furcation problem. Etiology, pathogenesis, diagnosis, therapy and prognosis. J. clin. Periodontol. 7: 73–95, 1980

**Walsh, F. T., Glenwright, H. D.:** Relative effectiveness of a rotary and conventional toothbrush in plaque removal. Community Dent. oral Epidemiol. 12: 160–163, 1984

**Ward, H. L., Simring, M.:** Manual of Clinical Periodontics. 2nd ed. Mosby, St. Louis 1978

* **Watts, E. A., Newman, H. N.:** Clinical effects on chronic periodontitis of a simplified system of oral hygiene including subgingival pulsated jet irrigation with chlorhexidine. J. clin. Periodontol. 13: 666–670, 1986

* **Watts, T., Palmer, R., Floyd, P.:** Metronidazole: A double-blind trial in untreated human periodontal disease. J. clin. Periodontol. 13: 939–943, 1986

**Wennström, J. L.:** Keratinized and attached gingiva. Regenerative potential and significance for periodontal health. Thesis, Göteborg 1982

**Wennström, J. L.:** Regeneration of gingiva following surgical excision. A clinical study. J. clin. Periodontol. 10: 287–297, 1983

**Wennström, J. L., Lindhe, J.:** Role of attached gingiva for maintenance of periodontal health. Healing following excisional and grafting procedures in dogs. J. clin. Periodontol. 10: 206–221, 1983 a

**Wennström, J. L., Lindhe, J.:** Plaque-induced gingival inflammation in the absence of attached gingiva in dogs. J. clin. Periodontol. 10: 266–276, 1983 b

**Wennström, J. L.:** Status of the art in mucogingival surgery. Acta parodont., in Schweiz. Mschr. Zahnmed. 95: 343/47–352/56, 1985

**Wennström, J. L.:** Lack of association between width of attached gingiva and development of soft tissue recession. A 5–year longitudinal study. J. clin. Periodontol. 14: 181–184, 1987

**Wennström, J. L., Lindhe, J., Sinclair, F., Thilander, B.:** Some periodontal tissue reactions to orthodontic tooth movement in monkeys. J. clin. Periodontol. 14: 121–129, 1987 a

**Wennström, J. L., Heijl, L., Dahlén, G., Gröndahl, K.:** Periodic subgingival antimicrobial irrigation of periodontal pockets. J. clin. Periodontol. 14: 541–550, 1987 b

○* **Wennström, J. L.:** What is a clinically healthy periodontium? Periodontology Today. Int. Congr., Zürich. Karger, Basel 1988 (pp. 1–5)

* **West, T. L., King, W. J.:** Toothbrushing with hydrogen peroxide-sodium bicarbonate compared to toothpowder and water in reducing periodontal pocket suppuration and darkfield bacterial counts. J. Periodontol. 54: 339–346, 1983

**Westfelt, E., Nyman, S., Socransky, S., Lindhe, J.:** Significance of frequency of professional tooth cleaning for healing following periodontal surgery. J. clin. Periodontol. 10: 148–156, 1983

**Westfelt, E., Bragd, L., Socransky, S. S., Haffajee, A. D., Nyman, S., Lindhe, J.:** Improved periodontal conditions following therapy. J. clin. Periodontol. 12: 283–293, 1985

**WHO:** Epidemiology, etiology, and prevention of periodontal diseases. WHO techn. Rep. Ser. 621: 1978

**Widman, L.:** The operative treatment of pyorrhea alveolaris. A new surgical method. Svensk tandläk.-T. Dec. 1918

**Winkler, J. R., Murray, P. A.:** Periodontal disease – Potential intraoral expression of AIDS may be a rapidly progressive periodontitis. J. Calif. dent. Ass. 15: 20–24, 1987

* **Wirthlin, M. R.:** The current status of new attachment therapy. J. Periodontol. 52: 529–544, 1981

* **Wirthlin, M. R.:** Review of bone biology in periodontal disease. J. West. Soc. Periodontol. 34: 125–143, 1986

○ **Wirz, J.:** Die Transfixation im Dienste der Teilprothetik. Quintessenz, Berlin 1983

* **Wiskott, H. W. A.:** Technical note on the statistical analysis of one longitudinal peridontal study. Schweiz. Mschr. Zahnmed. 98: 607–610, 1988

**Wolf, H. F., Rateitschak, K. H.:** Einfache temporäre Schienungsmöglichkeiten. Dtsch. Zahnärztebl. 17: 525–533, 1965

**Wolf, H. F.:** Der CPITN – schon wieder ein neuer Index? Schweiz. Mschr. Zahnmed. 97: 61–63, 1987 a

**Wolf, H. F.:** Technik der konservativen Parodontalbehandlung: Scaling – Deep scaling – Wurzelglättung. Schweiz. Mschr. Zahnmed. 97: 1135–1143, 1987 b

**Wolf, H. F., Rateitschak, K. H., Rateitschak-Plüss, E. M.:** Parodontitis bei juvenilem Diabetes (ein Fallbericht). Schweiz. Mschr. Zahnmed. 97: 1291–1294, 1987

**Wolf, H. F.:** Zwei Makroblitzgeräte im Test: Nikon Macro Speedlight SB-21 und Minolta Macro-Flash 1200 AF. Photomed 1: 111–124, 1988

**Wolff, L. F., Pihlstrom, B. L., Bakdash, M. B., Schaffer, E. M., Jensen, J. R., Aeppli, D. M., Bandt, C. L.:** Salt and peroxide compared with conventional oral hygiene – II. Microbial results. J. Periodontol. 58: 301–307, 1987

* **Wright, W. E.:** Success with the cantilever fixed partial denture. J. prosth. Dent. 55: 537–539, 1986

# Y

**Yukna, R. A.:** A clinical study of healing in humans following the excisional new attachment procedure in Rhesus monkeys. J. Periodontol. 47: 701–709, 1976

**Yukna, R. A., Bowers, G. M., Lawrence, J. J., Fedi, P. F., Jr.:** A clinical study of healing in humans following the excisional new attachment procedure. J. Periodontol. 47: 696–700, 1976

# Z

* **Zafiropoulos, G. G., Flores-de-Jacoby, L., Pappas, A.:** Einfluß der Parodontaltherapie auf spezielle Funktionen der Lymphozyten und Granulozyten. Dtsch. zahnärztl. Z. 41: 565–568, 1986

* **Zafiropoulos, G. G., Eldanassouri, N., Flores-de-Jacoby, L., Havemann, K.:** Bestimmung der ELP (Elastase-ähnliche Proteinase) bei Patienten mit rasch fortschreitender und mit juveniler Parodontitis. Dtsch. zahnärztl. Z. 42: 1056–1060, 1987

* **Zambon, J. J., Reynolds, H. S., Slots, J.:** Black pigmented bacteroides spp. in the human oral cavity. Infect. Immun. 32: 198–203, 1981

* **Zambon, J. J., Christersson, L. A., Slots, J.:** Actinobacillus actinomycetemcomitans in human periodontal disease. Prevalence in patient groups and distribution of biotypes and serotypes within families. J. Periodontol. 54: 707–711, 1983

* **Zambon, J. J.:** Actinobacillus actinomycetemcomitans in human periodontal disease. J. clin. Periodontol. 12: 1–20, 1985

* **Zambon, J. J., Reynolds, H. S., Chen, P., Genco, R. J.:** Rapid identification of periodontal pathogens in subgingival dental plaque. J. Periodontol., Spec. issue: 32–40, 1985

* **Zander, H. A., Polson, A. M.:** Zum gegenwärtigen Stand der Okklusionstheorien und Therapie okklusaler Störungen in der Parodontologie. Quintessenz 12: 83–88, 1978

* **Zappa, U. E., Polson, A. M.:** Factors associated with occurrence and reversibility of connective tissue attachment loss. J. Periodontol. 59: 100–106, 1988

# List of Materials

## Instruments, Devices, Medicaments

In response to requests from readers, this second edition of the *Color Atlas of Periodontology* includes a listing of the many "materials" that are depicted and mentioned in the text.

The authors wish to emphasize, however, that success in data gathering, diagnosis, therapy and maintenance for periodontitis patients depends only in small measure upon the type or manufacturer of the materials or instruments used. The most important goal in "causal" periodontitis therapy is, quite simply, cleaning the teeth and their plaque-covered root surfaces. This can be accomplished with many different instruments from numerous manufacturers. Each practitioner should select the instruments and materials that serve him/her best, and which make it possible to achieve the desired goals.

This list makes no claim of completeness. It is divided into two sections:

**Section 1** (pp. 386–389)
*Materials and manufacturers* (without addresses; see Section 2), presented with the page number on which they appear, under the main chapter headings such as Diagnosis, Therapy etc.

**Section 2** (pp. 390–391)
*Manufacturers* and *addresses,* presented alphabetically.

The reader has the authors' permission to reproduce for use in practice any of the forms for diagnosis and data collection that appear in this *Atlas.*

## Section 1: Materials and Manufacturers

| Page/Item | Manufacturer |
|---|---|
| **Diagnosis** | |
| **116  Periodontal probes** | |
| – Michigan-O | *Deppeler |
| – CPITN modif. | *Hu-Friedy |
| – Williams PQW | *Hu-Friedy |
| – CP 12 | *Hu-Friedy |
| – Probe CV 4 | *GC – American |
| **118  Furcation probes** | |
| – CH 3 | *Hu-Friedy |
| – Nabers no. 2 | *Hu-Friedy |
| – Zappa ZA 3 | *Deppeler |
| **120  Iodine solutions** | |
| – Schiller | Pharmacy |
| – Lugol | Pharmacy |
| **121  Electronic tooth mobility measurement** | |
| – Periotest | *Siemens |

| Page/Item | Manufacturer |
|---|---|
| **125  DNA bacterial test** | |
| – DMDx-Test | *Bio Technica Diagnostics |
| **126/ Charts** | |
| **127**  – Modifications of existing charts (without copyright!) | |
| **Oral Hygiene – Patient** | |
| **146  OHI, motivation** | |
| – Dental Atlas | * Quintessence Publishers |
| – Esroskop | * Profimed |
| **149  Disclosing agents** | |
| – Erythrosin solution | Dental supplier, pharmacy |
| – Dis-Plaque | *Pacemaker |
| – Esroblue | *Profimed |
| – Plak-lite, Set | *Brilliant |
| – Fluorescein solution | Pharmacy |

\* Manufacturers with an asterisk appear in alphabetical order in Section 2, with addresses.

| Page/Item | Manufacturer |
|---|---|
| **151 Dentifrices** | |
| – many brands | Many manufacturers |
| **152 Toothbrushes** | |
| – many brands | *Lactona/Tanrac |
| | *Oral-B |
| | *Profimed |
| | and many others |
| **154 Dental Floss** | |
| – Super-Floss | *Educational Health Products |
| – Brush and Floss | *Esro |
| – Dental Floss | *Johnson & Johnson |
| – POH Dental Floss | *Oral Health Products |
| **155 Toothpicks** | |
| – Te Pe | *Eklund & Peterson |
| – Stim-u-dent | *Johnson & Johnson |
| – Medical toothpick | *Blendax |
| – Elite (for Perio-Aid) | *Forster |
| **155 Interdental brushes** | |
| – with separate handle | *Butler |
| | *Curaden |
| | *Oral-B |
| | *Profimed |
| – without separate handle | *Macol |
| (with metal core) | |
| | *Profimed |
| | and many others |
| **156 Marginal brushes** | |
| – Jordan no. 2 | *Jordan |
| – Lactona no. 27 | *Lactona/Tanrac |
| **156 Stimulator** | |
| – Lactona no. 26 | *Lactona/Tanrac |
| **156 Handle for Elite toothpick** | |
| – Perio-Aid | *Marquis |
| **156 Threader** | |
| – EEZ-Thru Floss Threaders | *Butler |
| **157 Electric toothbrushes** | |
| – Rota-dent | *Rota-dent |
| – Touch Tronic | *Teledyne |
| **157 Irrigators** | |
| – Broxojet | *Walther |
| – Water Pik | *Teledyne |
| – Braun | *Braun |
| – Blend-a-Dent | *Blend-a-Med |
| **157 Subgingival irrigator** | |
| – Periodontal Pik | *Teledyne |
| **157 Canula with lateral orifice** | |
| – Max-i-Probe | *MPL |
| **158 Chlorhexidine rinsing solutions** | |
| – Peridex 0.12% | *Procter & Gamble |
| – Corsodyl 0.2% | *ICI |
| – Chlorhexamed 0.1% | *Blendax |
| – Plak-Out 0.1% | *Hawe-Neos |
| – Plak-Out Concentrate (10%) | *Hawe-Neos |

| Page/Item | Manufacturer |
|---|---|
| **158 Chlorhexidine gel** | |
| – Plak-Out 0.1% | *Hawe-Neos |
| – Corsodyl 1.0% | *ICI |
| **159 Chlorhexidine powder** | |
| – Pure CHX 100% | *ICI |

## Oral Hygiene – Dentist/Hygienist

| Page/Item | Manufacturer |
|---|---|
| **162 Sonic + Ultrasonic devices** | |
| – Prophy-Jet | *De Trey/Dentsply |
| – Cavitron | *De Trey/Dentsply |
| – Titan-S | *Star Dental |
| – Sonicflex | *KaVo |
| **164 Hand instruments, debridement** | |
| – Chisel ZI 10 | *Deppeler |
| – Scalers ZI 11, 11 L + R | *Deppeler |
| – Lingual Scaler ZI 12 | *Deppeler |
| – Universal curettes ZI 15, | *Deppeler |
| ZI 15 S, ZI 15 SS | |
| – Anterior curettes GX 4 | *Deppeler |
| – Posterior curettes M 23 A | *Deppeler |
| **164 Prophy paste, RDA grades** | |
| – Prophy pastes, | *Svenska Dental (SDI) |
| CCS-Color Coded System | |
| **166 Restoration polish** | |
| – Amalgashape | *Intensiv |
| – Disks, graded abrasiveness | *Hawe-Neos |
| | *3M |
| **166 Overhanging margins** | |
| – EVA handpiece | *Dentatus |
| – Proxoshape (diamond files) | *Intensiv |
| – EVA plastic files | *Dentatus |
| (many types) | |
| **166 Interdental polishing, tooth separation** | |
| – Strip holder | *LM |
| | *Bilciurescu |
| – Steel strips (graded) | *GC Dental |
| – Linen strips (graded) | *Hawe-Neos |
| **172 Odontoplasty, Contouring, Scaling** | |
| – Perio-Set | *Intensiv |
| (Diamonds, 12-set) | |

## Therapy – Scaling, Root Planing

| Page/Item | Manufacturer |
|---|---|
| **182 Scaling and root planing** | |
| – Hoes TC 210–213 | *Ash (De Trey) |
| – Universal curette ZI 15, | |
| ZI 15 S, ZI 15 SS | |
| – Anterior curette GX 4 | *Deppeler |
| – Posterior curette M 23 A | *Deppeler |
| – Gracey curettes GE 5/6, | *Deppeler |
| 7/8, 11/12, 13/14 | |
| (reduced set, cf. pp. 186–190) | |
| – Colgrips | *Colgrip |
| **184/** – Gracey curettes | *Hu-Friedy |
| **185** GRA 1–14 (complete set) | |

| Page/Item | Manufacturer |
|---|---|
| **192 Sharpening stones, natural + artificial** | |
| – Carborundum no.309 | *Carborundum |
| – India | *Norton |
| – Arkansas: | |
| HS 14 | *Fickert/Becker (Deppeler) |
| No. 4 | *Hu-Friedy |
| **192 Sharpening oil** | |
| – Acid-free mineral oil SSO | *Hu-Friedy |
| **192 Test rod** | |
| – Acrylic rod PTS | *Hu-Friedy |
| **198 Application of tissue adhesive** | |
| – Plast-O-Probe | *Maillefer |

## Therapy – Flap Surgery

| | |
|---|---|
| **214 Scalpels – Blades** | |
| – Nr. 11 | *Martin |
| – Nr. 15 | *Martin |
| – Nr. 12B or D | *Bard-Parker |
| – Nr. 15C | *Bard-Parker |
| see also p. 219 | |
| **214 Elevators** | |
| – FK 300 (6 mm wide) | *Aesculap |
| – VT 24, 22, 23 (5 mm wide) | *Deppeler |
| – VT 27 (4 mm wide) | *Deppeler |
| – Zabona (2 mm wide) | *Zabona |
| **214 Needle holders** | |
| – "Mathieu" | *Aesculap |
| (1500 g closure) | |
| – "Boyton" | *Hu-Friedy |
| (1200 g closure) | |
| – "Castrovieijo" | *Aesculap |
| (500 g closure) | |
| – "Gillis" (without lock) | *Dufner |
| **216 Needles, suture material** | |
| – Atraumatic needle/suture | *Davis + Geck |
| combinations | *Ethicon |
| | *SSC |
| **219 Special scalpels** | |
| – Nr. 6500 pointed | *Beaver |
| – Nr. 6700 rounded | *Beaver |
| – Handles (e.g., no. 1350) | *Beaver |
| **232 Bone, bony pockets** | |
| – Round bur | *Komet/Brasseler |
| Nr. 014, 018, 023 | |
| – Bone bur with internal | *Jota |
| cooling 4 mm ø, No. 473 | |
| (RS/040) | |
| – Bone forceps: | |
| "Luer-Friedmann" FO 409 | *Aesculap |
| "Cleveland" 5 S | *Hu-Friedy |
| **245 Bone replacement, pocket implants** | |
| **Tricalcium phosphate – TCP** | |
| – Ceros 82 | *Mathys |
| – Synthograft | *Miter |

| Page/Item | Manufacturer |
|---|---|
| **Hydroxyapatite – HA** | |
| – Alveograf | *Cook-Waite |
| – Allotropat | *Heyl |
| – Calcitite | *Calcitek |
| – Ceros 80 | *Mathys |
| – Interpore 200 | *Interpore |
| – Osprovit | *Feldmühle |
| – Periograf | *Cook-Waite |
| – Bio-Oss | *Geistlich/Hall |
| **245 Implant carrier** | |
| – Amalgam carrier F-10-11 | *Hu-Friedy |
| **252 Tissue adhesive** | |
| cf. p. 276 | |
| **260 Removal of autologous bone** | |
| – Bone filter No. 4320 | *Gelman |
| – Trephine 2.3; 2.8; | *Jota |
| 5.0 mm | |
| – Hand trephine | *Bovard |
| (with mm + inch markings) | |

## Therapy – Gingivectomy/GP

| | |
|---|---|
| **274 Pocket marking** | |
| – Marking forceps (paired) | *Deppeler |
| **274 Gingivectomy knife** | |
| – "Kirkland" knife GX 7 L+R | *Deppeler |
| – Papilla knife | *Depeler |
| – "Orban" ZI 14 L+R | |
| – Universal gingivectomy | *Deppeler |
| knife ZI 19 | |
| **274 Electrosurgery** | |
| – Electrotome | *Martin |
| | *Ellman |
| – attachments no. 2, 12, 14 | *Martin |
| **276 Dressings + Tissue adhesives** | |
| – Peripac | *De Trey/Dentsply |
| – Coe-pak | *Coe |
| – Histoacryl-N-blue | *B.Braun-SSC |
| – Bucrylat | *Ethicon |

## Therapy – Mucogingival Surgery

| | |
|---|---|
| **292 Mucotome for tissue harvesting** | |
| – Hand mucotome | *Deppeler |
| PR 1, 4, 2, M (holder) | |
| – Blades | *Deppeler |
| – Mörmann mucotome | *Aesculap |
| (12, 16, 20 mm) | |
| – Gillis hook (2 mm) | *Aesculap |
| **297 Free gingival graft, aids** | |
| – Metal foil | *Produits Dentaires |
| – Antihemorrhagic gauze: | |
| Sorbacel (sterile) | *Wander |
| Tabotamp (sterile) | *Johnson & Johnson |

Page/Item                    Manufacturer

## Therapy – Medicaments

**316  Topical application**
- CHX cf. p. 158/159
- Hextril                    Warner-Lambert
- Amosan                     Cooper
- Kavosan                    Cooper
- Aureomycin ointment 3%     Lederle
- Aureomycin ophthalmic
  ointment 1%                Lederle
- Terracortril               Pfizer
- Locacorten                 Ciba
- Dontisolon                 Hoechst

**317  Systemic medications**
- Hostacyclin                Hoechst
- Ledermycin                 Lederle
- Vibramycin                 Pfizer
- Flagyl                     Specia
- Tiberal                    Roche
- Rodogyl                    Specia
- Rovamycine                 Specia

## Therapy – Negative Results

**324  Gingival mask**
- Acrylic (hard)             Many manufacturers
- Gingivamoll (soft)         *Molloplast-Regneri

## Adjunctive Therapy – Function

**335  Diamond burs**
- Wheel ca. 3.5 mm           Many manufacturers
- Flame ca. 5.0×2.3 mm
- Ball ca. 2.3 mm

## Therapy – Quo Vadis?

**368  Regeneration membranes**
- Gore-Tex periodontal
  membrane                   *W. L. Gore

# Section 2: Manufacturers and Addresses*

**AAP – American
Academy of Periodontology**
Suite 1400
211 East Chicago Avenue
Chicago, IL 60611
USA

**Aesculapwerke AG**
Postfach 40
D-7200 Tuttlingen
West Germany

**Ash/Dentsply, Ltd.**
Ash Instrument Division
Hamm Moor Lane, Addlestone
Weybridge Surrey, KT 15 2 SE
England

**Bard-Parker**
Division of Becton,
Dickinson & Co.
Rutherford, NJ 07070
USA

**Beaver Surgical Products**
P.O. Box 589
Waltham, MA 02154
USA

**Dr. A. Bilciurescu**
Kaiserstrasse 3
D-5300 Bonn 1
West Germany

**BioTechnica Diagnostics, Inc.**
61 Moulton Street
Cambridge, MA 02138
USA

**Blendax-Werke/Blend-a-Dent**
Blend-a-med-Forschung
Rheinallee 88
D-6500 Mainz
West Germany

**M. Bovard**
Fabrique d'objets des
pansements à l'ambulance
16, place des Philosophes
CH-1211 Genève 4
Switzerland

**Gebr. Brasseler (Komet)**
Postfach 160
D-4920 Lemgo
West Germany

**Braun AG**
Postfach 1120
D-6242 Kronberg
West Germany

**B. Braun-SSC AG**
Carl-Braun-Strasse 1
D-3508 Melsungen
West Germany

**Brilliant International, Inc.**
137 Montgomery Avenue
Bala Cynwyd, PA 19004
USA

**John O. Butler Company**
4635 W. Foster Ave.
Chicago, IL 60630
USA

**Calcitek Inc.**
4125-B Sorrento Valley Boulevard
San Diego, CA 92121
USA

**Carborundum Comp. Ltd.**
Trafford Park
Manchester 17
England

**Coe Laboratories, Inc.**
3737 W. 127th Street
Chicago, IL 60658
USA

**Colgrip AB**
Sandelsgatan 31
S-11533 Stockholm
Sweden

**Cook-Waite Laboratories, Inc.**
90 Park Avenue
New York, NY 10016
USA

**Cooper Care, Inc.**
Palo Alto, CA 94304
USA

**Curaden AG**
Postfach 74
CH-6010 Kriens
Switzerland

**Davis + Geck International**
American Cyanamid Co.
One Cyanamid Plaza
Wayne, NJ 07470
USA

**Dentsply International**
570 W. College Ave.
P.O. Box 872
York, PA 17405
USA

**AB Dentatus**
Jakobsdalsvägen 14–16
S-12653 Hägersten
Sweden

**A. Deppeler SA**
12, rue des Petites Buttes
CH-1180 Rolle
Switzerland

**H. Dufner**
Medical Instruments
Föhrerstrasse 9
D-7200 Tuttlingen
West Germany

**Educational Health Products, Inc.**
P.O. Box 24
New Canaan, CN 06840
USA

**Eklund & Peterson**
P.O. Box 4305
S-2121 Malmö
Sweden

**Elida-Cosmetic AG**
Förrlibuckstrasse 10
CH-8031 Zürich
Switzerland

**Ellman International
Manufacturing, Inc.**
Ellman Building
1135 Railroad Avenue
Hewlett, NY 11557
USA

**Esro AG**
Böhnirainstrasse 13
CH-8800 Thalwil
Switzerland

**Ethicon**
see Johnson & Johnson
Dental Products Co.

**Feldmühle AG**
Produktbereich Humanmedizin
Fabrikstrasse 23–29
D-7310 Plochingen
West Germany

**K. Fickert/H. Becker**
Steinschleiferei
Hochwaldstrasse 4
D-6581 Bruchweiler
West Germany

**Forster Manufacturing, Inc.**
Wilton, ME 04294
USA

**Gaba AG**
Grabetmatsweg
CH-4106 Therwil
Switzerland

**GC Dental Industrial Corp.**
76-1 Hasunuma-cho
Itabashi-ku
Tokyo 174
Japan

**GC – American Int. Co.**
7830 East Redfield Road, Nr.12
Scottsdale, AZ 85260
USA

**Ed. Geistlich Sons/
Hall Reconstructive Systems**
1055 Cindy Lane
Carpinteria, CA 93013
USA

**Gelman Sciences, Inc.**
Ann Arbor, MI 48106
USA

**W. L. Gore & Assoc., Inc.**
Periodontal Division
P.O. Box 1350
Flagstaff, AZ 86002
USA

**Hawe-Neos Dental**
Dr. H. v. Weissenfluh AG
CH-6925 Gentilino
Switzerland

**Heyl – Chemical/Pharma-
ceutical Co.**
Goerzallee 253
D-1000 Berlin 37
West Germany

**Hu-Friedy**
Immunity Steel Instruments
3232 N.Rockwell Street
Chicago, IL 60618
USA

**ICI-Imperial Chemical
Industries PLC**
Pharmaceuticals Division
Alderley House, Alderley Park
Macclesfield, Cheshire
England

**Intensiv SA**
Via Molinazzo 22
CH-6962 Viganello
Switzerland

**Interpore International**
18005 Skypark Circle
Irvine, CA 92714
USA

# Manufacturers and Addresses

**Johnson & Johnson**
Dental Products Co.
20 Lake Drive
East Windsor, NJ 08520
USA

**A/S W. Jordan, WdM**
Thranesgate 75
Oslo/Norway

**Jota AG**
Postfach 56
CH-9464 Rüthi/SG
Switzerland

**KaVo**
Dental & Medical
Instruments
D-7950 Biberach/Riß 1
West Germany

**Lactona**
201 Commerce Drive
Montgomeryville, PA 18936
USA

**LM-Dental**
Lääkintämuovi Oy
Humalinstonkatu 11
Turku 10, SF 20100
Finland

**3M Dental Products**
P.O. Box 33600
St. Paul, MN 55133-3600
USA

**Maillefer SA**
3, chemin Verger
CH-1338 Ballaigues
Switzerland

**Marquis Dental Mfg. Co., Inc.**
2005 E
17th Avenue
Denver, CO 86206
USA

**Martin Bros.**
Ludwigskalerstrasse 132
D-7200 Tuttlingen
West Germany

**R. Mathys & Co.**
Güterstrasse 5
CH-2544 Bettlach
Switzerland

**Macol**
Fournitures Dentaires
22, rue L. Ruchonnet
CH-1337 Vallorbe
Switzerland

**Miter Inc.**
6550 Singletree Drive
Columbus, OH 43229
USA

**Molloplast-Regneri
GmbH & Co. KG**
Roonstrasse 23 A
D-7500 Karlsruhe 1
West Germany

**MPL, Inc.**
1820 W. Roscoe Street
Chicago, IL 60657-1079
USA

**Norton International Inc.**
Worcester, MA 617 853-1000
USA

**Oral-B Laboratories GmbH**
Rebstöcker Strasse 33–39
D-6000 Frankfurt am Main 1
West Germany

**Oral Health Products**
Box 45623
Tulsa, OK 74145
USA

**Pacemaker Co.**
P.O. Box 16160
Portland, OR 97216
USA

**Procter & Gamble**
P.O. Box 599
Cincinnati, OH 45201
USA

**Produits Dentaires SA**
18, rue des Bosquets
CH-1800 Vevey
Switzerland

**Profimed AG**
Böhnirainstrasse 13
CH-8800 Thalwil
Switzerland

**Quintessence Publishing Co.**
870 Oak Creek Drive
Lombard, IL 60148
USA

**Rota-dent AG**
Allmendstrasse 9
CH-8700 Küsnacht
Switzerland

**Safident AG**
5, chemin de la Combe
CH-1196 Gland
Switzerland

**SDI – Svenska Dental
Instrument AB**
Axel Johnson Instrument AB
Box 1432
S-17127 Solna
Sweden

**Siemens AG**
Medical Technology
Dental Branch
Fabrikstrasse 31
D-6140 Bensheim
West Germany

**SSC**
see B. Braun – SSC AG

**Star Dental
Manufacturing Co., Inc.**
A Syntex Dental Company
P.O. Box 896
Valley Forge, PA 19482
USA

**Tanrac (Lactona) Ltd.**
Box
S-80590 Gävle
Sweden

**Teledyne Aqua Tec.**
1730 East Prospect Street
Fort Collins, CO 80521
USA

**Walther AG**
Köllikerstrasse 45
CH-5036 Oberentfelden
Switzerland

**Wander AG**
Pharma Schweiz
Monbijoustrasse 115
CH-3007 Bern
Switzerland

**Zabona AG**
Labortechnik
Mattenstrasse 16 A
CH-4058 Basel
Switzerland

# Index

## D

## E

## F